FOUNDATIONS OF COMMUNITY HEALTH PRACTICE

Prof. (Dr.) Sujata K. Das

ALLIED HEALTH PRESS

Foundations of Community Health Practice

Author: **Prof. (Dr.) Sujata K. Das**

Allied Health Press
4164 Lakeshore Road
Burlington ON L7L 1A4
Canada
www.alliedhealthpress.com
Email: orders@arclereducation.com

ISBN: 978-1-77956-831-1

ABOUT THE AUTHOR

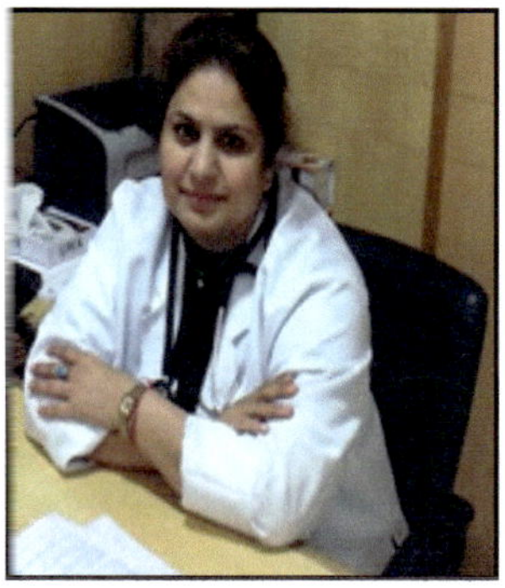

Prof (Dr) Sujata K. Dass, M.B.B.S, D.N.B, Ph.D. (Medicine) is a distinguished neuro-physician and academician, currently serving as an Attending Consultant in the Department of Neurology, B.L. Kapur Hospital, a renowned super-specialty medical institution in the New Delhi. Her illustrious career in medicine and research spans over three decades, characterized by her profound contributions to neurology and her unwavering commitment to medical education.

Dr. Dass began her educational journey at Flushing High School in New York, USA, and completed her High School Diploma thereafter she joined Queens College of the City University of New York as an undergrad student. With a passion for medicine, she pursued her MBBS degree at King George Medical College, Lucknow, U.P., India. Her academic prowess and dedication to medicine were evident early on, setting the stage for a remarkable career. Dr Dass worked under the supervision of Dr M.S. Bains, M.D. as a Visiting Fellow in cardio-thoracic surgery at Memorial Sloan Kettering Cancer Research Center, New York, USA.

Dr. Dass furthered her medical training by obtaining a D.N.B. (Family Medicine) and conducted significant research on hematological changes in malaria. Her quest for knowledge and excellence led her back to New York, where she completed her Ph.D. (Medicine) at the Department of Obstetrics & Gynecology, The New York Hospital-Cornell University Medical Center under the mentorship of Prof. Brij B. Saxena. Her groundbreaking work on Sn-Proto and Sn-Mesoporphyrin and the chemoprevention of neonatal jaundice culminated in the award of her D.Sc. (Medicine).

Dr. Sujata Dass joined as the BR Ambedkar Chair Professor in July 2002 in the Institute of Biomedical Sciences, Faculty of Medicine, Bundelkhand University, Jhansi. Her tenure was marked by her dedication to advancing medical research and education. She also served as UGC National Research Award (Professor) at V.P. Chest Institute, University of Delhi.

Throughout her career, Dr. Dass has received numerous awards and accolades on a global level. Notable among these are the UGC Research Award, the Fast Track Young Scientist Award from the Department of Science and Technology (DST), and the Women's Award of Highest Honour from Soka University, Japan. She has also received numerous research grants from DST, DBT and ICMR, UGC etc. These awards and grants underscore her exceptional contributions to medical science and research.

Dr. Dass is a respected member of various scientific and administrative bodies like Planning Board (IGNOU), Executive Council - Bhagat Phool Singh Mahila Vishwavidhlaya, Haryana (2008-2011) where she continues to influence the medical community with her insights and expertise. Her commitment to guiding and mentoring students in their master's and doctoral thesis highlights her dedication to nurturing the next generation of medical professionals. Dr. Dass remains a beacon of excellence and a role model for aspiring medical professionals worldwide.

Brief Table of Contents

Detailed Table of Contents

CHAPTER 7

Evaluation of Community Health Programs 225

CHAPTER 8

Health Communication and Social Marketing 261

CHAPTER 15

Emerging Trends and Future Directions in Community Health 511

LIST OF FIGURES

PREFACE

Health is more than the absence of disease but also a reflection of the overall well-being of individuals, families, and societies. The broader vision of health consists of economic stability, social harmony, education, physical environment, and accessibility of healthcare services. When all these factors converge, they create conditions in which individuals can thrive. Community health here is not just a public service concern but a shared responsibility based on collective behavior, civic action, and support systems. Community health workers' role is to help identify and solve the special problems of locally generated, culturally tailored, and sustainable measures that increase quality of life and reduce preventable sickness.

The practice of community health is centered on preventive interventions, population-based practices, and commitments to social justice and health equity. It is guided by multiple disciplines—public health, sociology, nursing, psychology, education, and political science—to gain knowledge about the impact of personal behaviors and system factors on health outcomes. In our times today, communication of infectious diseases, non-communicable diseases, mental illnesses, and social disparities is all at once. The needs for strong health infrastructure for communities have never been higher. It is through collaboration that communities can strengthen health systems, prepare to respond to health crises, and support lifelong well-being for all members.

Foundations of Community Health Practice is a comprehensive guide for professionals, practitioners, and students committed to promoting and protecting health in populations. The book aims to provide an integrated picture of the principles, practices, and policies shaping effective community health interventions. From inner-city neighborhoods, rural areas, to international health initiatives, the book provides background knowledge as well as practical strategies. It is meant to benefit those who work in designing, implementing, and evaluating programs that lead to healthier communities by evidence-informed, evidence-based, and contextually appropriate means.

Chapter 1 presents the core concepts of community health with definitions, historical foundation, and differences between individual and population approaches to health. It further presents the roles and activities of community health workers and the essential need for intersectoral collaboration.

Chapter 2 addresses the theoretical models guiding community health practice. The chapter discusses behavioral, social, and ecological theory used to explain and predict health behavior. The chapter underscores the significance of theory in intervention planning that is consistent, well-structured, and culturally sensitive.

Chapter 3 addresses the systematic community health assessment process. It introduces tools and techniques for data collection and analysis for identifying health priorities, including quantitative and qualitative methods, community surveys, epidemiological profiles, and participatory assessments.

Chapter 4 is dedicated to the planning phase of community health programs. It outlines how to establish goals, build measurable objectives, recognize priorities, allocate resources, and formulate strategic action plans. Special focus is given to logic models, stakeholder participation, and feasibility analysis.

Chapter 5 looks at implementation strategies in community health. It lays out the operational day-to-day requirements of putting a health plan into action, such as mobilizing partnerships, service coordination, staff training, and logistics. It also discusses expected challenges and adaptive strategies to support delivery.

Chapter 6 shifts attention to prevention of disease and promotion of health as core objectives within community-based practice. It explains how to encourage healthy behaviors, reduce risk factors, and enhance wellness through educational campaigns, screening services, immunization programs, and supportive environments.

Chapter 7 outlines how community health program success can be evaluated. Chapter 7 discusses types of evaluation, such as process, outcome, and impact evaluations, and methods of data collection, indicators, analysis, and reporting. The chapter discusses how findings might influence future practice.

Chapter 8 focuses on the contribution of health communication and social marketing. This involves message design principles, segmentation of audiences, media choice, campaign strategy, and assessing effects of communication. The emphasis is on reaching various populations and enhancing public participation.

Chapter 9 presents the principles and practices of Community-Based Participatory Research (CBPR). Community members need to be involved as equal partners in the research process to ensure interventions account for the local realities and values. Methodologies, ethics, and examples are also addressed.

Chapter 10 discusses policy development and advocacy in community health. It explains the process of developing public health policies, the political process, and the involvement of health professionals in bringing about change through policy. Examples include measures controlling tobacco, environmental health policy, and access to health care.

Chapter 11 addresses global and environmental dimensions of community health. Chapter 11 outlines how transnational health issues—pandemics, water sanitation, air quality, and climate change—affect communities worldwide. The chapter describes ways to develop partnerships and adapt interventions to suit global environments.

Chapter 12 addresses health disparities and the social determinants that are fueling unequal health outcomes. It reviews structural barriers of income, education, housing, racism, and geography and outlines strategies for attaining equity through specialized programs and policy change.

Chapter 13 discusses community resilience in emergency preparedness. Chapter 13 takes into account public health responses to natural disasters, disease outbreaks, and other emergencies. Preparedness planning, risk communication, resource coordination, and post-event recovery are stressed in the chapter.

Chapter 14 addresses the special population requirements in community health, which span from children to the elderly, migrants, Indigenous Australians, and those with disabilities. It emphasizes culturally inclusive and responsive practices that recognize the unique status of these groups.

Chapter 15 outlines future opportunities and challenges in community health. Topics of discussion are cross-sector collaboration, workforce development, care innovations, and digital health technology. This chapter raises questions about how professionals can get ready for emerging needs of communities and global trends.

This book is valuable reading for undergraduate and graduate students of public health, nursing, social work, and health education and early career practitioners who want to advance their skills in community health. It is also for health professionals, program planners, and policy advocates who want an evidence-based, easy-to-use reference that mirrors best practice. Instructors and trainers will find it helpful in mapping curriculum to community health competencies, while researchers can draw from its combined viewpoints for study design and applied health improvement projects.

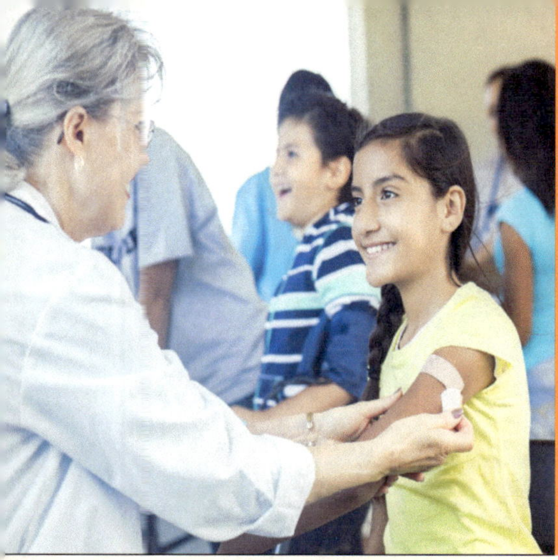

Chapter 1

INTRODUCTION TO COMMUNITY HEALTH

Contents

Introduction

Definition of Community Health

Community health is a multifaceted concept describing the wide range of physical, mental, and social factors influencing population well-being. Central to its definition is the understanding that community health encompasses more than just individual health status but is inclusive of the total health of a particular group of individuals, typically defined by geographical, cultural, or social ties. It emphasizes the interactions between individuals and their environment, highlighting the manner in which socioeconomic status, environmental hazards, and exposure to healthcare significantly affect health outcomes. Thus, community health calls for an integrated approach to health promotion, wherein approaches are developed to address disparities and enhance the well-being of each member within the community. Efforts to progress community health are as much about enabling individuals as they are about constructing shared community action that unites resources and knowledge to target shared health problems in an effective manner. In addition, the implementation of community health interventions is commonly a collaborative effort that touches on an assortment of sources of evidence. Such initiatives are often planned through the integration of top-down strategies, which may be derived from public health policy, and bottom-up interventions that address the needs and demands of the community. Most notably, literature identifies the importance of engaging local stakeholders so that interventions are culturally sensitive and contextualized. For instance, evidence-based interventions may be utilized to create programs that can promote health equity for vulnerable populations. This partnership of evidence and community involvement not only raises the effectiveness of health interventions but also facilitates a concordance between health providers and community members, ultimately empowering individuals to become active participants in their health and well-being (Anderson et al., 2020). The concept of community health also involves a strong emphasis on prevention, which is critical in addressing health inequities that disproportionately burden specific populations. Successful community health interventions foster an integrated risk factor agenda, one which seeks to unearth and tackle the multiple social determinants of health disparities. Through the solving of underlying issues of poverty, illiteracy, and insufficient access to healthcare, community health interventions can transform health environments in revolutionary ways. Additionally, the promotion of preventive interventions can lead to significant decreased economic spending in terms of health costs through reduced need for more complicated treatment measures in the future. In this respect, community health is not just a reactive framework but an active framework toward establishing sustainable health improvement and encouraging overall resilience within the community (Freeman et al., 2020) (Figure 1.1).

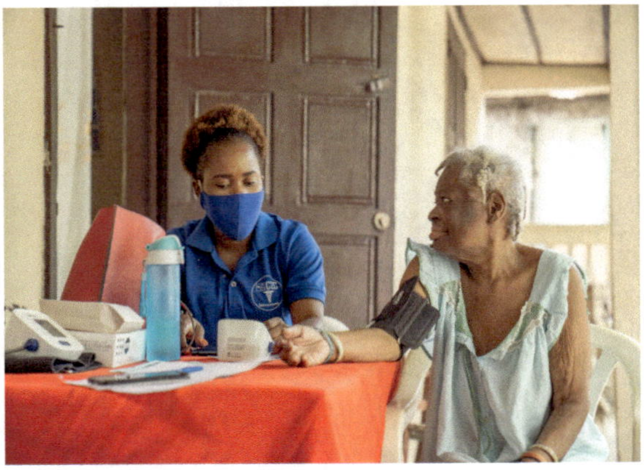

Figure 1.1. Community health.

Source: https://devex.shorthandstories.com/community-health-workers-delivering-frontline-health-innovations/assets/HaXbCtiCWM/c2c-august-2020-452-4096x2731.jpeg.

Explanation of Community Health Concepts

The concept of community health is a wide array of interventions aimed at enhancing the overall well-being of communities. It demands collective action by individuals, organizations, and governments to tackle social determinants of health like socio-economic status, education, and the environment. Effective community health interventions not only aim to combat health disorders but also emphasis the importance of preventive measures and health education. For example, healthy food habits promotion has become crucial in dealing with rising obesity and non-communicable diseases, as observed in research conducted among young adults in Greece. This research indicates the necessity of understanding eating behavior and the contextual determinants that govern it, showing how community health interventions must adapt to local circumstance and challenges for populations in given areas (Bandura et al., 2014). The partnership function is also key in constructing community health. Area-based initiatives (ABIs) are the type of collaborative frameworks that aim to bring in health service delivery into socio-economically disadvantaged areas. These programs place emphasis upon the requirement for collaborative efforts from various stakeholders, from the medical practitioners to the local government and community-based organizations. Nevertheless, research indicates that despite the requirement for such collaborations in order to provide integrated services, these end up being insufficient due to provider interdependencies. For instance, the 'organizational pull' theory can deter organisations from working together, and hence policymakers should consider these forces while designing community health frameworks. This discovery is able to inform better planning that focuses on ongoing collaboration, ultimately improving health in communities (Bartlett et al., 2014). Aside from partnerships, community health principles must also leverage health education and outreach to enhance their reach. Community education about the dangers of health and encouraging access to resources can empower people to make relevant decisions, ultimately enhancing their health status. Strategies aimed at addressing barriers to healthy living, such as time constraints, exposure to fast food, and social context, are at the forefront of this approach. Identifying discrete challenges faced by various populations and crafting focused interventions, proponents can create supportive environments that facilitate healthier choices. Engaging stakeholders, including communities and residents' groups, in such an effort not only helps to secure community buy-in but also facilitates the change that leads to better public health outcomes (Bandura et al., 2014).

Importance of Community Health in Public Health

Interconnected nature between community health and public health highlights the significance of paying attention to local health concerns within a larger system. Community health programs are crucial since they have direct implications on overall public health outcomes. As an example, community preparedness for natural disasters, including floods, has a key bearing on local health. Successful flood disaster mitigation to promote resilience at the community level calls for active engagement and knowledge among the community.

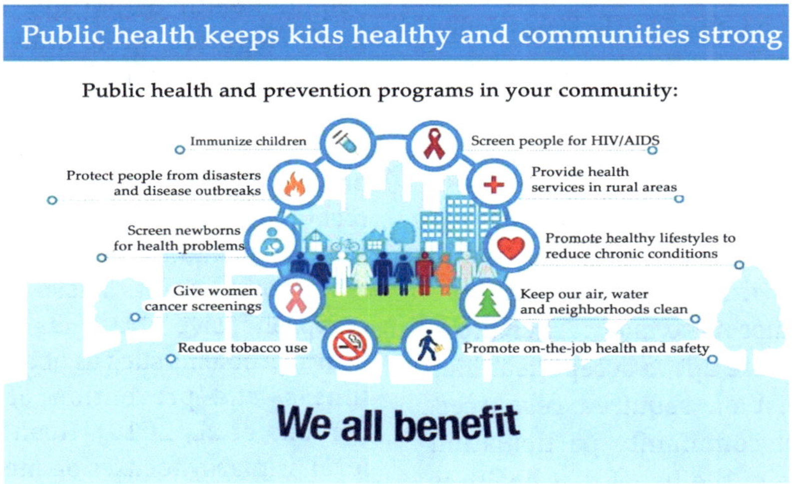

Figure 1.2. Importance of community health in public health.

Source: https://2.bp.blogspot.com/-oQXIuKlPlVs/UHxm8r8N4II/AAAAAAAAAJA/mldEzeAVFWY/w1200-h630-p-k-no-nu/apha_infographic.gif.

Research indicates that 75.6% of the participants in a study revealed a high level of understanding of flood disaster risk-reduction measures as a result of readily available information through the mass media (Widyanty et al., 2024). This suggests that enhancing public awareness and preparedness not only makes communities resilient but also facilitates an integrated attitude towards public health aimed at prevention and safety. Also of importance is the role of education in the care of chronic disease in communities. Educational programs for health have a great potential to raise public awareness about diseases like hypertension and stroke, which are prevalent in a number of populations. Including members of a community in health education programs offers greater opportunities for behavior change. An effective program at raising awareness of hypertension and risk factors for stroke utilized lectures and discussion sessions. Interestingly, post-intervention assessments revealed a tremendous boost in participants' awareness of healthy lifestyle choices and risk reduction practices (Wijayanti et al., 2024). Not only does this kind of education cement the knowledge of a subject, but it also establishes a proactive community health culture that makes efforts to prevent disease occurrence right at the forefront of public health intervention. Beyond this, community ownership of health issues is directly pertinent to improved health outcomes. When individuals within a community are engaged in health discourse and participatory activities, they are more apt to accept healthier behaviors and insist on required resources. This mechanism of community participation is the manifestation of the belief that health is not an individualistic issue but a community responsibility. The success of community-based programs is a testament to the worth of grass roots work in developing successful public health interventions. Therefore, prioritizing community health within the public health system not only ensures the health of individuals but also reinforces the collective capacity of the population to cope with health challenges, thereby creating sustainable public health progress (Figure 1.2).

Differences Between Community Health and Individual Health

The distinction between individual and community health is mostly in scope and intervention focus. Individual health focuses on personal wellbeing by intervening upon determinants of health that affect populations, groups, or the entire community. This will often include the consolidation of public health programs aimed at reducing health disparities and improving health equity on a broader scale. Individual care is focused on the needs of one patient, with stress on personalized intervention and treatment. It usually gives top priority to diagnosis, treatment, and management of particular health problems that directly impact the individual, sometimes not considering the greater social and environmental causes behind health disparities at the population level. Therefore, while individual care aims for the optimal health of one person, community health aims for systems change that can be replicated in many people. Community health programs often draw on a gigantic reservoir of resources and include involvement from several sectors, including health care, education, and local government. These programs focus on comprehensive strategies in managing public health problems such as obesity, smoking, mental illness, and prevention of substance abuse (Brooks et al., 2010). Health at the individual level primarily focuses on medical care provided by medical professionals in clinical settings. This clinical model can lead to an overreliance in defining health since patients are only given reactive care as opposed to preventive measures for promoting and maintaining health. Therefore, without a broad perspective, important health determinants such as socio-economic status and environment may be overlooked within localized paradigms of health. The consideration of such broader determinants of health is vital to truly enhancing overall community health outcomes. Ethical principles also vary quite dramatically between paradigms of community health and individual health. Individual medicine involves the medical ethics of autonomy, beneficence, and non-maleficence that advise healthcare providers to behave in the best possible interests of their patients. Community health involves a more complex ethical landscape that must balance personal privacy with the public good of public health. Public health programs usually involve policy choices that can paternalistically value group welfare at the expense of individual liberties and so create conflicts and tension (Coupland et al., 2006). Such ethical nuances are heightened when dealing with health inequalities in heterogeneous groups, calling for culturally informed intervention that is respectful of individual rights and yet promotes public health advantages. Understanding these fine points is significant for practitioners in both individual and community health settings, offering a globalized perspective to the provision of health care that respects individual rights but also promotes more universal community health needs.

1.1. Historical Context of Community Health

Community health history cannot be divorced from its historical context, and it has had a long-reaching influence on an understanding and provision of health services through the centuries. Historical practices and policies have often reflected broader social values, political structures, and economic conditions. The response to public health crises, such as pandemics, has consistently highlighted the need for collective action and community engagement. For example, the emergence of the public health movement in the late 19th century marked a paradigm shift toward preventive care, emphasizing the importance of sanitation and environmental factors in promoting health. This emphasis has served to fuel present discussions of health equity and access, as underprivileged groups have often borne the brunt of inadequate health care and institutional neglect. Recognition of such long-term trends is critical to building today's issues and interventions in community health. Understanding how socioeconomic determinants influence health outcomes has been at the core of community health practice for decades. As inequalities in health were increasingly apparent, and particularly within the cities in which populations were more diverse, researchers began to look into the reasons behind these inequalities. Place has now been the central idea in arguments over the determinants of health, revealing how individuals experience illness and health based on the environment in which they are located. For instance, studies that have investigated food insecurity in specific areas have indicated the recursive processes of food access and local resources that indicate nutrition is well embedded within regional social and economic processes (Bleecker et al., 2017). With such contextual factors understood, practitioners of health are capable of taking more targeted measures toward alleviating the multifaceted problems that face communities, hence creating a more equitable health setting. In addition, the development of grassroots movements has been a determining factor in shaping the discourse concerning community health, particularly with reference to women's empowerment and leadership. The participatory dynamics that one can observe in various health promotion initiatives, such as those in Lima, Peru, demonstrate the changing nature of community participation in health programs. These movements reveal how grassroots processes converge with worldwide trends and discourses, and how the intricacies of grassroots activism are uncovered (Jenkins et al., 2011). As community health continues to be formed, the historical background of the movements is useful for lessons on continued negotiations of power and representation. By being aware of the past, current leaders and health champions are in a stronger position to tackle the challenges of contemporary health promotion and to involve communities appropriately.

1.1.1. Evolution of Community Health Practices

Community health practice history has been primarily shaped by various social, political, and environmental determinants that have shaped public health policies over time. Traditionally, community health grew out of the need to respond to infectious diseases, and thus a fixation on sanitation and hygiene in urban settings was necessary. The growth of public health departments and vaccination campaigns were mile markers in such growth. What is worth pointing out is that these early interventions laid the groundwork for intersectoral collaboration between local communities, health practitioners, and municipal governments. Along with the evolving concept of health shifting toward a broader framework that embraces mind and social factors, community health practice expanded. Preventive care, health education, and advocacy were included in the field, reflecting more widespread recognition of individual and group health needs among diverse populations. In the last several years, community practice has increasingly valued the interdependence of ecological and human health and the necessity to integrate sustainable practices into health programs. The trend identifies the necessity for community programs to adhere to ecological resilience values, including self-regulation, diversity, and interdependence. As witnessed by Transition Networks initiatives towards constructing resilient local economies, communities are attempting novel approaches to tackling challenges such as climate change and resource limitations.

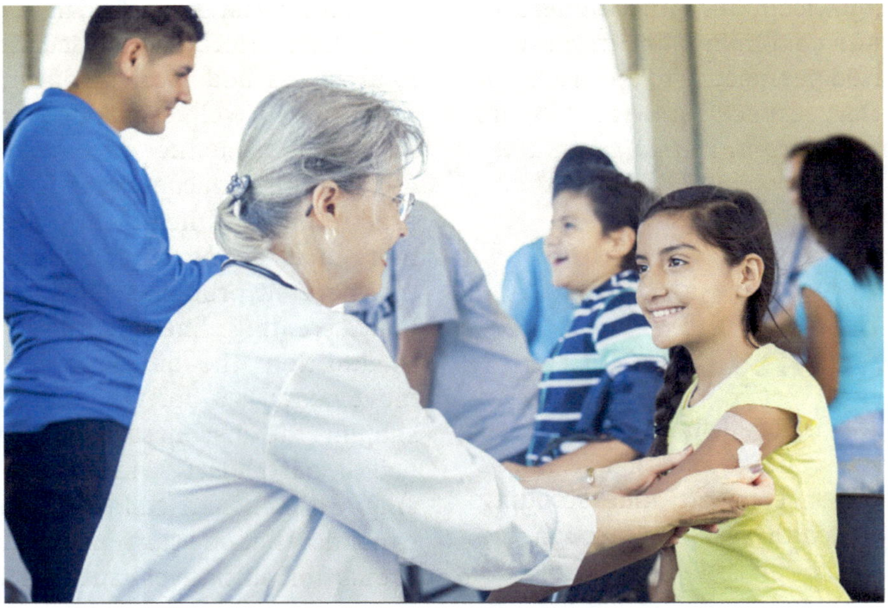

Figure 1.3. Evolution of community health practices.

Source: Evolution of community health practices.

These projects endorse localized solutions in sectors such as food, energy, and health, in a manner that ensures sustainable development through grassroots mobilization. By highlighting community and creativity, these practices seek to make people healthier while at the same time re-establishing ecological balance, highlighting the close nexus between environmental sustainability and the enhancement of public health. Additionally, the recognition of marginalized communities in forming community health practices has become increasingly common. This Emergence has contributed to incorporating diverse voices and, in particular, historically disenfranchised groups' voices into health policymaking. Scholars and practitioners like Gail Hornstein promote the complexity of experience and identity in community health interventions, particularly with mental health issues. When reconsidering the classical discourses for their mental health constructs, there is a commitment to embracing a more inclusive method in regard to the experiences of people and challenging the structural inequalities in health. This not only subverts the paradigms of mental health but provides an avenue for the enfeeblement of the cohesion within communities. As the practice of community health and public health evolves, embracing and recognizing these complex identities will be required to develop holistic interventions that resonate with the lived reality of all members in the community, building a more equitable health setting for future generations (Figure 1.3).

1.1.2. Key milestones in Community Health History

The history of community health has been characterized by major events that have transformed public health policies and interventions. One of the most crucial turning points was during the mid-19th century, when sanitation reforms were initiated, particularly in cities worst affected by infectious diseases. Key leaders, including Edwin Chadwick, highlighted the link between squalor and public health, resulting in government intervention to correct urban living conditions. These reforms spanned the creation of comprehensive sewage and clean water supply initiatives, revolutionizing community health's face. The ripple effects of these reforms not only slowed the advance of disease but formed a foundation on which to base future public health legislation, establishing a model for community-based health management that would continue to evolve during the decades. The late 19th and early 20th centuries marked another critical milestone in community health history as the germ theory of disease gained widespread acceptance. Scientists like Louis Pasteur and Robert Koch provided compelling evidence that microorganisms were responsible for many diseases, which radically transformed health education and practices. This paradigm shift led to the implementation of vaccination programs, disinfection methods, and improved hospital care, significantly reducing mortality rates. Public health organizations increasingly committed to educating communities about hygiene, prevention, and the importance of immunization. As public health practice improved, so did knowledge, leading to community health initiatives whose focus was to promote wellness as a means of preventing illness on a broader level, beyond individualistic medical care to encompass environmental and social determinants of health. Over the past decades, the community health field has shifted to a more comprehensive one that recognizes the complex interplay of factors affecting health outcomes. Some of the highlights of the new era include the development of the World Health Organizations Health for All strategy in the 1970s, which emphasized equity and social justice in health. Moreover, health education, access to healthcare, and community participation have been accorded significant significance. The increasing awareness of the role of social determinants in the health conditions has resulted in efforts directed toward bridging inequalities and ensuring inclusiveness in the delivery of healthcare. An example is the integration of services for the vulnerable, indicating an awareness of the necessity of multilateral interventions in community health. These interlinked milestones emphasize the ongoing advancement of community health, emphasizing environmental factors and community involvement in creating healthier communities.

1.1.3. Influential Figures in the Development of Community Health

The evolution of community health has been shaped by prominent figures whose innovative work has transformed healthcare delivery. One of the leading scientists in this field is Sir Michael Marmot, whose research into social determinants of health showed the large effect of social conditions on health outcomes. His hugely influential work culminated in the Marmot Review that provided irrefutable proof that inequality in health rests on social conditions such as education, income, and social status. Through the encouragement of health equity and the necessity of dealing with the broader determinants of health, Marmot has shifted community health policymakers and leaders to develop strategies which build healthier environments. This shift in mindset towards a wider approach of understanding health has led to the creation of a variety of community programs for bridging gaps, thereby signifying the active role played by social determinants in community health. In addition to the likes of Marmot, advancements in community health have also been guided by the efforts of grassroots champions like Dr. Paul Farmer.

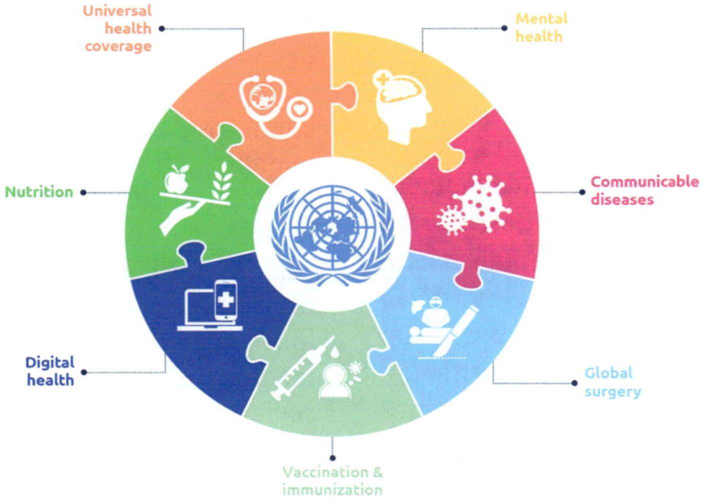

Figure 1.4. Influential figures in the development of community health.

Source: https://unitar.org/sites/default/files/media/image/PHD_circle_1_1.jpg.

By virtue of his work as a co-founder of Partners In Health, Farmer has played a leading role in demonstrating that accessible healthcare is a human right. His commitment to quality health care among poor populations challenged paradigms of health care delivery, particularly the engagement of health systems with marginalized communities. Through interprofessional solutions and community engagement, Farmers' practice has indicated the need for social justice inclusion in health care systems. Farmers work extends its influence beyond direct medical intervention to the social, economic, and political systems that drive health outcomes, challenging community health initiatives to shift towards more comprehensive, patient-centered approaches. Further, the introduction of Clinical Commissioning Groups (CCGs) in the United Kingdom is a testament to the forward vision of community health leaders who believe in clinical leadership for service redesign. The evolution of CCGs, according to the Health and Social Care Act 2012, was aimed at providing general practitioners with more autonomy in decision-making to enhance service delivery on the community level (Abbott et al., 2018). It shifts the emphasis from a fragmented health system towards one that encourages intersocietal cooperation between various sectors of healthcare. Among the successful examples of such leadership was the establishment of chronic disease care strategies that were coordinated. By struggling with the differences between which CCGs use clinical leadership, it is possible to observe that engaging clinicians in such activities can lead to significant improvements in health services. This is a serious point of consideration for understanding the evolution of community health and why constant innovation in healthcare processes is a necessity (Figure 1.4).

1.2. Determinants of Community Health

Understanding the community health determinants is crucial in reducing disparities in outcomes as well as in building healthier populations. Social determinants of health, which involve the social and economic conditions in which people are born, live, learn, work, and age, play important roles in influencing health behaviors and access to healthcare. Determining the determinants allows for targeted interventions that can improve health equity among various populations.

For instance, socioeconomic status, education, and social support structures directly correlate with health outcomes such that communities of low socioeconomic status develop higher rates of chronic diseases. Use of standard measurement protocols, e.g., by the PhenX Working Group, provides a general framework to measure such social determinants and enables systematic collection of data that enhances scientific understanding of their impact on health inequities (Breen et al., 2023). The role of community health workers (CHWs) becomes more important than ever to bridge the gap between excluded groups and the health system. Through close collaboration with communities, CHWs are able to overcome barriers to health service utilization, hence enhancing usage rates among hard-to-reach groups. Systematic review evidence identifies that CHWs can promote the equity of health access by modifying interventions that suit the specific requirements of the community, such as geographical location, gender disparities, and socio-economic status (Gomez et al., 2016). Furthermore, CHW programs have also been shown to enhance empowerment at the community level, which enables more participation of people in the management of their own health. Care and attention are, however, required; poorly planned CHW programs might actually perpetuate existing inequities rather than helping to reduce them. Lastly, determinants of community health need to be addressed through a multi-faceted approach that includes social, economic, and environmental determinants. Public health programs must not only target medical care but also the determinants of health outcomes at the structural level. Public health interventions must involve stakeholder engagement, including policymakers, healthcare providers, and community leaders. By embracing a holistic view of the socio-environmental settings affecting health, public health practitioners can implement effective interventions that not only increase access to health but also trigger overall system shifts. This wide vision is necessary in order to guarantee sustainable health improvement and closing inequalities, leading to healthier communities overall (Breen et al., 2023; Gomez et al., 2016) (Figure 1.5).

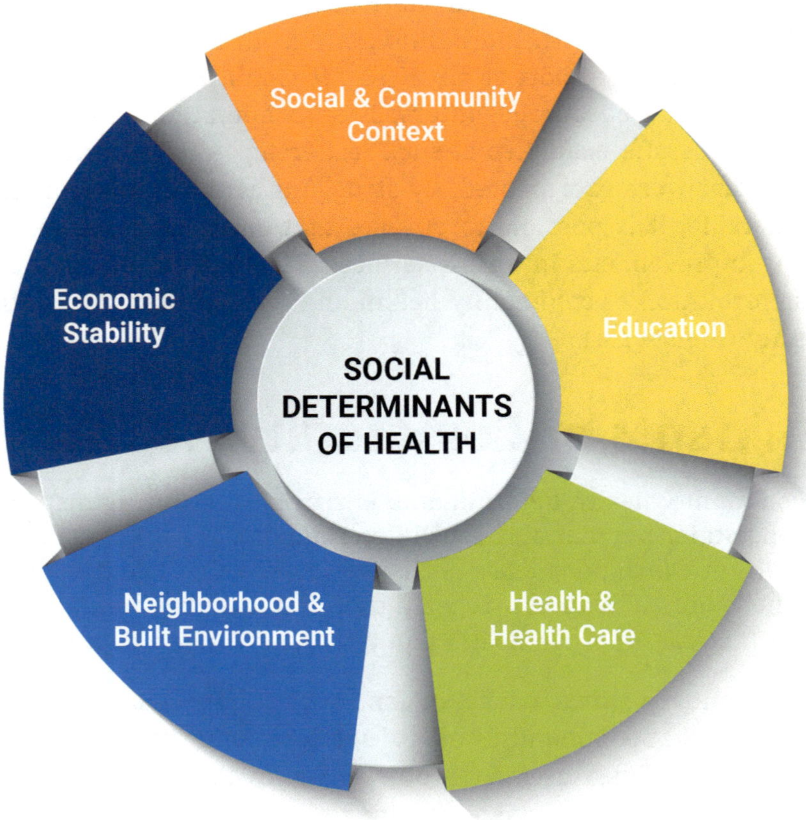

Figure 1.5. Determinants of community health.

Source: https://external-content.duckduckgo.com/iu/?u=https%3A%2F%2Fwww.iirp.edu%2Fimages%2Fimages%2FSocial_Determinants_of_Health_20_04_15.jpg&f=1&nofb=1&ipt=605520a5c78f652767382809cd7cab578b14e6771c6324d9df996d9b19105522.

1.2.1. Social Determinants and Their Impact

Social determinants must be familiar to interpret community health because these determinants have a significant impact on health outcomes in populations. Social determinants involve where and how individuals are born, grow up, live, work, and age, and the circumstances through which these factors affect behavior and access to resources determining health maintenance. Economic stability, education, and social environment, for instance, play strong roles in determining health disparities. In Nevada state, the examination of health outcomes proves the differing disease prevalence among affluent and impoverished communities, and the manner in which socio-economic conditions directly convert into markers of health. Research reveals that as much as 60% of disease risk is modifiable and comes from social factors, thus the importance of specific interventions to target these determinants to close health disparities (Millar et al., 2017). Additionally, the association of social determinants with community health can be further shown through an analysis of particular incidents, like the Ferguson, MO, unrest. Social, economic, and political dynamics within communities have a significant impact on their health consequences. In underserved populations, systemic inequalities are often manifested in limited access to good healthcare, which is tantamount to elevated levels of morbidity and mortality among marginalized groups. The analysis reveals how policies affect determinants of health, exacerbating the vulnerability of communities and creating significant health inequalities. From the perspective of social determinants of health, the stakeholders can examine the public policy implications and identify pragmatic public policy strategies to improve community well-being (Blessett et al., 2017). The effect of social determinants necessitates consideration under a multidisciplinary approach that integrates public health measures with social equity efforts. Effective community health interventions must include economic, educational, and environmental aspects to be able to deliver integrated solutions addressing root causes rather than symptoms.

For instance, increasing quality education access can empower individuals with information and resources, and in the long term, better health outcomes and healthier lifestyle decisions. Interventions that foster community action and enhance social connections can also reverse the negative effects of social determinants, enabling resilience and collective effort. Developing policy responses that target marginalized communities is central to establishing a fair health environment, and each person has an opportunity for optimal health (Millar et al., 2017).

1.2.2. Economic Factors Affecting Community Health

Economic factors are to blame for being central to shaping community health, influencing a number of social determinants of overall health. Provision and quality of health care are usually directly related to the economic situation of the community. The high unemployment communities lag behind in ensuring well-stocked health facilities, as a result of which they experience substandard health outcomes.

Additionally, inhabitants of economically disadvantaged neighborhoods may be constrained by factors such as scarce transport and means of accessing preventive health care—a situation that aggravates health disparities. Lack of financial capability for financing health programs can lead to the degeneration or decline in health standards, a situation indicating the need for targeted economic intervention aimed at promoting equitable access to health care services. Community-based economic interventions can thus reinforce health outcomes through direct access to care as well as longer-term systemic change. Investments in targeted areas can also stimulate local economies while public health is improved concurrently. For example, initiatives that generate jobs in health and social care have been shown to advance community health outcomes. The successful case studies reviewed across several EU Member States—e.g., Denmark and the Netherlands—show that job creation initiatives well-structured to meet the employment demands not only respond to the needs but also encourage the provision of quality healthcare services. Such economic interventions can fundamentally enhance the community members' quality of life, especially for vulnerable groups like adults with disabilities.

Hence, stimulating economic growth through job provision in the health sector can enable a virtuous circle that enhances community resilience and health outcomes and introduces new skills to the health sector (de Klaver et al., 2013). Additionally, addressing deeper economic determinants can lead to improved public health interventions. In recent arguments about primary prevention of illness, especially within communities, understanding the economic context is critical. For instance, in the case of addressing partner violence or alcohol consumption, adding economic assets like job security and education programs can create a support setting for reducing such issues. That is particularly crucial among immigrant groups, where economic integration can be used to establish better health norms and community cohesiveness. Policymakers must connect economic development and health policy in creating sustainable paths to better community health. This approach not only requires short-term healthcare interventions but also long-term economic stability as the foundation for creating healthier communities (Cohen et al., 2007) (Figure 1.6).

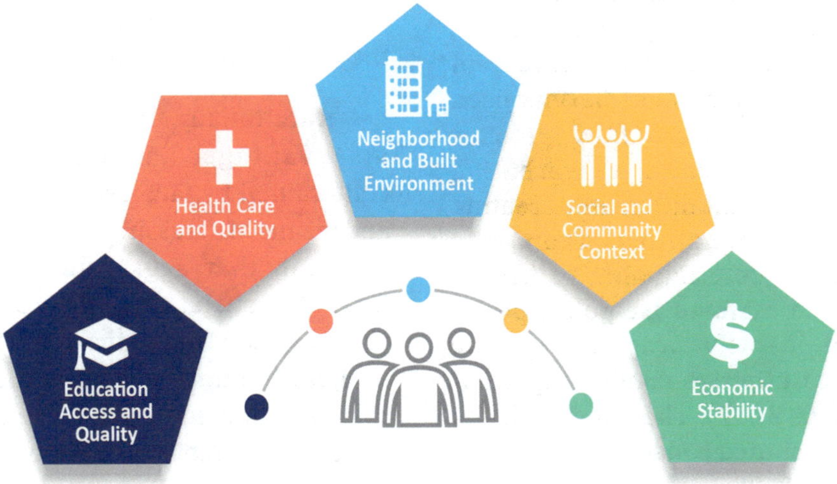

Figure 1.6. Economic factors affecting community health.

Source: https://www.cdc.gov/public-health-gateway/media/images/images/sdoh/SDOH-icons.png.

1.2.3. Environmental Influences on Health Outcomes

Environmental factors play an important role in determining outcomes of health, particularly when it comes to the health of communities. A number of determinants, including social, economic, and physical environments, converge to influence individual and population well-being. For example, access to clean water, healthy nutrition, and safe housing have a significant effect on health behavior and outcome. Resource-poor populations have higher chronic disease prevalence, necessitating an understanding of how environmental determinants converse with social determinants of health. Social enterprises are, through research, shown to be effective at enhancing health outcomes by addressing issues related to lifestyle at community levels, revealing the potential of grassroots action to end inequalities and facilitate individuals to take action on their health through healthier behavior and social relationships (Gordon et al., 2017). In addition, environmental impact reaches even the marginalized groups who are more likely to experience cumulative disadvantage. Vulnerable groups tend to be at heightened risk from their environment, such as pollution and lack of infrastructure. This calls for extensive knowledge about how broader socio-environmental circumstances affect children's development as outlined by the Children's Ground project. The projects' place-based approach emphasizes the need for joined-up services in addressing acute issues and system barriers that hinder the optimal health outcome. By examining the multiplex determinants of health, such as socioeconomic status and community engagement, we can design more effective interventions that are targeted at a community's needs (Lorains et al., 2025). Finally, health equity is only achieved through thoughtful interventions that are attuned to the interdependency of environmental determinants and resultant health outcomes. Policymakers and public health professionals must approach the issue with a holistic strategy that addresses both foreground and background determinants that affect the health of a community. This requires encouraging collaboration between various actors towards the development of governance systems that regulate resources in an efficient way. Through embracing approaches rooted in community-driven needs, as demonstrated by successful community food projects, resilience to health inequities becomes a reality. In summary, understanding effects of environment on health outcomes is essential to create long-lasting public health progress and allow all individuals in a community to thrive irrespective of the status (Gordon et al., 2017; Lorains et al., 2025) (Figure 1.7).

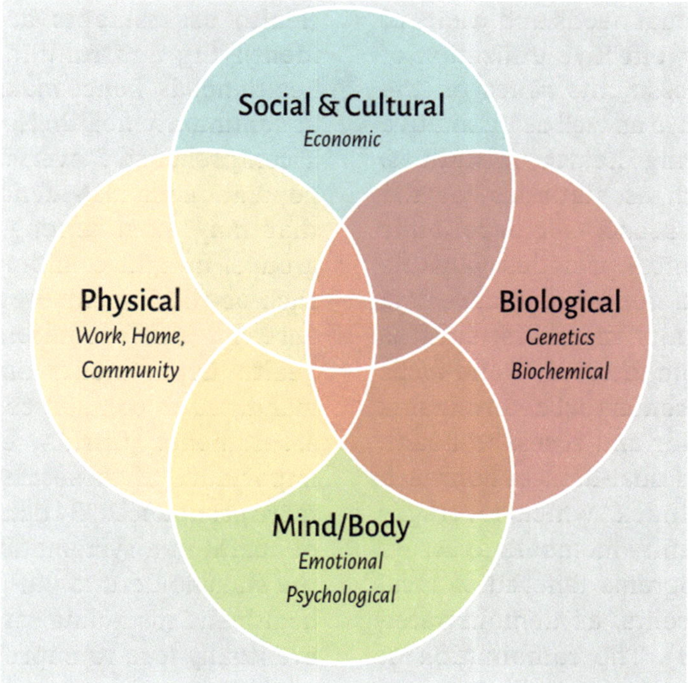

Figure 1.7. Environmental influences on health outcomes.

Source: http://box5233.temp.domains/~earthro4/wp-content/uploads/2022/10/Environmental-Influences-on-Health.png .

1.3. Community Health Assessment

Community health assessment is a key component of building effective health policies and interventions in practice. It involves a systematic process that involves data collection and analysis pertaining to the health status, needs, and resources of a community. By engaging a broad group of stakeholders, ranging from members of the community and health care providers to local health authorities, assessments form a comprehensive vision of the health reality that comes into play among a population. Such collaborative endeavors can be exemplified by efforts such as the interprofessional education (IPE) efforts cited in Blum et al., (2016), which show how collaborative efforts among health professionals tend to significantly increase the depth of community health projects. Effective identification and response to health disparities become possible when several perspectives are employed in the analysis, such that interventions become grounded in actual needs and wants of the public. Additionally, effective utilization of community health assessments relies on the application of quantitative as well as qualitative information in planning health initiatives. Quantitative data, such as statistics for the burden of chronic disease, socioeconomic status, and demographics, provides valuable information about health trends. Qualitative data obtained from community members, such as verbatim comments from interviews and focus groups, illustrates how contextual determinants influence health behavior and access to health care. An example of this dual-dataset approach is the School Health Index, which leverages school staff and community members to assess and build wellness programs tailored to local populations of adolescents, as demonstrated in Austin et al., (2010). The combination of these data types allows the possibility to build targeted interventions, optimally fitting into their respective relevance and potential influence. In the end, the continued cycle of community health assessment produces a constantly evolving model of health improvement. With the frequent renewal of the assessment process, communities can respond to shifting health trends and newly developing threats by revising their strategies in response. Through the repetition of the process, interventions remain timely and effective in the long run. For example, as has been observed in the case of the School Health Index, the use of external facilitators can play a crucial role in maximizing collaborative efforts in schools and subsequently, better health outcomes through collaboratively developed action plans. These regular assessments give power to communities by enabling them to own their health futures, which ultimately results in a healthier environment that ensures well-being and promotes resilience among its constituent members.

1.3.1. Purpose and Importance of Health Assessments

Health assessments are a critical factor in identifying and fulfilling populations' public health needs, hence making them a crucial part of community health. Not only do they provide a comprehensive overview of the health of a population but also identify specific inequalities that may exist among different population groups. In light of more recent developments, such as the Patient Protection and Affordable Care Act (ACA) requirements that local public health departments and hospitals must be mandated to conduct community health needs assessments (CHNAs) every three years, the importance of these assessments has become more pronounced. By data collection and analysis of health in a systematic way, it is possible for the stakeholders to pin-point priority issues of health and formulate certain interventions that eventually lead to improving the overall health of the public based on vital considerations of health literacy and availability of care (Robinson et al., 2017). Moreover, the assessment of health serves to facilitate collaboration among different stakeholders, including government agencies, healthcare professionals, and community organizations. These partnerships are central to enforcing successful public health measures and in establishing a comprehensive approach to health promotion. Incorporation of health screening within community settings has encouraged dialogue between such stakeholders, allowing them to recognize communities' needs better. Such communication by these assessments can help bridge perception and knowledge gaps related to health risks, particularly for groups suffering from environmental contaminants and other public health issues (Caron et al., 2011). The health assessments thus serve as a channel through which individuals within the community are engaged and their contributions received, thereby making public health programs more effective and useful. Finally, ongoing review and optimization of health evaluations maintain the beat of applicability in the face of ever-changing public health dynamics. As communities evolve with time, so do their health needs, and regular checks ensure that health interventions remain in sync with current issues. Moreover, trends revealed through these evaluations stand the chance to guide resource allocation and policymaking, optimizing return on investment for public health. For instance, emerging issues such as mental illness, drug addiction, and chronic disease can be made priorities from assessment findings, facilitating timely interventions for pressing health conditions. Thus, health assessment is not merely a snapshot of community health at one moment in time but provides actionable information in driving systemic change towards healthier and more resilient communities (Robinson et al., 2017) (Figure 1.8).

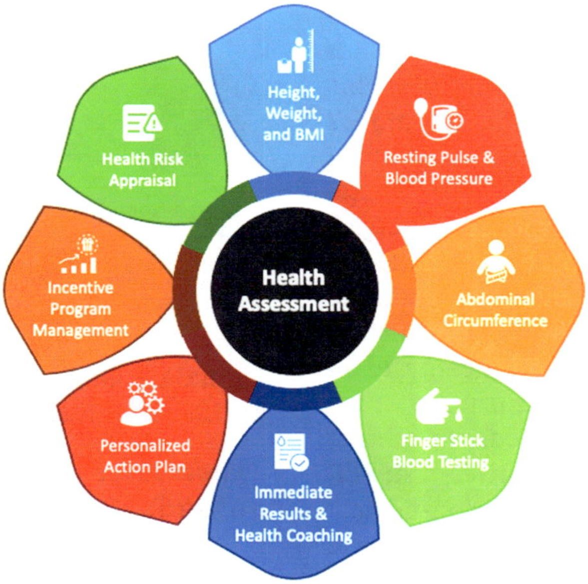

Figure 1.8. Purpose and importance of health assessments.

Source: https://cdn.sketchbubble.com/pub/media/catalog/product/optimized1/a/8/a8fb2f35d621a507cdb7b60a9b107cce40d6 9c0f85b46fd2b840c2a59a4934db/health-assessment-mc-slide2.png.

1.3.2. Methods for Conducting Community Health Assessments

Conducting successful community health assessments requires a systematic process that integrates various methodologies and frameworks in order to gather inclusive health information. Among the methodologies are qualitative and quantitative, which provide different information on community health needs. Qualitative research, including interviews and focus groups, allows a rich overview of attitudes and experiences of communities regarding health. Quantitative research, for example, surveys and health metrics, provides numerical findings that can detect public health trends and disparities. This combination permits the ability of health workers to gain more extensive and in-depth information, to inform interventions and policy making and to address the specific health concerns within the community. The application of a mixed-methods design offers not only data-driven evaluations but also responsive responses to the lived experience of community members, and this actually makes health initiatives much more effective and applicable. One extremely powerful model for community health assessment is the Community Assessment for Public Health Emergency Response (CASPER). Developed by the Centers for Disease Control and Prevention, CASPER applies standardized instruments to rapidly capture data on basic needs and health status following emergencies or disasters. This technique applies sound statistical techniques to obtain information systematically from households, thus enabling rapid collection of data with the ability to inform response strategies effectively. CASPER's adaptability makes it applicable not just in crisis but also in routine community health assessments, permitting public health administrators to concentrate on responses to health concerns in priority order based on actual community needs. In uniting citizens with public health agencies, CASPER lays groundwork for informed decision-making and resource planning in both emergency and non-emergency situations in achieving improved public health outcomes for communities. Assessment of partnerships in community health ventures is pivotal to establishing their effectiveness and sustainability over the long term. As contextualized by newer studies, the difference between effectiveness in projects versus partnership is essential in capturing the multifaceted dynamics in collaborative healthcare ventures. This is necessary not just to examine the outcome of health interventions but also the quality and durability of partnerships formed in the process. An analysis of factors such as relevance, coherence, and sustainability in such partnerships can illuminate the options for enhancing community health programs. Ultimately, this view underscores the value of formulating approaches that measure both project outcomes and partnership processes because the effectiveness of community health programs is contingent on durable, effective partnerships and not isolated project success. Development of strong relationships can lead to long-term health benefits, once more supporting the role of community health assessments to develop resilient health systems (Dokova et al., 2022; National Center for Environmental Health (U.S.) Division of Environmental Hazards and Health Effects. Health Studies Branch, 2025) (Figure 1.9).

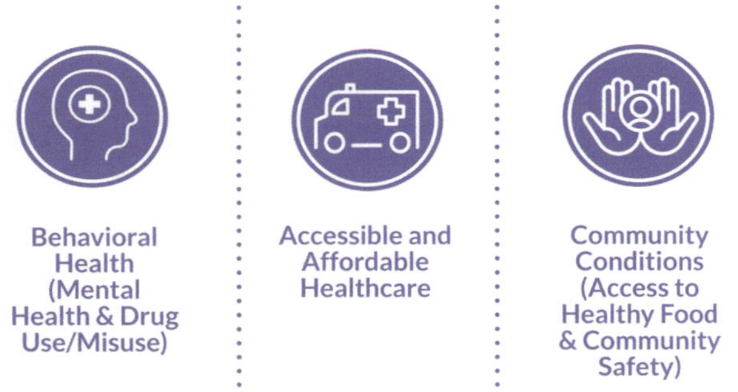

Figure 1.9. Methods for conducting community health assessments.

Source: https://hipcuyahoga.org/wp-content/uploads/2022/10/Cuyahoga-County-Prioritized-Health-Needs-Visual-1.png.

1.3.3. Analyzing Data and Identifying Health Needs

Data analysis in community health is crucial in identifying the various health needs that arise among various populations. Data analysis involves rigorous review of numeric as well as textual information, which can reveal unsuspected patterns and trends among health outcomes. With the application of quantitative techniques, such as community health surveys and prevalence studies, researchers can gain insights into some health concerns among various groups. Use of tools like the Alcohol Use Disorders Identification Test-Consumption (AUDIT-C) is one method through which specific tools can be utilized most effectively to measure risk behaviors and the need for interventions. The responses collected with the aid of such tools are more appropriate for elaboration on the effects of socio-environmental factors on health, especially among marginalized communities, and why culturally sensitive approaches are necessary in public health programs (Conigrave et al., 2019). Diagnosis of health needs is unavoidably linked with understanding the multifactor determinants of community health issues. Treatment of pressure injury, for instance, exemplifies how health needs are influenced by an interaction between socio-economic status, access to health care, and the presence of support systems. By way of comprehensive data collection, community health researchers can evaluate the effectiveness of existing care models and access barriers to receiving necessary treatments, namely within chronic care environments. Leveraging the use of interdisciplinary teams and gathering qualitative data through clinician conversation, a greater understanding is obtained, revealing gaps in practice and opportunities for improvement. Identification of such gaps requires the development of intervention that not only covers immediate needs for health but, significantly, enhances ultimate health gain in community settings (Rose et al., 2016). Moreover, implications of the health needs identification extend beyond provision to include policy and organizational change in health systems. Through the integration of information from various sources, public health practitioners and health workers can advocate for evidence-based change that addresses the actual needs of the community. To illustrate, the creation of community-led health services can be critical in making care accessible, equitable, and responsive to cultural expectations. As shown through initiatives to increase alcohol screening and treatment among Indigenous populations, the emphasis on local data can inform intervention that is tailored to the local setting and optimizes resource utilization. Such ongoing surveillance and responsiveness are essential as it serves to address urgent health concerns while also contributing to the development of resilient health systems that are more capable of adapting to emerging community demands (Conigrave et al., 2019; Rose et al., 2016).

1.4. Community Health Programs and Interventions

The integration of community health programs and interventions is an essential component in increasing public health results. The interventions have the tendency to concentrate on the management of chronic diseases, which have brought about numerous challenges to health care systems across the entire United States. Recent studies have presented an enhanced understanding of the capabilities for cooperation between health care systems and public health practitioners to drive effective interventions. For instance, in one survey, 84% of state-level chronic disease public health professionals reported collaborating with health care systems to work on diverse areas such as tobacco control and cardiovascular health. This collaboration not only foster a more holistic approach but also emphasizes the need to utilize evidence-based tools, including the Community Guide, as a source of guidance in developing more comprehensive intervention strategies that crosscut both the health care and public health systems (Allen et al., 2014). Community health programs also consist of specific interventions designed to mitigate health threats associated with tobacco smoking, a primary causant of morbidity and mortality. The Task Force on Community Preventive Services has reviewed systematically various interventions attempting to lessen tobacco-related health issues. Interventions involve decreasing exposure to secondhand smoke, preventing initiation, and promoting cessation in current users. In offering support for such recommendations, communities are better positioned to mobilize resources and take programs tailored to their settings. Such targeted approaches both improve the individual health status and the general health setting by lowering social costs associated with tobacco smoking (Task Force on Community Preventive Services (U.S.), 2025). How well community health intervention programs and strategies perform relies heavily on ongoing monitoring and adaptability to changing health problems. As public health needs evolve, so too do the strategies used to meet them. Regular feedback and data gathering are essential to establishing the impact of programs deployed and suggesting areas of change. Utilization of community feedback is essential as it makes interventions culturally appropriate and attuned. Additionally, involvement of partnerships among various stakeholders like local institutions, health agencies, and members of the community has the potential to optimize resource mobilization and distribution. Lastly, the synergy created because of all these synergistic actions can be converted into sustainable gains in health and move communities toward the control of their own health (Allen et al., 2014).

1.4.1. Types of Community Health Programs

Community health programs play an important role in enhancing the overall well-being of populations by addressing various issues involving health at the community level. One of the most apparent types is the preventive health program, whose aim is to avoid illness prior to its occurrence.

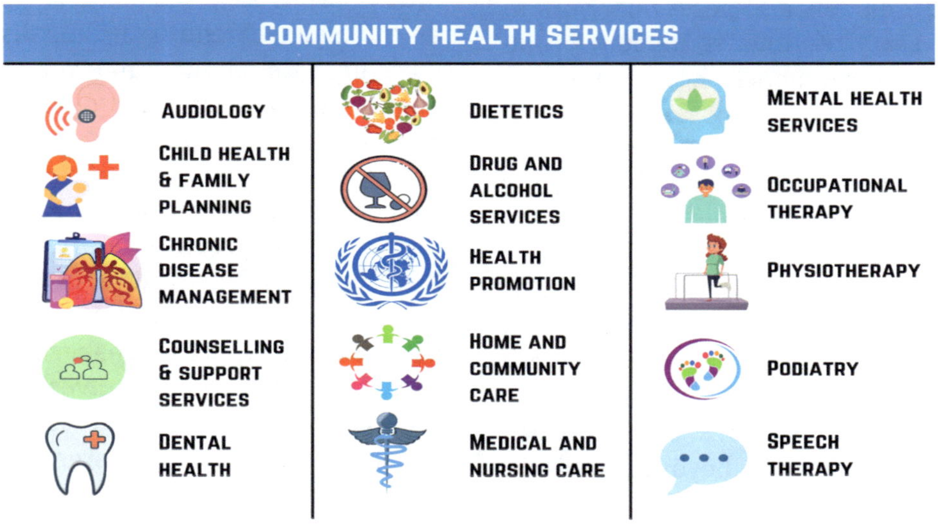

Figure 1.10. Types of community health programs.

Source: https://myknee.trekeducation.org/wp-content/uploads/sites/14/2021/12/Community-health-services-1500x1061.png.

These programs typically provide their agenda for vaccination campaigns, screenings, and educational programs designed to increase the ability of individuals to make healthy decisions. Through emphasis on prevention, communities can ease the burden of healthcare systems and improve quality of life. For instance, successful immunization drives not only protect individuals but also confer herd immunity to those who cannot be vaccinated. Such a pre-emptive measure is required in order to prevent infectious diseases as well as chronic diseases and demonstrate that effective community health programs can have far-reaching impacts on public health outcomes. Another significant type of community health programs is directed towards maternal and child health because they address the unique healthcare requirements of women and children. These programs often consist of essential services such as prenatal and postnatal care, nutrition counseling, and family planning education.

By focusing on mother and child health, these types of programs aim to reduce mortality rates and improve health metrics in a population. Programs that educate parents on breastfeeding, immunizations, and regular check-ups are essential to healthy populations. Review of children's insurance health reveals shifts in coverage patterns, wherein it may be said that governmental health programs are also capable of addressing disparities in access to care. Public insurance among children has increased, reflecting a response to needs of vulnerable populations, with the contribution of government-sponsored programs to robustness of community health (Bean et al., 2011). Furthermore, the role of community health programs extends to environmental health also, as initiatives are made in decreasing health risks present in the environment. Health impact assessment programs demonstrate how extensive environmental policies can be in influencing community health outcomes. Through the examination of potential health impacts of projects pertaining to transportation, energy, and waste management, communities are able to make well-informed decisions that serve public health. Inclusion of HIAs in community planning points out the importance of inter-sectoral collaboration in addressing complex health-related issues. By effectively incorporating health outcomes and environmental policies, communities are able to create sustainable, healthy environments, ensuring an integrated public health approach that favors the whole population. It is a balanced strategy that is important since it assists in the construction of a strong problem-solving community with respect to both short-term and long-term health issues (Corbett et al., 2012) (Figure 1.10).

1.4.2. Strategies for Effective Health Interventions

To effectively intervene in health disparities among communities, one should use a comprehensive approach that combines individual and environmental strategies. Far-reaching health interventions must consider the complex interaction between social determinants and their impact on health outcomes. For instance, population-level interventions should be designed in such a way that they encompass educational outreach, resource availability, and cultural nuances of the target community. This is particularly important while designing health communication campaigns for populations at risk of health disparities, such as lesbian, gay, bisexual, and transgender (LGBT) populations, who are not going to take messages of health well. Involving community voices in the intervention process and tailoring messages for targeting specific needs enables health interventions to achieve better participation and build an ecological orientation that supports long-term health benefits (Drabble et al., 2003). Empirical consideration of environmental determinants of health is also crucial for successful intervention. Ecological orientation emphasizes the requirement of modifying the near environment and social circumstances to promote healthier habits and outcomes. For Indigenous groups, this might involve targeted interventions like improved housing, enabling physical activity infrastructure, and food security. Effective interventions are found to incorporate local knowledge and community opinion to ensure maximum uptake and salience. Intervening at various levels—individual, interpersonal, community, and policy—health programs can get the environment ready to facilitate ease of making it easier for people to enhance their health behavior effectively (Leah Johnston, 2025). These changes amplify the impact of interventions at the individual level, culminating in increased health benefits. Health interventions must be complemented by robust mechanisms for evaluation if they are to reach their potential. Routine monitoring and evaluation of health programs are required for impact assessment and improvement areas. Both quantitative and qualitative forms of evaluation should be employed to capture the intricacies of the outcomes of community health programs. Engagement of community members in the evaluation process can yield essential information that is used to inform program design in real-time. Furthermore, provision of continuous feedback loops facilitates adaptive plans flexible to changing needs and circumstances in a community. A cyclical process ensures that health interventions continue to be relevant and responsive to those whom they are meant to serve, ultimately boosting health literacy and outcomes for diverse populations (Leah Johnston, 2025).

1.4.3. Evaluation of Program Effectiveness

Program effectiveness evaluation is crucial in community health programs, particularly because it informs policy development and optimizes the use of resources. Evaluators apply different methodologies for measuring the impact of various health programs. These methodologies of evaluation are qualitatively and quantitatively varied. Collectively, they aid in evaluating the process and impacts of the programs. For example, the Sierra Health Foundations Clinic Capacity Building Program is a systematic assessment approach to developing operating capacity of community health centers. Launched as a response to the increasing need for health care services after the Affordable Care Act, the efficacy of the programs was thoroughly tested by the Center for Community Health and Evaluation. By the systematic evaluation of clinic leadership, quality of care, and economic sustainability data, the review had tangible proof of the programs contribution toward improving Federally Qualified Health Centers in the region (N/A, 2015). Secondly, economic review of community health programs is an important element in proving their worth and feasibility. Cost-effectiveness analyses (CEA) and cost-benefit analyses (CBA) are vital frameworks for the identification of the cost implications of healthcare interventions. New South Wales's Brighter Futures program is a prime example of the analytic evaluation approach. The program, focused on giving support to disadvantaged families and children, has its effectiveness tested by a consortium led by the Social Policy Research Centre, which conducts economic appraisal and measures long-term effects for the target group.

Through the application of CEA and CBA, the appraisers are not only able to identify the economic effectiveness of such programs, but also their overall social impacts, effectively further strengthening the argument to maintain investment in preventative health care (Gallego et al., 2025). In the case of community health, applying evaluation methods maintains focus on the big picture of program performance and allows for successive improvements. Evaluation should consider multiple measures including outcomes in health, user satisfaction, and community engagement. Outcomes from evaluation not only do no more than justify the diversion of resources but also guide scaling up good practice. For instance, the Clinic Capacity Building Programs evaluation highlighted strengths and weaknesses, providing a model for the next programs designed to enhance access and quality in health care. In general, good evaluation is the foundation for propelling progress in community health, where programs are not just implemented but also modified according to empirical findings and changing needs of the populations they are working with.

1.5. Role of Healthcare Professionals in Community Health

Roles of healthcare professionals in community health involve patient care directly, education, and contact with various stakeholders. Nurses, physicians, and pharmacists have a pivotal role in delivering preventive services and managing chronic conditions. Healthcare professionals have an imperative role in shaping the health behavior of individuals and communities through their participation in health promotion and disease prevention programs. For example, community pharmacists have been at the center of public health interventions in public health programs such as immunization and screening services for health. Research shows that the involvement of pharmacists can augment public health outreach, indicating their ability to work collaboratively with other health providers to solve health issues in communities (Agomo et al., 2017).

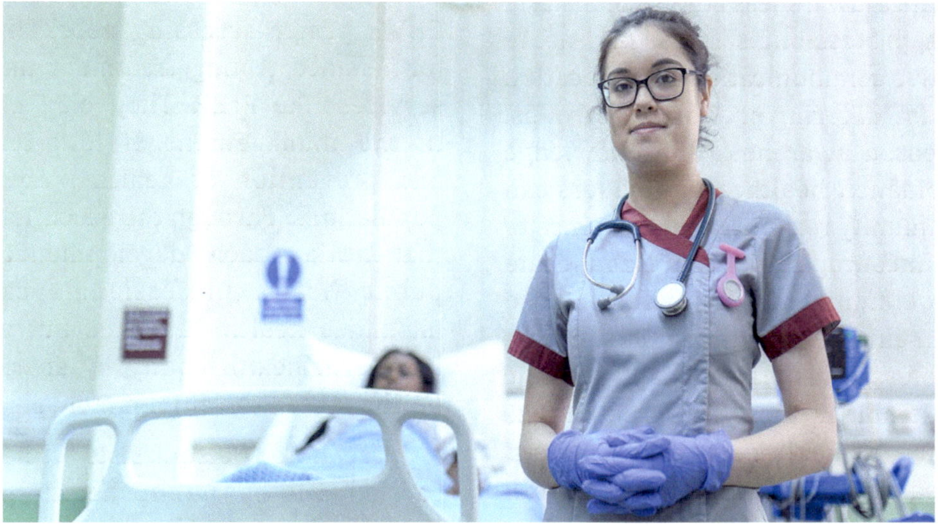

Figure 1.11. Role of healthcare professionals in community health.

Source: https://healthplan.co.uk/wp-content/uploads/2023/01/explaining-the-role-of-healthcare-professionals.jpg.

Such a multidisciplinary approach is vital in solving health disparities and ensuring effective healthcare delivery among underserved populations. Moreover, education and training of healthcare professionals significantly influence their performance while working in community health. Good foundation in the fundamentals of public health is very important for professionals who hope to carry out community health programs successfully. Evidence indicates that interprofessional learning in which medical students learn together can potentially enhance teamwork and improve service provision in public health environments (Agomo et al., 2017). This training not just puts the required skills in the hands of health professionals but also creates a full understanding of diverse health issues among populations. Cooperative and collaborative efforts by health professionals can create a culture of health literacy, thus enabling citizens to take control of their health. In the long term, professionally trained health personnel are likely to be engaged in community health activities that are effective, leading to high positive health outcomes in the population. Moreover, the role of healthcare practitioners is not confined to straightaway care and teaching alone; they have a significant role in conducting research and health policy promotion for the benefit of communities. Public health practitioners must anticipate trends in health, such as infectious disease incidence, and come up with education and intervention plans. For instance, awareness studies of malaria among health professionals stress the acute need for effective communication and education interventions for differing professional groups. Through increased awareness and knowledge of disease avoidance, healthcare providers can maximize community response and resilience to health crises. Encouraging policies that allocate resources to community health programs is also required, again emphasizing the important role healthcare professionals play in shaping public health policy. Combined, these efforts emphasize the importance of healthcare professionals' input into healthy communities and overall wellness (Figure 1.11).

1.5.1. Responsibilities of Public Health Workers

Public health professionals occupy a pivotal role in advancing and protecting community health through several responsibilities that go beyond education, advocacy, and provision of services. They work with multitudes of populations, sometimes acting as cultural brokers who help bridge healthcare systems with vulnerable populations. In the context of chronic diseases and infectious diseases like HIV, the benefits of CHWs can't be overemphasized. They contribute positively by offering health education and consciousness, which ultimately helps individuals to make an informed choice regarding their health. By holding outreach programs, public health professionals establish trust and credibility among members of the community, making them have a setting where proper interventions for health and overall population well-being can be effective (Nunez et al., 2024). In addition to education and outreach, public health workers also perform coordination of care services, ensuring that individuals receive coordinated care tailored to their specific needs. This involves collaboration with different stakeholders like healthcare providers, social service agencies, and community organizations.

For instance, when addressing HIV care, CHWs prefer accessing necessary resources, for instance, testing, treatment, and prevention services like PrEP. They play a crucial role in the management of long-term diseases and prevention of health inequities among populations. Through the execution of activities that entitle capacity development and advocacy, public health professionals can not only maximize health outcomes but also increase long-term health equity by sparking changes on the system level (Himmelweit et al., 2010).

Technology also assists with the activities carried out by public health professionals has also been an important factor in recent healthcare delivery. Technology enables CHWs to gather data, monitor health trends, and use evidence-based interventions more efficiently. The use of technology in their practice enhances the interaction between public health workers and members of the population and the availability of health information. This transition into technology-based practice proves the need for ongoing training and assistance to CHWs due to the constantly evolving healthcare system. As they continue to adapt and innovate, the work of public health professionals is paramount in building the resilient communities and addressing the multifaceted challenges of public health today (Nunez et al., 2024).

1.5.2. Collaboration with Community Organizations

Effective community organization collaboration is a cornerstone in community health promotion, which guarantees significant linkage between various stakeholders and facilitates public health outcomes. These collaborations leverage unique resources, skills, and abilities a single organization may lack. One example is the Mental Health Services Act (MHSA), where it focuses on public-private partnerships, i.e., the Respite Partnership Collaborative (RPC) in Sacramento County, which brings together community members and organizations to improve mental health services. With the coming together of opinions and experience from various sectors, collaborations like the RPC are able to establish new solutions that are a direct response to local healthcare preferences and needs and, ultimately, establish a more responsive health system and community resilience, as witnessed through the RPCs community-based approach and its firm drive to improve respite service choices, as presented in the project's evaluation report (Poon et al., 2016). Multisector community partnerships (MCPs) are another critical strategy for developing enhanced community health by strategic partnership. Through the engagement of stake-holders like governmental public health agencies, non-profit agencies, and neighborhood groups, MCPs are positioned to intervene in the social determinants of health (SDOH) impacting community well-being. Health departments have been found to play an essential role in these efforts through the provision of resources such as funds, technical assistance, and data sharing, which improve the collaborative work among such agencies. MCPs' collaborative structure provides holistic insights into health issues within the community and the development of meaningful interventions designed to promote health equity. When plans for uniting the assets of health departments and the work of community organizations come to fruition, stakeholders are able to work together towards closing gaps and building a culture of health in their communities, recent evaluation results of MCPs show (N/A, 2025). Collaborations involving community groups will not only succeed with resource sharing but also through trust and communication among the partners. Building robust connections among community organizations requires prolonged contact, sensitivity, and common vision for enhancing health. Initiatives like RPC illustrate how effective partnerships can enable local stakeholders to influence health policy and practice by having their voice heard in decision-making. Furthermore, building robust networks enhances the capacity of community organizations to mobilize resources effectively, addressing pressing health needs in communities. While communities struggle to address sophisticated health problems, enduring partnerships are vital in developing distinctive strategies towards long-term improvement in health and building frameworks that prioritize the health of all members of the community, demonstrating the invaluable contribution of partnership in community health.

1.5.3. Advocacy and Policy-making in Community Health

Policy and advocacy are crucial components of community health because they aid in addressing the system barriers that confront health outcomes. Effective advocacy is not just about raising awareness for health concerns, but also advocating for stakeholders and community members to influence policy decision-making. Such involvement is critical because policies are likely to affect the allocation of resources, access to healthcare, and implementation of health programs. For instance, health programs aimed at improving community welfare can be supported or hindered by public policies.

In this context, the intricacies of policy-making procedures are supposed to be familiar and comprehensible to advocates interested in establishing meaningful improvements. With health systems as an instrument of change through well-informed decision-making, advocacy serves as a viable mechanism for achieving equal health outcomes among populations with diverse needs. The role of foundations in policy making and advocacy is more and more recognized as a means of maximizing impact in community health. In incorporating public policy into their grantmaking, foundations can leverage their investment to bring about system change. Advocacy campaigns, when connected with funding efforts, enable foundations to not only provide funding for intervention-specific health efforts but also to invest in long-term sustainable solutions.

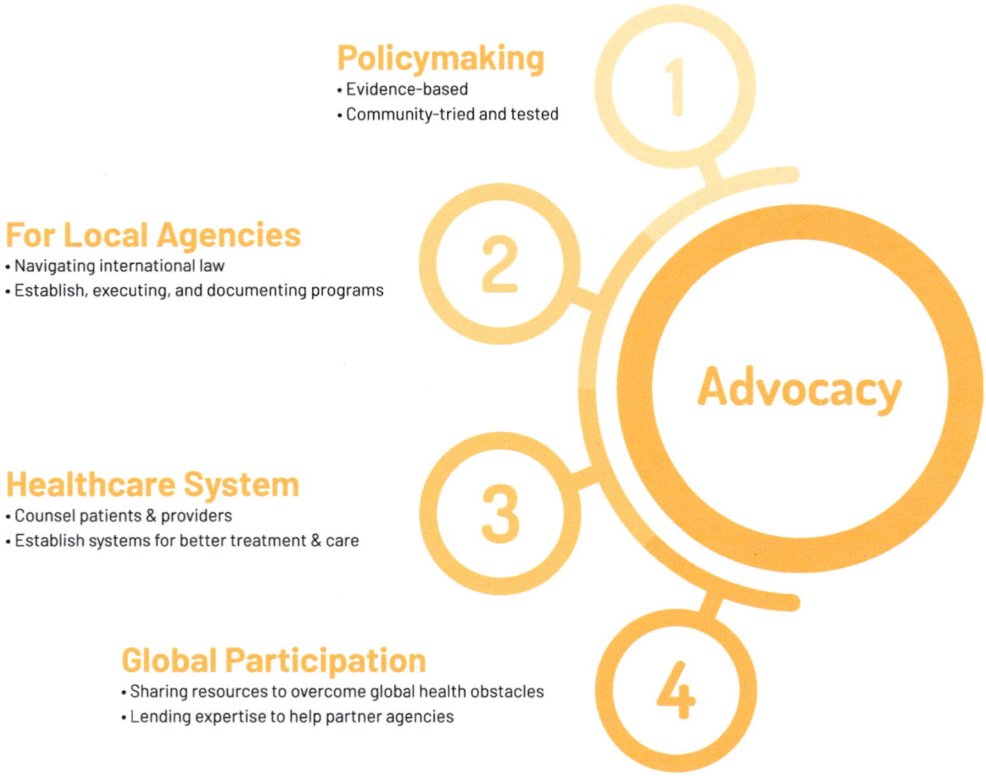

Figure 1.12. Advocacy and policy-making in community health.

Source: https://www.basichealth.org/wp-content/uploads/2020/11/BHI-Advocacy@300x-2048x1597.png.

Evidence indicates that effective public policy grantmaking has the potential to generate higher returns for society, connecting private philanthropic efforts with public investment strategies. Nevertheless, the application of policy advocacy as part of foundational efforts remains constrained with the majority of organizations yet to regard exploring this as an option. In order to use their maximum value, foundations must grasp the challenge to become change agents of policy, upholding health system improvements for alignment with community health and well-being (Coffman, 2008). Multifield environmental change strategies are equally important to the promotion of healthier communities due to their approach towards the determinants of the inter-related outcomes of health. The Health Eating Active Living Convergence Partnership is interested in creating integrated frameworks that convene several sectors so that healthy promotion activities are synergistic and not fragmented. Through this, various stakeholders like government, non-profits, and community groups are convened to work together towards the creation of policies that can facilitate healthy environments. These models enable the establishment of policies that assist in expanding access to healthy food and active lifestyles, thus mitigating health disparities. Through engaging in advocacy activities seeking environmental and policy-level changes, community health programs are able to reap benefits that carry far beyond to improve the quality of life for all members of the community (Morganstern et al., 2009) (Figure 1 12).

1.6. Challenges in Community Health

Community health is faced with numerous challenges resulting from the complexity of social, economic, and environmental determinants affecting populations. Some of the significant challenges are a lack of access to healthcare services, particularly in rural or disadvantaged urban communities. The people in such communities have increased chronic diseases in consideration of the low level of access to medical facilities and specialists. Moreover, socioeconomic disparities exacerbate health inequities because poorer communities may lack access to necessary treatments or preventive care. Initiatives such as the EPA's Community Action for a Renewed Environment (CARE) program have highlighted the key role played by community-led processes in addressing these inequalities through multi-stakeholder collaboration. By establishing local action and participation on priority environmental risks, CARE aims to increase sustainable health improvements while promoting marginalized communities' participation and engagement in health planning initiatives (John et al., 2009). Another issue in community health is the link between the environment and public health. Health conditions are greatly influenced by environmental factors such as air and water quality, food safety, and toxicant exposure. For instance, degradation of the environment can lead to respiratory diseases, waterborne diseases, and starvation, which call for an integrated response in public health interventions. People from communities need to be made aware of the link between environmental management and health. One Health approach programs incorporating human, animal, and environmental health are particularly applicable.

They promote a comprehensive consideration of environmental effects on community health and unsafe or unsecure food habits. The issue is making the best use of educational models that have the potential to address varied community needs concerning these complicated interrelationships (Angelos et al., 2017). To address these challenges to community health, more coordination between healthcare providers, government agencies, and community organizations is necessary. Multi-sector partnerships are able to leverage different resources and competencies in the development of niche interventions that cater to the unique health priorities of various populations. Networks that facilitate data sharing and resource allocation are crucial for successful implementation of community health programs. In addition, community empowerment through health literacy interventions can enhance individual and collective agency and ultimately healthier outcomes. Active participation of residents in decision-making promotes ownership of the health interventions, and hence they become more effective. Continued campaigning for policies in support of equitable access to healthcare, conservation of the environment, and community engagement will consolidate these efforts, contributing to a healthier future in diverse communities and reconciling the numerous problems inherent in community health (Angelos et al., 2017; John et al., 2009).

1.6.1. Barriers to Accessing Healthcare Services

Access to healthcare services is progressively being restricted by a range of barriers that disproportionately affect specific groups. Of these challenges, location stands out as especially relevant, namely for the people residing in rural and remote regions of the globe. Research has indicated that such populations will have poor health infrastructure, leading to long waiting times and a general lack of available services. In a study on Newfoundland and Labrador, the respondents pointed out the shortage of local health practitioners, inadequate transport, and limited opening hours for essential services as some of the prevalent issues that cumulatively impede timely access to care (Heath et al., 2014).

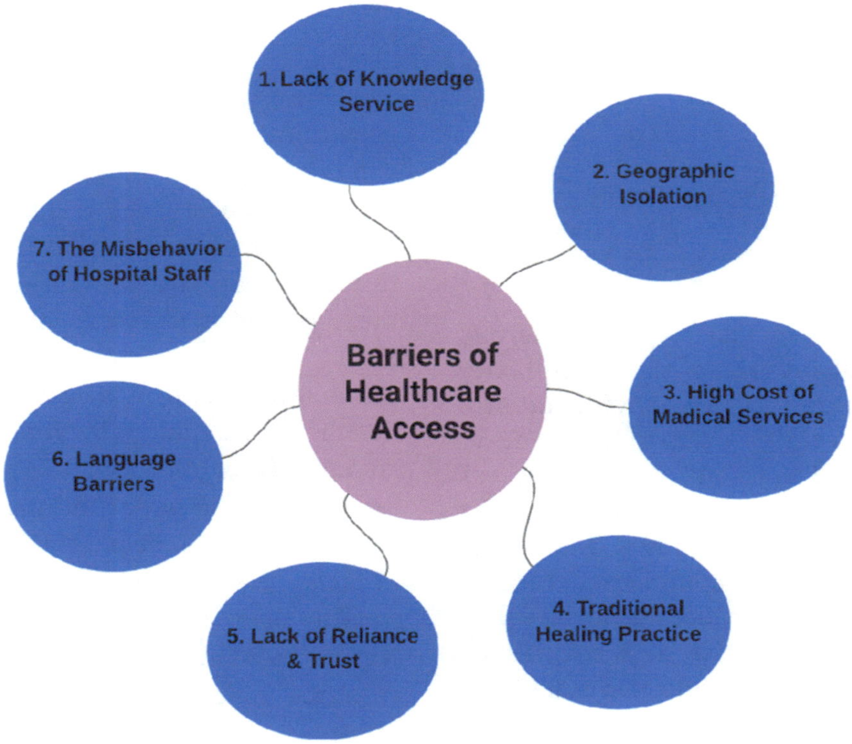

Figure 1.13. Barriers to accessing healthcare services.

Source: https://www.researchgate.net/publication/373130775/figure/fig1/AS:11431281181614824@1692106994470/Barriers-to-healthcare-access.png.

Thus, geographical deficits and system flaws pose severe challenges to ensuring that individuals can access healthcare services in their locality efficiently. Socio-economic conditions also contribute significantly to the barriers in accessing healthcare. Economic constraints, including medical insurance non-coverage, may deter individuals from seeking necessary medical treatment. For vulnerable populations, such constraints are often compounded by social stigma and health-related cultural attitudes. In a qualitative study in Southeast England, black and minority ethnic (BME) patients explained not wanting to discuss their mental illness conditions since they did not wish to risk discrimination or being misunderstood (Cooper et al., 2016). The study also established that economic pressures could lead to the inability to recognize or accept mental illness conditions, which could culminate in a denial cycle of necessary healthcare services. The understanding of these socio-economic determinants is vital in offering equal access to medical care across the various populations. Lastly, communication barriers between the patients and health workers also contribute to the hurdles of accessing care. Language differences and unhealthy literacy may cause miscommunications, which result in mistrust and substandard care. Among BME communities, the study demonstrated that cultural insensitivity and misperception by healthcare professionals discouraged them from accepting help. In addition to this, unreasonable delays and poor communication strategies are often left to leave patients helpless within a framework meant to benefit them effectively (Cooper et al., 2016). Enhanced training among healthcare professionals to cultivate culturally sensitive practices can fortify such relationships. Through a concerted strategy focused on patient-provider interaction, healthcare systems are in a position to address the issues that bar patients from quality care in their communities (Figure 1.13).

1.6.2. Health Disparities Among Different Populations

Health disparities constitute a key issue in community health, reflecting systematic differences in health outcomes among diverse groups of individuals. Various factors contribute to these disparities, for instance, geographic location, gender, socioeconomic status, and race. For instance, individuals from minority racial and ethnic groups are likely to have disproportionate health outcomes and suffer from such obstacles as limited access to healthcare, inadequate health insurance, and discrimination in the health care system. As discussed in available literature, the problems of these disparities impact severely ill patients, resulting in preventable disease and mortality. The need for targeted interventions to decrease these disparities is imperative because they affect not only individual health but also increase healthcare expenditure across the board (Carlson et al., 2016). Decreasing these disparities requires a multidimensional approach involving policy reform as well as community-based initiatives for ensuring equal access to health. Technology's role in mitigating health disparities cannot be downplayed, particularly in terms of expanding access to health information. Historically disadvantaged communities have limited access to valid health sources, thereby expanding disparities. Through participatory research methods with communities, researchers have begun exploring how different populations are accessing the internet for health information. For example, research among American Indian groups has documented significant variation in the use of the internet and searching for health information. Respondents signaled the need for culturally appropriate health material that best captures their respective experiences and traditions. As the study indicates, a modified approach to leveraging online health resources can play a powerful role in addressing health literacy and engagement among such communities, thus playing a vital role in counteracting health disparities (Begaye et al., 2014). Lastly, the journey to health equity within community health requires an understanding of the persistent barriers that impact diverse populations. Plans for setting systemic change in motion must address the core social determinants of health that create disparities, including education, income levels, and secure housing. The cooperative system among local, state, and national parties must serve in order to institute strong interventions that can say a lot to the specific character of diverse communities. With increased awareness and dedication to equity, stakeholders can construct sustainable solutions that extend health outcomes for all populations. As we continue to learn about and fix these disparities in health, it only becomes clearer that it cannot be done alone but as a concerted, community-led endeavor (Carlson et al., 2016) (Figure 1.14).

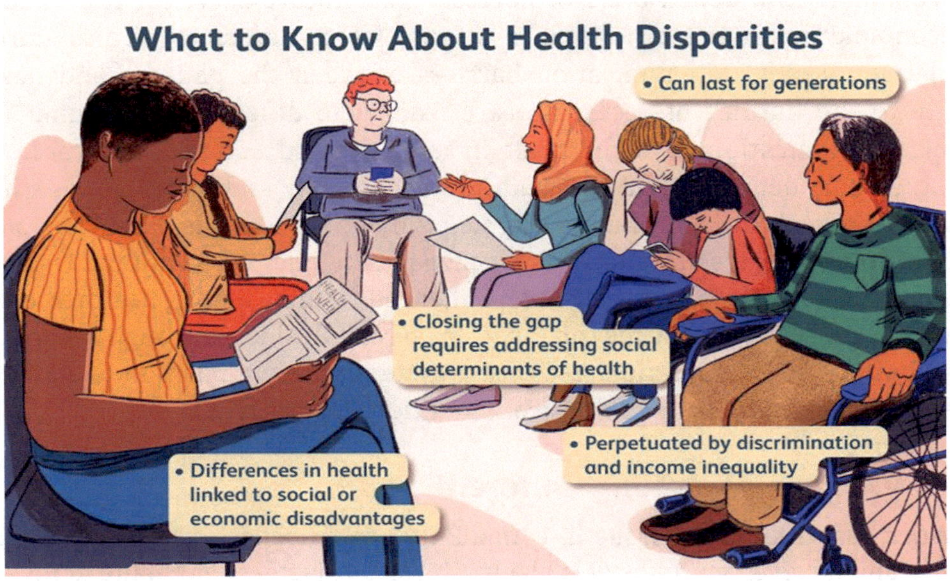

Figure 1.14. Health disparities among different populations.

Source: https://www.verywellhealth.com/thmb/28zhufSBRwb6RpQo2TPPie9tu8U=/750x0/filters:no_upscale():max_bytes(150000):strip_icc()/health-disparities-4173220_v1-e8914773af574e3d9f02b08d86835de5.jpg.

1.6.3. Impact of Policy Changes on Community Health

The social health impacts of policy change are usually viewed through the lens of targeted health interventions in relation to specific local priorities. For example, in the Born in Bradford study, a large cohort illustrated the value of 'embedding' research evidence in local health policy, particularly regarding maternal and child health. Provision of systematic interventions, such as a paperless maternity data system and enhanced interlinking of child, secondary, and primary health services, is an indication of the potential of the integration of research into practice to facilitate organizational change. Apart from making it easier to collect data, these changes also make it possible to reconfigure health services to address special needs of the populace, thereby improving population health outcomes in populations with diverse backgrounds, especially among vulnerable groups (Hadjar et al., 2015). Policy adjustments can also generate significant advancements in vaccine strategies, such as the example of the UK's introduction of rotavirus vaccine to its child immunization program. Before the introduction of the vaccines, the healthcare system had significant burdens, and rotavirus caused about 750,000 episodes of diarrhea yearly among children under the age of five years. Through an ecological study to quantify the vaccines' effect, researchers can provide a systematic evaluation of disease outcomes, hospitalization, and health visitation after vaccination. Not only do such reviews inform country immunization policies but they can also inform other countries who plan for similar implementations, thereby underscoring the global implications of local policy adjustments on public health (Cunliffe et al., 2014). Besides, community involvement plays a central role in successful implementation of policy grounded in empirical research. For instance, findings regarding the genetic implications of consanguinity in the Pakistani population in Bradford enabled significant local educational programs on genetic counseling. This illustrates how policy-making, research, and community involvement engage in favoring a health-promoting environment responsive to local issues. Since communities are engaged in the process of policy implementation, they become engaged actors in fighting for their health, demonstrating that policy reforms are optimal when they are grounded in, and answerable to, the unique cultural and social arrangements of the populations they are aimed at (Hadjar et al., 2015) (Figure 1.15).

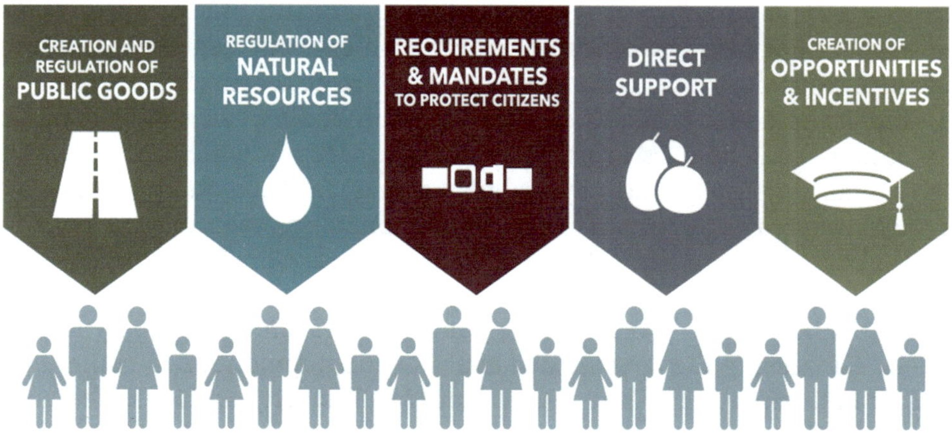

Figure 1.15. Impact of policy changes on community health.

Source: https://sycamoretn.org/wp-content/uploads/2024/05/5-ways-policy-impacts-health-e1532716467411.png.

SUMMARY

In total, the issue of community health involves a complex environment in which social determinants play key roles in contributing to or hampering health. Local-level integration of services must be used in order to promote better health and well-being. Community health initiatives must address barriers to care that arise from geography and societal context, particularly for at-risk populations. For instance, LGBTQ+ individuals from rural settings may encounter additional barriers when accessing affirming mental health care, ultimately impacting their overall health status and integration with community (Bettergarcia et al., 2021). An understanding of these dynamics is necessary to the development of effective interventions that are purpose-built to meet the needs of various communities. Integrated Community Care (ICC) is also a conceptual framework for health disparity. ICC promotes co-operation across sectors between health and social services, adopting an integrative process that not only treats acute medical problems but also engages with wider social determinants. The integrated model aims to create support networks that enhance communities' resilience and capacity to address health concerns (Thiam et al., 2021). By placing health care in the community setting, stakeholders are able to design spaces in which individuals can thrive—to a point—emotionally, mentally, and physically, and thus enhance quality of life overall. Lastly, the results of this research highlight the necessity of ongoing research and policy creation for community health. With the constantly changing socio-political climate, new issues and challenges to care continue to emerge. The evidence-based practices that result from these research studies hold the potential to guide health professionals, policy-makers, and community leaders in crafting effective solutions. Addressing the specific needs of diverse populations in community health not only contributes to individual health but also to society. Ultimately, it will be the unlocking of the power of inclusive practices that will lead to healthier, more just communities in the future.

The multimodal nature of community health requires an understanding of diverse factors contributing to it, chiefly the contribution of physical activity. A significant volume of research indicate that widespread physical inactivity is a leading global risk factor for mortality, a condition that is driven by stabilized physical activity levels since 2001. World Health Organization emphasizes that adults need to engage in a minimum of 150 minutes of moderate-intensity or 75 minutes of vigorous-intensity physical exercise weekly to stay in optimal health. However, concerning reports reveal over a quarter of adults worldwide are falling short of these guidelines, and there is an urgent need for quality public health interventions to promote active living and limit sedentary behavior. This review highlights that promoting physical activity is not only a healthy program but a part of societal welfare that warrants immediate attention and seriousness (Draim et al., 2024). In addition to physical activity, the ethical principles of community health research are essential to fostering trust and partnership among stakeholders. Involvement in community-based participatory research (CBPR) enhances intervention quality and responsiveness by incorporating community partners into the research process. But for this collaboration to be successful, the participants must have a good understanding of research ethics as well as human subject safeguards. Innovative approaches, such as the Research Ethics Jeopardy™ Game, offer stimulating possibilities for the education of community members, particularly youth, on such key ethical considerations. Placing contemporary case studies within context and using interactive learning, such initiatives not only enhance knowledge retention but also encourage active participation in community health research (Guerrero et al., 2014). Lastly, the overcoming of physical activity barriers and ethical understanding promotion in community health studies reaffirms the necessity for targeted interventions. Effective community health interventions must incorporate awareness campaigns, education materials to raise awareness on ethical behavior, and physical activity opportunities to foster a culture of health. Investments in active recreational spaces, policy to promote active transport, and health programs at a community level can all contribute to fighting the effects of inactivity and the promotion of healthier living. Meanwhile, establishing an educated population with knowledge of persons rights and dignity ensures that health programs are respectful of persons rights and dignity. These integrated measures are an inclusive plan for enhancing community health outcomes, which eventually result in a healthier and better-educated population (Draim et al., 2024; Guerrero et al., 2014).

KEY TERMS FROM THIS CHAPTER

- Advocacy
- Area-based initiatives (ABIs)
- Chronic disease
- Collaboration
- Community-based organizations
- Community ownership
- Community voices
- Data collection
- Drug addiction
- Economic stability
- Educational programs
- Equity
- Health care
- Healthcare services
- Health disparities
- Affordable Care Act (ACA)
- Behavior change
- Climate change
- Community-based health management
- Community health
- Community participation
- Data analysis
- Discrimination
- Economic development
- Education
- Employment
- Evidence-based interventions
- Healthcare expenditure
- Health communication

CLOSER LOOK

CLINICAL COMMISSIONING GROUPS (CCGS)

Clinical Commissioning Groups (CCGs) were statutory NHS bodies introduced by the Health and Social Care Act 2012, formally replacing Primary Care Trusts and Strategic Health Authorities from 1 April 2013 Reddit+13Wikipedia+13NHS England+13. They were "clinically led" organisations composed of groups of GP practices, supported by nurses, secondary care consultants, and lay members. CCGs were responsible for assessing local health needs, setting priorities, and commissioning most NHS services in their local areas, including elective hospital care, urgent and emergency services, community health, mental health, and services for people with learning disabilities — managing around 60–66 % of the NHS England budget, which amounted to approximately £60–80 billion annually National Audit Office (NAO)+3NHS Confederation+3public-sector.co.uk+3.

Each CCG had a governing body composed of clinicians, an accountable officer, and lay participants. They drew support from Commissioning Support Units (CSUs) that provided operational services such as contract negotiation, data management, finance, and HR public-sector.co.uk+1NHS Confederation+1. Though primary care commissioning remained the responsibility of NHS England initially, from 2014 onwards many CCGs assumed delegated or joint responsibility over GP contracts and primary care performance management

Performance varied substantially across organisations. A National Audit Office review found that over 50 % of CCGs were rated "good" or "outstanding", while around 42 % were judged as "requires improvement" or "inadequate". Many struggled to stay within budget or attract leadership talent, prompting mergers and consolidation into larger commissioning footprints over time National Audit Office (NAO).

By April 2020, the number of CCGs had fallen from 211 at inception to approximately 135, and by early 2021 the count was about 106 due to further mergers Wikipedia. All CCGs were legally abolished on 1 July 2022, with their commissioning responsibilities assumed by Integrated Care Systems—namely Integrated Care Boards (ICBs) and Partnerships (ICPs)—under the Health and Care Act 2022, shifting the NHS towards greater regional integration and collaboration

In essence, CCGs marked a decade of clinician-led, localized NHS commissioning—shaping local care delivery—until their functions transitioned into a more integrated NHS structure in mid 2022.

REFERENCES

1. Abbott, S., Aveling, E. L., Battilana, J., Bourgeault, I., British Medical Association, Care Quality Commission, Checkland, K., et al. (2018). Clinical leadership in service redesign using Clinical Commissioning Groups: A mixed-methods study. https://core.ac.uk/download/146487437.pdf (accessed on 26th June 2025).
2. Agarwal, A., Das, M., Pradhan, S., Singh, A., et al. (2023). Assessing the knowledge and awareness of malaria disease among healthcare professionals and community workers of Meerut District: A hospital-based study. https://core.ac.uk/download/588567200.pdf (accessed on 26th June 2025).
3. Agomo, C., & Agomo, C. (2017). Strategies enhancing the public health role of community pharmacists in the UK. https://core.ac.uk/download/573852072.pdf (accessed on 26th June 2025).
4. Allen, P., Brownson, R. C., Elliott, L., Jacob, R., et al. (2014). Health care system collaboration to address chronic diseases: A nationwide snapshot from state public health practitioners. https://core.ac.uk/download/70383689.pdf (accessed on 26th June 2025).
5. Anderson, I., Beaton, L., Coles, E., Freeman, R., et al. (2020). Promoting inclusion oral-health: Social interventions to reduce oral health inequities. https://core.ac.uk/download/305118180.pdf (accessed on 26th June 2025).
6. Angelos, J. A., Arens, A. L., Cadriel, J. L., Johnson, R., et al. (2017). One Health in food safety and security education: Subject matter outline for a curricular framework. https://core.ac.uk/download/323068605.pdf (accessed on 26th June 2025).
7. Austin, S. B., Cheung, L., Cohen-Bearak, A., Fung, T., et al. (2010). Facilitating change in school health: A qualitative study of schools' experiences using the School Health Index. https://core.ac.uk/download/28934675.pdf (accessed on 26th June 2025).
8. Bandura, A., Carroll, A., Drewnowski, A., Kafatos, A., Kirmani, A., Papadaki, A., Richards, A., et al. (2014). Social marketing and healthy eating: Findings from young people in Greece. https://core.ac.uk/download/29843393.pdf (accessed on 26th June 2025).
9. Bartlett, D., Berkeley, D., Bradford, N., Carlisle, S., Charmaz, K., Department for Communities and Local Government, Department of Health, et al. (2014). Local status and power in area-based health improvement partnerships. https://core.ac.uk/download/20072931.pdf (accessed on 26th June 2025).
10. Bean, J. A., Staley, M. J., & Ulrich, J. D. (2011). Rates of public health insurance coverage for children rise as rates of private coverage decline. https://core.ac.uk/download/72048278.pdf (accessed on 26th June 2025).
11. Begaye, J., Choi, W. S., Crosthwait, R. J., Daley, S. M., et al. (2014). Internet use for health information among American Indians: Facilitators and inhibitors. https://digitalscholarship.unlv.edu/cgi/viewcontent.cgi?article=1174&context=jhdrp (accessed on 26th June 2025).
12. Bettergarcia, J., Wedell, E., Shrewsbury, A. M., & Thomson, B. R. (2021). "There's a stopgap in the conversation": LGBTQ+ mental health care and community connection in a semi-rural county. *Journal of Gay & Lesbian Mental Health, 26*, 48–75. https://www.semanticscholar.org/paper/35b5bfa3c5a5bb573a439afd77fd211846ec5e6d (accessed on 26th June 2025).
13. Bleecker, M., Krause, C., Linder, K., Moffett, M., et al. (2017). Situating food insecurity in a

historic Albuquerque community: The whorled relationship between food insecurity and place. https://digitalscholarship.unlv.edu/cgi/viewcontent.cgi?article=1675&context=hdrp (accessed on 26th June 2025).

14. Blessett, B., & Littleton, V. (2017). Examining the impact of institutional racism in Black residentially segregated communities. https://core.ac.uk/download/231127761.pdf (accessed on 26th June 2025).

15. Blum, J. M. S., & DeMarco, J. (2016). Implementing IPE in community college health professions programs: Challenges and rewards. https://core.ac.uk/download/83049780.pdf (accessed on 26th June 2025).

16. Brackenridge, C., Faulkner, L., Hills, L., Kay, T., et al. (2013). Child exploitation and the FIFA World Cup: A review of risks and protective interventions. https://core.ac.uk/download/29140656.pdf (accessed on 26th June 2025).

17. Brand, C., Jordan, J., Nankervis, J., Osborne, R., et al. (2006). Chronic disease self-management programs: Perspectives on enablers and barriers to GP and patient engagement. http://hdl.handle.net/10536/DRO/DU:30025237 (accessed on 26th June 2025).

18. Breen, N., Cullen, T., Darity, W., Entwisle, B., et al. (2023). The PhenX Toolkit: Measurement protocols for assessment of social determinants of health. https://core.ac.uk/download/617033193.pdf (accessed on 26th June 2025).

19. Brooks, F., Bunn, F., Gage, H., Kendall, S., et al. (2010). The nursing contribution to chronic disease management: A whole systems approach: Report for the National Institute for Health Research Service Delivery and Organization programmed. https://core.ac.uk/download/30707929.pdf (accessed on 26th June 2025).

20. Campbell, M. M., Lyons, A., McEwan, B. J., Swain, N., et al. (2013). Pleasure, profit and pain: Alcohol in New Zealand and the contemporary culture of intoxication. https://core.ac.uk/download/29201720.pdf (accessed on 26th June 2025).

21. Carlson, C., Sholk, J., Nanni, J., Peterson, K., Smith, L. A., & Bhavaraju, N. (2016). Breaking the barriers to specialty care: Practical ideas to improve health equity and reduce cost–Striving for equity in specialty care. https://core.ac.uk/download/75785769.pdf (accessed on 26th June 2025).

22. Caron, R. M., Dionne, D., & Rezaee, M. E. (2011). Community ecology and capacity: Advancing environmental communication strategies among diverse stakeholders. https://core.ac.uk/download/72051469.pdf (accessed on 26th June 2025).

23. Coffman, J. (2008). Foundations and public policy grantmaking. https://core.ac.uk/download/71340682.pdf (accessed on 26th June 2025).

24. Cohen, L., Parks, L. F., & Kravitz-Wirtz, N. (2007). Poised for prevention: Advancing promising approaches to primary prevention of intimate partner violence. https://core.ac.uk/download/71346855.pdf (accessed on 26th June 2025).

25. Conigrave, J. H., Conigrave, K., Dobbins, T., Gray, D., et al. (2019). Supporting Aboriginal Community Controlled Health Services to deliver alcohol care: Protocol for a cluster randomized controlled trial. https://core.ac.uk/download/587393686.pdf (accessed on 26th June 2025).

26. Cooper, M., de Visser, R., Memon, A., Mohebati, L., et al. (2016). Perceived barriers to accessing mental health services among Black and minority ethnic (BME) communities: A qualitative study in southeast England. https://core.ac.uk/download/46523728.pdf (accessed on 26th

June 2025).

27. Corbett, A., Fuse, E., Hodge, J., & Scanlon, M. (2012). Legal review concerning the use of Health Impact Assessments in non-health sectors. https://core.ac.uk/download/71358594.pdf (accessed on 26th June 2025).

28. Coupland, A., Day, F., El-Arifi, K., Griffin, G., et al. (2006). Public policies, law and bioethics: A framework for producing public health policy across the European Union. https://core.ac.uk/download/42625276.pdf (accessed on 26th June 2025).

29. Cunliffe, N., French, N., Hungerford, D., Iturriza-Gomara, M., et al. (2014). Ecological assessment of the direct and indirect effects of routine rotavirus vaccination in Merseyside, UK using data from multiple health systems: A study protocol. https://core.ac.uk/download/80774672.pdf (accessed on 26th June 2025).

30. de Klaver, P., Grijpstra, D., Snijders, J., van der Graaf, L., et al. (2013). More and better jobs in home-care services. https://core.ac.uk/download/16749544.pdf (accessed on 26th June 2025).

31. DeWitt John, E., Hollander, E., & Hansell, W. (2009). Putting community first: A promising approach to federal collaboration for environmental improvement: An evaluation of the Community Action for a Renewed Environment (CARE) Demonstration Program. https://core.ac.uk/download/71345950.pdf (accessed on 26th June 2025).

32. Dokova, A. (2022). Effectiveness of health partnerships. https://core.ac.uk/download/559511035.pdf (accessed on 26th June 2025).

33. Drabble, L. A., Keatley, J., & Marcelle, G. (2003). Progress and opportunities in lesbian, gay, bisexual and transgender health communications. https://core.ac.uk/download/70410107.pdf (accessed on 26th June 2025).

34. Draim, M., Dzierzgowska, W., Kosowska, M., Kupisiak, A., et al. (2024). Physical inactivity–Do we hit rock bottom? The epidemiology and impact of physical activity and sedentary behavior in adults. https://core.ac.uk/download/636385585.pdf (accessed on 26th June 2025).

35. Freeman, R. (2020). Promoting inclusion oral health: Social interventions to reduce oral health inequities. https://core.ac.uk/download/286356190.pdf (accessed on 26th June 2025).

36. Gallego, G., Katz, I., Tannous, K., van Gool, K., & Haas, M. (2025). *Framework for the Cost Benefit Analysis of the NSW Department of Community Services Brighter Futures Program. CHERE Working Paper 2009/4*. https://core.ac.uk/download/pdf/6376810.pdf (accessed on 26th June 2025).

37. Gienapp, A., Reisman, J., & Stachowiak, S. (2012). A handbook of data collection tools: Companion to "A guide to measuring advocacy and policy." https://core.ac.uk/download/84911833.pdf (accessed on 26th June 2025).

38. Gilgoff, J., & Ginwright, S. (2015). Toward more equitable outcomes: A research synthesis on out-of-school time work with boys and young men of color. https://core.ac.uk/download/75786240.pdf (accessed on 26th June 2025).

39. Gomez, W., McCollum, R., Taegtmeyer, M., Theobald, S., et al. (2016). How equitable are community health worker programmers and which programmed features influence equity of community health worker services? A systematic review. https://core.ac.uk/download/74363669.pdf (accessed on 26th June 2025).

40. Gordon, K., Shaw, E., Tonner, A., Wilson, M., et al. (2017). How can social enterprises impact

health and wellbeing? https://core.ac.uk/download/77036381.pdf (accessed on 26th June 2025).

41. Guerrero, J., Madrigal, D. S., & Minkler, M. (2014). What is ...? A research ethics jeopardy" game to help community partners understand human subjects' protections and their importance https://core.ac.uk/download/323310442.pdf (accessed on 26th June 2025).

42. Hadjar, A., & Samuel, R. (2015). Policy and practice change at local, regional and international levels: Impacts from Born in Bradford. https://core.ac.uk/download/153514072.pdf (accessed on 26th June 2025).

43. Heath, S., Hippe, J., Jesso, B., Maddalena, V., et al. (2014). Access to health services in Western Newfoundland, Canada: Issues, barriers and recommendations emerging from a community-engaged research project. https://core.ac.uk/download/213625635.pdf (accessed on 26th June 2025).

44. Heckmann, H. C. (2017). An internationally adopted child's transition: A family story. https://core.ac.uk/download/84120682.pdf (accessed on 26th June 2025).

45. Himmelweit, S., & Land, H. (2010). Who cares: Who pays? A report on personalization in social care. https://core.ac.uk/download/106316.pdf (accessed on 26th June 2025).

46. Huxley, A., Komaromi, A., Sinfield, A., Sweeney, A., Woods, A., Woods, A. D., Smith, A., et al. (2018). Madness decolonized? Madness as transnational identity in Gail Hornstein's *Agnes's Jacket*. https://core.ac.uk/download/42369304.pdf (accessed on 26th June 2025).

47. Jenkins, K. (2011). Depoliticization and the changing trajectories of grassroots women's leadership in Peru: From empowerment to service delivery? https://core.ac.uk/download/4150285.pdf (accessed on 26th June 2025).

48. Johnston, L. (2025). A review of programs that targeted environmental determinants of Aboriginal and Torres Strait Islander health. https://core.ac.uk/download/pdf/30676074.pdf (accessed on 26th June 2025).

49. Lorains, J., Green, J., Hopkins, L., Fry, R., & Moore, T. G. (2025). Review of the evidence base in relation to early childhood approaches to support children in highly disadvantaged communities for the Children's Ground Project. https://core.ac.uk/download/pdf/30672649.pdf (accessed on 26th June 2025).

50. Main Morganstern, A., & Putnam-Walkerly, K. (2009). Making the case and getting underway: A funder toolkit to support healthy people in healthy places. https://core.ac.uk/download/75778427.pdf (accessed on 26th June 2025).

51. Millar, R., & Yamashita, T. (2017). Disease prevalence and health determinants in Nevada. https://digitalscholarship.unlv.edu/cgi/viewcontent.cgi?article=1064&context=social_health_nevada_reports (accessed on 26th June 2025).

52. N/A. (2015). Impact of the Sierra Health Foundation's Clinic Capacity Building Program: Final evaluation report. https://core.ac.uk/download/80510503.pdf (accessed on 26th June 2025).

53. N/A. (2025). *J Public Health Manag Pract*. https://core.ac.uk/download/556254503.pdf (accessed on 26th June 2025).

54. National Center for Environmental Health (U.S.), Division of Environmental Hazards and Health Effects. Health Studies Branch. (2025). *CASPER Toolkit*. https://core.ac.uk/download/144202570.pdf (accessed on 26th June 2025).

55. Nunez, V. A. (2024). Community health workers to strengthen HIV care continuum and PrEP delivery in the US/HICs: A scoping review. https://core.ac.uk/download/604291164.pdf (accessed on 26th June 2025).

56. Poon, A., Gilmore, D., Lumby, E., Wang, G., & Koester, L. (2016). Respite Partnership Collaborative (RPC) Innovation Project Evaluation: Final Report. https://core.ac.uk/download/80511006.pdf (accessed on 26th June 2025).

57. Richardson, J. (2012). Economic resilience: Including a case study of the global transition network. https://commons.ln.edu.hk/cgi/viewcontent.cgi?article=1005&context=southsouthforum (accessed on 26th June 2025).

58. Robinson, B. (2017). Evaluating the role of health literacy in communities: A review of community health needs assessments of Georgia hospitals. https://core.ac.uk/download/71427930.pdf (accessed on 26th June 2025).

59. Rose, A. J. (2016). Pressure injury management: An exploration of current practice within New South Wales and Victorian health services. https://core.ac.uk/download/212686550.pdf (accessed on 26th June 2025).

60. Task Force on Community Preventive Services (U.S.). (2025). Strategies for reducing exposure to environmental tobacco smoke, increasing tobacco-use cessation, and reducing initiation in communities and health-care systems: A report on recommendations of the Task Force on Community Preventive Services. https://core.ac.uk/download/144168269.pdf (accessed on 26th June 2025).

61. Thiam, Y., Allaire, J. F., Morin, P., Hyppolite, S. R., Doré, C., Zomahoun, H., & Garon, S. (2021). A conceptual framework for integrated community care. *International Journal of Integrated Care, 21*. https://www.semanticscholar.org/paper/e6922de3908d046811a88b589e688019ac03c890 (accessed on 26th June 2025).

62. Widyanty, B., & Putri, M. D. (2024). Overview of the level of community knowledge about flood disaster mitigation in Village X. *Indonesian Journal of Community Health Nursing*. https://www.semanticscholar.org/paper/fc195743d7d57b91b0daa6fd6be677305f384bda (accessed on 26th June 2025).

63. Wijayanti, Y. T., Sumiyati, S., & Tira, D. S. (2024). Health education for the community in the prevention of hypertension and stroke. *Journal Pengabdian Masyarakat Edukasi Indonesia*. https://www.semanticscholar.org/paper/8b1e0f7035abc2cdfce4851f412ddeeb763b5d66 (accessed on 26th June 2025).

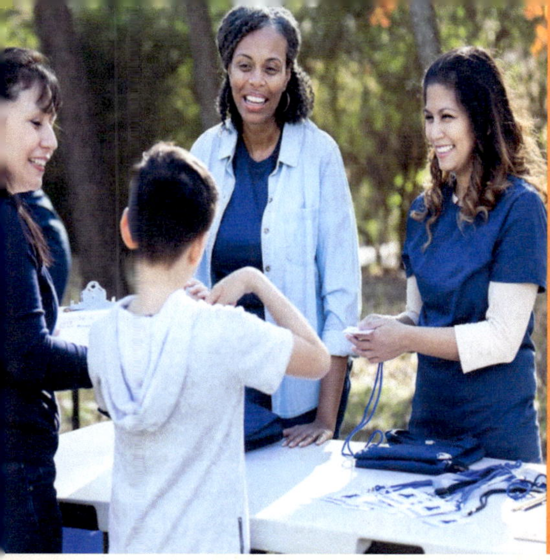

Chapter 2

THEORIES AND MODELS IN COMMUNITY HEALTH

Contents

Introduction

Community health is a multifaceted discipline that aims at the improvement of health outcomes by concentrating on populations and the various systems influencing their health. It is a discipline that has numerous theories and models that inform the practice and interventions that aim at the promotion of health and prevention of disease among communities. Here, an understanding of social determinants of health is essential since socioeconomic status, education, environment, and access to health care are determinants that play a vital role in health production. Using theoretical models, like the socio-ecological model, researchers and practitioners can better grasp the interdependence of individual behaviors, community resources, and structural arrangements. This approach allows for an integrated study of health disparities and offers innovative solutions tailored to emergent community needs. Critical assessment of community health calls for the application of effective methodologies that inform strategic planning and application. A useful instrument that can be applied is the SWOT analysis, which analyzes the strengths, weaknesses, opportunities, and threats relative to specific health initiatives. As noted in recent studies, this analysis is critical in guiding regional plans in addressing prevailing challenges, for example, digital health disparities and underserved care access. For example, the analysis can illuminate the internal strengths and external pressures that healthcare systems will have to navigate, and allow for community health organizations to develop adaptive improvement plans for services. Through the utilization of such analysis models, community health workers are better positioned to handle the complexities of health promotion and respond appropriately to newly emerging public health concerns, finally developing enhanced resilience in communities. Social entrepreneurship has emerged as an innovative approach to the solution of community health issues, over and above conventional interventions in health. Social entrepreneurs utilize business principles to generate social value by formulating solutions that can tackle immediate health inequalities. They must accurately describe, measure, and report their social effects, which are vital for keeping investors and programs going in the long term. Drawing on the principles as specified in community health theories, these entrepreneurs contribute to our knowledge of how collaborative practices can yield long-term change. Particularly among marginalized groups, the integration of social entrepreneurship into paradigms of community health could lead to revolutionary developments, both advancing health and economic empowerment. At the nexus of health, social innovation, and economic planning lies a watershed moment in terms of the potential for communities to come together to address system-level health and well-being problems (Figure 2.1).

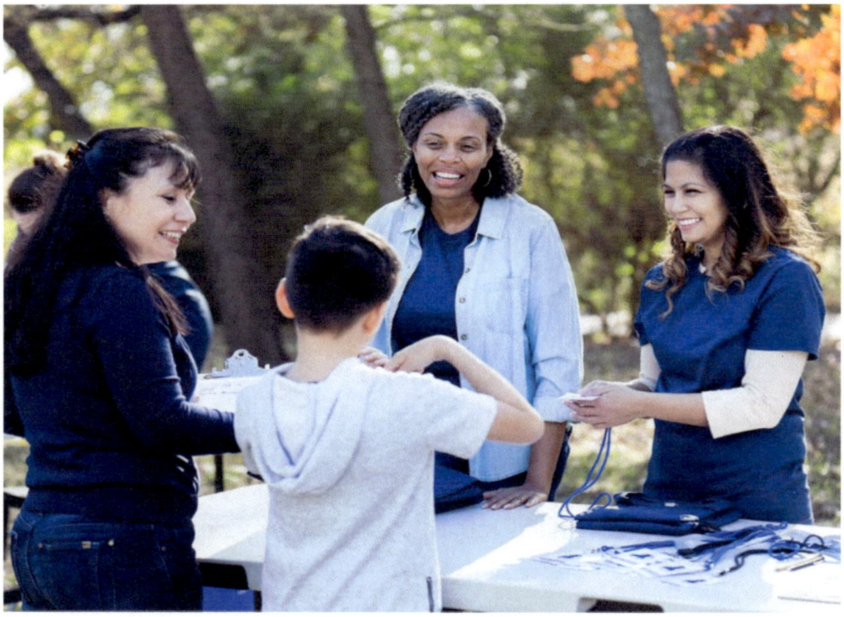

Figure 2.1. Community health is a multifaceted field.

Source: https://idahofoodbank.org/wp-content/uploads/2022/07/community-health-worker-opt.jpg.

Definition of Community Health

Community health takes a holistic approach to health with regard to the physical, mental, and social state of members in a community. The definition is extended to encompass collective consequences of health based on shared resources, values, and environmental determinants. Effective community health intervention relies on the assumption that health is influenced by a variety of determinants including socioeconomic status, education, and access to healthcare services. By establishing a context in which a participatory stake for the community people in health decision-making can be fostered, public health practitioners are able to respond to the unique needs of targeted groups and eventually attain improved health results as well as greater equity in the community environment. The relevance of community health is also emphasized through various models and theories that serve as a source of understanding the complex interplay between health systems and structures in the community. The Whole Community Approach, for instance, in the New York City Department of Health's 2018 jurisdictional risk assessment pilot, where inclusivity is emphasized through the expansion of the definition of expertise to include lived experience. This participatory model of involvement not only enhances the strengths of community members but also facilitates a richer response to public health disaster preparedness. By engaging heterogeneous members in decision-making, these initiatives are able to offer more inclusive risk assessments that better reflect the realities facing different communities and therefore enhance their resilience and effectiveness of health interventions (Ray et al., 2023). Moreover, interventions for specific health issues, such as overweight and obesity, emphasize context as the most important in community health interventions. In a study in rural Ghana, the transtheoretical model demonstrated the successful development of a nutrition education program based on regional needs with the aim of lowering awareness of overweight and obesity. This approach highlights the manner in which culturally appropriate architecture can serve as key mechanisms in engaging residents and encouraging sustainable health behaviors. Each of the program's components, such as lessons regarding body image, diet, and exercise, demonstrates the synergy between community engagement and health education, ultimately resulting in healthier lifestyles and stakeholder ownership (Kushitor et al., 2023) (Figure 2.2).

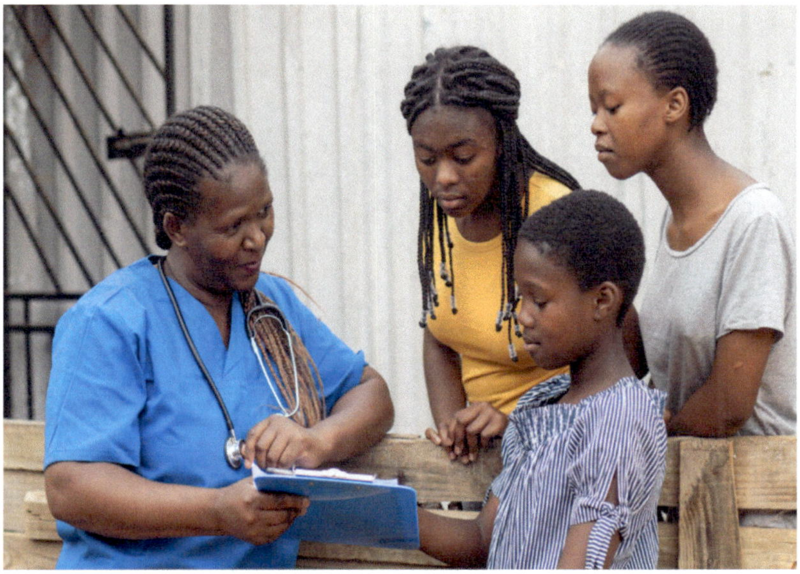

Figure 2.2. Community health.

Source: https://www.newyorkfed.org/medialibrary/media/newsevents/events/regional_outreach/2023/062323/community-health-workers-06232023event-eventpage.

Importance of Community Health

Understanding the function of community health is the core for the effective application of the majority of theories and models in public health programs. Community health emphasizes the common well-being of populations with a realization that conditions of health are most likely to arise from prevalent environmental, social, and economic factors. Thus, interventions guided by principles of community health are likely to advance more equitable health outcomes by eliminating causes of health disparities. The settings perspective, as discussed in the literature, acknowledges that there are determinants of health in specific settings, hence allowing for the building of health promotion strategies at the community level. The localized approach allows interventions that, in addition to addressing short-term health issues, enhance the health-supportive culture in communities (Armstrong et al., 2014).

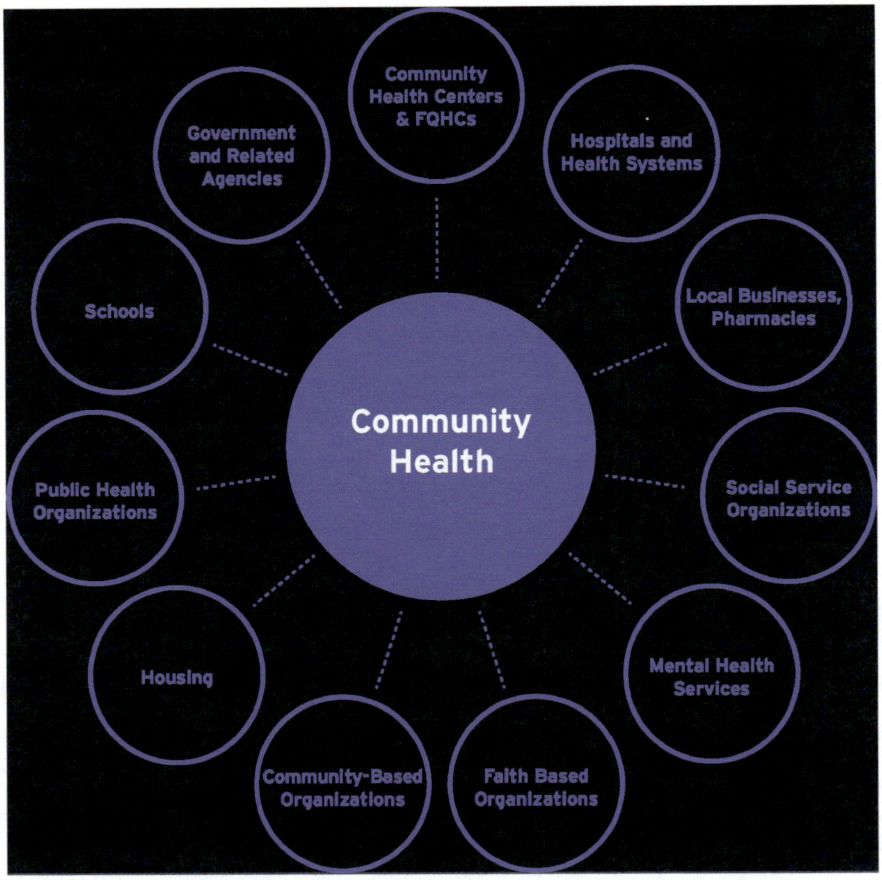

Figure 2.3. Importance of community health.

Source: https://www.nm.org/-/media/northwestern/images/about-us/community/community%20program%20initiatives/manifesto%20health%20communities%20diagram.png?hash=9197E145C1EAE8E124D6ABDCFCA1169B3696375F.

Moreover, the application of behavioral theory in community health models enhances understanding and effective management of health behaviors. For instance, research conducted in Greece shows how contextual factors, such as peer influence and access to unhealthy foods, are what shape eating behavior among young adults (Bandura et al., 2014). This research highlights the necessity of bringing behavioral knowledge into community health interventions and reinforcing that interventions must be attractive to the specific problems and incentives of target groups. Through examining how communities function, health programs can be built to create healthier habits, which will in return lead to improved public health outcomes. This emphasis on environment and behavior concurs with numerous theoretical frameworks that are focused on fostering sustainable change in communities (Armstrong et al., 2014). Lastly, the integration of multiple theoretical perspectives to guide community health practice is paramount in order to advance comprehensive health strategies. As noted in the scoping literature review, models like the socio-ecological model and systems thinking facilitate understanding of the interplay of variables influencing health (Armstrong et al., 2014). These models encourage multi-level interventions since they recognize that behavior at an individual level cannot be effectively addressed without consideration of the broader social and environmental context. Through the usage of these frameworks, health workers can design more inclusive plans that recognize the interconnectedness of factors dealing with health. As such, such informed strategies could go a long way in enhancing general community health, making it obvious why well-designed models and theories play a crucial role in working towards healthier populations (Bandura et al., 2014) (Figure 2.3).

Overview of Theories and Models

Theories and models are central to the understanding and addressing problems of community health. They provide the structures through which health practitioners are able to interpret data, form interventions, and measure outcomes. For instance, the Health Belief Model predicts that individuals would be more likely to engage in healthy behaviors if they perceive themselves to be susceptible to a health problem, see the severity of the problem, and believe that engaging in a specific behavior would reduce their risk. This model stresses awareness and perception in health behavior, and it is argued that educational interventions to alter perceptions will be effective in affecting healthier choice among community members. Also, integrating models such as the Social Ecological Model, which tackles more than one level of influence on health, allows the practitioner to operate at not only individual behavior but at community norms and institutional practice that affects outcomes of health. Furthermore, the application of theory-of-change methodology has gained widespread acceptance in health program evaluation. This process emphasizes causal connections between activities and intended outcomes and moves the process of evaluation from the measures of success to grasping the underlying processes within the final outcomes. It is from such frameworks, as per emerging developments in Health Technology Assessment (HTA), that the importance of a holistic comprehension of how decisions affect health outcomes is emphasized, given the complexity of actual world interactions between health systems and population behaviors. These frameworks can provide the bridge from improved decision-making to enhanced health outcomes, incorporating local factors into the assessment process. Through the measurement of wider impacts, like the less obvious, more intangible effects of health programs, such models encourage greater, longer-term stakeholder engagement, ultimately encouraging policy-makers commitment to interventions in health (Briggs et al., 2017). Community health requires the approach of a lifespan when considering health behavior theory and models. This perspective takes into account not only the proximal impacts on health outcomes but also the distant developmental trajectories of individuals and families. From an integrated framework incorporating precepts of individual and family development, as defined in educational standards, health professionals are better able to comprehend how crises and other environmental factors affect health across life stages (Fawcett et al., 2012). By integrating development-focused theory and resilience frameworks, practitioners can tailor interventions that address the unique challenges faced by different demographic groups. Under this holistic framework, health strategies are responsive and inclusive, resulting in a community that is enlightened and empowered to pursue better health outcomes throughout the lifespan.

2.1. Historical Perspectives on Community Health

There is a need to comprehend the historical contexts of community health in order to appreciate existing health models and theories. The history of community health illustrates a reaction to shifting interactions between societal needs and environmental circumstances. Conventionally, public health programs emerged as reactions to epidemics, demanding coordinated community effort against disease outbreaks. This visionary approach led the way towards modern community health interventions, with prevention of disease being only one aspect of targeting the need to address social determinants of health. Through the different paths of history, the shift in paradigms from reactive social responses to proactive participation in health illustrates how the role of collaborative action at the level of a community is crucial in determining health outcomes. History education answers to the imperative of appreciating prioritizing collective action in ensuring public health, with individuals as agents rather than as mere passive recipients of interventions for health. Insertion of social justice in community health has also borne witness to its historical roots. History has shown that marginalized groups have had unequal burdens of health, and therefore it is important to highlight equity as a key component of public health initiatives. An analysis of history's trajectory of health disparities will be able to uncover the patterns of marginalization and exclusion that have shaped contemporary health models. Feminist and justice models have come to dominate this debate, advancing a pluralistic model based on the interdependence of social and environmental determinants. Defined by various academic paradigms, such as the debate for ecological economics, the evolving definition of justice in health disciplines indicates the need for interprofessional collaboration to advance community health. Resolving past injustices is then necessary, with a resultant environment in which fair health outcomes become accessible to all in the community (Erickson et al., 2018). The complex dynamics of past cultural factors also form community health models in every multiple population. The Indian example is the best proof of how local cultural narratives affect health communication and community mobilization. Traditional health paradigms exist side by side with Western notions of modernity, forcing into the open critical divergences that reinforce the role of context in deciding on health theories. An appreciation of these layers of culture enables one to go deeper into community health, ruling out the applicability of a one-size-fits-all model in favor of a participatory one. Recent developments in community health studies emphasize the significance of successful strategies based on indigenous practices and knowledge that correspond with the values and perceptions of individual communities. With the application of a historical focus along with existing practices, community health can be transformed into a more unified and culturally relevant discipline that is ultimately more effective and sustainable (Chaparro et al., 2016).

2.1.1. Evolution of Community Health Practices

Community health practice is firmly rooted in historical thinking, from the classical models to modern approaches emphasizing holistic and participatory strategies. Early community health programs were built around infectious disease control, led by medical professionals who were the spokesmen. Top-down approach typically neglected social determinants of health as well as muted the voices of community members. Over the decades, increased sensitivity to such differences led to the incorporation of community voice into planning and execution for health. The developments exemplify the call for adaptive models that are responsive to local settings, as articulated in recent theories like Ken Wilbers Integral view. This change represents an articulation of a broader consciousness that healthy community practice must be ethically responsive as well as dynamically adaptive to the needs of diverse populations (Burns et al., 2008).

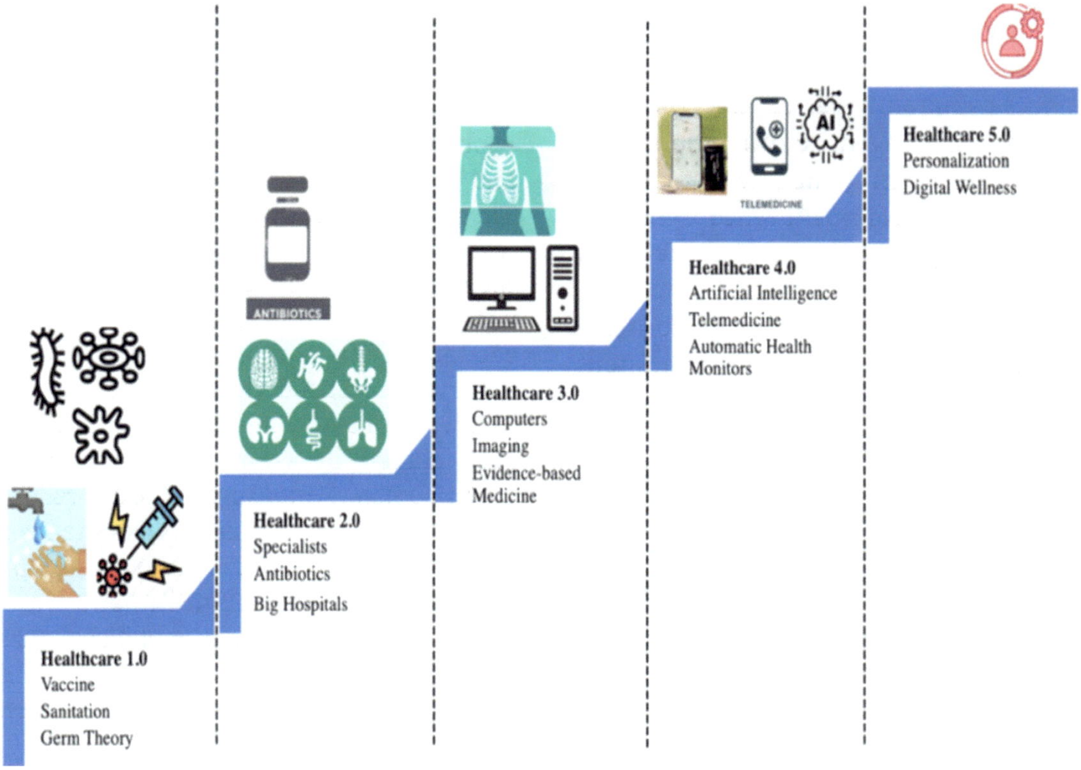

Figure 2.4. Evolution of community health practices.

Source: https://www.researchgate.net/publication/363499887/figure/fig1/AS:11431281084121379@1663039375289/Timeline-of-Healthcare-evolution.ppm.

In contemporary dialogue, holistic leadership emerges as a dominant theory that guides community health practice. This model emphasizes self-leadership and citizen involvement in decision-making, empowering individuals to take ownership of their health futures. Dr. Candis Best's research explains how holistic leadership develops personal capacities for self-determination, eventually enabling an more open environment for making health decisions. Community health practice increasingly employs this model now, recognizing that leadership needs to be shared, not hierarchical. This model works in concert with modern paradigms in health, promoting resilience and flexibility among members as they navigate through complicated health environments. Through the intersection of both leadership and participatory approaches, communities can develop responsive sustainable health strategies that are most suitable to meet their unique challenges and strengths (Best et al., 2012). As the evolution of community health practice continues, mature theories' interaction with developing models is necessary in shaping future initiatives. The integration of holistic paradigms and participatory approaches not only enhances community participation but also addresses long-standing structural inequalities that have become entrenched within health systems. On-going development reflects growing recognition of the dynamic interactions between determinants of health and health outcomes, and emphasizes the importance of context-informed interventions. Besides, commitment to ongoing practitioner reflection, as elaborated in Integral Futures approaches, captures the urgency of ongoing learning and adaptation in community health practice. As such, advances in such practices signify not only a shift in strategy but an essential transformation in how communities understand and valued health, so that all members can engage and gain from communal wellness interventions (Burns et al., 2008) (Figure 2.4).

2.1.2. Key Historical Figures in Community Health

Historical figures have been central to the evolution of community health, whose contributions still shape theories and models employed today. Among the key figures is Florence Nightingale, who is typically remembered not just for her work in nursing but also as a pioneer in public health. Nightingale emulated the worth of statistical measurement and physica environments in health, introducing the idea that sanitation and hygiene actually made a difference in mortality rates. Her healthcare work during the Crimean War introduced the necessity for appropriate healthcare systems serving as a precedent for subsequent public health efforts to address the conditions of living. Nightingales legacy continues in contemporary community health policies and asserts the value of employing holistic approaches and introducing environmental considerations into health policy. John Snow, the father of epidemiology, is another such moment in community health history. His investigation of the cholera outbreak of 1854 in London shed light on the need to immunize exposed populations and discover the spatial and social contexts for the spread of diseases. Through diligent tracing of choleral cases, Snow was able to identify a polluted water supply and thereby provide empirical evidence conflicting with the prevailing miasma theory of disease causation. His approach illustrated the role of evidence-based decision-making in health interventions and highlighted the fundamental role played by community participation in effective health measures. Snow's research laid the groundwork for the development of public health models that consider the importance of community and environmental factors in accounting for the dynamics of disease, a concept that continues to be central to contemporary theories of health. The work of Paul Farmer has also significantly influenced community health, particularly on the basis of his emphasis on eradicating health inequities for low-income populations. Farmers' view is centered on the intersection of health and social justice and advocates for the availability of healthcare as a human right. His experiences in Haiti revealed the sophistication of healthcare delivery within socio-political contexts and explained how poverty and education are inextricably linked with health outcomes. Informed by such theories as Critical Race Theory, Farmers model incorporates the need for culturally relevant healthcare interventions that empower people through the use of local resources and knowledge. This perspective holds that health policy must be integrative and address the economic, political, and cultural influences over health experiences, which is in very close alignment with existing paradigms of social determinants of health and community health (Allotey et al., 2010; McKie et al., 2019).

2.1.3. Impact of Historical Events on Community Health

The interface of past events with communal health is a complex tapestry, often marked by the socio-political context of the time. Wars, natural catastrophes, and large-scale public health crises have had lasting effects on communal buildings and patterns of health. In the midst of and in the aftermath of the Industrial Revolution, rapid urbanization built up closely packed housing situations, which readily spread infectious illness. The following public health reactions provided the foundation for contemporary health systems, demonstrating the way past problems can stimulate community health advances. This historical context is crucial when considering present-day health issues, as communities tend to look to the past when tackling present predicaments.

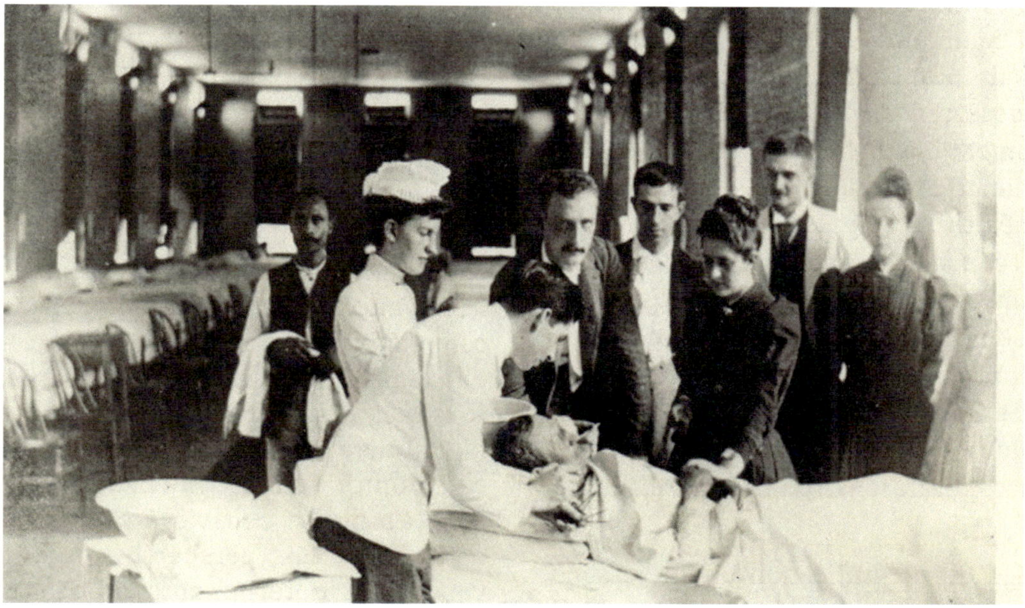

Figure 2.5. Impact of historical events on community health.

Source: https://19thcentury.us/wp-content/uploads/navigating-the-19th-century-health-care-landscape-a-historical-perspective.jpg.

Additionally, using these lessons within models of community health ensures greater responsiveness to emerging threats, making an analysis of history a critical building block in community health planning. Historical events also possess the ability to profoundly affect the mental health of populations, demonstrating the value in possessing a sensitive conceptualization of trauma and resilience. For instance, exposure to potentially traumatizing experiences (PTEs) such as violence, displacement, or socio-economic insecurity is correlated with severe mental health impacts. Empirical evidence indicates that the burden of traumatic events results in heightened levels of PTSD and depression among the exposed populations, supporting the dose-response model of trauma. Yet, some of them remain resilient despite recurrent exposures to PTEs, indicating the subtlety of stress-inoculation theory. This duality highlights how historical traumas can jeopardize community health but simultaneously promote collective resilience.

Therefore, effective models of community health must take into account the negative and positive responses of individuals when formulating interventions and support mechanisms that challenge the lingering effects of historical happenings on mental health. The Vermont Climate Assessment brings to light the crucial connection between environmental issues and community health, particularly the issue of climate change—a contemporary historical occurrence with far-reaching effects. The assessment highlights the degree to which changed climatic trends threaten not only the physical health of populations but also the social and economic rural community fabric. For instance, impacts on tourism, agriculture, and natural resources in turn affect the livelihoods and health of communities directly. As health threats emerge through climate change, it is increasingly important that community health models incorporate environmental resilience strategies.

Through the identification of the lessons of history of previous epidemics or natural catastrophes, health policymakers will be able to develop inclusive frameworks targeting current and future health needs. As societies confront climate change reality, the intersection of historical reflection and planning in health will be essential to delivering long-term and equitable health outcomes for diverse populations (Baker et al., 2014; Brown et al., 2018) (Figure 2.5).

2.2. Theoretical Frameworks in Community Health

Theoretical frameworks used in community health are key instruments for the comprehension and solution of complex health issues arising in diverse populations. By providing uniform methods through which to examine data and take action, these frameworks allow researchers and practitioners to identify the underlying determinants of health. For instance, such models as the socio-ecological model emphasize the multidimensional nature of health, appreciating that individual behavior, social networks, and the environment are all intertwined. What this does is bring to the forefront how health promotion activities need to deal with more than one level of influence, ranging from personal choice to organizational strategy. Furthermore, applying models like the PARiHS model, emphasizing evidence, context, and facilitation, can enhance the effectiveness of health intervention implementation in particular community needs, resulting in higher successful outcomes in community health interventions (Grandos et al., 2008). The settings approach is another vital theoretical framework in community health, which deals with where people's health behaviors take place in their daily lives. This perspective appreciates the value that determinants of health operate within the context of specific settings, such as schools, workplaces, and communities, which significantly influence individual and community health outcomes. While promising, the settings approach has been criticized for lacking a strong theoretical foundation, which is essential to guide research, policy, and practice in an effective manner. A scoping review is reported to have identified that a number of theoretical models have been employed in some settings, for example, Healthy Universities, such as the Ottawa Charter and system thinking, setting the significance of having a solid theoretical framework for better application and evaluation of health interventions (Armstrong et al., 2014). This reveals that gaining knowledge regarding the intricate dynamics of different environments is pivotal to promote health more effectively. The synthesis of theoretical models comes to ultimately assist in the refinement of community health strategies that are responsive to the evolving reality of public health issues. Effective frameworks allow researchers and practitioners to navigate the complexities of health promotion, and make sure interventions are not only evidence-informed but contextually adapted. As an example, the application of salutogenesis in models of community health enables the stakeholders to reflect on factors that enhance health and well-being rather than simply reacting to sickness. Further, the inclusion of multidimensional theories aids in creating a proper understanding of the system issues affecting health inequity among people. By provoking discussion among various theoretical models, community health practitioners can provoke creative solutions based on an integrative knowledge of the determinants of health and the complex interdependencies between them, maximizing the effectiveness of community health programs (Armstrong et al., 2014; Grandos et al., 2008) (Figure 2.6).

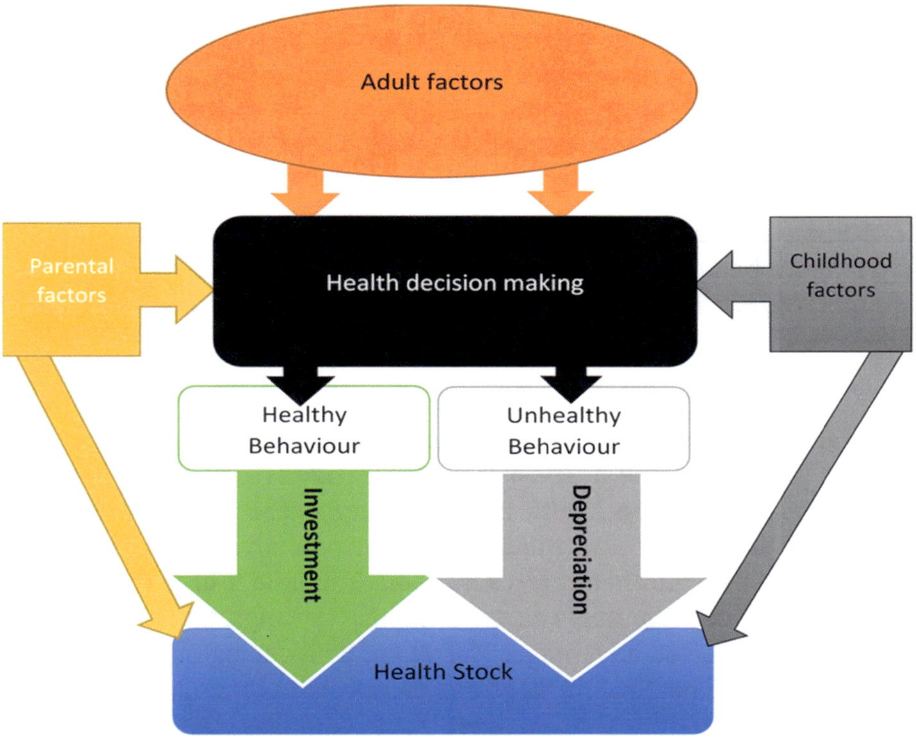

Figure 2.6. Theoretical frameworks in community health.

Source: https://www.researchgate.net/publication/362660337/figure/fig1/AS:11431281084984219@1663552634258/Theoretical-framework-health-decision-making-Source-Authors-construct.png.

2.2.1. Social Ecological Model (SEM)

The SEM is a guiding structure for comprehending the dialogue between specific behavior and the complex social environments that define health outcomes. Drawing from the assumption that health behavior is both sculpted by personal decision but also guided by more pervasive societal forces, SEM places emphasis on numerous levels of influence—spanning from intrapersonal to interpersonal, organizational, community, and policy levels. It is possible to adopt a holistic approach to public health intervention through the use of this model, with attention to structural determinants responsible for health inequity. For instance, SEM will provide insight into how socioeconomic status social determinants and values in a culture control food choices and physical activity, highlighting intervention pathways for effective community health interventions (Bandura et al., 2014). In community health, SEM is particularly insightful in addressing health issues such as obesity and chronic conditions. The Athens study shows that food consumption among young adults is driven by numerous factors ranging from peers and pressure from family members to the availability of fast food (Bandura et al., 2014). Such instances mean that when creating interventions for changing them specifically, the broader environment has to be considered. Through engagement with the SEM, public health programs can inform policy intervention in favor of healthier food environments and greater access to healthy foods, thereby strengthening reinforcement for healthy lifestyle behaviors. Eventually, incorporation of SEM in community health frameworks can enhance the effectiveness of public health interventions in the prevention of spread of non-communicable diseases. Further, the SEM's strengths also include its power to resolve wicked problems in community health such as public health crises and environmental sustainability. As argued in recent critiques, there are different constructivist views pointing towards the need for adaptive solutions to address intricate health-and-wellness-targeted societal problems. Such congruence with SEM underscores the necessity of confronting health problems multi-dimensionally, appreciating how an individual's behavior is ingrained in complex systems of social interaction and environmental impact. Through the application of SEM, public health professionals are able to craft interventions that not only address individual health behavior but also engage community resources, promote system change, and construct supportive environments to a more resilient health promotion approach.

2.2.2. Health Belief Model (HBM)

HBM is a core model of health behavior study in community health contexts. Basically, the HBM indicates that people tend to pursue health-promoting behaviors more when they possess a high level of perceived susceptibility to a health issue, supplemented by a high perceived severity of potential consequences. This dual acknowledgment induces individuals to proactively implement measures in disease avoidance and health preservation. The model brings into focus the presence of perceived obstacles because individuals have a tendency to weigh the effort involved in acquiring new behavior against its perceived advantage. Therefore, by focusing on efficacy maximization and barrier reduction, community health interventions can provide an environment in which persons are more likely to adopt healthy lifestyle changes, thus leading to improved health outcomes for diverse populations. A synergistic application of the HBM can be seen in persuasive game design in which underlying principles guide motivation for health behavior change. Through understanding various gamer archetypes, interventions can be tailored to match motivations and barriers towards healthy behaviors. Research highlights that most of the current persuasive games lack a theoretical foundation for incentivization of behavior, thus weakening their ability to facilitate actual change (Barrett et al., 2013). By developing many types of gamers, as studied in contemporary research, designers can craft solutions that address specific groups while encouraging broader adherence to health guidelines. These tailored approaches enable interventions that are engaging on a large scale to also deal with the nuances of individual experience and expectation in health behavior theory. Also, the applied conceptualizations of the HBM come to fruition in interventions against specific health challenges, such as preventing diabetes among adolescents. A study implemented a day camp for diabetes awareness and healthy lifestyles for preadolescents in a rural community, demonstrating the viability and impact of such interventions on the targeted settings (Mead et al., 2012). This HBM-based intervention used activities to change the antecedents to health behavior, demonstrating that positive attitude changes and procedure changes are possible by applying structured interventions. It also highlighted, however, the longer time it takes to actually feel changes in behavior, stressing the complexity of health interventions. This highlights the necessity of grounding community health interventions on formal theoretical foundations such as the HBM in order to respond effectively to public health issues (Figure 2.7).

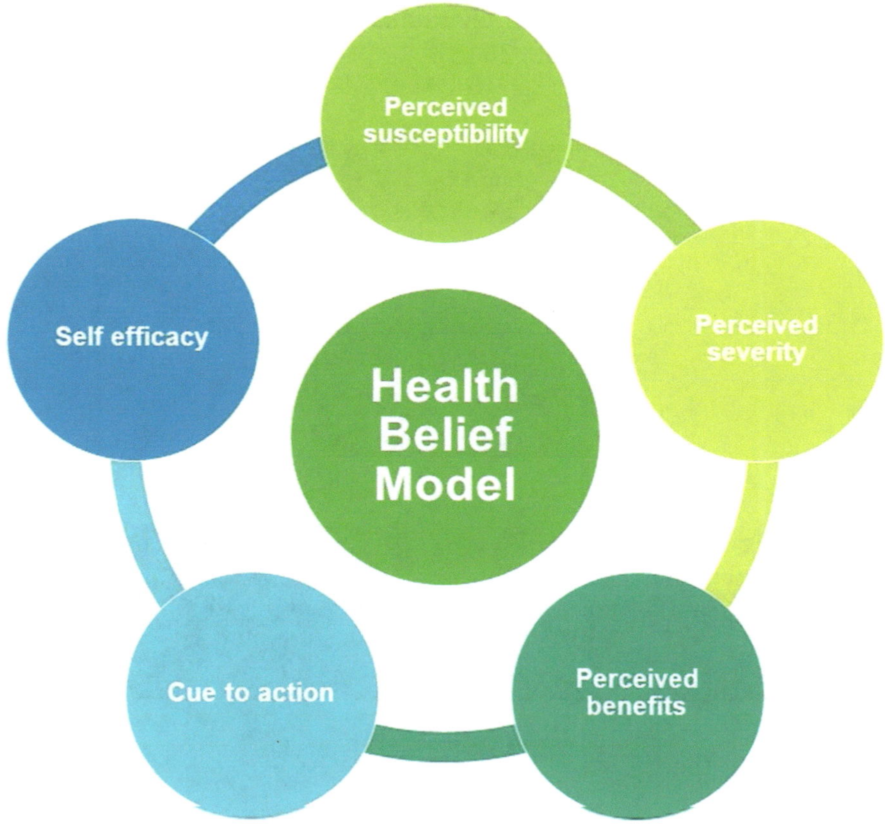

Figure 2.7. Health belief model.

Source: https://static.wixstatic.com/media/a27d24_7f854cb97fbd4d8f80645a07b6d0af3c~mv2.jpg/v1/fill/w_568,h_566,al_c,q_80,usm_0.66_1.00_0.01,enc_avif,quality_auto/a27d24_7f854cb97fbd4d8f80645a07b6d0af3c~mv2.jpg.

2.2.3. Social Cognitive Theory (SCT)

SCT seems a powerful model in accounting for health behavior change among community health programs. Derived from Albert Bandura's theory, SCT postulates that personal, behavioral, and environmental factors interact to determine an individual's behavior. The theory emphasizes the function of observational learning, wherein people learn behaviors and consequences from observing others. In public health, such a phenomenon can have real effects. For instance, if individuals see other individuals performing health behaviors, they will imitate them. This mutually interactive connection between cognition, behavior, and environment makes it critical to establish supportive community networks that promote healthy desirable health practices, thus supporting the general purposes of community health promotions and interventions. The application of SCT in community health programs demands comprehension of the varied determinants of behavior. For example, social norms and cultural beliefs are pivotal factors in defining the actions of people, especially in regard to such behaviors as female genital mutilation (FGM). The World Health Organization has promoted the use of behavior change strategies in FGM combating campaigns due to the realization that interventions should be contextualized to fit within the targeted communities. It appears that an inability to understand how to integrate individualistic and community-focused approaches has stalled progress in this area (Barrett et al., 2013).

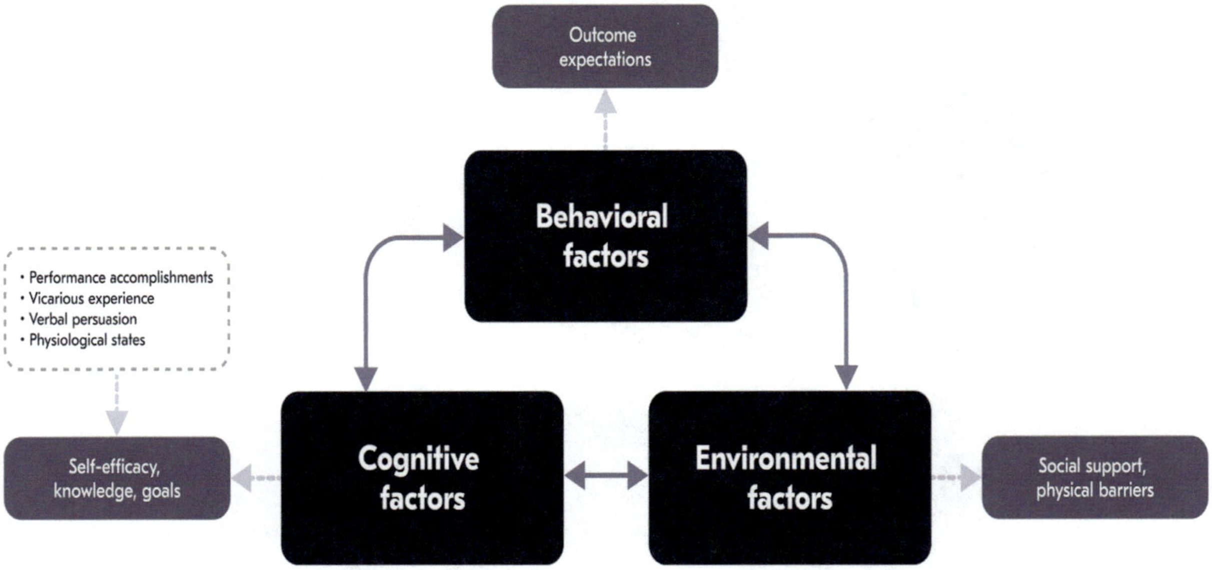

Figure 2.8. Social cognitive theory.

Source: https://cdn.prod.website-files.com/5df525c935688cef3b0a9c79/655a559a37035711c4e95a6c_Social%20Cognitive%20Theory%20(SCT)%20-%20Simple%2C%20Monochrome.jpg.

Utilizing the principles of Social Cognitive Theory, health initiatives can design more nuanced approaches that not only educate people but also engage community influencers and leaders to support and promote healthy behaviors while mitigating unsafe ones. In addition, SCT emphasizes the function of self-efficacy—the belief in a person's ability to perform a behavior—most explicitly as a fundamental determinant of behavior change in health. Intervention that successfully builds self-efficacy can bring about lasting health improvements, demonstrating the relevance of the theory to community health environments. For example, an experiment that implemented a diabetes prevention program through a day camp for children in a rural setting had positive outcomes on behavioral precursors, although long-term behavioral change would require longer participation

(Mead et al., 2012). These findings suggest that implementation of the concepts of Social Cognitive Theory in program development can enhance participants confidence to embrace healthier lifestyles and, in turn, attain better health outcomes. With its integral strategy, SCT is a fundamental part of community health programs in asserting the significance of environmental support and agency on behalf of the individual for enhancing health (Figure 2.8).

2.3. Models of Health Promotion

Health promotion models are critical frameworks that guide the development and implementation of strategies to maximize the health effects of policies at the community level. Models of health promotion provide a structured approach to understanding how various factors influence health behavior and assist in the formulation of successful interventions. Among the most famous frameworks is the Ottawa Charter for Health Promotion, which puts significant focus on creating conducive environments, enabling individuals, and mobilizing community. This framework not only presents a theoretical basis for health promotion activities but also stresses on addressing social determinants of health. Because several models illustrate distinct thinking and application, each contributes uniquely to the discussion of community health, giving insight into how health can be best fostered within varying settings, such as the workplace, school, and neighborhoods (Armstrong et al., 2014). When considering health promotion models, it is also significant to recognize the adaptability of models across different populations and settings. For instance, the socio-ecological model focuses on the relationship between individual behavior and the global social and environmental determinants of health. Therefore, this system outlines where interventions are most likely to succeed and observes that it needs multi-level interventions that consider individual, social, and policy-level factors. Importantly, health promotion interventions must be formulated to suit specific cultural and situational demands of target groups. The success of such models is commonly based on a rigorous evaluation of their impact in particular settings, which is a testament to the dynamic nature of community health promotion programs and the requirement of ongoing research and contextuality (Bandura et al., 2014). Furthermore, the application of health promotion models has become to encompass newer theoretical concepts that advance our understanding of multi-dimensionality of complex health behaviors.

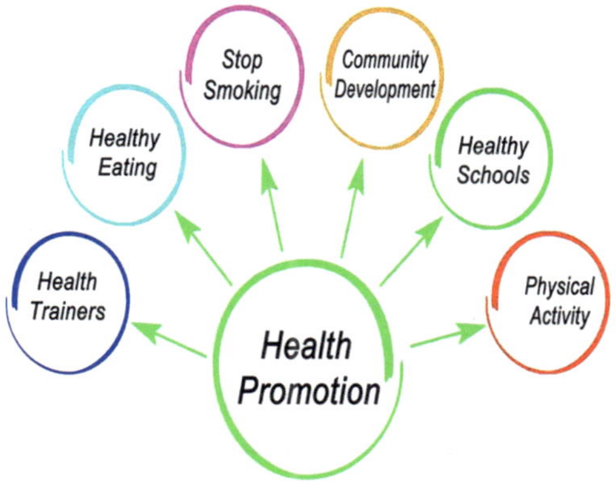

Figure 2.9. Models of health promotion.

Source: https://c8.alamy.com/comp/2BHNNN1/six-targets-of-health-promotion-2BHNNN1.jpg.

For example, the use of behavior theory to promote health, such as in qualitative research that explores young adults' diet, reveals important data regarding motivation and barriers to diet. This research illustrates how psychological and social determinants, such as environmental and peer support, must be considered when intervening in health. In addition, integrating social marketing principles with health promotion has proved effective in addressing public health problems such as obesity and unhealthy eating. Employing a comprehensive model that consolidates numerous diverse models and theoretical frameworks, interventions in health promotion will be in a better position to treat overarching health issues in communities (Bandura et al., 2014) (Figure 2.9).

2.3.1. PRECEDE-PROCEED Model

PRECEDE-PROCEED Model is a comprehensive planning and evaluation model for health promotion interventions, spanning between theory and practice. The name suggests a two-step approach; the PRECEDE step deals with the evaluation of health needs and determinants of behavior change, and PROCEED focuses on implementation and evaluation of such interventions. Through a systematic approach, the model allows for the recognition of predisposing, enabling, and reinforcing factors that ultimately determine health outcomes. This is central to the development of targeted programs that are tailored to the distinctive nature of a specific population so intervention can target both proximal health conditions as well as the determinants of health. Such a comprehensive assessment supports the models usability in developing effective health strategies in complex community settings. In an actual case, the PRECEDE-PROCEED Model has proved valuable across various healthcare settings, particularly in chronic disease management and in the augmentation of care delivery. Scholars have made its usability clear in case studies, setting the models effectiveness in responding to the needs of specific patient populations, such as patients with complicated health challenges. For instance, in the development of an oncology patient-centered medical home, the model guided the analysis of existing health resources and patient needs for evaluation so that interventions were evidence-based. An analysis of emergency room patterns of use determined health service use and comorbidities' correlations, ultimately resulting in more complex care planning. These evidence-based approaches illustrate mechanisms by which the PRECEDE-PROCEED Model can guide innovative action to address pressing health concerns, ultimately enhancing patient outcomes and public health. The strength of the PRECEDE-PROCEED Model lies in its ability to adapt to a wide range of health settings and to accommodate stakeholder involvement throughout the planning process. By engaging the people, health practitioners, and policymakers, the model instills collaboration that optimizes both effectiveness and applicability of health interventions. Participatory process in the model guarantees establishment of determinants at the community level to provide room for conceptual frameworks for solutions that are developed to suit target populations. This is particularly important in health disparity or resource-poor areas where applicability of single-common approaches will be low. By ensuring interventions are appropriate to the culture and individualize to the diverse needs of the population, the PRECEDE-PROCEED Model fosters long-term health benefits and empowers populations to take responsibility for their own health (Davidson et al., 2012; Rosiecki et al., 2015).

2.3.2. Transtheoretical Model (TTM)

The TTM offers a comprehensive approach within the field of behavior change, particularly in community health environments. This model categorizes the process of change into five phases: precontemplation, contemplation, preparation, action, and maintenance. Each is a measure of how prepared a person is to change their behavior, which makes TTM very appropriate for tailored interventions. For instance, precontemplators may not know they need to change, whereas contemplators know they need to but are not yet committed. This understanding enables the building of appropriate strategies that resonate with the person's state of mind at the time, not just maintaining motivation but also enhancing adherence to health-promoting behaviors (Hughes et al., 2006). Thus, the TTM is central to developing effective community health interventions attuned to the fluctuation of readiness among individuals. One traditional application of the Transtheoretical Model is in exercise counseling interventions for encouraging physical activity in patients with cardiovascular disease. The interventions utilize a systematized approach with the assessment of the individual's level of change and the development of individually customized action plans. Client-centered, the model comprises an array of strategies such as decisional balance, goal setting, and relapse prevention to cause long-term behavior change. Through the knowledge of the psychological barriers to adopting habits, the exercise consultation can encourage patients to embrace increasingly moderate-intensity activities in their daily lives, thus contributing to long-term health results (Hughes et al., 2006). This practice application of TTM not just acts as a blueprint for physical activity programs but also emphasizes the facile implementation of behavioral theories to community health practice. Further, the flexibility of Transtheoretical Model allows it to be easily integrated with other behavioral change theories, thus becoming more efficient in health in other domains. For example, TTM can be used together with mobile health interventions aimed at educating individuals on nutrition and diet behaviors. By employing a phase-change strategy to user needs analysis, software developers can ensure that TTM principles are followed by technical applications, thus creating scenarios for promoting behavior change. This collaborative approach enables the merging of multi-disciplinary insights and interventions addressing the intricacies of behavior intervention. An integrated approach of this kind not only completes gaps in practice and knowledge across disciplines but also ensures that health interventions are founded on theoretical models that enable sustainable lifestyle changes among populations.

2.3.3. Community-Based Participatory Research (CBPR) Model

The CBPR model is increasingly viewed as a vital strategy under models of community health, with an emphasis on collaboration between researchers and community participants. This strategy not only demystifies research but also ensures a guarantee that the produced knowledge is as relevant and helpful to the affected community as possible. By engaging the community at all levels of the research process—problem definition, research design, data collection, and knowledge dissemination—CBPR fosters ownership among the participants. This participatory mechanism produces more culturally appropriate and sustainable responses to health issues, as it incorporates the voices and experience of the very same people who are most affected by health disparities. It also enhances the capacity of community members to address their own health issues, which is central to empowering communities that are at times on the periphery or overlooked. Furthermore, the incorporation of negotiation skills, which have been brought to the forefront by Sharkey et al. (2008), emphasizes the effectiveness of CBPR. Good negotiation skills in dealing with stakeholders can facilitate more open and more productive processes throughout the research process. This comprises emotionally solving situations, building rapport, and employing creativity in problem-solving, all of which are important constituents necessary for successful collaboration. By equipping researchers and community activists with negotiation skills, the CBPR model has the ability to bridge communications gaps and foster mutual understanding. This fosters a climate of trust, which is a critical component for the effective use of health interventions co-designed with the people. Participative decisions that come from diverse groups, as research indicates, yield more robust, credible health outcomes. In the context of issues like FGM, a pressing global concern, the CBPR model identifies its role in influencing behavioral change in these affected communities. Research in Barrett et al. (2013) suggests that conventional methods for challenging FGM have failed quite often. Using CBPR approaches to involve members of the community is likely to foster intervention that is specifically designed, leading to ownership of the problem and stimulating community-led solutions. Through the usage of individualistic and community-change models, CBPR takes advantage of the efficacy of managing the complexity of social norms around FGM. The model not only educates but also enables communities to shun unwholesome behavior in solidarity, showing the effectiveness of participatory action in re-shaping health behaviors and outcomes. The model of CBPR, therefore, is presented as a vital approach in alternative health paradigms and resilience building in communities (Figure 2.10).

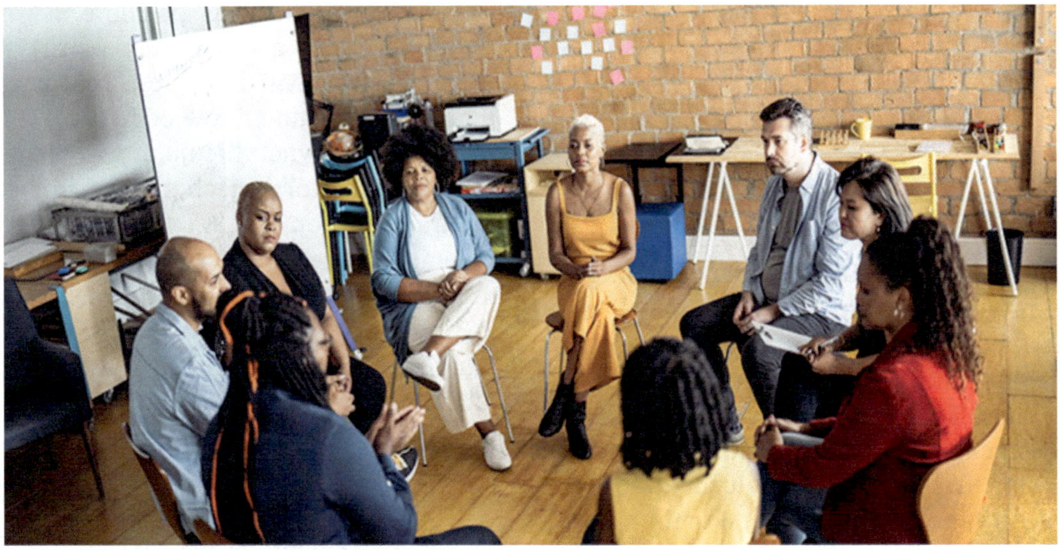

Figure 2.10. Community-based participatory research model.

Source: https://www.uab.edu/medicine/palliativecare/images/Community-Banner_750x350.png

2.4. Role of Social Determinants in Community Health

Identifying the role of social determinants within community health is important in the eradication of health inequalities and encouragement of equal health results. Social determinants are numerous factors, including socioeconomic status, education, living conditions, and social support systems, that together influence the health of communities and individuals. Social determinants dictate access to health resources like healthy food, secure housing, and quality healthcare services. Theoretical frameworks emphasizing these determinants—e.g., the Social Ecological Model—emphasize the dynamic interaction between individual actions and broad-scale social circumstances. Under this understanding, community health interventions that address such factors can be more effective at fostering resilience and overall levels of health in populations that are both heterogeneous and widespread. Housing is a key social determinant that has a substantial influence on outcomes for community health. Evidence suggests that housing quality improvements can impact both health and socioeconomic status in ways that lead to better health outcomes. For instance, studies reference the connection between proper housing conditions—energy efficiency and warmth—to improved health indicators. Intervention study models demonstrate this connection, illustrating a logic model accounting for how changes in environmental factors can lead to better health. The research into such mechanisms provides helpful information about the preventative value in community health programs and hence the policy need to address housing upgrades as a pathway towards enhancing public health outcomes. Indeed, addressing housing-related issues can have long-term payoffs that much surpass the immediate impact of the upgrades to residential settings (Thomas et al., 2015). In addition, environmental education is a key component of tackling social determinants through public engagement and awareness. Environmental conservation organizations normally seek to educate individuals about local and global matters, but effective change involves a deeper grasp of models of behavior. Psychosocial determinants and knowledge acquisition play roles in interaction towards the formation of pro-environmental behaviors that end up influencing community health. Evidence has shown that the congruence of educational materials with established theories of behavior change will be stronger in enabling individuals to change their habits and developing a healthier environment. Thus, the integration of psychosocial knowledge in community programs will enhance the effectiveness of education campaigns, leading to long-term health improvements through the development of awareness and action culture for social determinants (Bolt et al., 2017) (Figure 2.11).

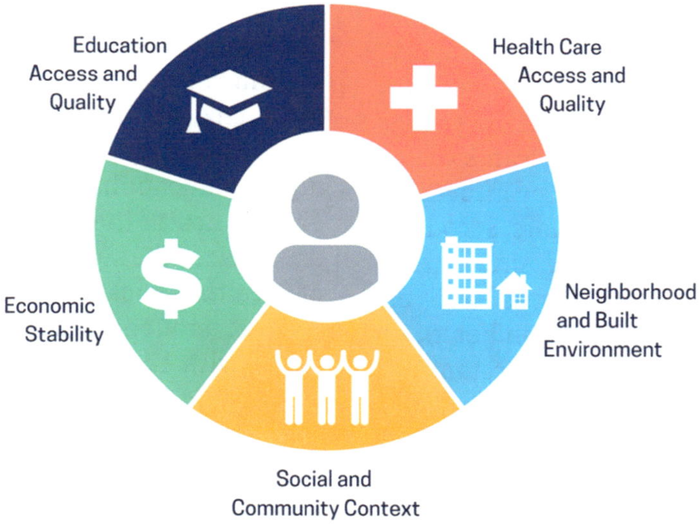

Figure 2.11. Role of social determinants in community health.

Source: https://external-content.duckduckgo.com/iu/?u=https%3A%2F%2Ftse1.mm.bing.net%2Fth%3Fid%3DOIP.nAIB6UhrIeEal89S7dfBVgHaII%26pid%3DApi&f=1&ipt=3e4d8d624aa20f1c4dfadc56d344d93a1ad6a3a77c8f966992683df2f2915044.

2.4.1. Economic Factors

Economic factors significantly impact the determination of community health outcomes by influencing the accessibility of health resources and the availability of services to populations. A community's wealth or lack of it directly influences the investment in healthcare infrastructure, preventative care, and health education. Economically constrained societies may not be in a position to have adequate healthcare systems, leading to disparities in treatment access and outcomes across different socioeconomic strata. This may be particularly heightened in urban areas where disparities in wealth are acute, illustrating how the economic connects with social determinants of health. Understanding these economic determinants is critical to create effective models to address disparities in health and improve overall health of the community, increasing the relevance of integrative models that consider fiscal as well as social influences. Economic forces also have a direct impact on individual health behaviors and choices. Individual economic conditions can restrict their ability to pursue healthy lifestyles, e.g., purchasing healthy food or going to recreation facilities. Economic hardship has a tendency to lead individuals to place current money ahead of future health requirements, making decisions that can harm their health, such as dependence on fast foods or forgetting about preventive care. This relationship points toward the relevance of economic frameworks that illustrate how money security or insecurity can affect community health behaviors. Secondly, effective interventions must be integrated, addressing economic difficulties as well as developing awareness and literacy on health at the community level. Therefore, understanding the economic factors becomes important while developing community health interventions that are sustainable and responsive. Lastly, the integration of health technology assessments (HTA) into economic frameworks presents a golden opportunity to improve the decision-making around community health. Through a theory of change-based methodology, HTA can assure the evaluation of health intervention economic impacts, contributing to better resource allocation. It targets the linkage between health investment and resulting health improvement, enabling policymakers to visualize not only the cost consequences but also the qualitative effects of health interventions. As described in current research, these frameworks promote an integrated vision of local circumstances and structures that determine health results and measure the connection between choices and real improvements in health. By effectively bridging economic models and health outcomes, HTA provides critical insights with the ability to enhance the provision of quality healthcare services to populations, ultimately contributing to a healthier society as emphasized in the recent debate on strategies for the improvement of community health (Agarwal et al., 2011; Briggs et al., 2017).

2.4.2. Education and Health Literacy

Education plays a central role in deciding health literacy, which is becoming an essential component of community health. Health literacy encompasses the skills and knowledge necessary for individuals to make informed health decisions, navigate the healthcare system, and understand health information. As such, the intersection of education and health literacy is critical; individuals with higher educational attainment tend to exhibit greater health literacy levels. This relationship emphasizes the significance of the incorporation of health education in educational systems so that students get to study health issues along with the basics. Also, the participation of teachers in advocating health literacy can employ the school environment to promote overall conditions of community health, which indicates the connection between education and public health interventions. Incorporation of health literacy within the educational system can significantly support community health. Schools not only offer places for traditional learning but also play key roles as agents of social habits and attitudes to health. Drawing on research evidence, the quality of schooling has been shown to correlate with outcomes in terms of rates of crime, tolerance, and social coherence, and it is generally assumed that educated individuals are more likely to facilitate collective health action (Green et al., 2003). While teachers attempt to connect the curriculum with longer-term health objectives, there is opportunity to construct synergies that will empower the learner. By promoting an understanding of health issues and a healthy practice within schools, learners can be change agents for their local communities, generating increased health gain beyond the classroom. Furthermore, the work of developing successful education programs for enhancing health literacy is complicated by outside factors that impact both education and health systems. The need for a curriculum that is sensitive to contemporary health issues and community needs is evident, given the changing nature of public health challenges. As noted in attempts at aligning teacher preparation with national health goals (Cooper et al., 2010), educational policy and community health initiatives must be thoughtfully considered together. Schools of education need to modify their practices to develop a curriculum that not only transfers knowledge but also enables students to have practical abilities to manage health self-assuredly. This interlinkage is central to creating a health-literate population that can successfully navigate medicine's subtleties and meaningfully contribute to the well-being of populations. Through such interlinkages, education systems can become important catalysts towards health literacy, ultimately changing the health environment in general (Figure 2.12).

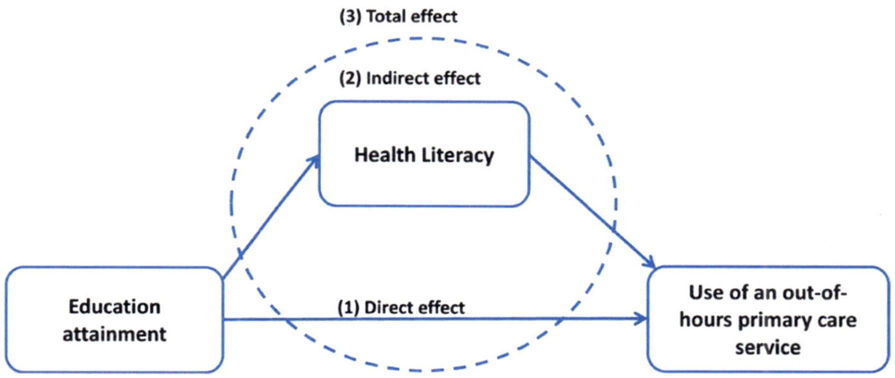

Figure 2.12. Education and health literacy.

Source: https://media.springernature.com/lw1200/springer-static/image/art%3A10.1186%2Fs12913-018-3197-4/MediaObjects/12913_2018_3197_Fig1_HTML.png.

2.4.3. Access to Healthcare Services

Availability of healthcare services continues to be a problem in community health, influencing the general health of populations. There are multiple barriers that make it difficult for one to receive the appropriate medical attention, which is likely to create dominant health disparities. Socioeconomic status, geography, and culture are key determinants that influence one's ability to access healthcare. For example, native groups are often subject to systemic issues that affect their access, as seen in recent governmental changes geared toward prioritizing intercultural healthcare in countries such as Bolivia. Though attempts have been made to enact policies that promote indigenous rights and equality in healthcare, people tend to report minimal benefit in their interactions with the healthcare system. This divide signals the necessity for critically appraising and refining existing healthcare policy and interventions to better address the needs of vulnerable groups and facilitate equal access to essential medical care (DeLoge et al., 2012). Behavior change in healthcare practice demands sophisticated uses of theoretical frameworks to ensure efficient intervention. As a component of health improvement approach implementation, it is necessary to understand the driving behavior and belief of healthcare practitioners. The Theoretical Domains Framework (TDF) has also been an essential resource in this direction, offering a systematic way of comprehending behaviors through the categorization of these into various explanation constructs. The theoretical model assists in the identification of the barriers to behaviors that healthcare professionals face, and therefore facilitates individualized interventions that can enhance healthcare provision. By attacking specific constructs of behavior change, researchers can develop targeted strategies that not only increase healthcare service access but also positively affect healthcare providers' behaviors. Therefore, the inclusion of the TDF in community health interventions aligns with the overall mission of closing access gaps and improving health outcomes (McCluskey et al., 2012). Further, the utilization of the knowledge of healthcare access via behavior change theories underscores continuous research and applied practice. Although models like the TDF indicate processes whereby healthcare behavior may be influenced, practical application often presents limitations in efficacy as well as application. As evidenced in ongoing research, there is a definite need for a more critical analysis of how such theoretical paradigms operate among different communities, specifically among indigenous communities that are unique in their experience of challenges. Sensitivity to these barriers is essential in designing interventions that will resonate with the unique cultural and social contexts of different populations. Lastly, enhancing access to health care is not merely a case of policy formulation but also requires profound insight into human behavior, belief systems, and the systemic processes that underlie health inequities (DeLoge et al., 2012; McCluskey et al., 2012).

2.5. Community Health Assessment

Community health assessment is an essential process of examining the health needs of the population and acting as a foundation for good health policy and program development. The process uses a number of methods including surveys, focus groups, and analysis of health data to acquire information on health indicators and determinants of health in a community. By involving stakeholders such as members of the community and health care providers, the assessment promotes a participatory process that can promote validity and relevancy in the findings. In addition, the collaborative process can shed light on health disparities and social determinants of health that public policy needs to target to enhance overall community health outcomes. By integrating local understanding and knowledge, community health assessments help in ranking health issues and point to areas where targeted intervention and utilization of resources are needed. Public health policy-making is significantly impacted by the findings of community health assessments, emphasizing research-informed decision-making. Recent studies have demonstrated how the successful utilization of data garnered through community assessment contributes to public health success due to it enabling policymakers to best address confirmed health needs. Information garnered through such assessments, for instance, can be able to effectively guide resource allocation towards health interventions and services tailored to the unique needs of vulnerable populations. Furthermore, evidence indicates that if the evaluation process involves direct participation by communities, there are greater opportunities for sustained health improvement. That the intervention is participatory not only provides scope for more in-depth analysis of local health problems but also enhances public trust in health interventions, making community involvement in health programs stronger

(Buxton et al., 2010). Besides, inclusion of community health assessments in broader health systems can create equity and close disparities in health. Through the mechanism of determining the state of health needs translated into policy action, the assessment role itself points to resources and services gaps areas that affect marginalized communities. For instance, improved conditions of housing have been shown in studies to affect smoking cessation among health behaviors in marginalized communities (Bond et al., 2012). It is thus important that policymakers consider the socio-economic drivers revealed through community health assessments while designing interventions for health. Ultimately, the assessment acts as a motivation to tackle immediate as well as systemic health issues, affirming the importance of context-specific interventions and regard for how individual actions blend with broader socio-political realities in community health frameworks (Figure 2.13).

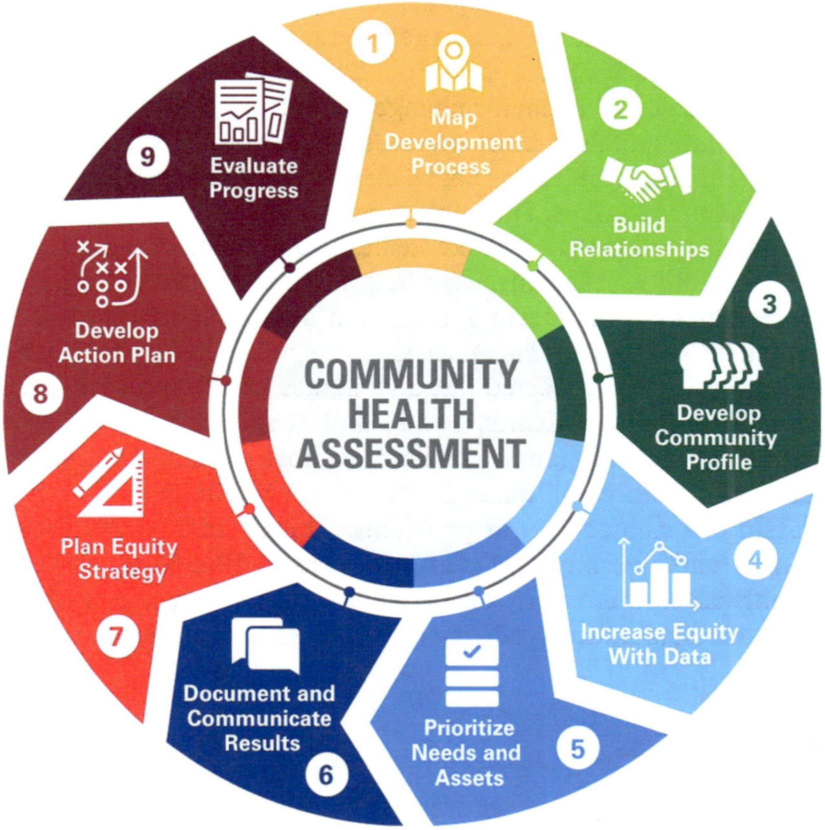

Figure 2.13. Community health assessment.

Source: https://www.healthycommunities.org/sites/default/files/2023-05/AHA-CHA-Toolkit_Home_Graphic.jpg.

2.5.1. Importance of Community Health Assessments

Community health assessments are the foundation of learning and improving public health. By methodically compiling and analyzing data, these assessments provide the general health status and needs of a community. These assessments are most critical in the determination of health disparities because they consistently provide discrepancies in health outcomes among different segments of the population. In doing this, community health assessments ensure well-informed decision-making for stakeholders ranging from public health workers to local agencies. This evidence-based approach not only raises awareness among communities for leading health issues but also lends support to collective action of various constituents striving for improved health. The use of such assessments in health planning ensures that resources are allocated effectively and interventions created to address the specific needs of communities. Finally, such assessments establish a baseline against which to judge the success of public health programs. Moreover, by grounding practice in tested theories and models, community health assessments are more effective at describing interventions and policy recommendations. For instance, application of models like the Community Health Improvement Process emphasizes organized assessment of community needs. This is also important in understanding the larger contextual factors that influence health, such as socioeconomic status and access. Incorporating models such as the Transtheoretical Model can even provide insight into stages of behavior change within the community, allowing for targeted interventions that address individuals at different levels of readiness to engage in healthier behaviors. It assists stakeholders in making predictions based on such theories and models, thereby facilitating a more strategic allocation of resources. Thus, the alignment of assessment practice with theoretical models generates effective strategies that make health programs in the community more effective as a whole. Community health assessments also help in strengthening community empowerment and participation. Involvement of the local population in the evaluation process creates a feeling of ownership and guardianship of the health concerns of their daily lives. This participatory approach not only strengthens the evidence collected but also makes health interventions more applicable. A better knowledge of the unique cultural, social, and economic contexts of the community is brought about through such participation, which leads to more effective health promotion strategies. Secondly, assessments offer a site for dialogue between stakeholders to facilitate collaborative strategies for addressing calculated health problems. The common strategy is in line with the principles of community empowerment, in that local leaders lead health initiatives. Last but not least, community health assessments provoke an active participation of residents in community health policy and program formulation, endorsing the importance of their perspectives in fostering healthier communities.

2.5.2. Methods of Conducting Assessments

For the context of community health, procedures for carrying out an assessment are invaluable in establishing individuals' health needs and evaluating the effectiveness of interventions in facilitating health. Surveys, interviews, focus groups, and observational studies are categories of assessments that can be broadly listed here, all meant to obtain some information that is utilized in preparing health plans. For instance, questionnaires may provide quantitative data regarding health behavior and outcomes, while qualitative instruments like focus groups can demonstrate indications of the perceptions and issues regarding health within the community. All these different tools of assessment enable health practitioners to triangulate data, thereby gaining an overall picture of health issues. Also, placing these assessments within a theoretical framework can enhance the maximum potential by aligning the aggregated data with the desired health outcomes within the community. Lastly, the longitudinal study design is a critical method for assessing shifts in health behavior over time, particularly within disadvantaged neighborhoods. As is evident from the research on housing improvement in Glasgow, longitudinal assessments enable the researcher to observe changes in smoking patterns and wants among those residents who were subjected to housing improvement. It is a reliable model for determining the impact of environmental alteration on health since it can adjust for confounding variables using baseline adjustment. The findings indicated support for a significant relationship between home renovation and stronger quit smoking intentions, indicating the potential for environmental impact on health habits. However, the lack of quitting among several residents suggests that environmental renovations do prompt consideration of behavior but are maybe not strong enough in themselves to sustain long-term health changes, hence requiring supportive interventions. The integration of technology such as HTA can also enhance the process of conducting community health assessments. The proposed theory of change-framework by the iDSI points out that there must be a systemized approach to evaluate health decision-making effects. Through linking causes and consequences of health interventions, experts can have a better understanding of the determinants of health outcomes. Through the use of economic models in combination with qualitative analysis, this framework supports quantifiable measurement of health impacts and the reasons for observed changes. Through such an integrated methodology, not only is the importance of informed decision-making emphasized but continuous improvement in health metrics is guaranteed, and ultimately more effective community health programs. The crossing of data collection techniques and theoretical structures is essential to realizing the highest health outcomes in multicultural community settings since it aims assessment efforts towards bigger health targets.

2.5.3. Utilizing Data for Health Improvement

In community health, the use of data is at the heart of decision making for health improvement programs. By systematic collection of, analysis, and interpretation of information, public health practitioners are in a position to guide the needs of communities and allocate interventions in priority. By way of illustration is the Scotland's National Health Service program, Childsmile, which is concerned with early years dental health by prioritized intervention. By Theory-Based Evaluation (TBE) strategies, stakeholders were in a position to map program implementation against central goals, thereby maximizing intervention efficacy. The process involved comparing program divergences and bringing them into conformity with pre-conceived Programme Theory before ultimately shaping action adjustments to deliver better outcomes in community health programs (Blamey et al., 2013). This systematic surveillance loop signals how data implementation makes health policy responsive and adaptive. Also, the use of data-driven models such as the Consolidated Framework for Implementation Research (CFIR) emphasizes the importance of determining contextual determinants that contribute to health program success. Mostly, CFIR combines significant constructs from dominant implementation theories to provide a systematic typology for evaluating health interventions across various settings. By clustering major elements such as intervention characteristics, external and internal environments, and individual processes, community health workers may identify barriers and facilitators to implementation. Such information not only supports formative evaluation but also fosters ongoing health improvement by making certain interventions are designed to meet specific community needs (Bandura et al., 2009). Lastly, systematic frameworks enable more insightful comprehension of how factors interact with one another in health improvement efforts. Combined with theoretical models, following data collection and utilization throughout the life cycle of health programs enhances the potential for beneficial change. Formative evaluations that actively incorporate knowledge derived from data enhance continuous reflection and enhancement of program design and implementation. For instance, Childsmiles approach to conducting discussions on implementation results is an illustration of how ongoing data dialogue can lead to enhanced program effects. Furthermore, the returned feedback from qualitative and quantitative data allows for participation of all levels of stakeholders, thereby creating an inclusive environment allowing for mutual learning. With an iterative process of utilization of data, community health interventions can respond to new threats and address them accordingly, hence fostering public health outcomes as well as health equity (Bandura et al., 2009; Blamey et al., 2013) (Figure 2.14).

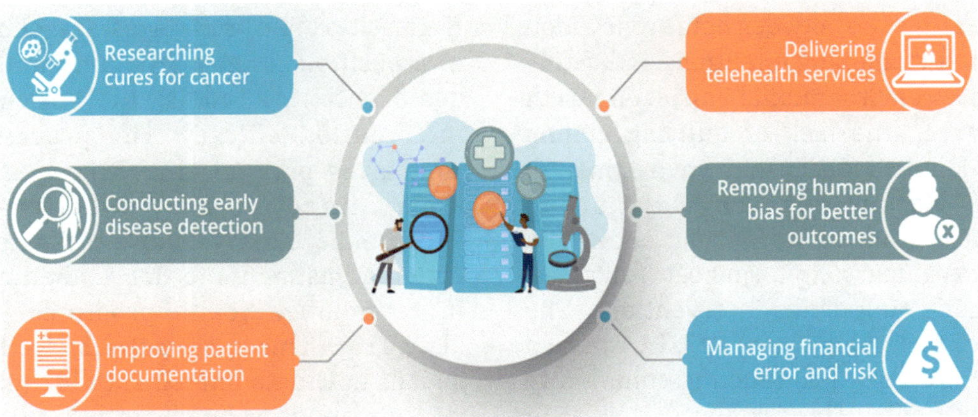

Figure 2.14. Utilizing data for health improvement.

Source: https://www.truenorthitg.com/wp-content/uploads/Data-Driven-Healthcare-Explained-Image3-1024x628.png.

2.6. Challenges in Community Health

Community health programs also experience a myriad of challenges that undermine their efficiency and sustainability. One of the primary challenges is the lack of accessible resources, not just financial aid but also human resources, like well-trained staff. This scarcity makes organizations rely heavily on contract or temporary staff, creating inconsistency in the delivery of services. For instance, New Zealand's Rape Prevention Education: Whakatu Mauri faced great challenges in maintaining a regular force of instructors for their BodySafe program. The necessity to recruit and train instructors numerous times within a year not only strained resources but also impacted the regularity of education programs against sexual violence (Good et al., 2015). These logistical issues demonstrate the means through which resource constraints can disrupt community-based health interventions, retarding their overall penetration and impact. Targeted communication and interventions that address targeted populations are also a challenge in community health. Where there are diverse cultural and socioeconomic determinants of health practice, one model is seldom adequate. The role of knowledge brokers (KBs) in low- and middle-income countries serves to demonstrate the best this complexity; they act as intermediaries between producers of evidence and users of health policy. Success for such KBs is defined by whether they are able to make communications align with local context and the particular needs of the community (Howell et al., 2021). This is why adaptability is a key element in enhancing the uptake of evidence-based practice. Mastery of these barriers involves new approaches that involve active citizen engagement, making it possible to create more relevant and targeted health interventions. Furthermore, the practice of health policy is often hindered by systemic shortcomings that stem from ineffective inter-agency collaboration. Organizations function in silos, lacking the synergistic interaction necessary for effective community health interventions. As highlighted by the activities of RPE among others, such isolated activities may lead to lost opportunities and wasted efforts in terms of overall gains in community health (Good et al., 2015). In particular, harmonizing knowledge translation approaches, as illustrated by the activity of KBs, could foster collaboration across organization boundaries. This would not only be advantageous to the delivery of health care but also help to create a united front against pervasive health issues. Such challenges have a nature that calls for well-coordinated effort with pooled expertise and means, ultimately toward an integrated public health model.

2.6.1. Health Disparities

Health inequities, or systematic difference in health status between different population groups, are significant indicators of social and economic inequities in populations. These inequities are often the outcome of the interaction of numerous variables that have to do with socioeconomic status, access to healthcare, and environmental health. The implications of such inequities are multifaceted in the sense that they hinder community-level health and limit economic productivity. As an illustration, American Indian communities suffer from vast health disparities related to obesity as a consequence of having very poor access to policy and environmental measures that support healthy practices. Interventions based on the community that acknowledge the unique infrastructural and cultural conditions of these groups are crucial in bridging these health disparities as brought out by measurements of community readiness for implementing obesity prevention practices. The study accentuates the need for tailored approaches that prioritize community engagement and participation in creating effective health interventions (Jernigan et al., 2016). The ecosocial model provides a methodical method of understanding the intricate determinants of health disparities, particularly for chronic illnesses like asthma. Research has revealed significant gaps in the management of asthma prevalence and treatment effectiveness between African Americans and White Americans.

The model brings together determinants at multiple levels—individual, family, healthcare, community, and sociocultural—and realizes that outcomes of health are influenced not only by the behavior of the individual but also by broader systems. For instance, socioeconomic status such as poverty and availability of good-quality healthcare have been reported to exacerbate asthma management inequalities. By taking into account the interrelationalities among these determinants, community health professionals can design multilevel interventions targeting barriers at all levels simultaneously, hence attempting to reduce inequities among marginalized groups in managing chronic diseases like asthma (Evans-Agnew et al., 2012). Additionally, the eradication of health disparities requires a shared effort transcending clinical care to incorporate broader social determinants of health. Particularly, community-based interventions will have to address enhanced access to nutritious food, stable shelter, and clean environmental conditions, together combining to drive improved health outcomes. Stakeholder engagement at the community level to determine constraints and formulate practical solutions is critical. For example, American Indian reservation stakeholders named making healthy food options available as a critical way to reduce obesity risk, and the potential of community involvement in guiding good health policy. Engaging local people not only ensures that interventions are culturally acceptable but also enhances ownership and accountability to health improvement. Thus, the integration of community inputs into health plans is crucial to alleviating health inequities and enhancing overall community health (Jernigan et al., 2016) (Figure 2.15).

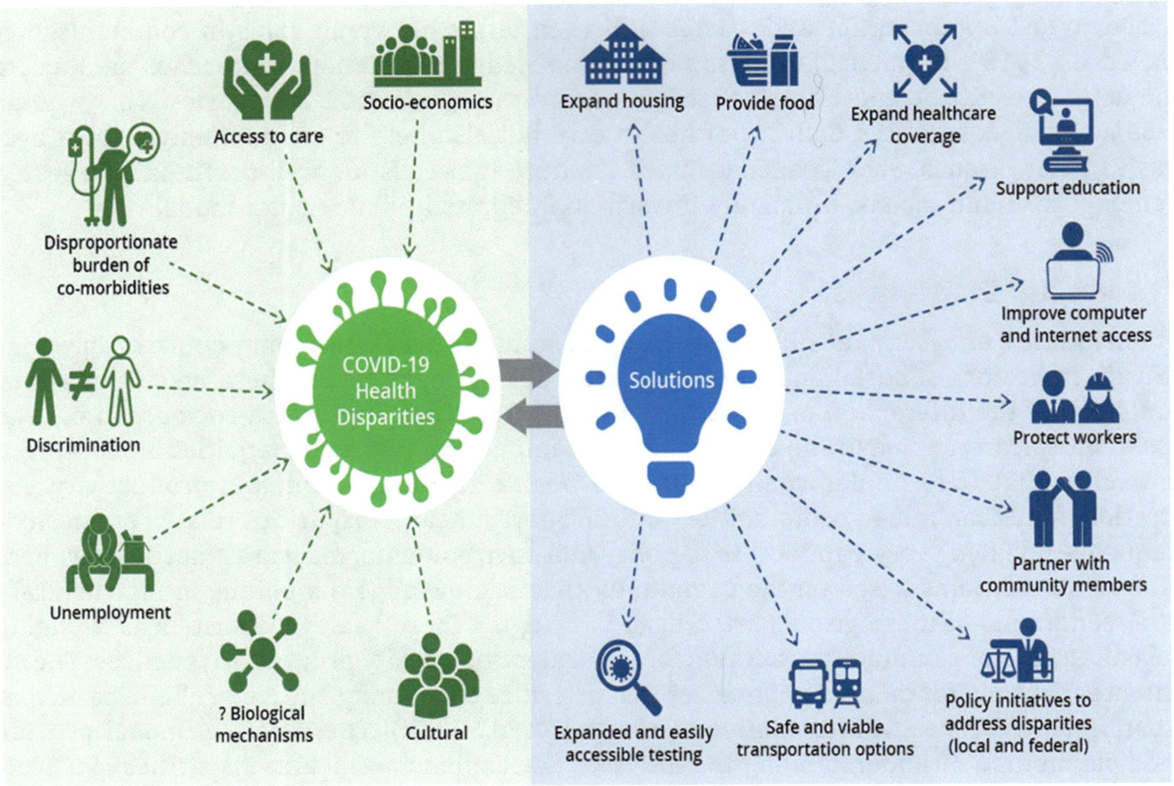

Figure 2.15. Health disparities.

Source: https://ucsfhealthcardiology.ucsf.edu/sites/ucsfhealthcardiology.ucsf.edu/files/inline-images/COVID-19%20Health%20Disparities%20and%20Solutions.jpg.

2.6.2. Policy and Funding Issues

Policy and funding issues in community health are crucial to the definition of the effectiveness of interventions in alleviating gender-based violence. An examination of existing frameworks shows a need for sweeping reforms that consider the socio-economic forces behind this kind of violence. By analyzing critically the existing legislative framework, specifically attempts like the Violence Against Women Act (VAWA), scholars have identified the limitations of the available legal frameworks in addressing the complexities of domestic violence. For instance, prevailing paradigms are prone to disregard structural dimensions of gendered inequality and economic insecurity upon which domestic violence dynamics critically depend. By repositioning the conversation about these intersections, advocates may be able to develop a more nuanced model that fosters legislative transformation and resource investment that is responsive to these broader socio-economic realities (Weissman et al., 2013). Funding mechanisms also complicate these policy systems, and they affect the sustainability and availability of programs at the community level. Organizations that work to prevent sexual violence, such as New Zealand's Rape Prevention Education (RPE) program, often struggle with budget constraints that impact their capacity to deliver comprehensive education programs. Insufficient resources can mean that they have to employ casual contract teachers, leading to high staff turnover and inefficiencies in running the show, which undermine programs such as BodySafe. Consequently, the agencies must not just search for prevention funding, but also new program delivery models that would maximize resource use.

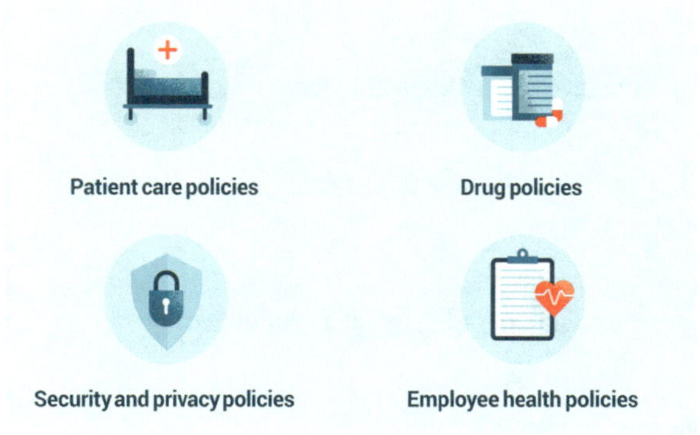

Figure 2.16. Policy and funding issues.

Source: https://www.usa.edu/wp-content/uploads/2021/10/healthcare-policy-examples.png.

A study on behalf of RPE points to the urgency of a re-evaluation of the approaches to funding in order to make the community health efforts in violence prevention stable, robust, and effective (Good et al., 2015). Solving the intricate policy and finance problems in community health necessitates a method that addresses multifaceted aspects across various stakeholders. Policymakers have to take action to facilitate authentic collaboration with community-based organizations addressing gender-based violence for purposes of building holistic and effective strategies. These partnerships are instrumental in unifying resources, skills, and campaigns in a way that addresses the real needs of the affected populations. Strategies to align funding mechanisms with evidence-based interventions can also increase the sustainability of community health programs, so they remain beneficial in the future. In pushing stakeholders to engage with one another across sectors, opportunities for innovative solutions are high, facilitating an environment for solving pressing gendered health issues in communities (Weissman et al., 2013; Good et al., 2015) (Figure 2.16).

2.6.3. Community Engagement Barriers

Effective community outreach is an indispensable intervention towards enhanced health outcomes, but there are numerous constraints towards this, particularly for vulnerable groups. The candidacy theory, which accounts for the way individuals perceive their acceptability and candidacy for service, becomes a useful theoretical orientation in accounting for the constraints. The majority of individuals in marginalized communities withdraw from health services due to socioeconomic issues, cultural diversity, or previous negative experiences with the healthcare system. These barriers pose a complex setting in which outreach programs struggle to establish rapport and trust. Lack of engagement problems range from unawareness to deep-seated distrust, meaning that recognizing such engagement barriers is critical to improving health interventions for hard-to-reach groups (Cameron et al., 2011). Further, the integration of patient engagement strategies into community health models makes it more challenging to engage people. In ACO studies, patient activation through effective patient education and involvement in their own care through mechanisms such as shared decision-making and motivational interviewing is brought up as imperative. However, frontline clinicians and managers indicate towards an occasional level of awareness of such strategies, which implies that there is a disconnect between theory and practice. This disconnect can undermine the effectiveness of interventions aimed at enhancing community health participation. Without proper training and support, healthcare professionals are unlikely to effectively utilize such participation approaches in their interaction with patients, which leads to negative outcomes and minimal involvement from the community (Elwyn et al., 2018). Addressing the barriers to community participation requires a multi-faceted approach that incorporates education, outreach, and advocacy. Services that are based solely on traditional models of care are likely to exclude unintentionally those people who could be most assisted by them. Thus, health organizations need to adopt a more inclusive and culturally sensitive model of community engagement. Taking learnings from outreach practices and an understanding of the candidacy nuances can guide the development of targeted interventions that take hold among disparate populations. Ultimately, an appreciation of how engagement is not a uniform approach will enable health professionals to create spaces in which individuals feel empowered and supported to activate their health, resulting in enhanced health outcomes and reduced disparities (Cameron et al., 2011) (Figure 2.17).

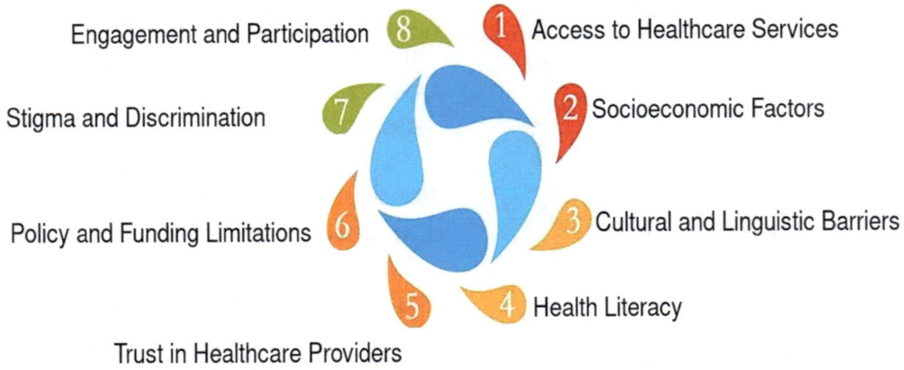

Figure 2.17. Community engagement barriers.

Source: https://fastercapital.co/i/Community-engagement--Community-Health--Promoting-Well-Being-Through-Community-Health-Initiatives--Challenges-and-Barriers-in-Community-Health-Engagement.webp.

SUMMARY

In conclusion, discussion on diversified theories and models in community health brings to fore the complexity of the link between individual actions and determinants of health in the environment. As studies in Greece have shown, young adults face numerous challenges in adopting healthy eating habits, which range from time constraints, peer influence, and environment without support. They highlight the need for holistic approaches that transcend the realm of individual responsibility to consider systemic issues. Such an awareness aligns with social marketing interventions that customize interventions in accordance with local contexts and motivations of target populations, thereby laying the ground for enhanced community health programs (Bandura et al., 2014). Also, measuring the impact of community health programs entails collaboration to identify the public will and how it results in public health outcomes. Engaging diverse stakeholders within policy-making decisions can activate community receptivity and produce enduring behavior change. Connecting conceptual frameworks with real-life experiences offers an outline for implementing campaigns that resonate with members within a community. With the employment of social movements and media advocacy theories and models, health practitioners can mobilize resources and create awareness on key health challenges, thereby creating collective action to tackle underlying social determinants of health (Salmon et al., 2003). Finally, the outcome of this evaluation of theories and models of community health reveals that effective health interventions must be holistic in nature, taking into account behavioral in addition to socio-political aspects. It is essential that follow-up research continues to question the mechanics of changing health behavior while simultaneously advocating on behalf of policies that increase healthier environments. Integrating theoretical bases with evidence-based interventions should hopefully yield comprehensive health strategies that enable populations to be the masters of their own destiny. Thus, by making investments in community health infrastructure and intersectoral collaboration, we can lay the groundwork for improved health and overall well-being in communities.

From recognition of the complexity of community health, a number of theories and models are found to be key frameworks wherein to investigate how health is conceived, governed, and delivered in varying populations. A key model that is relevant here is the Health Trainer model, which places emphasis on the role of using members of the community to be health advocates and educators. Introduced in 2005, this model has gained popularity across different environments, especially within offender health schemes, where it aims to empower individuals to become responsible for their health paths. The collaboration of Health Trainer Hubs with education institutions has helped establish resources such as the educational workbook established in 2008 to enhance the training process of instructors and learners of health-related professionals. This model points out the critical element of community engagement for health education, resulting in a more responsive and culturally competent health care delivery system (Davidson et al., 2009). A second concern among community health paradigms involves the influence of cultural constructs on health behavior. Lay explanatory models, particularly in low- and middle-income environments, demonstrate the ways in which traditional practices and beliefs shape health-seeking behavior. A qualitative study in Indonesia, for instance, discovered that local populations view strokes as conditions caused by reversible occlusions, something that deviates considerably from biomedical conceptions of strokes as acute clinical emergencies. This locally generated understanding guides health responses and highlights the importance of education strategies that are locally centered and congruent with indigenous beliefs. The identification and use of these lay models in health education can effectively bridge the gap between clinical practice and community health needs and eventually lead to more effective health interventions (Allotey et al., 2010). The confluence of existing health models and community-held beliefs leads to the overarching necessity of a multilayer approach in community health interventions. Effective provision of health interventions must consider the interaction of dynamic relationships among formal systems of care and traditional cultural norms. Developing educational materials respectful and inclusive of these beliefs is challenging, but crucial to support health promotion and disease prevention at the community level. By understanding the fundamental principles guiding various theories of health, the stakeholders can design more holistic strategies that enhance the health of varied populations. Beyond this inclusion empowering the individuals, it also creates a healthcare environment that is inclusive, flexible, and in accordance with the day-to-day experiences of individuals (Allotey et al., 2010; Davidson et al., 2009).

KEY TERMS FROM THIS CHAPTER

Academic paradigms	Advocacy	Asthma
Behavioral theory	Behavior change	Chronic disease
Community resources	Crime	Curriculum
Data collection	Disease outbreaks	Displacement
Economic empowerment	Epidemiology	Health inequity
Housing quality	Human resources	Marginalization
Nutrition	Nutritious food	Obesity
Physical activity	Poverty	Public engagement
Resource allocation	Sanitation	Social Ecological Model
Social justice	Social marketing	

CLOSER LOOK

COMMUNAL WELLNESS INTERVENTION

Communitybased or communal wellness interventions are locally rooted strategies designed to promote health by engaging community members in collective behavior change, health education, and social support. These interventions often involve peer-led models—such as *Care Groups* where volunteers teach neighboring households—or community hygiene clubs that foster dialogue around hygiene, sanitation, nutrition, and WASH (water, sanitation, and hygiene) practices. In Africa, Community Health Clubs—meeting weekly for dialogue sessions—help communities adopt low-cost hygiene habits, build communal nutrition gardens, and establish savings or incomegeneration groups, yielding measurable reductions in disease and improvements in women's empowerment. Peerled group interventions, such as India's women's group programs, combine maternal and child health education with livelihood support, leading to higher service uptake and improved socioeconomic resilience among marginalized communities.

Systematic reviews confirm that community interventions outperform individual approaches in primary health care: they are effective in reducing cardiovascular risk, promoting physical activity, preventing falls, and enhancing selfcare in chronically ill patients. Importantly, interventions that are sustained, multi-component, and culturally tailored—incorporating mutual goalsetting and participatory planning—tend to outperform one-off education programs. Reviews in South Asia show that maternal health interventions relying on community mobilization modestly increased antenatal attendance and facility births, although effects on mortality were limited. In urban lowincome settlements, behavior change communication combined with WASH improvements and socioeconomic components (e.g., income support, home treatment kits) significantly reduced infectious disease burden—including TB, diarrheal illness, and influenza—by improving hygiene behaviors, treatment adherence, screening uptake, and immunization coverage.

The *Care Group* model—a scalable peereducation approach where volunteers cascaded health messages and supervised small household cohorts—has expanded globally to address nutrition, parenting, WASH, tuberculosis, and mental health challenges in vulnerable settings. Another example, *Whole Health Action Management (WHAM)*, combines peer coaching with goal setting and selfmanagement support for individuals with chronic conditions or behavioral health diagnoses. Across interventions, community involvement in design and delivery enhances acceptance, ownership, and sustainability, while promoting empowerment and social cohesion. Although outcomes vary based on context and intensity, communal wellness approaches consistently deliver improvements in health knowledge, preventive behaviors, and access to services—particularly when sustained, participatory, and adapted to local cultural contexts.

REFERENCES

1. Agarwal, R., Benbasat, I., Eisenhardt, K. M., Fishbein, M., Mijinyawa, K., Kwan, S. K., Lincoln, Y. S., et al. (2011). A theory-grounded framework of Open-Source Software adoption in SMEs. https://core.ac.uk/download/20496319.pdf (accessed on 26th June 2025).
2. Alam, K., Erdiaw-Kwasie, M., Ryan, B., Shahiduzzaman, M., et al. (2018). Assessing regional digital competence: Digital futures and strategic planning implications. https://core.ac.uk/download/211503258.pdf (accessed on 26th June 2025).
3. Allotey, P., Barrett, G., & Norris, M. (2010). "I feel like half my body is clogged up": Lay models of stroke in Central Aceh, Indonesia. https://core.ac.uk/download/20496346.pdf (accessed on 26th June 2025).
4. Alrøe, H. F., & Noe, E. (2012). Observing environments. https://core.ac.uk/download/10932845.pdf (accessed on 26th June 2025).
5. Armstrong, R., Baríc, L., Bronfenbrenner, U., Checkland, P., Coats, D., Davies, J. K., Davies, J. K., et al. (2014). Theorizing healthy settings: A critical discussion with reference to Healthy Universities. https://core.ac.uk/download/42136826.pdf (accessed on 26th June 2025).
6. Baker, D. V., Carlson, S., Ford, S., Galford, G., et al. (2014). Considering Vermont's future in a changing climate: The first Vermont climate assessment. https://core.ac.uk/download/215155341.pdf (accessed on 26th June 2025).
7. Bandura, A., Carroll, A., Drewnowski, A., Kafatos, A., Kirmani, A., Papadaki, A., Richards, A., et al. (2014). Social marketing and healthy eating: Findings from young people in Greece. https://core.ac.uk/download/29843393.pdf (accessed on 26th June 2025).
8. Barrett, H., Beecham, D., & Brown, K. (2013). The applicability of behavior changes in intervention programmers targeted at ending female genital mutilation in the EU: Integrating social cognitive and community level approaches. https://core.ac.uk/download/323060331.pdf (accessed on 26th June 2025).
9. Berry, D., Bults, R. G. A., de Wijk, R., Franch, M., et al. (2011). Requirements for a nutrition education demonstrator. https://core.ac.uk/download/pdf/11481114.pdf (accessed on 26th June 2025).
10. Best, K. C. (2012). Holistic leadership: A model for leader-member engagement and development. https://core.ac.uk/download/144550648.pdf (accessed on 26th June 2025).
11. Blue Bird Jernigan, V., Boe, G., Buchwald, D., Carroll, M., et al. (2016). Assessing feasibility and readiness to address obesity through policy in American Indian reservations. https://digitalscholarship.unlv.edu/cgi/viewcontent.cgi?article=1428&context=jhdrp (accessed on 26th June 2025).
12. Bolt, C. A. (2017). Environmental education in the public sphere: Comparing practice with psychosocial determinants of behavior and societal change. https://core.ac.uk/download/129153482.pdf (accessed on 26th June 2025).
13. Bond, L., Clark, J., Egan, M., Kearns, A., et al. (2012). Smoking and intention to quit in deprived areas of Glasgow: Is it related to housing improvements and neighborhood regeneration because of improved mental health? https://core.ac.uk/download/16460995.pdf (accessed on 26th June 2025).

14. Briggs, A., & Grieve, E. (2017). A methodological approach for measuring the impact of HTA. https://core.ac.uk/download/80697121.pdf (accessed on 26th June 2025).

15. Brown, L. A., Contractor, A. A., Dranger, P., Frankfurt, S., et al. (2018). Influence of multiple traumatic event types on mental health outcomes: Does count matter? https://core.ac.uk/download/216809067.pdf (accessed on 26th June 2025).

16. Burns, A., Floyd, J., & Ramos, J. (2008). A challenging conversation on integral futures: Embodied foresight and trialogues. https://core.ac.uk/download/10827496.pdf (accessed on 26th June 2025).

17. Buxton, M. J., Gonzalez-Block, M. A., Hanney, S., Kogan, M., et al. (2010). The utilization of health research in policy-making: Concepts, examples, and methods of assessment. https://core.ac.uk/download/336631.pdf (accessed on 26th June 2025).

18. Cameron, A., Sowden, A., Tod, A. M., Corr, C., Davison, C., O'Donnell, C., O'Donnell, C., et al. (2011). What is the 'problem' that outreach work seeks to address and how might it be tackled? Seeking theory in a primary health prevention programmed. https://core.ac.uk/download/1437084.pdf (accessed on 26th June 2025).

19. Chaparro, M., Das, B., & Landaburu, A. (2016). Epistemología de la comunicación en India: Una aproximación histórica más allá del "desarrollo." https://core.ac.uk/download/288159360.pdf (accessed on 26th June 2025).

20. Clark, C., Long, D., Olsen, S., & Rosenzweig, W. (2004). *Double Bottom Line Progress Report: Assessing Social Impact in Double Bottom Line Ventures, Methods Catalog*. https://core.ac.uk/download/71350848.pdf (accessed on 26th June 2025).

21. Cooper, B., Cowie, B., & McGee, C. (2010). Initial teacher education and the New Zealand curriculum. https://core.ac.uk/download/29199940.pdf (accessed on 26th June 2025).

22. Davidson, J., & Wilkinson, K. (2009). Evaluation of the content and delivery of the student workbook for RIPH Level 2 award in understanding health improvement for health trainer champions in prisons and the wider community. https://core.ac.uk/download/16669924.pdf (accessed on 26th June 2025).

23. Davidson, P. M., Phillips, J. L., & Rolley, J. X. (2012). Developing targeted health service interventions using the PRECEDE-PROCEED model: Two Australian case studies. https://core.ac.uk/download/18719492.pdf (accessed on 26th June 2025).

24. DeLoge, A. (2012). Impressions of interculturality and health care in Bolivia: Three cases from Cochabamba. https://core.ac.uk/download/12211765.pdf (accessed on 26th June 2025).

25. Elwyn, G., Fisher, E., Mishra, M. K., Rodriguez, M., et al. (2018). How do healthcare professionals working in accountable care organizations understand patient activation and engagement? Qualitative interviews across two time points. https://core.ac.uk/download/323081191.pdf (accessed on 26th June 2025).

26. Erickson, J. D., Perkins, P. E. (Ellie), & Spencer, P. (2018). Re-establishing justice as a pillar of ecological economics through feminist. https://core.ac.uk/download/287659734.pdf (accessed on 26th June 2025).

27. Evans-Agnew, R. A. (2012). Asthma management: An Eco social framework for disparity research. https://digitalscholarship.unlv.edu/cgi/viewcontent.cgi?article=1011&context=jhdrp (accessed on 26th June 2025).

28. Fawcett, M. (2012). CE 611 Syllabus: Development over the lifespan. https://core.ac.uk/download/524877040.pdf (accessed on 26th June 2025).
29. Gerling, K., Mandryk, R., Rita, M., et al. (2013). Tailoring persuasive health games to gamer type. https://core.ac.uk/download/20320900.pdf (accessed on 26th June 2025).
30. Gienapp, A., Reisman, J., & Stachowiak, S. (2012). *A Handbook of Data Collection Tools: Companion To "A Guide to Measuring Advocacy and Policy."* https://core.ac.uk/download/84911833.pdf (accessed on 26th June 2025).
31. Good, G., Julich, S. J., Oak, E., Terrell, M., et al. (2015). The sustainable delivery of sexual violence prevention education in schools. https://core.ac.uk/download/148643123.pdf (accessed on 26th June 2025).
32. Grandos, A., Kitson, A., Loftus-Hills, A., Oxman, A., Titchen, A., Titchen, A., Van de Ven, A. H., et al. (2008). Evaluating the successful implementation of evidence into practice using the PARiHS framework: Theoretical and practical challenges. https://core.ac.uk/download/48947.pdf (accessed on 26th June 2025).
33. Green, A., & Preston, J. (2003). *The Macro-Social Benefits of Education, Training and Skills in Comparative Perspective* [Wider Benefits of Learning Research Report No. 9]. https://core.ac.uk/download/pdf/83568.pdf (accessed on 26th June 2025).
34. Howell, C., Norton, T., Reynolds, C., Rodriguez, M., et al. (2021). 'Maybe we can turn the tide': An explanatory mixed-methods study to understand how knowledge brokers mobilize health evidence in low- and middle-income countries. https://core.ac.uk/download/237011937.pdf (accessed on 26th June 2025).
35. Hughes, A., & Mutrie, N. (2006). Maintaining physical activity in cardiac rehabilitation. https://core.ac.uk/download/9020260.pdf (accessed on 26th June 2025).
36. Kushitor, S. B., & Colecraft, E. (2023). Development of a facilitator guide for nutrition education on overweight and obesity in the eastern region of Ghana. *African Journal of Food, Agriculture, Nutrition and Development*. https://www.semanticscholar.org/paper/0a99574983270700e8498dbdcc5ed6ba831ad292 (accessed on 26th June 2025).
37. McCluskey, A., Kitson, A. L., Weiner, B., Cuthbertson, B. H., Helms, C., O'Connor, D., Zhu, D. Q., et al. (2012). Theories of behavior change synthesized into a set of theoretical groupings: Introducing a thematic series on the Theoretical Domains Framework. https://core.ac.uk/download/9559515.pdf (accessed on 26th June 2025).
38. McKie, R. E., & Nwalozie, C. J. (2019). An examination of the experiences of BAME students in the Community and Criminal Justice Division. https://core.ac.uk/download/287585159.pdf (accessed on 26th June 2025).
39. Mead, A. S., Nagy, M. C., & Nagy, S. (2012). Utilizing community resources to reduce the presence of type 2 diabetes in rural youth. https://digitalscholarship.unlv.edu/cgi/viewcontent.cgi?article=1060&context=jhdrp (accessed on 26th June 2025).
40. Ray, M., Tornello, A. R., Pickart, F., Stripling, M., Ali, M., & Vargas, L. (2023). A jurisdictional risk assessment for the whole community: A new, systematic approach to participatory decision-making in public health emergency preparedness using the analytic hierarchy process. *Journal of Multi-Criteria Decision Analysis*. https://www.semanticscholar.org/paper/ef4d145f73dd04ec5970c2a81724c9de2db02b91 (accessed on 26th June 2025).

41. Rosiecki, J. (2015). Needs assessment for a patient centered medical home model of care at the Providence Alaska Cancer Center. https://core.ac.uk/download/162578511.pdf (accessed on 26th June 2025).

42. Salmon, C. T., Post, L. A., & Christensen, R. E. (2003). Mobilizing public will for social change. https://core.ac.uk/download/71340672.pdf (accessed on 26th June 2025).

43. Sharkey, S., & Sharples, A. (2008). From the beginning: Negotiation in community evaluation. https://core.ac.uk/download/76704.pdf (accessed on 26th June 2025).

44. Thomas, S., & Thomson, H. (2015). Developing empirically supported theories of change for housing investment and health. https://core.ac.uk/download/42357280.pdf (accessed on 26th June 2025).

45. Weissman, D. M. (2013). Law, social movements, and the political economy of domestic violence. https://core.ac.uk/download/62560159.pdf (accessed on 26th June 2025).

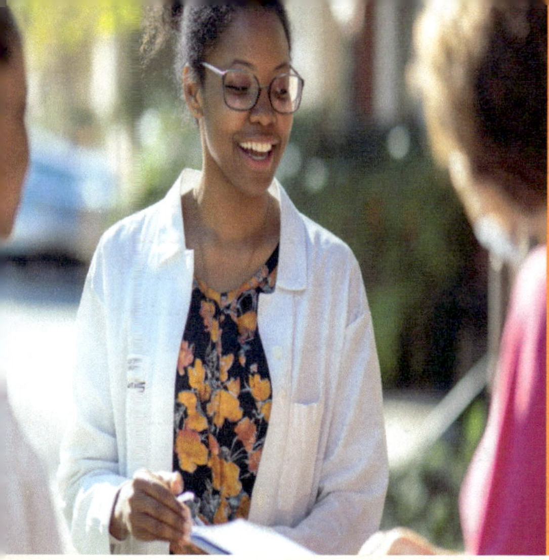

Chapter 3

COMMUNITY HEALTH ASSESSMENT

Contents

Introduction

Community health assessment is an essential piece in the quest to improve public health outcomes at the local and overall level. Through collecting data, analyzing, and interpreting systematically the health status and needs of a population, community health assessment strives to identify significant health issues and disparities in a target area. It is not only a numerically based introduction, i.e., morbidity and mortality figures, but also one that incorporates qualitative findings in the form of feedback from the community members. Such common knowledge helps to inform public health practitioners and policy makers to devise intervention methods aimed at the specific ailments. Second, the use of more than one source of information makes the validity of assessment results stronger so that they are guided by the intricate reality of the focus community. Therefore, good community health assessment is a good stimulant for actual health improvement. A key aspect of community health assessment is that the identification of environmental determinants with significant impacts on health outcomes is a critical component. These are air and water quality, access to recreation sites, and access to health care, which characterize members' overall health in a given society. Measuring these in the surroundings allows for detection of areas that should be addressed with policy measures or infrastructural expansion to be carried out. For instance, environmental information is highly ranked by the Environment Agency in evaluating management of water resources, requiring analyses that improve environmental impact sensitivity and regulatory performance (N/A, 1996). Same models apply to community health assessment, which allows for the determination of socio-environmental determinants with differential impacts on vulnerable populations. Therefore, the inclusion of environmental factors in health evaluation not only broadens the scope of analysis but also indicates the mutual dependence of community health and environmental sustainability. Additionally, the findings of the community health assessment are not merely identification of health issues; they prompt strategic planning and resource mobilization for public health interventions. The analysis helps stakeholders like the health workers, government officials, and community organizations to prioritize decisions and plan resources appropriately. Issues still exist, including how to prevent biases in the collection of data and engage the community throughout the stages of the analysis process. Of specific interest, problems with genetically modified food have exposed the requirement for robust methodologies that address ecological and socio-economic issues (Andersen et al., 2012). With stakeholders and robust assessment instruments involved, community health screenings can contribute towards a more balanced health in the environment. In total, methodical use of community health assessments provides a strong background for fact-based decision-making, in turn facilitating the vital integration of health, environment, and community involvement (Figure 3.1).

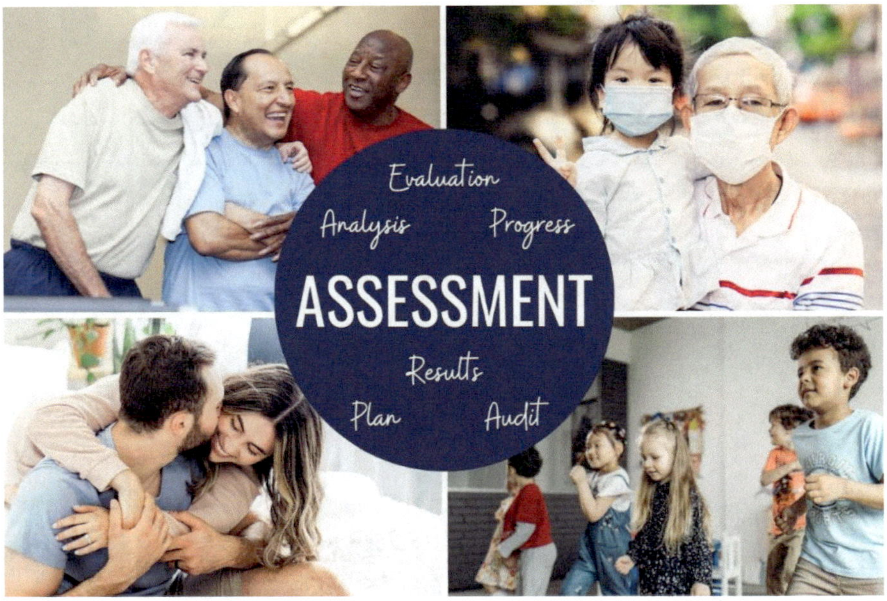

Figure 3.1. Community health assessment (CHA).

Source: https://www.capecountyhealth.com/cmsAdmin/uploads/2/ch-assessment_1200x800.jpg.

Definition of Community Health Assessment (CHA)

A CHA is a systematic data collection and analysis process used to become aware of the health status and health needs of a specific community. It is accomplished by engaging members and stakeholders in the community to identify the health problems they are facing, and therefore obtaining results that reflect their values and beliefs. CHAs integrate multiple dimensions like socio-economic status, health habits, and health service accessibility in an attempt to achieve a holistic picture of local health dynamics. The intention extends to gathering quantitative data but also to appreciate the qualitative experience of life for individuals in populations. An in-depth CHA enables public health organizations and governments to formulate evidence-based interventions that are tailored to the needs of the community, promoting increased health equity and the success of resource distribution for the population. Second, a community health assessment becomes more effective when it recognizes health disparities among subgroups. For example, an understanding of various populations' differences in health literacy can go a long way in helping them plan for interventions to improve health. Literature has proven that low health literacy significantly affected health outcomes, particularly for risk groups such as Spanish-speaking immigrants who may be disenfranchised with current health resources due to language barriers or inadequate access to information (Hund et al., 2016). Drawing on such information, a CHA can identify vulnerable groups and provide tailored health education interventions to empower them. Lastly, these disparities must be identified to enhance the role of health policy and programs that can even further strengthen community health as a whole. For making the assessments in community health work effectively and efficiently, different stakeholders with a diverse population from the very start of the assessment process are needed. They are local agencies, healthcare providers, policymakers, and community members who will present different perspectives while addressing pressing health issues. Involvement of stakeholders not only generates a cooperative environment but also establishes trust and facilitates the implementation of recommended measures. In addition, community involvement in the CHA process has the potential to improve community capacity and ownership of health projects, which ultimately reflects in enhanced health outcomes in the long run. Evidence indicates that citizens' involvement in such participatory processes is a means of empowering them to improve their action capacity for promoting their health requirements and acting constructively for improving community resilience (King et al., 2010). Participatory involvement through CHAs can better shape public health policies responsive to the complexities of health in the context of the community.

Importance of Community Health Assessments (CHAs)

CHAs are effective tools used in the assessment of health outcomes and needs of particular populations. By systemically collecting and analyzing data, they provide a snapshot of the general health status of the community, its strengths and weaknesses. This involves not only measuring health outcomes but also the social determinants of health contributing to health disparities among the population. As has been contended in literature in existence, the effectiveness of such assessments is weakened to some extent by weak monitoring and assessment systems, reducing strategic planning (N/A, 2010). Thus, proper appraisal has the ability to shed light on resource use, guide policy choices, and eventually lead to improved interventions for specified health issues. Through participatory approaches, people in the community are engaged, facilitating ownership and collaboration that is required for long-term improvement in health. In addition, co-operation between public health and local government is key in successful implementation of community health assessments. Local government possesses unique leadership roles in constructing the public health infrastructures required to assess and ultimately enhance community well-being. After the critique of literature, effective local governance is essential to act upon the social determinants of health and develop healthy environments that promote equity in health (Gamsu et al., 2014). All these assessments direct local policymakers to formulate interventions according to the requirements of the citizens. Through the application of evidence-based interventions from assessment findings, local governments are able to effectively mobilize resources to offer assistance to vulnerable populations. The key is at the intersection of community outreach and local government, ensuring assessments are translated into real health gains. Last but not least, the impact of community health assessments goes beyond enhanced immediate health; they play a critical role in creating long-term public health outcomes. By regular conduct of these surveys, communities are able to track trends over time, thus identifying new developments and issues in health. Not only does this serve to make health providers and policymakers accountable but it also generates the public's trust in health programs. Moreover, regular involvement via such surveys forces communities to assume the activist role for health, thus presenting a platform via which health promotion becomes everyone's cause. Lastly, when community health assessments are implemented and used in public health planning, they have the predominant function of comprehending the complex interrelation of various determinants of health, thereby laying the groundwork for constructing healthier communities (Figure 3.12).

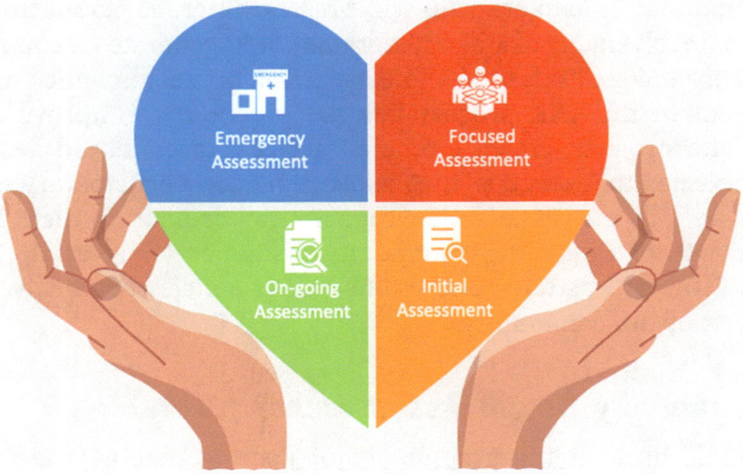

Figure 3.2. Importance of community health assessments.

Source: https://cdn.sketchbubble.com/pub/media/catalog/product/optimized1/1/1/11510df9eec9c85aa78c2395c792c27d552cf3eafe01a77574120d1d26658b09/health-assessment-mc-slide1.png.

3.1. Purpose of Community Health Assessment (CHA)

CHAs are central to defining and evaluating the health needs of targeted populations. CHAs provide a snapshot of the general health of a community by gathering and analyzing data on many health indicators, social determinants of health, and the environment. By structured analysis of the trend in health, access to health care, and existing health inequities, CHAs enable public health leaders and officials to realize the potential of the comprehensive picture of community health. The central analysis underpins evidence-based decision-making and resource prioritization for public health and ultimately enables communities to focus interventions. In addition, as part of an integrated public health response, evidence generated by CHAs can be used to inform policy and enhance public services supporting well-being and addressing priority community health concerns. Further, CHAs do not only raise awareness on health matters but also promote community empowerment and inter-stakeholder dialogue. Through the involvement of a wide range of stakeholders including the local departments of health, community residents, and advocacy organizations, CHAs promote a culture of conversation and shared understanding of health issues. The participatory process does enhance timeliness in the assessments and developing relationships with stakeholders, which facilitates a sense of ownership in working on issues in health. In addition, through active participation of community members, there is the possibility for incorporating feedback from the most affected into the assessment, paving the way for culturally and contextually responsive interventions.

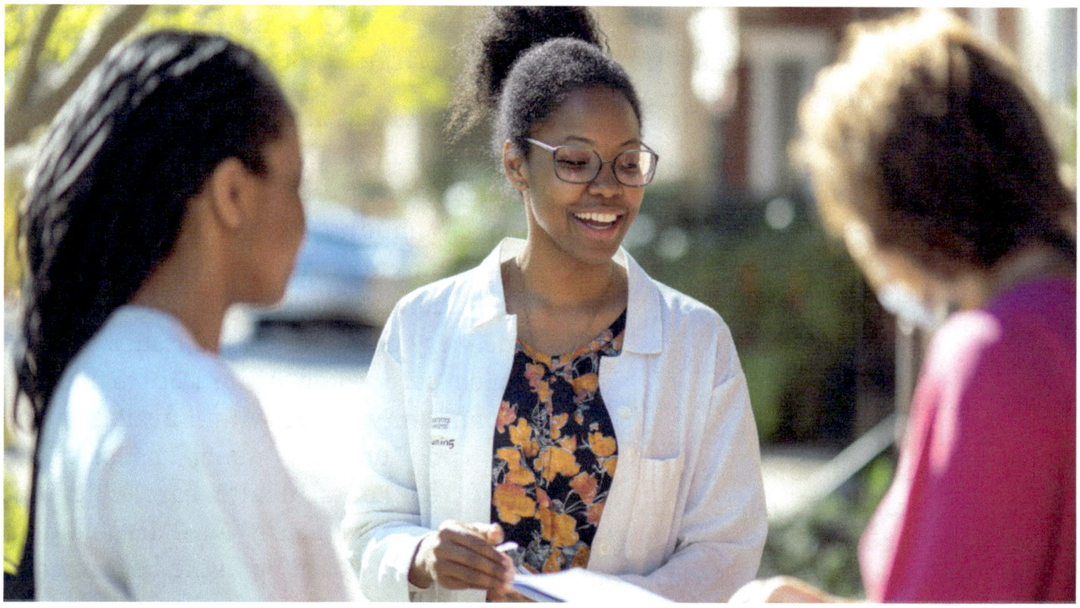

Figure 3.3. Community health assessments (CHAs) serve.

Source: https://blogger.googleusercontent.com/img/b/R29vZ2xl/AVvXsEgTDHlrNxhNq8iLghWrzTHxvMipZkBzVmhCofGD1q5lcozZETeuD6aNozOa5CKnFSMaBAzfuVDgBG0pOe46kobwWrF4WNdcObIdqhzES89eNDId-DJLQao0b3Sh5c3m1j932s9sFK3An_xdf5A9-0kompSKGogpVu5FaSTW4-tHu0jQfU84NLKQyzKXzCY/s1200/CHA%20FAQ%20Blog.jpeg.

This type of participation is helpful in developing credibility and buy-in from the community and in maintaining public health programs based on CHA findings. Finally, with evolving public health settings, the function of CHAs is to monitor progress and review the impact of interventions conducted. Continued monitoring provides an opportunity for health workers to redesign approaches based on evolving community needs, new trends in the data, as well as newly emerging health hazards. For instance, by taking advantage of advances in public health information systems, it is possible to make the process of evaluation more robust so that analysis and data collection are in real-time. It is such adaptability that is essential when handling the dynamicity of public health challenges, particularly in relation to the situation of an event such as pandemics or natural calamities where quick and well-informed action is necessary. The use of innovative technology, like developing the Public Health Information Technology Maturity Index, is the last way to enhance systems in a bid to further guarantee CHA effectiveness and consequently attain healthier outcomes among people (Agarwal et al., 2016). Continued innovation of CHAs is thus crucial to guarantee they remain effective and relevant in the development of community health (Figure 3.3).

3.1.1. Identifying Health Needs

Identification of health needs in a community is a vital first step of any thorough comprehensive community health assessment. It is not merely an additional step to document existing health issues but more so to illuminate potential gaps in care and services that require remediation. An example of determining the needs of community mental health is provided, for example, by a coordinated specialty care (CSC) model of care for individuals with first episode psychosis (FEP). A recent Ohio study reported extensive variations in services offered to such a high-risk group by community mental health centers (CMHCs). Utilizing mixed methods in the measurement of service availability and administrative attitudes, the study revealed that in rural settings, despite robust administrative infrastructure, subjective deficiencies in treatment capacity remain, which are particularly rooted in rural settings. Addressing such weaknesses through focused measurements, in turn, can empower stakeholders to develop effective, population-targeted interventions. In addition to information regarding mental health needs, identification of social determinants of health is an important component of community health needs assessments. Inclusion of social needs screening in academic health systems (AHS) emphasizes the importance of identifying and responding to non-medical determinants that can affect health outcomes. An Association of American Medical Colleges study points out challenges in the incorporation of social needs screening in an existing healthcare system. While AHS have indeed taken great strides in the provision of services to reach populations at risk and in collaboration with community-based agencies, resource constraints and regulation complexities are still persisting challenges. These also reflect on the importance of addressing the systemic change towards more holistic integration of social services into healthcare provision.

Thus, health needs assessment must address both the clinical and also the social dimensions to facilitate an integrated response to community health. Effective health need assessment strategies also have to involve consideration of strengthening models of service delivery that address the issues of the day. One such care being calibrated to meet evolving community needs within available constraints is a mix delivery model of face-to-face visits and telemental health care. The Ohio study reported that nearly all CMHC administrators believed it would be in the best interest of FEP patients to expand telemental health services. The recognition of potential gains indicates a possible potential among stakeholders to reconsider traditional models of care and leverage technology in order to increase access to care. Besides, successful implementation of such hybrid models also involves recasting existing organizational structures of resources and processes in the bid to enhance their accessibility and efficiency. With populations continuing to struggle to make sense of the complexity of the delivery of health services, ongoing assessment of actualized health needs will be crucial in informing adaptive and responsive healthcare interventions.

3.1.2. Informing Public Health Policy

In addition to informing public health policy, comprehensive community health assessments significantly contribute, and the identification and solving of key health problems are amongst them. By bringing in both quantitative and qualitative data, the public health professionals will be capable of determining the health disparities and unmet need of the population. One such example would be measuring childhood obesity in Kentucky that brought to light a dire public health problem affecting a significant proportion of children and adolescents. The research synthesized data from multiple sources, including the Centers for Disease Control and Prevention (CDC), and engaged community members to examine systemic hindrances to healthy behavior. Through embracing evidence-based interventions—such as school and family-centered programs—public health policy can be tailored to work effectively against obesity, improve health outcomes, and promote fairness of access to health in the community (Hasan et al., 2025). In addition to child overweight, maternal and child health (MCH) greater issues on which there is meaningful policy change can be founded are presented by community health assessments with meaningful data.

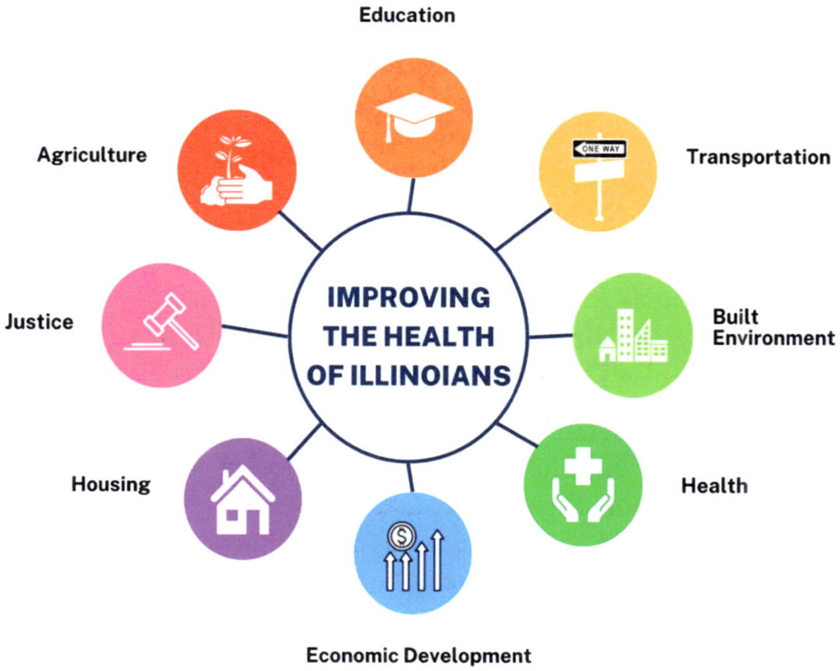

Figure 3.4. Informing public health policy.

Source: https://publichealth.uic.edu/wp-content/uploads/sites/302/2023/06/health-in-all-policies-framework.png.

A CHNA in Pakistan found dramatic rates of child malnourishment and maternal anemia that pointed to the need for critical action. The above systematic research design, for example, collection of socio-demographic data and health needs assessment of mothers and children, formed the foundation of identifying social determinants of health. However, the findings support a pressing need for community interventions in rural areas, including improved maternity care and more family planning services. Therefore, the establishment of specialized health centers can be one of the most important policy recommendations that are aimed at targeting known states of health and encouraging partnerships with the community for increased public health levels (Zakar et al., 2025). Lastly, integrating community health surveys into policy-making ensures interventions are sensitive to the needs and issues of the people. The policymakers must recognize the importance of ongoing working relationships with stakeholders at the local level in order that the programs may be provided effectively and ongoing engagement in health activities is guaranteed. Partnership-building ensures public health policies are enriched by various perspectives that make them more useful and efficient. Best practices from successful models, such as those built in Kentucky and Pakistan, highlight the value of contextualizing global solutions to suit regional realities. This two-pronged approach—taking account of local patterns of health and evidence-based worldwide best practice—gives communities the ability to develop health policy that is not just evidence-based but also specifically aimed at their own unique health issues and cultural backgrounds (Figure 3.4).

3.1.3. Engaging Community Stakeholders

Community stakeholder engagement is a key component of conducting a thorough community health assessment. Stakeholders also constitute a broad range of individuals and organizations such as healthcare providers, government officials at the local level, special interest groups, and citizens who possess individual understanding of the health resources and needs in the community. Through establishing relationships with stakeholders, healthcare providers are in a position to gain beneficial information that emanates from the priority and requirements of the community. Such collaboration not only enhances the validity of the survey but also creates openness and trust among the stakeholders by ensuring that their voices are heard and given weight. Additionally, as illustrated in the National School Climate Center's work, effective stakeholder collaboration forms the basis for having sustainable change in health and wellness programs that ultimately contribute to an environment shared and that promotes good health outcomes (Dary et al., 2013).

Applicability for community health needs assessments requires the use of outreach methods that are appealing to numerous stakeholders. The utilization of focus groups or forums for the community is, for instance, a method by which stakeholders are given the opportunity to discuss important health issues, share experiences, and aid in data collection processes. Efforts at outreach, specifically to defined groups, can also significantly boost participation rates among historically marginalized communities. As has been shown through the Enroll Americas model of mobilizing neighborhood volunteers and accessing neighborhood resources, careful communication and outreach lead to greater awareness of the health services and programs provided within the community (Orfield et al., 2014). Through this method, stakeholder involvement becomes a two-way conversation which not only enhances the assessment but also generates a sense of shared responsibility towards the health of the population. In addition, engaging stakeholders is crucial in developing useful health strategies and policies in eliminating the root causes of health inequalities. By including community members in the decision-making process and by giving their view top priority, health agencies are forced to design programs that answer back and are attuned to the community's unique needs. This inclusive process engenders sustained stakeholder participation, instilling a sense of duty to foster health activities beyond the project's end. By experiencing the concrete impact of what they do, stakeholder engagement is most likely to be converted into partnership, allowing prolonged dialogue and collaboration towards improved health. Long-term community stakeholder participation therefore not only strengthens the evaluation process but also improves overall community health infrastructure (Dary et al., 2013) (Figure 3.5).

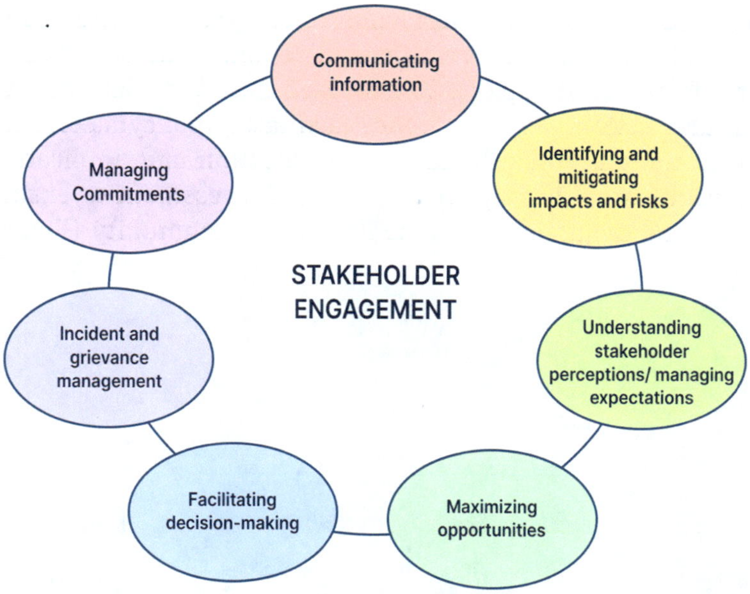

Figure 3.5. Engaging community stakeholders.

Source: https://creately.com/static/assets/guides/stakeholder-engagement/Stakeholder-Engagement.png.

3.2. Methods of Data Collection

Methods of gathering data in community health assessment are key in deciding whether the assessment was successful or if the results are valid. A mix of methods guarantees that what is gathered is reflective of the complexity of community health requirements. Surveys, interviews, focus groups, and observational studies are typical methods of data collection. For instance, questionnaires can be sent to a wide sample of the population to gather quantitative data, while interviews and focus groups provide qualitative data about members' experience and perceptions of community health. Observational studies reinforce understanding by reporting real-time behavior and environmental determinants on health. This multi-pronged approach enables health professionals to paint a clear picture of the community health situation, informing evidence-based interventions and resource planning. In addition, specific techniques can be adapted to suit specific community environments to render the data collected more pertinent. For example, combining laboratory analysis with questionnaires in certain community health screenings enables one to research health issues more intensively, particularly in epidemiological studies. In their research, scholars have utilized combinations of qualitative and quantitative methods, for instance, in certain studies in which data were gathered from surveys, laboratory experiments, and field observation to establish biogas technology uptake, stressing the importance of diversified methods in obtaining vast knowledge of the activities of communities and health effects (Tarimo et al., 2024). This flexibility in approaches is reflective of the need for community assessments to be dynamic and adaptive, to meet the specific nature and needs of various populations. In addition, the selection of data gathering methods may substantially shape the collective findings and their relevance to community health programs. For instance, regional health service financial performance analysis, as conducted by the study of Siti Fatimah Hospital, utilized interviews, observation, and document data collection methods to obtain relevant financial data (Parita et al., 2024). The focused nature of data collection guarantees not only valid findings but also actionable ones, hence facilitating policymakers to embrace evidence-based interventions in community health. Lastly, the selection and application of data collection methods must be congruent with the objectives of health assessment to ensure data is reliable as well as representative of the dynamics of the health of the community (Figure 3.6).

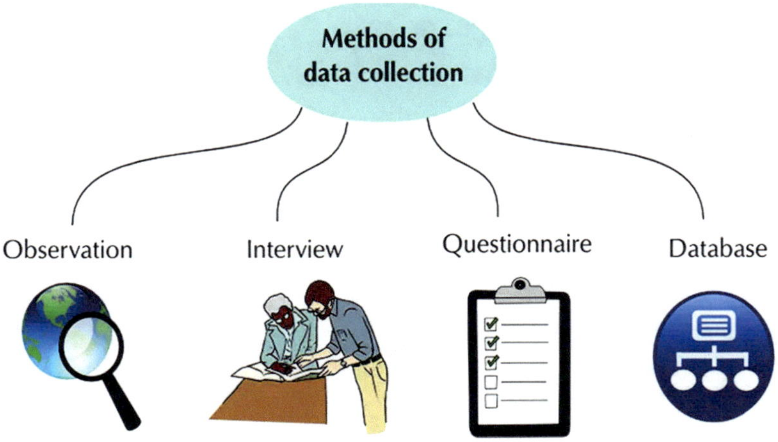

Figure 3.6. Methods of data collection.

Source: https://image-static.collegedunia.com/public/image/7ff4c6b3d0510e38255cfe97bb8c63f2.png.

3.2.1. Surveys and Questionnaires

Surveys and questionnaires are simple tools applied during community health assessment, offering a systematic approach to gathering useful information regarding corresponding perceptions, actions, and needs in populations. Through the structuring of such tools, researchers can obtain quantitative as well as qualitative data collection, contributing to a comprehensive understanding of the dynamics of community health. For instance, employing a Self-Assessment Survey (SAS), as has been done in the farmers-centric study, enables us to gain faint evidence on various dimensions of occupational health such as the severity of work environment factors and health habits. Such evidence is crucial to detect gaps in service delivery and comprehend the distinct requirements of various portions of the population, thereby rendering health interventions that are targeted. The success of surveys relies on their development and on the clarity of questions, which ultimately determines participation rates and accuracy of resultant data. The role of online platforms in enhancing the success of surveys and questionnaires is increasingly apparent in community health measurements. Recent studies have indicated that the application of a data management platform can significantly improve response rates and completion times for mental health screening, e.g., from 45%–71% after adopting an online measurement data management platform (OMDMP) by a sexual assault crisis center. This shift to electronic methods not only streamlines data gathering processes but also addresses the demands of the time for real-time data collection effectively, especially during challenging periods like the COVID-19 pandemic. Additionally, the use of technology in surveys provides respondents with a more comfortable method of participating, thereby increasing levels of engagement and improving the quality of gathered data, which is critical for enlightened decision-making in public health. Despite the benefits of questionnaires and surveys in community health assessments, numerous challenges exist that may dilute their effects. In the case of farmers' occupational health needs assessment, the key concerns generally include poor response rate, data collection biases, and misinterpretation of survey questions. Secondly, while technology has the ability to increase participation, digital disparities and literacy problems can create representational gaps in certain groups of the population. It is therefore important for community health practitioners to be cognizant of these challenges and use interventions that promote greater inclusivity in data collection. Continuous training and support for respondents can also increase data reliability, as can be seen in the farmer study results, where addressing knowledge gaps led to enhanced health outcomes. By recognizing these challenges, community health assessment projects can be more robust and effective (Figure 3.7).

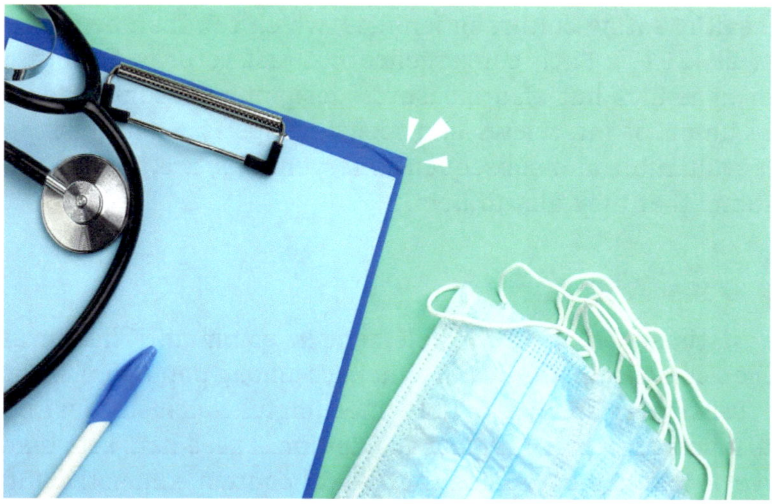

Figure 3.7. Surveys and questionnaires.

Source: https://external-content.duckduckgo.com/iu/?u=https%3A%2F%2Ffile.forms.app%2Fsitefile%2F20-Amazing-health-survey-questions-for-questionnaires.jpg&f=1&nofb=1&ipt=1cbe7a4fc08eb20e9c7fc22369ba1dcb1720ea173ee6afb07f78c427c23e2f84.

3.2.2. Focus Groups and Interviews

Effective community health evaluation then relies on the application of qualitative methods such as focus groups and interviews to produce deep information from representative members of various communities. Group discussions through focus groups enable researchers to probe for common experiences and perceptions about health issues. Not only do group discussions elicit common health concerns of communities, but they also reveal what dissuades health interventions. For instance, in addressing childhood obesity, focus groups can uncover parent attitudes and lack of knowledge regarding nutrition and exercise that need to be tackled when designing interventions targeted at them. Through this process of tapping key informants, researchers learn about available local resources and needs and ensure that health programs are within the context and accessible. This is particularly apt in groups with specific social structures, as it allows for the adaptation of health messages and interventions based on community-specific features. Interviews also complement focus groups as a venue through which to comprehensively explore personal experiences and the perceptions of experts. Stakeholder qualitative interviews from such stakeholders as health workers and community leaders can provide insight into issues and possibilities within the healthcare environment. For example, in a childhood obesity community readiness assessment study, semi-structured key informant interviews provided essential information on what the community is aware of regarding the health issues and resources (Cameron et al., 2013). Thematic analysis of the interviews guides researchers on how to rank intervention steps, showing where the maximum perceived need lies. This strategy not only enriches the database but also builds a more solid relationship between community residents and researchers, with greater trust and collaboration for future health projects. Blending a mixed-methods approach, where focus groups and interviews are utilized together, strengthens community health surveys. This strategy allows for triangulation of data, where findings from one method can support and provide background to findings from another. For instance, feedback from families through focus group might show an underdeveloped healthy eating culture in families, which can then be further explored through interviews (Brook et al., 2017). Such convergence not just records an improved understanding of community health dynamics but also measures designing person-centered health promotion programs. Lastly, the union of interviews and focus groups is what gives power to community voices so that health evaluation, and subsequent interventions, are grounded on actual needs and wants of the populations that they aim to help.

3.2.3. Secondary Data Analysis

Secondary data analysis is still a significant element in community health assessment where it supports the comprehension of complex health dynamics among populations. Through the utilization of existing data sets, researchers are able to draw meaningful conclusions without the considerable resource investments involved in primary data acquisition. These data sets tend to incorporate key statistics, health surveys, and demographic reports that contain exhaustive information regarding conditions of the community. The ability to conduct cross-population comparative analysis facilitates nuanced understanding of health disparities since it is possible to analyze social determinants such as gender and wealth, and their impact on school enrollment as well as levels of achievement in various communities. This not only extends the range of investigation but also allows for the detection of specific interventions against established health inequities, thus fostering healthier communities (Filmer et al., 2025). Moreover, secondary data analysis makes it possible to study longitudinal relationships and trends that are impossible through primary studies. With the help of existing data, researchers can analyze past health trends, track over time trends, and assess the effects of public health interventions. This is particularly relevant in the context of chronic disease, where long-term information is required for understanding progression of disease and of factors influencing health outcomes. For instance, in a study among older adults, researchers learned that preclinical disability was a significant predictor of falls based on data collected by longitudinal studies covering greater than one geographic region (Beck et al., 2017). These findings highlight the worth of secondary data in informing effective public health policies that engage at-risk groups. Secondary data use also responds to the ethical aspect of the research by lessening participant burden but enhancing the utility of existing information. Populations are likely to face challenges with healthcare evaluation since they lack resources, which can be counterproductive to conducting massive-scale primary research. By employing secondary data analysis, these shortcomings can be rectified by researchers so that there is a more holistic approach to health need determination and prioritization of resources. In addition, integrating numerous datasets can reveal hidden patterns and relationships in order to inform good community health policy. Finally, secondary data analysis is not merely a methodology but also an adaptive strategy for enhancing community health assessments in order to make them evidence-based and attuned to the populations they are trying to serve (Figure 3.8).

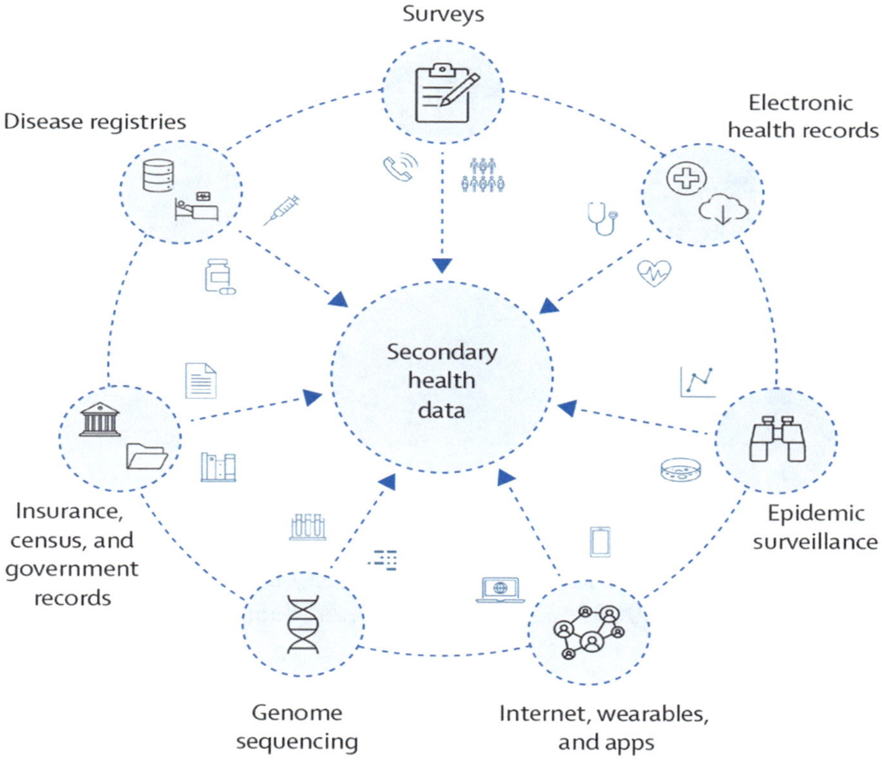

Figure 3.8. Secondary data analysis.

Source: https://www.thelancet.com/cms/asset/6f5be09b-acdc-48e6-a037-133a4876ef48/gr1.jpg.

3.3. Key Indicators of Community Health

A full understanding of community health relies on establishing the key indicators that reflect general population well-being. These indicators are usually dimensions pertaining to health status, access to healthcare, and socio-economic status. Indicators of health status include occurrences of diseases, mental health evaluations, and mortality rates, which are key measures used in assessing the performance of a specified community. Healthcare availability, one of the crucial elements quantifies availability of services, insurance coverage, and hindrances residents encounter while accessing care. Besides, socio-economic indicators, such as employment status and educational levels, can significantly influence both health status and availability of services.

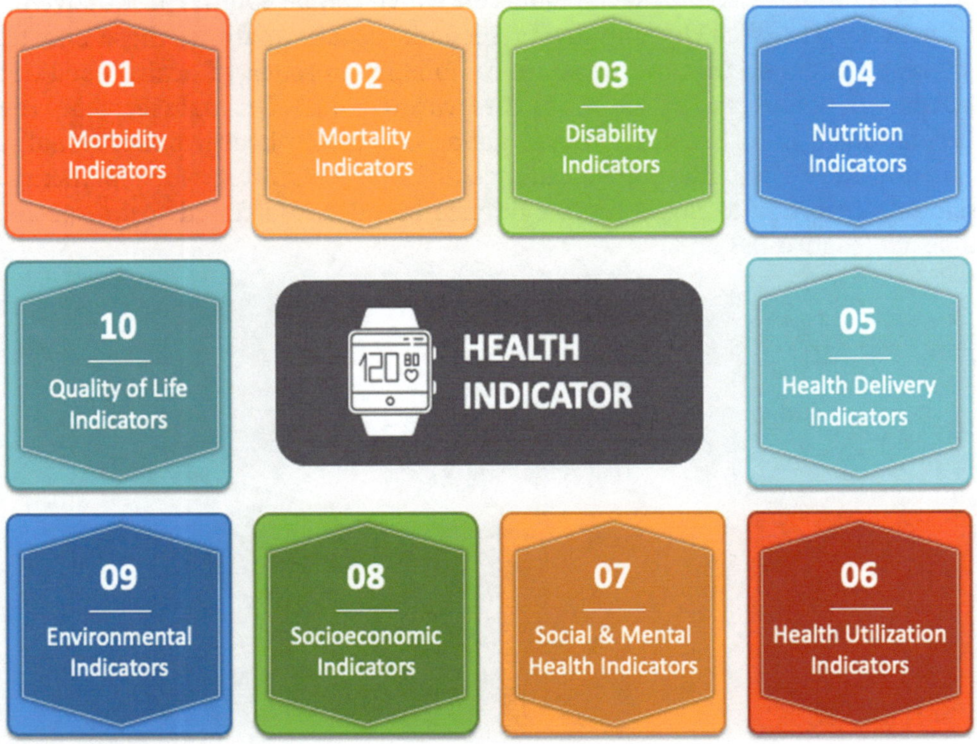

Figure 3.9. Key indicators of community health.

Source: https://www.collidu.com/media/catalog/product/img/d/9/d9364d94b79b494d8e53e24f13e0095a2a17554048114aa88e5a04ffb7d8c951/health-indicators-slide1.png.

By careful analysis of these factors, stakeholders can improve the tailoring of interventions and resources to address special needs, and consequently enhance the overall health of the community. A key component of evaluating community health is the consideration of environmental factors that contribute to the well-being of people who inhabit it. Sustainable processes within the agrifood value chains (AVCs) have the capability of significantly influencing community health by affecting local economies and ecosystems. For example, connection with AVCs in the local community can provide job opportunities, resulting in improved income and social equity. On Reunion Island, research demonstrated the ways in which participatory methods enabled stakeholders to measure and diagnose the environmental effects of poultry AVC activities, evidence that showed the importance of local resources in ensuring the health of ecosystems (Acosta et al., 2019). Such observations provide insights into ecological-socio-economic trade-offs in terms of health, pointing to the complex interaction that exists. Hence, the interpretation of such indicators makes communities adopt not only public health-improving measures but also sustainability measures. Additionally, subjective well-being measures like empowerment and community integration are deserving of attention as factors indicating importance in health research. Empirical research indicates that individuals who have more empowerment levels report better recovery and participation rates within communities (King et al., 2010). This correlation suggests the importance of allowing community members to engage in substantial social, economic, and health-related activities. For instance, employed individuals with serious mental illnesses are likely not only to have improved financial well-being but also increased empowerment and social integration. As these subjective indicators receive increasing attention, they offer important reflections on the health and resilience of populations as a whole. Therefore, a multi-dimensional approach incorporating both objective and subjective indicators is crucial in order to conduct effective community health assessment (Figure 3.9).

3.3.1. Morbidity and Mortality Rates

One of the most important components of evaluating community health is the analysis of morbidity and mortality rates, which show very significant information about the health status of populations. Morbidity rates quantify the occurrence of disease within a population and the effectiveness of public health interventions in both disease loads as well as relief of disease. Mortality rates, in contrast, highlight the deaths that occur within a population and are a blunt measure of overall health outcomes. Increased morbidity and mortality rates in particular groups often signal underlying determinants of health, such as poverty, access to care, and environmental exposures. Health professionals are able to use the rates to identify high-risk communities, which in turn guides resource allocation and policy-making targeted at reducing disparities and improving the health of diverse populations. Furthermore, the interplay between environmental exposures and health outcomes is decisive in affecting morbidity and mortality. Environment-based policymaking with evidence from research on environmental health helps address these disparities. Urban dwellers, for instance, and particularly those with reduced socioeconomic status and ethnic minority concentration, are more susceptible to negative environmental exposures, such as air pollution. This relationship has shaped the environmental justice movement, which has demanded fair access to a cleaner environment. Interventions to reduce environmental harms can lead to improved health statistics among these underprivileged groups, as noted by the outcomes of the American Lung Association workshop on Urban Air Pollution and Health Inequities, which stressed targeted research and community-based interventions (American Lung Association, 2001). Hence, the recognition and response to the relationships between environmental determinants and health will go a long way in lowering morbidity and mortality rates among affected populations. In addition, certain demographic groups, the elderly being the most prominent one, pose specific challenges in controlling morbidity and mortality rates. Because cancer occurrences rise with increasing age, the value of thorough pre-surgical geriatric evaluations becomes clear. These assessments can stratify risk and optimize care for elderly patients, who experience excess morbidity and mortality secondary to comorbid disease and frailty. Utilization of these assessments remains suboptimal, however, largely secondary to time limitations in healthcare systems. Nevertheless, studies indicate that targeted interventions, for instance, medical staff education on the most predictive regions of geriatric screenings, can enhance quality of care for this group (Lampugnane et al., 2017). Targeting such programs, the healthcare sector can be able to advance overall treatment outcomes, thus reducing morbidity and mortality rates among the elderly, thus positively contributing to public health.

3.3.2. Access to Healthcare Services

A critical community health survey brings to the fore the general issue of access to health care services, a matter that still remains a core determiner of health outcomes. For the majority, access obstacles come in many different forms, from geographical, economic, to sociocultural barriers. For instance, communities located in rural areas tend to have monumental barriers in accessing health care facilities, creating drastic health outcome inequalities relative to their urban counterparts. The research on Primary Health Centers (PHCs) with a spatial and statistical examination suggests that patients' access to PHCs directly influences healthcare uptake rates among communities. Enhanced availability of PHCs is important not only for increasing utilization of health services but also for fostering equitable health outcomes among various populations. With the continued inequalities in access to healthcare, policymakers are forced to focus on enhancing infrastructure and reducing economic constraints so that quality healthcare is accessible to all members of society (Vinothini et al., 2025). The COVID-19 pandemic has further opened up existing gaps in access to healthcare even further, highlighting the necessity to understand the evolving nature of health services. As witnessed during this worldwide crisis, numerous people were subject to increased barriers such as limitations in time and information about existing healthcare resources. The application of Food is Medicine (FIM) initiatives, which offer healthy food as a way of enhancing health outcomes, was interrupted, highlighting the connection between food security and access to healthcare. Surveys of Federally Qualified Health Centers (FQHCs) clients revealed significant changes in healthcare accessibility, where the majority of them confirmed that it is becoming more challenging and costly to access care.

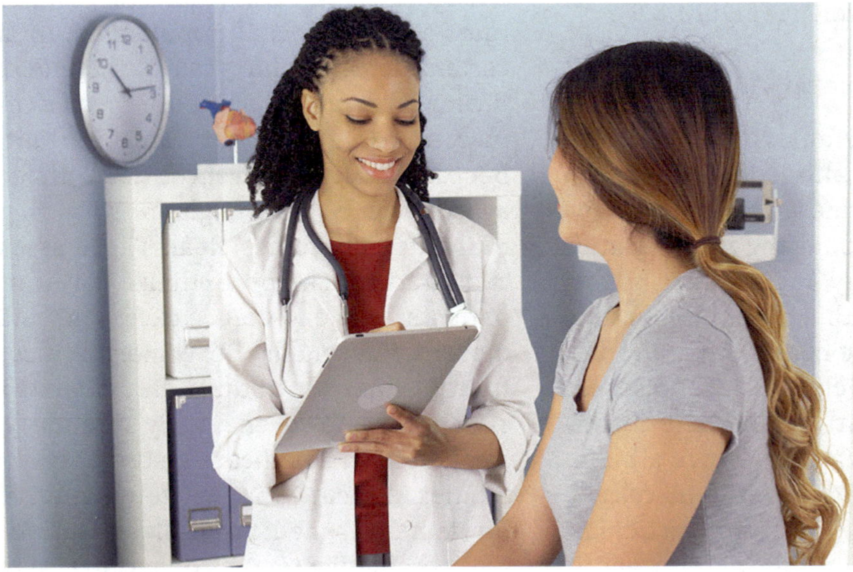

Figure 3.10. Access to healthcare services.

Source: https://www.ruralhealthinfo.org/assets/2632-9901/healthcare-access-fb.jpg.

These findings emphasize the critical imperative for community resilience through having resilient health programs that can stay strong and face future shocks while maintaining continued access to essential services (Franco et al., 2024). Addressing health care access as part of a community health assessment needs a multi-dimensional approach that takes into account both the health care infrastructure as well as social determinants of health. Economic stability, education, and community awareness can have an amazing effect on people's capacity to seek out and access care. Effective public health intervention should take on building increased community awareness of what resources are available as well as enhancing knowledge of health care navigation. Closing these gaps through bridging interventions is essential to promote health equity and improve collective population health. In prioritizing improving the delivery and affordability of healthcare, communities can move towards a more equitable healthcare system that prioritizes everyone's needs, particularly marginalized groups who are disproportionately impacted by access disparities. This consolidated approach can provide more just health outcomes as well as a more just health care setting (Vinothini et al., 2025) (Figure 3.10).

3.3.3. Socioeconomic Factors

Socioeconomic factors play a core role in shaping community health outcomes, across an expansive range of determinants including income, education, and employment status. Individuals from lower socioeconomic backgrounds are more likely to experience increased morbidity and mortality, usually due to limited access to healthcare and amenities. Poor education is among the determinants that may hamper the understanding of health-related information, leading to poor health literacy. This lack of knowledge tends to enhance health disparities, as individuals will fail to apply preventive measures or seek medical care in a timely manner. Moreover, socioeconomic status also affects lifestyle, such that economically disadvantaged groups trust less healthy sources of food and become less active, exacerbating conditions like obesity and heart disease. All these determinants must be comprehended in the case of effective community health assessments so that stakeholders are able to target interventions at overcoming specific socioeconomic barriers in the delivery of health care. Furthermore, integrating socioeconomic determinants in community health assessment has to be met with a multi-dimensional strategy appropriate to the unique conditions of every community. Marine Managed Areas (MMAs) are a good case in point; they strive to enhance ecological health, in addition to the socioeconomic determinants. Research has indicated that the success of MMAs relies significantly on local systems of governance and community involvement, which tend to be determined by socioeconomic conditions. Assessing these projects from a range of perspectives, including socioeconomic impacts, helps with the understanding of broader implications for well-being in communities. The inter-action between governance and socioeconomic processes evokes inclusive planning processes with the involvement of local communities such that their needs and views are incorporated in the decision-making process. This inter-action fosters ownership feelings and improved health outcomes through matching policies with community health priorities (Shank et al., 2010). Within indigenous populated communities, the interrelation of environment, culture, and socioeconomic factors is particularly complex. Native cultures have historically had eco-cultural systems that are closely integrated with human existence and the environment, and that include an integrated understanding of health. Socioeconomic disparities typically threaten such systems' viability, however, which subsequently exacts a cost on health. For instance, compounded environmental stressors combined with limited economic opportunity access impact health effects for these groups adversely. The specific difficulties these groups experience highlight the importance of culturally guided evaluations that recognize the compounded impacts on trust resources and customary ways of living. Implementing equity strategies that consider the intersection of culture health, and socioeconomic status is essential to creating effective interventions that appreciate and integrate indigenous knowledge systems (Harper et al., 1999). Addressing these factors in a holistic manner addresses the community's general resilience and health equity, which results in healthier and sustainable environments.

3.4. Community Engagement Strategies

Community engagement strategies are critical to increasing the effectiveness of community health assessments by creating genuine collaboration between health practitioners and community members. Such strategies are based on grasping the specific needs, perspectives, and dynamics within different communities, especially marginalized communities. One approach is the use of lay health workers (LHWs) who, because they are located within the communities and thus have local knowledge, can assist with bridging the gaps between community life and the evidence base.

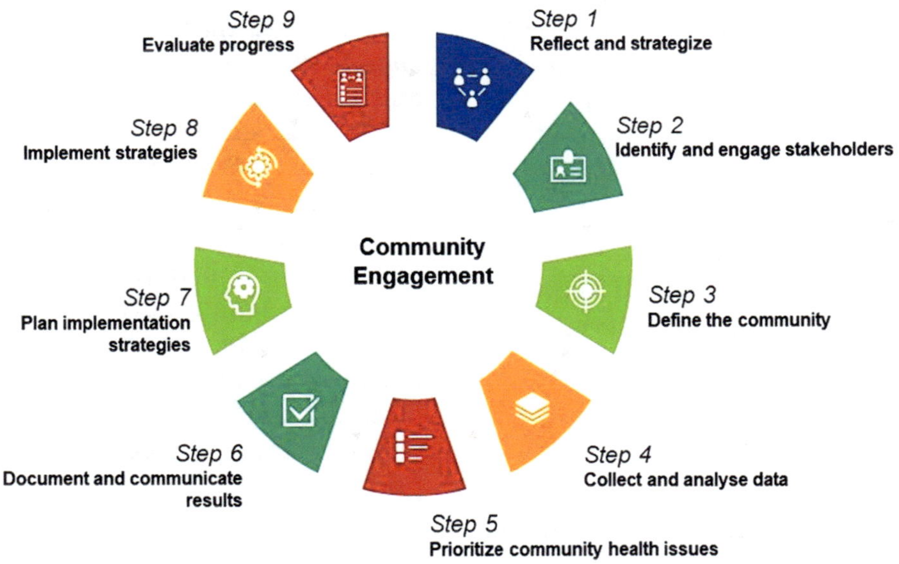

Figure 3.11. Community engagement strategies.

Source: https://www.slideteam.net/media/catalog/product/cache/960x720/9/_/9_step_model_of_community_engagement_slide01.jpg.

Mobilization of LHWs, for instance, has been shown to increase Latinx parents' involvement in behavioral parent training programs that are central to intervention for early-onset conduct problems and child maltreatment. Such community-based initiatives not only extend coverage for key health care but also allow evidence-based practice to be effectively utilized in regular settings, ultimately benefiting individual families along with society in general (Barnett et al.,

2019). Moreover, the necessity of involvement by the youth community in planning community health cannot be overstressed given that their unique voices normally fall on less attentive ears in traditional approaches.

Active engagement of youth is useful in making more comprehensive assessments and to ensure that health priorities are within the true needs of youth. Evidence indicates that although only 20% of Massachusetts Community Health Needs Assessments (CHNAs) actively engaged youths, a vast majority listed youth-specific health concerns as priorities. This gap indicates a fertile field for growth, as engaging with youth can illuminate important social determinants of health and raise their voice in decision-making about young people's health. Utilizing participatory resources such as focus groups and participatory photo mapping can encourage effective youth engagement, providing greater holistic insight into the context of communities and enabling more nuanced understanding of the concerns regarding the health of young people (Chen et al., 2017). By incorporating robust community participation strategies, there is a more responsive and just health assessment environment. When youth and other citizens are invited to the table, they can inform with insights and recommendations that more directly reflect their experiences. For example, the outcomes of youth engagement activities usually reveal nuanced health and community states that are not always captured by traditional measures, providing avenues for targeted interventions. In a bid by health agencies to develop effective community health improvement strategies, tapping into local knowledge through strategic engagement not only enhances the feasibility of health initiatives but also establishes trust and ownership among the population. By prioritizing these engagement strategies, health evaluations can more effectively match interventions with community needs to espouse a dynamic, inclusive model ultimately leading to improved health outcomes (Barnett et al., 2019; Chen et al., 2017) (Figure 3.11).

3.4.1. Building Trust with Community Members

The most important aspect of successful community health evaluations is the establishment of trust between health workers and community members. Establishing trust is not an added-on element but a fundamental requirement to effective health interventions. As seen from many studies, including those investigating the underserved, trust can play an important role in influencing people willingness to engage in health programs. The absence of knowledge regarding existing healthcare resources illustrates an open gap that can be filled through regular community interaction and outreach activities. Population-based programs are likely to increase participation rates and overall health outcomes since they foster a setting where the population is understood and valued. Lacking trust, efforts to improve the health of communities will be impeded, and unmet needs will be present, and populations will continue to be underserved, with the importance of trust in health advocacy being demonstrated (Ali et al., 2016). Effective communication is necessary in order to build this trust among the community. Transparent communication techniques let the choices be understood and what are the benefits of being included in health programs. Employing means such as participatory action research (PAR), where the residents of the community are directly involved in planning and implementing health programs, produces a sense of belongingness and empowerment. In Bangladesh, for instance, the "self-help for health" program effectively leveraged existing community systems to improve health literacy and participation (Ahmad et al., 2016). Such collaborative systems not only raise awareness among community members regarding available services but also motivate them to share experiences and suggestions. As such, communication is a co-creation tool to enable the health professionals to adapt their approach based on the individual needs and preferences of the community, further establishing trust.

The success of health projects, in the majority of cases, is contingent on establishing and constantly building the trust in the community. If the health professionals fail to persist in following up or respond appropriately to the initially given priority needs, the trust could be damaged. Regular contact, education, and capacity development are required to maintain such trust and indicate a commitment to community well-being. Such programs with built-in mechanisms of regular feedback have the ability to significantly enhance health indicators, such as programs that engaged community members in decision-making (Ahmad et al., 2016). By identifying community capacities and involving participatory approaches, health assessments can effectively address health disparities. Lastly, building and sustaining trust is not only beneficial for individual health outcomes but is also necessary in creating stable and empowered communities capable of negotiating their health needs.

3.4.2. Collaborating with Local Organizations

Collaboration with local organizations is fundamental in supporting community health assessments and follow-up interventions. Collaborating with local organizations has the advantage of ensuring that the unique needs and cultural understanding of various populations are addressed appropriately. For instance, community-based organizations generally have established trust within the community, which can significantly increase participation in health screenings and outreach activities.

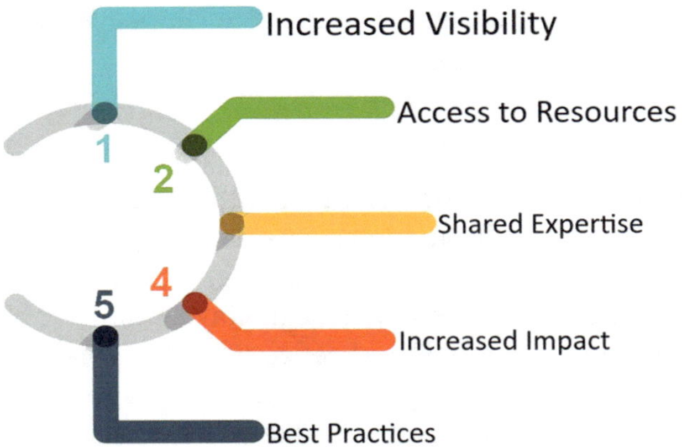

Figure 3.12. Collaborating with local organizations.

Source: https://fastercapital.co/i/Loan-Committee-Success-Stories--Celebrating-Positive-Outcomes-in-Lending--Collaborating-with-Local-Organizations.webp.

By drawing upon such relationships, community health assessors are better able to obtain more trustworthy information and establish an atmosphere conducive to health gain. Such partnerships not only enhance data collection activities but also set the platform for healthier amplification of the voice of marginalized individuals, resulting in greater knowledge about health disparities caused by ethnicity and race. Ultimately, healthier collaboration can be decisive in developing targeted interventions in health that are relevant to culture and are effective. The existence of health disparities among racial and ethnic minorities also requires the collaboration of health assessors with community-based organizations.

As proposed, despite controlling for variables such as income and insurance, they receive inferior care, the necessity for targeted initiatives thus highlighted. Collaborations with organizations catering to these groups can lead to the development of tailored programs meant to address specific health requirements, including access to quality care and health education. The Colorado Trusts Equality in Health Initiative is one good example of how such collaborations increase local organizations' cultural competency, hence their effectiveness in outreach to reduce health disparities (Lee et al., 2012)). This creates a feedback mechanism where the organizations modify practices based on community engagement, leading to enhanced health outcomes for underprivileged populations. Further, the effectiveness of such collaborations is also increased when organizations come together for shared agendas, particularly advocacy for policy change and quality service delivery. Some of the recent initiatives led by foundations and government institutions have actually brought together numerous partners and created harmony plans for health improvement. Collaborations target evidence-based approaches that guide practices and policies (Farley et al., 2012). Through sharing resources, information, and skills, local institutions can launch evidence-based programs that address not only immediate health problems but also advance long-term systemic change. This collaborative effort optimizes the sustainability of interventions within the health field by ensuring that programs are regularly monitored and improved to meet evolving community needs. Through this process, collaboration is an imperative model of addressing the complex interrelated problems characterizing the contemporary public health landscape (Figure 3.12).

3.4.3. Utilizing Social Media for Outreach

Social media has become a valuable tool for community health assessment as a key tool for mobilization and outreach. These websites, characterized by their widespread reach and accessibility, enable the release of information, facilitate social interaction, and support health promotion. By utilizing social media, health organizations can connect with diverse populations, specifically targeting underrepresented communities, thereby amplifying their voices in health discussions. Furthermore, the interactive nature of these platforms enables real-time feedback, allowing organizations to tailor their messages according to community needs. This dynamic relationship is more so in addressing public health concerns where data in real time can significantly influence community attitudes and actions towards health behaviors and, subsequently, help improve the success of health interventions. The COVID-19 pandemic demonstrated how social media was used as a vehicle for health information and community engagement. In this historic moment, digital platforms became stars for health communications, sharing real-time information and guidance on prevention, vaccination, and mental health services. Social media's ability to offer scalable interventions is particularly well-tailored in mental health environments, as individuals increasingly seek help online. As (Torous et al., 2021) highlights, mobile mental health technologies have been identified as having the potential to facilitate remote interventions. Social media not only serves to disseminate educational content but also to facilitate networks among community members. Thus, agencies engaging these platforms are able to promote greater awareness of services and resources, leading to improved outcomes in the health of populations. Nevertheless, the use of social media for outreach also poses challenges, such as vulnerability to misinformation and unequal access to technology. The digital divide is a big challenge, and the underprivileged groups typically face challenges that disqualify them from engaging on these platforms. Therefore, one has to engage with social media in a critical frame of reference that confronts these inequalities, as highlighted by Brewer et al., (2019). The interventions must be designed for specific individuals by recognizing their own contexts and needs. Successful outreach practices should thus set the greatest priority on community engagement to ensure content is relevant and available to all. Through direct engagement of the community in planning and implementing social media campaigns, health organizations can improve the targeting of disparities and promoting equitable health results, reinforcing the importance of digital public health practices being inclusive.

3.5. Challenges in Conducting Assessments

Conducting community health assessments has numerous challenges that can contribute significantly to the impact and quality of the evaluation process. One of the main challenges is that there are numerous health disparities in populations, which are aggravated by socioeconomic determinants that complicate data collection. Precisely recognizing and responding to these imbalances demands a thorough comprehension of community trends, which may differ significantly among disparate geographic and demographic groups. For instance, findings of a recent CHNA revealed that there existed an immediate need to address issues such as addiction and mental illness in some populations served by a regional burn center, illustrating how critical it is to design assessments that are sensitive to the unique needs and experiences of community members (White et al., 2025). Thus, thorough engagement of the population is required but can also prove to be difficult to achieve within a limited timeline. One of the other big challenges in making the assessments is data collection and analysis methods. Proper assessments must involve quantitative as well as qualitative data to develop a holistic view of community health. Application of diverse sources such as interviews, surveys, and accessible healthcare use data presents unique challenges in terms of getting participants to respond and eliciting credible responses. The recent CHNA attempted to integrate information from varied sources to determine priority health issues, but it necessitates methodological rigor to avoid potential biases that could arise from artificial bias in participant selection or response systems (White et al., 2025). Also, the achievement of appropriate representation of the community's health issues may be impeded by such barriers as literacy limitations, distrust in healthcare systems, or logistical challenges in reaching certain groups. Lastly, the need for interdisciplinary collaboration in carrying out the assessment may enhance and complicate the process. Engaging experts from various fields ensures that there is a broader perspective in considering challenges in community health; actionable objectives and priorities may, however, be conflicting and thereby give rise to tension and non-uniformity in action planning and data interpretation. Furthermore, inconsistencies in knowledge and practice by community health officers, as identified by a recent report, may reinforce disparities across appreciating critical health concerns like non-communicable diseases. This highlights the importance of training and education programs that enhance the capability of the people conducting health assessments. When community health assessments are conducted without the benefit of an objective framework that includes standardized training, the generated data may not be actionable, and major health issues may be poorly addressed or may go off the radar entirely (Figure 3.13).

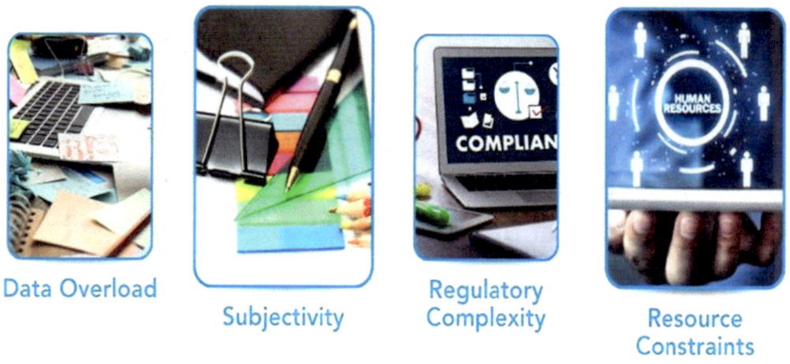

Figure 3.13. Challenges in conducting assessments.

Source: https://asterdocs.com/wp-content/uploads/2024/07/Challenges-of-risk-assessments.jpg.

3.5.1. Data Privacy and Ethical Considerations

At the time of conducting community health assessment, technology-based data collection often creates severe concerns about data privacy along with ethical concerns. As community health systems increasingly adopt mobile health technologies, the massive volume of behavior data captured by sensors and applications poses strong ethical standards for protecting people's rights. These technologies allow for constant tracking and personalized interventions, which can improve health significantly; however, they also carry risks of surveillance and data misuse. The outcome is that the development of guidelines to guarantee user consent and transparency in the management of data has become imperative.

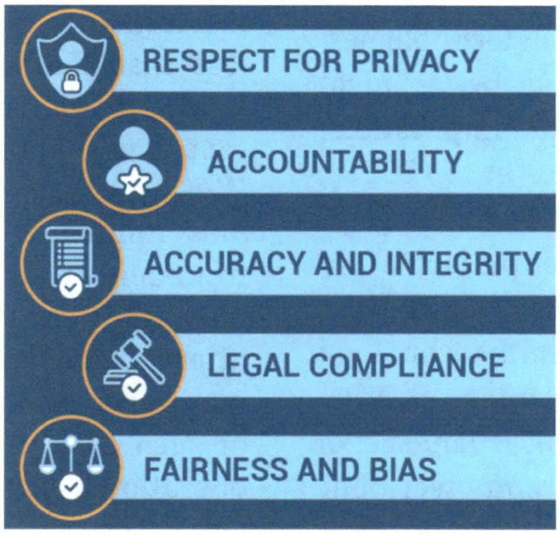

Figure 3.14. Data privacy and ethical considerations.

Source: https://www.quanthub.com/wp-content/uploads/Batch36_Image01-1-1024x538.png.

The ethical issues surrounding the compilation and utilization of health information underscore the importance of balancing policy to promote innovation with privacy protection at the individual level in community health assessment. Personal Health Monitoring (PHM) devices and software exemplify the manner in which the compilation of health data outside of the clinical environment has transformed the health assessment scenario. The use of such technologies creates serious ethical concerns, particularly related to privacy, autonomy, and the risk of stigmatization. It appears that PHM systems have a tendency to create a dualism where users are advantaged by enhanced monitoring of their health but, at the same time, might lose privacy and feel more anxious about being surveilled. Medicalization and social isolation themes found in addition bring more weight to the dynamic relationship between technology and individual identity within health environments. Through the analysis of the ethical aspects of PHM, it is clear that stakeholders have to factor in the possible effects of such devices on autonomy at the individual and societal levels, eventually leading to the ethical practice of health initiatives in populations (Mittelstadt et al., 2013). Furthermore, the intersection of ethics and health assessments in communities and technology usage requires constant interplay between influential stakeholders, such as healthcare professionals, technology innovators, and policymakers. While behavioral scientists develop further with mobile health technologies, thinking will need to shift beyond the technical feasibility to encompass the broader implications of their use in daily life (Nebeker et al., 2020). Developers are confronted with the challenge of creating systems that respect user privacy while exploiting data that enable public health action. Concurrently, the utilization of health technology must be policy-directed in a manner sensitive to the wide and interactive ethical landscape, especially that of consent and empowerment of users. Ultimately, creating an integrated strategy with ethics training for actors involved in rolling out health technologies is requisite for trust-building and upholding public health evaluations that are genuinely in the public good (Figure 3.14).

3.5.2. Resource Limitations

In community-level health assessment, restrictions of available resources are real hindrances that may undermine the effectiveness of health programs and interventions. One of the findings of the studies is that there exists a practice where evidence-based practices are restricted by available resources, most notably in community health centers. For instance, an adequate staff shortage is characterized in terms of available resources, namely levels of staffing, with a direct impact on the overall climate of learning and leadership engagement necessary to establish effective interventions (Lee et al., 2025). Correction of such resource deficits is essential as they have direct consequences for the availability of care and quality provided to disadvantaged groups and hence reinforce health inequalities in populations. Furthermore, economic evaluation of community-based health promotion (CBHP) interventions continues to reveal the intricacies of restrictions on resources. The majority of interventions targeting disadvantage groups fall short of being able to assess their economic elements because there exists no thorough cost examination. The instability of resource assessment—such that less than half of interventions quantify costs in depth—mirrors a degree of uncertainty that would make decision-making challenging (Weber et al., 2024). These limitations not only hinder evidence-informed interventions from being translated into operational systems but also constrain political acceptability interventions can realize, which is vital for long-term development. Finally, implications of such limitations extend beyond immediate operational issues to inform overall systemic processes that affect health equity. Traditional health economic evaluation procedures do not often allow for the complexity involved in CBHP interventions, such as intersectoral expenditures and the complexity of benefits they accrue to societies (Weber et al., 2024). The necessity for alternative innovative approaches, such as cost-consequence analysis (CCA), taking into consideration quantitative as well as qualitative findings, thereby enriching the evaluation process, becomes apparent. By reorganizing how we think of resource constraints in community health screening, stakeholders are well equipped to employ better techniques of harnessing the best use of health interventions and, as a result, better health outcomes among vulnerable populations.

3 5.3. Resistance from Community Members

Public resistance is a strong barrier to effective community health intervention and screening. Most of the resistance is created by perceived lack of transparency and credibility towards the intentions of health programs. When the public feels that programs are being imposed upon them without consent or consultation, suspicion of the health organizations' intent is created. Such suspicion could be invigorated with a history of previous injustice or bad experience of health systems. That is why community participation is the solution to breaking such resistance as it provides a collective platform where the voice of the people is heard and valued. The learning through such participatory platform not only makes interventions more acceptable but also guarantees that programs are suitable and desirable at a community level. Additionally, cultural disparities cannot be overemphasized while conducting research on resistance by the inhabitants of a population during the assessment process for health. Various populations have their own cultural practices and beliefs, and therefore misconceptions are sure to cause revulsion towards certain of the health interventions or tests. For instance, some practices can be not compatible with Western practice for health and cause mistrust or refusal to comply. Overcoming these cultural divides requires a reaction that has been modified to be responsive to difference and that includes local knowledge. With the use of strategies that reactivate different models of culture, health agencies can establish trust and enhance participation levels. As noted, the importance of developing the multicultural competency of health agencies, as proposed by Mayeno (2007), is paramount in achieving the effectiveness of community participation and eradicating resistance. The power of the effect of resistance by members of the community also has long-term effects on outcomes outside of direct health interventions, which affect longer-term public health outcomes. If populations resist participating in health surveys, valuable data may be lost, undermining the foundation of evidence-based interventions based on actual community intelligence. Resistance can even be found in public health program performance, especially in areas of WASH (Water, Sanitation, and Hygiene), such as was pointed out in N/A (2007). Setting the problems and obstacles of concern to the people of the community can lead to more effective policy and programming that addresses the real needs of the community. By incorporating the input of communities and solutions to their problems, health organizations can minimize resistance as well as create partnerships that build increased public trust and cooperation in future health efforts (Figure 3.15).

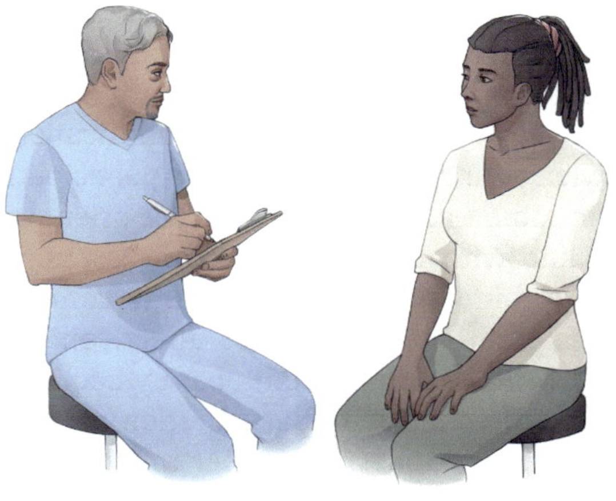

Figure 3.15. Resistance from community members.

Source: https://ecampusontario.pressbooks.pub/app/uploads/sites/455/2019/05/health-assessment.jpg.

3.6. Case Studies of Successful Assessments

With regards to case studies of successful assessment of community health, one of the most pertinent determinants is the understanding of the collaboration of partnerships whose aim is to enhance outcomes in health. One of the best examples of collaborative efforts, as described by Howarth et al., (2009), demonstrates the success of more than one institution combining efforts to combat challenges of community health. These partnerships support extensive data collection and analysis, which are a prerequisite for making rightful assessments of health needs. Through the engagement of different stakeholders like local institutions, universities, and community members, such programs establish a greater pool of knowledge and understanding that guides context-specific interventions. This partnership does not only improve the evaluation process, but ensures that solutions developed are culturally and contextually appropriate to the populations they will be serving. Quality assessments also have rigorous systems of evaluation that provide space for continuous feedback and improvement. The international experts' conference referred to in Campbell-Patton et al., (2009) emphasizes the significance of knowledge in relation to the civic participation role in community development. The orientation is in line with community health assessment to determine not just the health condition of communities but also the effectiveness of health promotion interventions. By sequential analysis of community participation activities, health assessments can determine the role of social determinants in influencing health outcomes. This style, thus, allows such health assessments to provide useful information that could inform policymakers and health experts to adjust interventions in an effort to make them more effective and pertinent to the target population. Finally, the conclusion derived from such case studies illustrates the importance of responsiveness and flexibility within health assessments. Successful programs realize that health needs of populations may evolve over time and, therefore, need the evaluation strategy to be dynamic. This is particularly so in longitudinal studies focused on engaging with communities at all times to monitor changes in health status and intervention outcomes. The partnership model introduced in Howarth et al., (2009) is a template for future evaluations that foster continuous dialogue between researchers and the community. Given that it is already established by the study in Campbell-Patton et al., (2009), including multiple perspectives in the evaluation process does not only enhance the data but also promotes participation and trust with communities and can lead to healthier and sustainable outcomes.

3.6.1. Example of a Local Health Initiative

A very good example of a local health program that has gained recognition under the hypothesis of community health evaluation is the development of food initiatives to promote greater access to fruit and vegetables in Health Action Zones (HAZs) in England. The developments were prompted by an acute sense of diet inequality and its relationship to public health outcomes. It was not just to improve the rate of diet nutritional intake among members of the population but also to treat underlying poverty and food access problems. The key informant interviews stressed that most of these programs focus on skill building, i.e., teaching people how to cook, which equips a person with information that they require in order to eat more healthful foods. Besides, integrating such projects typically involves setting strategies, such as work place and school interventions, thereby strengthening overall health interventions in the society (Caraher et al., 2004). Increasing complexity in these food projects highlights the necessity of standard policy models that will maintain them and be effective. Most of the local projects did not have specific data, which compromised their ability to monitor impact and decide on best practice. It was revealed in the assessment of the food projects in the HAZs, where locally strategically-targeted priority was more than integrative strategy on the regional front. Appropriate systems of evaluation were in the process of development, further exemplifying an emerging need in the next policy making that is supported by integrative strategies. Policy leadership clarity is the priority in addressing food access issues at their root (Caraher et al., 2004). Monitoring the aspects of health equity continues to highlight the need for local public health policy to promote better health among communities. The health equity movement, as in most reports, portrays the ongoing emphasis on narrowing health disparities with innovative solutions. Community-oriented, neighborhood-based initiatives can target problems of socioeconomic inequalities and restriction of access to healthy food. The reports indicate that successful programs need the participation of multiple stakeholders, including local authorities, health professionals, and community groups, in a bid to have a coordinated effort towards improving health. Lastly, these local health initiatives are the embodiment of the real spirit of the significance of local initiatives in helping to yield equitable health outcomes, thereby helping in creating a healthier and more equitable society (Figure 3.16).

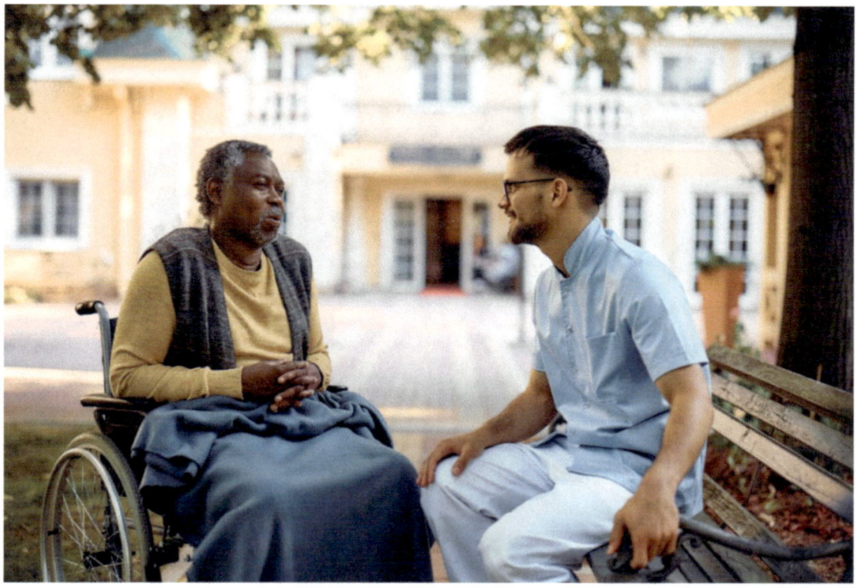

Figure 3.16. Example of a local health initiative.

Source: https://online-learning-college.com/wp-content/uploads/2024/01/Community-Health-Initiatives-Promoting-Wellness-Locally-1.jpg.

3.5.2. Lessons Learned from National Assessments

The national public health accreditation process has taught lessons regarding community health assessment, strengths and weaknesses of the public health districts. A classic case study in Georgia concluded that the accreditation process was successful due to diligent staff and supportive Board of Health, which are values related to community health assessment. These findings underscore the value of seasoned leadership and budgeting for forging a culture of quality improvement and comprehensive health assessment. Additionally, Georgia-wide accreditation readiness assessments have illuminated areas of priority in which local health departments can better streamline their functions and enhance community involvement, resulting in more effective public health interventions and greater adherence to national standards. Lastly, these lessons emphasize the necessity of long-term commitment at all levels in achieving effective community health assessment procurement (Alexander et al., 2015). Accreditation challenges found via national evaluation also introduce useful insight into the mix regarding challenges to public health districts.

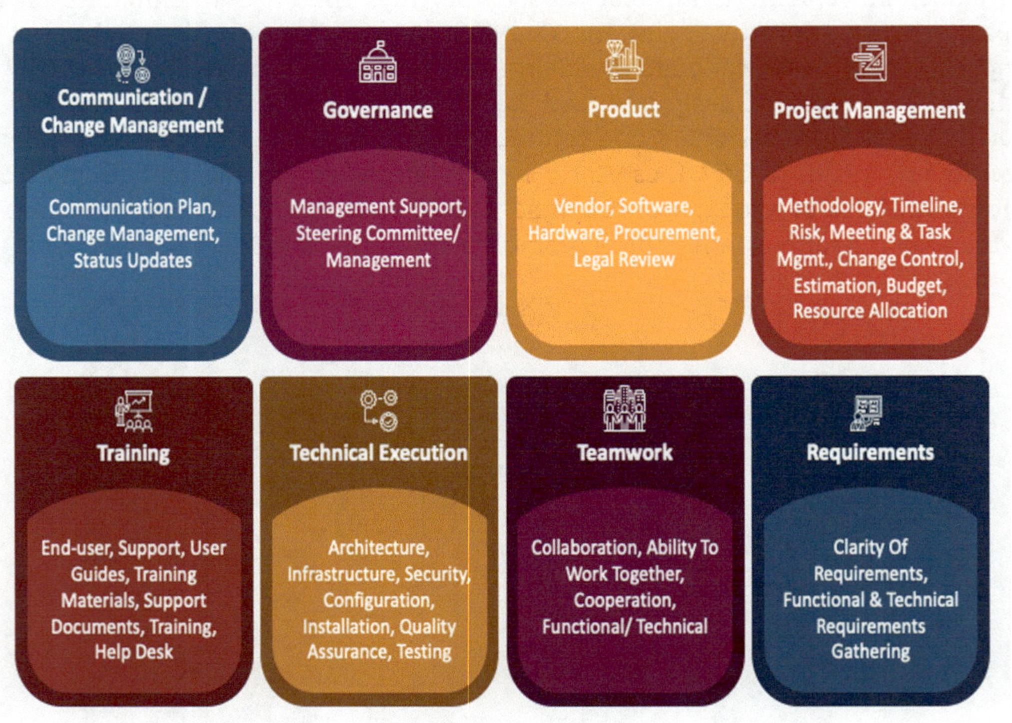

Figure 3.17. Lessons learned from national assessments.

Source: https://www.collidu.com/media/catalog/product/img/d/6/d6d72de07050ca0427545e3db8a862bed4e8e33897581c32bf50ecfd532a3c76/lessons-learned-slide4.png.

The research pointed out the financial implications of accreditation, where expense was a principal obstacle to most agencies in attempting to perform thorough community health assessments. Inadequate staff time also widens this condition, indicating a call for improved resource management and strategic labor planning. These challenges show that although the efforts towards national accreditation are commendable, actual-world issues must be taken care of to make sure the public health departments can effectively respond to community needs. Therefore, removal of such barriers is urgently required in defining perfect strategies for increasing activity in community health assessment and achieving needed resources for successful accreditation programs (Alexander et al., 2015). Moreover, the TA advice on pursuing national accreditation demonstrates a most valuable lesson in joint support interventions in community health assessments. Over 90% of the respondents to the PHAB Pre-application Technical Assistance Survey have shown a high level of interest in TA, and this is an indicator that there is a high demand for mentorship and guidance throughout the process of accreditation. This is an assumption that inter-agency coordination, in addition to establishing good support structures, can enhance the capacity for good health assessments even more. Therefore, the creation of partnerships among accredited and emerging health districts would facilitate the sharing of information as well as the best use of resources, ultimately leading to enhanced health outcomes among communities. By consolidating such collaborative platforms, public health agencies are able to better streamline their assessment processes not only but also make sure their strategies are nationally accredited, hence increasing wider public health impact (Alexander et al., 2015) (Figure 3.17).

3.6.3. Impact on Policy Changes

Community health assessments have been a key impetus for comprehensive policy reforms, particularly with the increasing mandate of health disparities. Assessments provide not only evidence-based data on community needs but also a key policy guide to respond to these needs. For instance, by placing in the front plan key public health determinants such as socioeconomic status and availability of healthcare resources, community health assessments give policymakers good decisions to work with. Integration of the qualitative and quantitative data also enhances the validity of the assessments since it places in spotlight the nuance experience of various groups of people in the community.

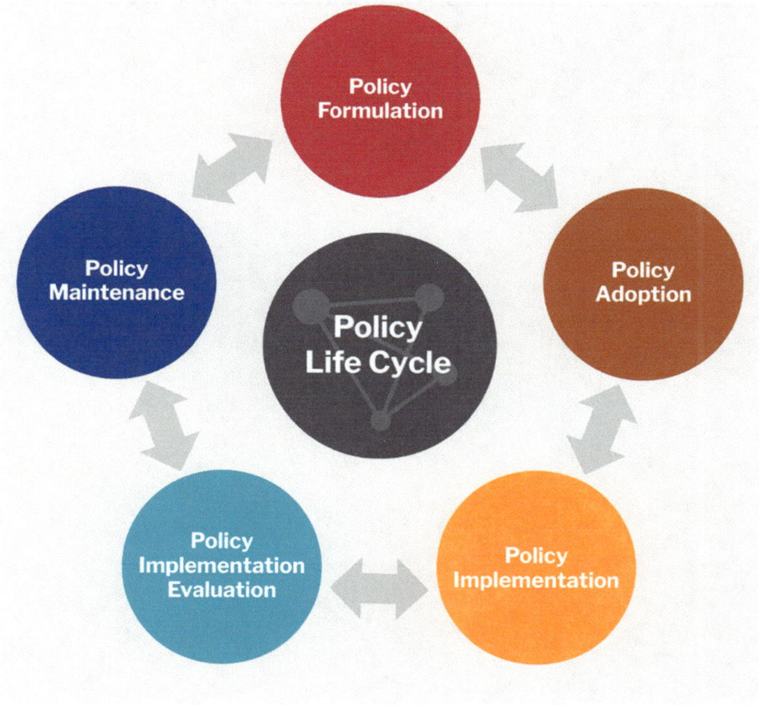

Figure 3.18. Impact on policy changes.

Source: https://catalyst.harvard.edu/wp-content/uploads/2021/07/Unknown.png.

Where populations are engaging with their health systems, this can create new policy responses that are attuned to local context and demand, following the trail of advance of health system organization and the pursuit of health equity (Seeman, 2025). Over the last few years, attempts to promote utilization of health equity impact assessments (EIAs) have served as a central approach to directing policy changes at the local government level. EIAs seek to evaluate the likely impact of policies on health equity and ensure that the interests of vulnerable groups are considered in making decisions. Results of research in Victoria, Australia, indicate that nearly all EIAs led to intended policy changes, particularly interventions for greater accessibility by vulnerable groups. The findings provide strong arguments for the use of EIAs as core components of community health assessment, going beyond information collection to engaging actively with communities in order to bring about equity-focused policy changes. This directs the need for local governments to embrace a health equity principle as a collective principal, which eventually leads to sustainable improvement in population health outcomes (Schultz et al., 2024). Embedding community feedback in policy-making provides a stage upon which health assessment can lead to meaningful and sustainable change. Engaging stakeholders, indeed, the underrepresented population allows one to grasp needs and concerns of the community more deeply. Such engagement can also power policies that are not only reactionary to current health problems but also reactive to future ones. When health systems react to people's voices, such information shapes a feedback loop necessary for ongoing policy development and upkeep. Lastly, the discussion of community health surveys and policy-making has a revolutionized approach to public health, remembering legislation as not necessarily top-down but rather inclusive and dynamic to the evolving nature of the health concerns faced by present-day communities (Seeman, 2025) (Figure 3.18).

SUMMARY

While concluding a community health assessment, one needs to understand the complex matrix of influences public health dynamics. The assessment is a key indicator of health trends, disparities, and needs in the community. By combining data gathered from multiple sources—clinical reports, survey questionnaires, and epidemiologic studies—the assessment gains an overall panorama of the health environment. A critical analysis not only illustrates usual health matters but also brings to the surface the socio-economic determinants of such matters. Augmenting the value of sustained observation, as seen brought forth through studies in Dlamini et al. (2024), can enhance the capacity of the community to resist imminent threats such as epidemic influenza. Thus, application of data to public health policy cannot be exaggerated since it forms the foundation for evidence-based targeted interventions that can be translated into positive health impacts. In addition, sophisticated methods must be incorporated into community health assessment in order to have a complete picture of public health and opinion. Social media and other open source data are available as an immediate reflection of the public opinion about health issues like vaccine resistance and opinion on health policy. Evidence in Daniore et al. (2024) prescribes the potential of open data to affect health programs but with caution to guarantee public concern regarding matters of privacy and ethical usage. With a focus on transparency and engaging individuals from the community, public health professionals can help build trust and partnership. These strategies permit active involvement by residents, required for the creation of interventions addressing and benefiting the population and eventually leading to health equity. Finally, effective implementation of community health assessments relies on the creation of implementable recommendations and careful follow-up. The operationalization of evaluation results should be given first priority by stakeholders for the purpose of filling gaps in health services and supplies as set. Regular reporting of findings and reaction can cement people's trust and ensure sustained participation in health programs. The learning acquired from measuring public opinion, like that noted in the findings of Daniore et al. (2024), can be utilized to inform policy adjustments and public health campaigns. By responding in an anticipatory manner to the mentioned expectations and concerns of the community, public health authorities can ensure that their programs are more effective and achieve the actual needs of the population. Overall, the product of a community health assessment need not be the culmination but rather the beginning of an endless loop of assessment, intervention, and modification that is by nature responsive to the community it is trying to serve.

Data on special education program effectiveness are especially relevant to community health assessments. One study details the advantages of learning communities in community colleges. Specifically, Kingsborough Community College freshmen entering a learning community made much greater gains in their course work than students in the regular environment. Not only did the students complete developmental English courses at a faster rate, but they earned more credits and had a greater likelihood of remaining in college two years down the road. This information shows the success of formal education and support systems within communities to support education attainment, eventually to healthier outcomes at the community level through increased attainment and readiness for employment (LeBlanc et al., 2008). In addition to educational advancement, mental health care assessments should be incorporated in assessments of community health. The primary care mental health specialist (PCMHS) pilot project is a valuable source of information regarding such tests. Conducted in six Clinical Commissioning Group (CCG) areas within Medway and Kent, the review aims to put patients' experience first alongside the influence of service providers at the operational level. By utilizing specially trained experts in the mental health sector, the program focuses on the evaluation of innovative mental health models' influence on various stakeholders like patients and health professionals. Knowledge of these dynamics is critical to the success or failure of community health assessments, and once again, stresses the interdependence of mental health care and community well-being (Brigden et al., 2015). Most importantly, pointing out key points from a multitude of sources of community health assessments illustrates complex population needs. Through the exploration of educational attainment and mental health service results, health assessment models can be enhanced in an attempt to address the unique requirements of diverse populations. Models need to be established in an effort to provide guidance for policy-making and resource allocation so that interventions can be targeted optimally to improve health status. The combination of educational and mental health services is also a reflection of the general style towards improving community health, such as improved academic achievement and enhanced patient outcomes in mental health programs. Consequently, ongoing evaluation and modification in community health assessment practice is not only necessary but also part of developing public health (Brigden et al., 2015; LeBlanc et al., 2008).

KEY TERMS FROM THIS CHAPTER

- Academic health systems (AHS)
- Cancer
- Community-based organizations
- Community organizations
- Community stakeholder engagement
- Coordinated specialty care (CSC)
- Demographic data
- Employment
- Environmental sustainability
- Ethnic minorities
- Federally Qualified Health Centers (FQHCs)
- Food is Medicine (FIM)
- Government institutions
- Agrifood value chains (AVCs)
- Child overweight
- Community involvement
- Community participation
- Community voices
- Cultural competency
- Educational attainment
- Empowerment
- Ethnicity
- Evidence-based interventions
- First episode psychosis (FEP)
- Food security
- Health advocacy

CLOSER LOOK

COMMUNITY MENTAL HEALTH CENTERS (CMHCS)

Community Mental Health Centers (CMHCs) play a vital role in delivering accessible and comprehensive mental health services to individuals within their local communities. Established primarily under the Community Mental Health Act of 1963 in the United States, CMHCs were designed to decentralize mental health care and shift the focus from institutionalization to community-based support. These centers offer a broad range of services, including crisis intervention, outpatient therapy, medication management, case management, and support for individuals with severe mental illnesses, substance use disorders, or co-occurring conditions. CMHCs are often staffed by multidisciplinary teams composed of psychiatrists, psychologists, social workers, nurses, and peer support specialists, allowing them to provide integrated and person-centered care. One of the key features of CMHCs is their commitment to serving vulnerable populations, including those who are uninsured, underinsured, or living in poverty, ensuring that mental health services are not limited by socioeconomic status. Many centers also engage in community outreach, education, and prevention programs to reduce stigma and encourage early intervention. In rural and underserved areas, CMHCs may be the only source of mental health care, making them essential for bridging gaps in access. Despite their importance, CMHCs often face challenges such as underfunding, workforce shortages, and increasing demand for services, which can limit their ability to provide timely and comprehensive care. Nevertheless, they remain a cornerstone of the public mental health system, striving to promote recovery, reduce hospitalizations, and improve the overall well-being of individuals and communities. Their emphasis on continuity of care, cultural competence, and recovery-oriented practices highlights the shift toward more humane and effective mental health care models. As mental health needs continue to grow globally, strengthening and expanding CMHCs will be critical to building equitable, resilient, and community-focused mental health systems.

References

1. Acosta, I., Thevenot, A., Tillard, E., Vayssières, J., et al. (2019). A participatory, territory-rooted and change-oriented approach to assess the multi-criteria contribution of an agrifood value chain to sustainable development. https://core.ac.uk/download/288641619.pdf (accessed on 26th June 2025).
2. Agarwal, R., Bandi, S., Crowley, K., Gold, M., et al. (2016). The Public Health Information Technology Maturity Index: An approach to evaluating the adoption and use of public health information technology. https://core.ac.uk/download/232572792.pdf (accessed on 26th June 2025).
3. Agrawal, S., Agrawal, R., & Verma, A. (2025). Strengthening pathways to prevention: Assessment of knowledge, attitude and practice for non-communicable disease screening among community health officers in Agra District. *Indian Journal of Applied Research*. https://www.semanticscholar.org/paper/a087739d537fdfe63591c6a267b727b47e94403f (accessed on 26th June 2025).
4. Ahmad, A., Bhuiya, A., Bhuiya, A., Bhuiya, A., Bhuiya, A., Bhuiya, A., Bhuiya, A., et al. (2016). Unlocking community capability through promotion of self-help for health: Experience from Chakaria, Bangladesh. https://core.ac.uk/download/286047961.pdf (accessed on 26th June 2025).
5. Alexander, D. S., Anderson, A., Jones, J. A., Marshall, J., et al. (2015). The state of accreditation readiness in Georgia: A case study. https://core.ac.uk/download/386167347.pdf (accessed on 26th June 2025).
6. Ali, H., Hardt, N., Hirpa, M., Ilyas, M., et al. (2016). Addressing health disparities among homeless in Alachua County through community-based participatory research. https://digitalscholarship.unlv.edu/cgi/viewcontent.cgi?article=1389&context=jhdrp (accessed on 26th June 2025).
7. American Lung Association. (2001). Urban air pollution and health inequities: A workshop report. https://core.ac.uk/download/323074325.pdf (accessed on 26th June 2025).
8. Andersen, E., Aslaksen, I., Bernard, J., Binimelis, R., et al. (2012). A framework for a European network for a systematic environmental impact assessment of genetically modified organisms (GMO). https://core.ac.uk/download/16386196.pdf (accessed on 26th June 2025).
9. Barnett, M., Kia-Keating, M., Landsverk, J., Lau, A., et al. (2019). Developing and evaluating a lay health worker delivered implementation intervention to decrease engagement disparities in behavioral parent training: A mixed methods study protocol. https://core.ac.uk/download/323062727.pdf (accessed on 26th June 2025).
10. Beck, J. C., Clough-Gorr, K. M., Erpen, T., Gillmann, R., et al. (2017). Multidimensional geriatric assessment: Back to the future—Preclinical disability as a risk factor for falls in community-dwelling older adults. https://core.ac.uk/download/85218696.pdf (accessed on 26th June 2025).
11. Bezold, C., Birnbaum, N., Masterson, E., Shoomaker, M., et al. (2011). *State of Health Equity Movement, 2011 Update: DRA Project Report No. 11–01*. https://core.ac.uk/download/pdf/18491810.pdf (accessed on 26th June 2025).
12. Bretsch, J. K., Wallace, A. S., & McCoy, R. (2024). Social needs screening in academic health systems: A landscape assessment. *Population Health Management*. https://www.

semanticscholar.org/paper/c5d6fec82b1bbbac0262f0142e46f4406b8fe816 (accessed on 26th June 2025).

13. Brewer, L. C., Fortuna, K. L., Jones, C., Walker, R. M., Hayes, S. N., Patten, C. A., & Cooper, L. A. (2019). Back to the future: Achieving health equity through health informatics and digital health. *JMIR Mhealth and Uhealth, 8*, e14512–e14512. https://doi.org/10.2196/14512 (accessed on 26th June 2025).

14. Brigden, C. L., Chisnall, N., Hamilton-West, K. E., Hedayioglu, H., et al. (2015). Evaluation of the Primary Care Mental Health Specialist role: Final report. https://core.ac.uk/download/30707993.pdf (accessed on 26th June 2025).

15. Brook, J., Deave, T., Novak, C., Salmon, D., et al. (2017). Evaluation of the Specialist Community Public Health Nursing Peripatetic Assessment Model. https://core.ac.uk/download/163076635.pdf (accessed on 26th June 2025).

16. Cameron, N., Griffiths, P. L., & Kesten, J. M. (2013). Assessing community readiness for overweight and obesity prevention in pre-adolescent girls: A case study. https://core.ac.uk/download/29026951.pdf (accessed on 26th June 2025).

17. Campbell-Patton, C., & Mattero, M. (2009). Measuring the impact of youth voluntary service programs. https://core.ac.uk/download/71342437.pdf (accessed on 26th June 2025).

18. Caraher, M., & Cowburn, G. (2004). A survey of food projects in the English NHS regions and Health Action Zones in 2001. https://core.ac.uk/download/2707830.pdf (accessed on 26th June 2025).

19. Chen, B. H. (2017). Engaging youth in community health needs assessments: What are the opportunities, methodological approaches, contributions, and feasibility? https://core.ac.uk/download/142080074.pdf (accessed on 26th June 2025).

20. Daniore, P., Sedlakova, J., Zavattaro, F., Huber, Z., Knieps, M., Wyl, V., Benhamou, Y., et al. (2024). Public views on open data health research in Switzerland: Implications for research and policy. *The European Journal of Public Health, 34*. https://www.semanticscholar.org/paper/83ff43516a6af6142afce3faa5f6e62094716d80 (accessed on 26th June 2025).

21. Dary, T., & Pickerel, T. (2013). School climate: Practices for implementation and sustainability. https://core.ac.uk/download/71361523.pdf (accessed on 26th June 2025).

22. Dlamini, M., Msolo, L., Ebomah, K. E., Nontongana, N., & Okoh, A. I. (2024). A systematic review on the incidence of influenza viruses in wastewater matrices: Implications for public health. *PLOS ONE, 19*. https://www.semanticscholar.org/paper/cb718695b745e075e30de59f7c458d9d9f8b3df9 (accessed on 26th June 2025).

23. Dufour, G. K., Yun, S. H., & Fiorini, L. (2024). Using an online measurement data management platform to improve survey response rates in a community sexual assault center. *Journal of Evidence-Based Social Work*. https://www.semanticscholar.org/paper/5ead929a10e8a7defc759036b282eaacc63cde6b (accessed on 26th June 2025).

24. Farley, C., Walker, K. E., & Polin, M. (2012). Using data in multi-agency collaborations: Guiding performance to ensure accountability and improve programs. https://core.ac.uk/download/71359978.pdf (accessed on 26th June 2025).

25. Filmer, D. (2025). The structure of social disparities in education: Gender and wealth. https://core.ac.uk/download/pdf/6644896.pdf (accessed on 26th June 2025).

26. Gamsu, M., Hunter, D. J., & South, J. (2014). Need to know review number two: What local government needs to know about public health. https://core.ac.uk/download/29018952.pdf (accessed on 26th June 2025).

27. Harper, B., & Harris, S. (1999). Environmental justice in Indian Country: Using equity assessments to evaluate impacts to trust resources, watersheds and eco-cultural landscapes. https://core.ac.uk/download/71342295.pdf (accessed on 26th June 2025).

28. Hasan, M. R., Sarker Rony, S. K., Muna, M. A., & Hassan, S. (2025). A descriptive study on childhood obesity: Examining research gaps, evaluating interventions, and informing policy for sustainable health outcomes. *Asian Journal of Public Health and Nursing*. https://www.semanticscholar.org/paper/5462a8434fa7c2051825c913cdd1e870c6a2bcac (accessed on 26th June 2025).

29. Howarth, M. L., & Warne, T. (2009). Explicating the role of partnerships in changing the health and well-being of local communities in urban regeneration areas: Evaluation of the Warn Warth conceptual framework for partnership evaluation. https://core.ac.uk/download/1664404.pdf (accessed on 26th June 2025).

30. Hund, L., Jacobson, H. E., & Soto Mas, F. (2016). Predictors of English health literacy among U.S. Hispanic immigrants: The importance of language, bilingualism and sociolinguistic environment. https://core.ac.uk/download/213627759.pdf (accessed on 26th June 2025)

31. King, R., Lloyd, C., & Moore, E. (2010). Subjective and objective indicators of recovery in severe mental illness: A cross-sectional study. https://core.ac.uk/download/10907546.pdf (accessed on 26th June 2025).

32. Lampugnale, C. A. (2017). Surgical assessment of the geriatric oncology patient. https://open.bu.edu/bitstream/2144/26707/5/Lampugnale_bu_0017N_13146.pdf (accessed on 26th June 2025).

33. LeBlanc, A., Rouse, C. E., Paxson, C., Sommo, C., Bloom, D., & Scrivener, S. (2008). A good start: Two-year effects of a freshmen learning community program at Kingsborough Community College. https://core.ac.uk/download/71340123.pdf (accessed on 26th June 2025).

34. Lee, K., & Woods, L. (2012). Addressing health disparities through organizational change–Evaluation report. https://core.ac.uk/download/71360286.pdf (accessed on 26th June 2025).

35. Lee, R. M., Daly, J. G., Gundersen, D. A., Lederman, R. I., Dargon-Hart, S., Winickoff, J. P., & Emmons, K. M. (2025). Assessing the inner setting among Massachusetts community health centers: Opportunities for multilevel investigation and expansion of influences on health equity. *Implementation Science Communications, 6*. https://www.semanticscholar.org/paper/c1d9fbb21e4d4e2f6abccf9d6b342ac3b977c14d (accessed on 26th June 2025).

36. Mayeno, L. Y. (2007). Multicultural organizational development: A resource for health equity. https://core.ac.uk/download/71353326.pdf (accessed on 26th June 2025).

37. Mittelstadt, B. (2013). The ethical implications of personal health monitoring. https://core.ac.uk/download/131214432.pdf (accessed on 26th June 2025).

38. Moraga Franco, C., Kuyper, E., & Engle-Stone, R. (2024). Formative assessment of community health center Food is Medicine programs during COVID-19 in Northern California. *Journal of Agriculture, Food Systems, and Community Development*. https://www.semanticscholar.org/paper/5b1efe4932fc3a9bcfa4ed98be6096ce8e7e6ac8 (accessed on 26th June 2025).

39. N/A. (1996). *Guidelines for the Scoping and Environmental Assessment of Water Resources Projects. The Environment and Water Resources Projects–Volume 2.* https://core.ac.uk/download/11023125.pdf (accessed on 26th June 2025).

40. N/A. (2007). Analysis of research on the effects of improved water, sanitation, and hygiene on the health of people living with HIV and AIDS and programmatic implications. https://core.ac.uk/download/71345778.pdf (accessed on 26th June 2025).

41. N/A. (2010). Gender and development: An evaluation of World Bank support, 2002–08. https://core.ac.uk/download/71360948.pdf (accessed on 26th June 2025).

42. Nebeker, C. (2020). mHealth research applied to regulated and unregulated behavioral health sciences. https://core.ac.uk/download/323082820.pdf (accessed on 26th June 2025).

43. Orfield, C., Orzol, S., & Hoag, S. (2014). Evaluation of Enroll America: An implementation assessment and recommendations for future outreach efforts. https://core.ac.uk/download/75781072.pdf (accessed on 26th June 2025).

44. O'Rourke, B. P., Hefner, J. L., Breitborde, N., Montesano, V. L., Knudsen, K., & Hogan, T. (2025). Understanding capacity to treat first episode psychosis with a hybrid tele mental health delivery model: A needs assessment of Ohio community mental health centers. *Administration and Policy in Mental Health, 52*, 584–593. https://www.semanticscholar.org/paper/c984f662579f31f8b007aa0969a34117694fb73b (accessed on 26th June 2025).

45. Parita, D. N., Adam, M., & Mu'izzuddin, M. (2024). Assessment of financial performance of Siti Fatimah Hospital, South Sumatra Province, in the application of the Regional Public Service Agency (PPK-Blud) financial management pattern. *Journal Indonesia Social Technology*. https://www.semanticscholar.org/paper/641599c940257b4e33d30bf1c5c0b7bf6a8296de (accessed on 26th June 2025).

46. Schultz, S., Beissmann, F., Zorbas, C., Yoong, S., Peeters, A., & Backholer, K. (2024). A realist impact evaluation of a tool to strengthen equity in local government policy-making. *International Journal for Equity in Health, 23*. https://www.semanticscholar.org/paper/bc8f3ab52b6fefd3ce9bdcb63e8533c8d228bf07 (accessed on 26th June 2025).

47. Seeman, N. (2025). Essential readings and continuous learning in healthcare policy. *Healthcare Quarterly, 27*(4), 14–16. https://www.semanticscholar.org/paper/c74783ed1998a421aa4d3a9fae158697abe05f3b (accessed on 26th June 2025).

48. Shank, B., Dalghren, C., Patel, H., Bertrand, J. F., Kaufman, L., Pomeroy, R., Gopal, S., et al. (2010). Global Management Effectiveness Study: Integrated social and ecological report for non-node and node sites. https://core.ac.uk/download/75777360.pdf (accessed on 26th June 2025).

49. Tarimo, D. L., Kimwaga, R. J., & Alexandera, A. (2024). Assessment of adaptation and diffusion of biogas technology in Dar es Salaam. *Tanzania Journal of Engineering and Technology*. https://www.semanticscholar.org/paper/5f60f6438434d1c2c5e3cbb8330b8b9f49e4f951 (accessed on 26th June 2025).

50. Torous, J., Bucci, S., Bell, I., Kessing, L. V., Faurholt-Jepsen, M., Whelan, P., Carvalho, A. F., et al. (2021). The growing field of digital psychiatry: Current evidence and the future of apps, social media, chatbots, and virtual reality. *World Psychiatry, 20*, 318–335. https://doi.org/10.1002/wps.20883 (accessed on 26th June 2025).

51. Utami, T. N., Manik, H. F., Acob, J. R., Aulia, D., & Sillehu, S. (2025). Needs assessment: Occupational health effort post in the informal sector in Pakpak Bharat District, Indonesia. *Journal of Community Empowerment for Health*. https://www.semanticscholar.org/paper/3393ccff5d957c4de76db74437b05a4738d84e97 (accessed on 26th June 2025).

52. Vinothini, C., Suja Rose, R. S., Vadivel, S., & Saravanabavan, V. (2025). Determinants of primary healthcare centers utilization: A geo-statistical study of healthcare access in Madurai district, Tamil Nadu. *International Journal of Science and Research Archive*. https://www.semanticscholar.org/paper/7c7d8b51451915e69c0c81743580df3a333dc152 (accessed on 26th June 2025).

53. Weber, P., Birkholz, L., Straub, R., Kohler, S., Helsper, N., Dippon, L., Pfeifer, K., et al. (2024). The limitations and potentials of evaluating economic aspects of community-based health promotion: A critical review. *Applied Health Economics and Health Policy, 22*, 165–179. https://www.semanticscholar.org/paper/505faddd2f9596babfaf6b578a1938e8e921ebb3 (accessed on 26th June 2025).

54. Wernham, A., Bauser, D., Bhatia, R., BLM (Bureau of Land Management), Burdge, R. J., California Department of Transportation, CEDA (Community Economic Development Agency), et al. (2009). Integrating human health into environmental impact assessment: An unrealized opportunity for environmental health and justice. https://core.ac.uk/download/pdf/8162498.pdf (accessed on 26th June 2025).

55. White, A., & Miranda, A. (2025). 956 Leveraging Community Health Needs Assessment (CHNA) data to inform burn outreach and prevention strategies. *Journal of Burn Care & Research: Official Publication of the American Burn Association, 46*, S366–S367. https://www.semanticscholar.org/paper/9f39042f366a980f626e0a5db22fdc77dad1dbeb (accessed on 26th June 2025).

56. Zakar, R., Zakar, N. M., Shahzad, R., Tekian, A., & Fischer, F. (2025). Community health needs assessment: Findings from a community-university partnership strengthening program on maternal and child health in Pakistan. *BMC Public Health, 25*. https://www.semanticscholar.org/paper/e3b3bb93dfe90d46b3d2109118dafc871ab10e46 (accessed on 26th June 2025).

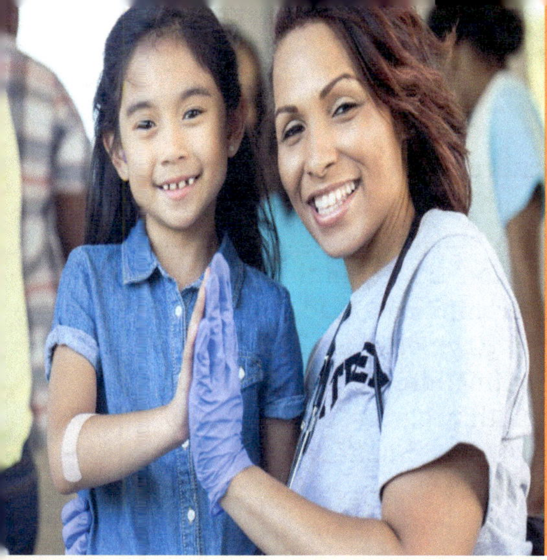

Chapter 4

PLANNING COMMUNITY HEALTH PROGRAMS

Contents

Introduction

Planning of community health programs is a critical undertaking that requires a strategic planning process to address the complex health requirements of the population. Effective community health programs must be founded on a thorough knowledge of the local environment, such as the population's demographics, existing health issues, and the local cultural background. These initiatives aim not only to improve health impacts, but also strengthen communities by engaging in cooperation and active stakeholder participation. Such collaboration is essential, as evidenced by initiatives like the EPAs Community Action for a Renewed Environment (CARE) Demonstration Program. CARE attempts through community-led process to prioritize environmental risks as well as create partnerships among business, government, and resident groups. By establishing a strong foundation of cooperation, community health programs can better address emerging issues and deploy resources to bring enduring improvements in health (John et al., 2009). Moreover, the role of maintaining effort cannot be overemphasized while designing community health programs. Continuous communication and relationship-building among stakeholders are imperative for effective implementation. Ensuring participants feel supported and connected through the planning and implementation stages fortifies the programs strength and effectiveness. This need is advocated in literature emphasizing employment retention strategies, where relationship building and continued contact with participants are indicated as critical to success. Similarly, community health programs are assisted by regular outreach activities that establish relationships within the community and permit trust-building among all parties. So long as stakeholders are engaged, the resulting partnerships can lead to collective responsibility and creativity, ultimately building a healthy community (Clymer et al., 2003). Finally, embracing community feedback during planning is essential in designing interventions tailored to fulfilling some specific needs of the local population. Community health programs need to employ evidence-based strategies to select priorities that are attractive to the population being served. Engaging the community members in the planning process not only leads to more effective health outcomes, but also introduces a sense of ownership and responsibility among the participants. Such inclusiveness practices can significantly enhance program effectiveness and confirm whether the health interventions are related to the values and expectations of the community or not. Lastly, by adopting participatory decision-making, planners can create a responsive and resilient community health setting that is capable of adequately addressing both current and emerging public health problems. Participation, collaboration, and community-level input together open the door to successful planning and implementation of sustainable health interventions (Figure 4.1).

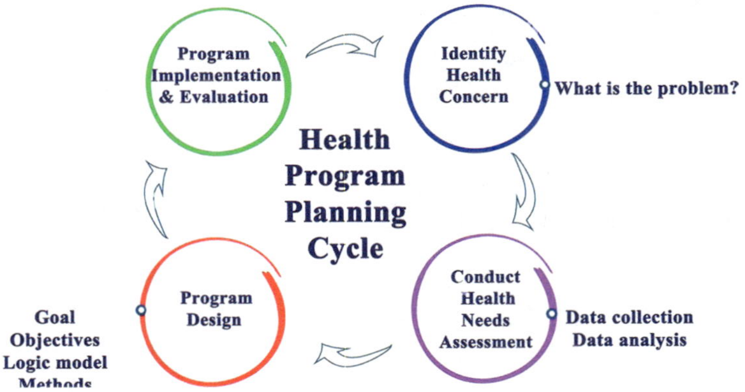

Figure 4.1. Planning community health programs.

Source: https://c8.alamy.com/comp/2AEPN7R/cycle-of-health-program-planning-2AEPN7R.jpg.

Definition of Community Health Programs

In its characterization of community health programs, stress must be laid on their ultimate intent: to serve the well-being and health of designated groups through concerted effort. Community health programs are typically an answer to a community's realization of prevalent health issues, chronic illness, infectious disease epidemics, or drug addiction. Participation by local members is necessary because they can offer information that would be lost on those who come in from outside. Through partnership and shared responsibility, community health programs encourage locally targeted interventions that address the unique cultural and social settings of the population in question. This participatory practice not only ensures ownership but also matches the services with community priorities, making a more sustainable impact on the health outcomes in the long term. Effective community health programs typically borrow models that emphasize communication, participation, and empowerment to harness collective efforts towards health gain. Active participation among the members of the community is one of the key components of effective community health programs. Describing a variety of activities in which individuals are engaged in determining health problems and impacting decisions regarding programs or policies, community participation provides an interactive environment that boosts solving health problems efficiently. Most notably, it happens at two levels that are significant: individuals being in control of their health and the community deciding together for health. Support for such participation relies on the contention that when individuals are engaged with the health system, services thereafter are likely to be appropriate and effective. Leibbrandt et al. (1997) affirm that shared responsibility-sharing, decision-making, and problem-solving ensure interventions are not imposed but are rather co-developed with the community to enhance their ownership of and commitment to health programs. Moreover, community health programs are grounded in structures that enable ongoing participation and evaluation. This shift from paternalism has given rise to new paradigms, such as Community Development and Participatory Research, which rest on shared decision-making and ownership. These paradigms acknowledge the rich and dynamic complexity of community existence and move beyond the typical arrangements of health services. For instance, through dialogue capacity-building activities and priority-setting by and among the community, programs are more capable of meeting changing health environments. As Arreola et al. (2014) suggests, despite growing awareness of the importance of community involvement, concerns around resource allocation and representation remain central to program success. Therefore, constructing successful community health programs involves not only empowering individuals but also systems that enable sustained feedback and responsiveness, so that programs remain relevant and effective over time (Figure 4.2).

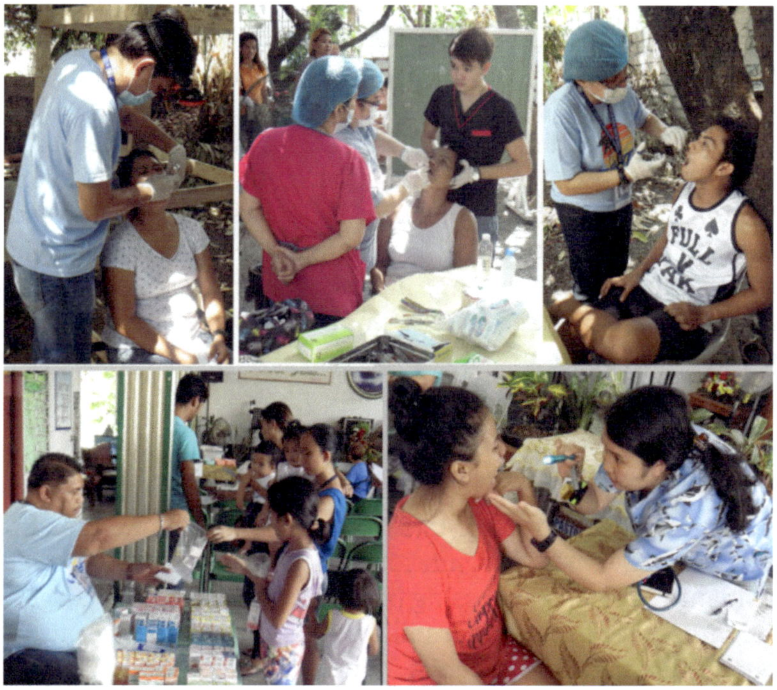

Figure 4.2. Community health programs.

Source: https://cavite.gov.ph/home/wp-content/uploads/2018/06/MD-Mission-in-Bayan-Luma-5.jpg.

Importance of Community Health in Public Health

The significance of community health within the larger scheme of public health cannot be overstated, as it is a foundation block that underpins the formulation of successful health programs. Strategically developed community health programs address the unique needs of the particular population, enhancing health status and resilience against public health threats. By addressing local populations and socio-economic status, such programs facilitate a concentrated approach that is more productive in rallying large amounts of engagement and activity. In addition, involving members of the community in the planning process of health programs assures that their concerns are addressed, leading to more culturally sensitive and effective interventions. As emphasized in community health initiatives, utilization of local knowledge plays an important role in ensuring the success of such programs because it ensures ownership and sustained investment in health improvement. Moreover, evidence-based practices as embedded in community health planning are essential in inducing systemic change in public health. Through the application of proven approaches for increasing physical activity, particularly among older people, planners can create enabling environments for healthier living. 50 and older targeted programs are the best examples of this model since they not only target physical health but also social connections and mental well-being. These types of programs respond to the growing need for age-targeted health programs that address some of the challenges faced by older adults, including mobility and isolation. Thus, through the successful application of these individualized measures, they significantly improve the living standards of the community members, particularly those at-risk ones, thus further entrenching the position of community health in public health discourse (N/A, 2001). Lastly, continued initiative in community health is significant in advancing the case for health equity, an underlying ethic in the practice of public health. By prioritizing problems of vulnerable populations, community health programs can cross over chasms that have a tendency to constrain the reach of good healthcare. By incorporating recommendations that aim at reducing health inequities—like those outlined in State of Health Equity Movement—community health programs can see to it that vulnerable populations receive adequate care and support (Birnbaum et al., 2011). Community health interventions with outreach, education, and prevention components tap into a multi-faceted approach to address determinants of social determinants of health, ultimately leading to greater equity in health outcomes. By supporting cooperation among stakeholders, including healthcare providers, government, and community organizations, program planning and implementation become more collaborative. This integrated framework not only enhances the effectiveness of public health interventions but also lays the ground for a healthier, more equitable society.

Overview of the Planning Process

Planned process of community health programs is critical since it provides the basis for effective interventions aimed at particular health conditions. As a first step, a thorough needs assessment must be conducted to identify the most pressing health issues among the target group. This process often involves partnerships with stakeholders like community members, local organizations, and representatives of public health. Involvement of these stakeholders ensures that the evaluation reflects true community needs and provides ownership of the program. As exemplified in a community health project strengthening women's and children's health, the handbook emphasizes the importance of assessing community needs before moving forward with planning, in order to facilitate the development of interventions tailored specifically to the population unique context (Assell et al., 1995). This process sets the stage for successful community involvement and the development of effective health projects. Following the needs assessment, the next step is the strategic planning of the interventions. This involves the articulation of clear goals and the selection of appropriate strategies to address the needs that have been identified. Health program planners must include evidence-based practice as they translate these strategies into the values of a community and available resources. The process further encompasses a precision description of logistics and an implementation template. According to the National Center on Health, Physical Activity and Disability, it is essential to integrate inclusion principles throughout this planning process, particularly for marginalized communities such as individuals with disabilities (N/A, 2025). By mirroring diverse feedback and ensuring programs are accessible, planners can achieve a high level of participation and engagement rate, which are important for the success of the programs. Such a strategic framework ensures that the planned interventions are both realizable and effective in the advancement of desired health outcomes. Finally, the implementation stage calls for keen execution and regular monitoring of the program. Successful community health programs entail ongoing communication among partners to respond to emerging community needs and challenges. In the execution stage, it is crucial to monitor the progress of programs and apply feedback mechanisms to determine its impact. Evaluating health programs not only involves measuring outcome but also gaining participant feedback to enhance and influence subsequent editions. The feedback collected can provide an indication of both what was challenging to execute as well as the overall impact on health outcomes. By embracing a culture of continuous improvement and responsiveness, health planners can enhance program sustainability and ultimately contribute to long-term well-being in communities. Through rigorous planning and evaluation, community health programs are better equipped to accomplish their goals and adapt to the evolving demands of public health (Figure 4.3).

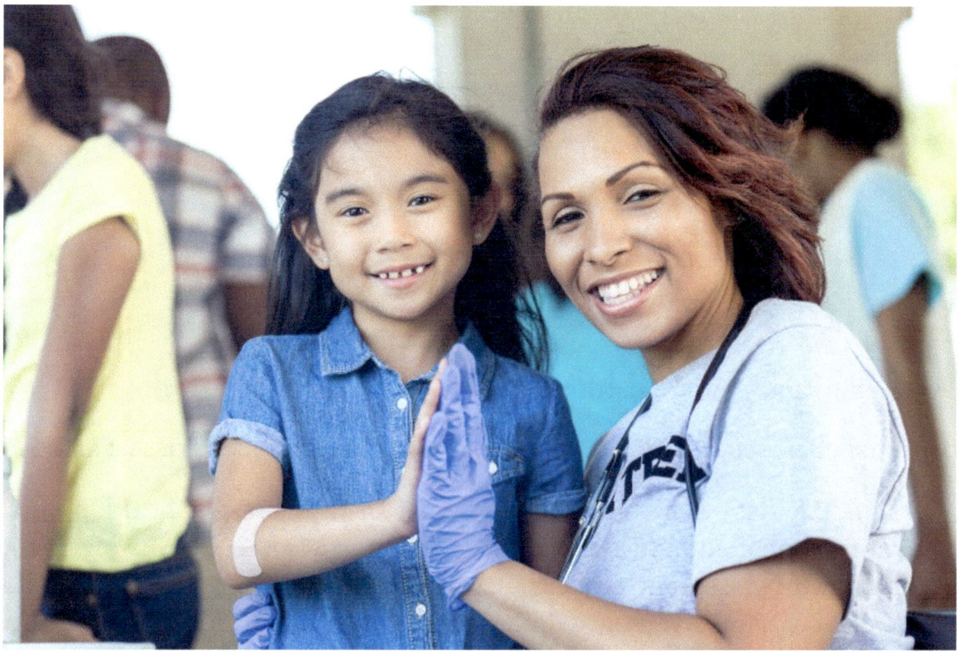

Figure 4.3. Overview of the planning process.

Source: https://ostrowonline.usc.edu/wp-content/uploads/2021/11/public-health-pyramid-and-community-oral-health-program-planning-feature.jpg.

4.1. Assessing Community Health Needs

Community health needs assessment is a key element of successful health program planning. Through careful evaluation of the specific health problems faced by various populations, health planners are able to develop interventions specifically targeting each group's unique needs. Technologies such as the SAVI Community Information System maximize the capacity for this assessment by providing access to a wide variety of data for social, physical, and economic conditions. This level of information facilitates health professionals to decide health disparities, understand their implication, and effectively allocate resources to meet these needs. Hence, the use of instruments like SAVI not only contributes to program planning but also fosters a participatory approach among community stakeholders and agencies, thus rendering interventions actionable and relevant to addressing community health outcomes (Derr et al., 2011). The influence of social determinants of health (SDOH) cannot be overstated when assessing the needs of community health. Economic stability, education, and health care access play a critical role in influencing health behaviors and outcomes. For instance, American Samoa studies illustrated the manner in which limited availability of cancer resources had a major impact on screening rates, illustrating continued disparity within provision of health due to more profound SDOH barriers. Assessment of these determinants allows health planners to determine the etiology of health issues and devise more impactful interventions. By including SDOH within their assessment, health programs can address not only acute health concerns but also the holistic socioeconomic factors that influence a person's overall level of well-being.

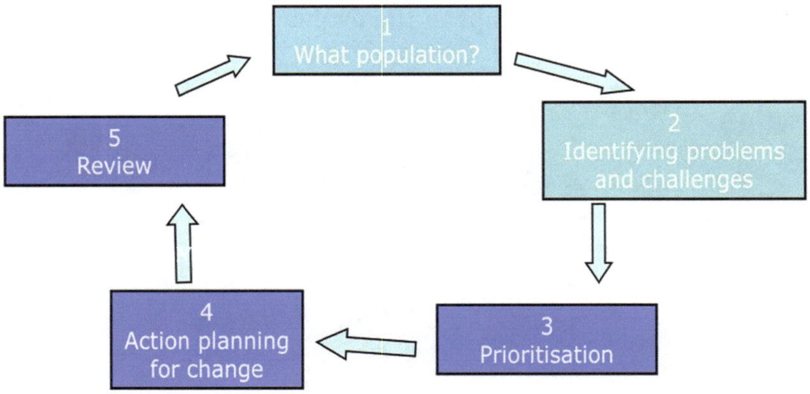

Figure 4.4. Assessing community health needs.

Source: https://image3.slideserve.com/6744110/cycle-of-health-needs-assessment-l.jpg.

Thus, understanding these dynamics is important in terms of crafting health programs that work towards long-term improvement and sustainability (Kaopua et al., 2019). Involvement of members from society during the assessment process also renders health programs more meaningful and effective. Local stakeholder involvement will lead to a more comprehensive vision for community needs, as evidenced by the collaboration in American Samoa to combat cancer disparities through the INSPIRE initiative. This collaboration between research institutions and community organizations demonstrates the importance of local involvement in identifying health priorities and available resources. Such participation not only fosters trust and candor but also allows members of the community to take ownership of their health outcomes. The integration of community feedback into the evaluation phase is thus pivotal, as it forms the platform for successful intervention strategies that are pertinent to the population they aim to affect. Together, health programming can more effectively respond and eventually be more effective in achieving health equity in communities (Kaopua et al., 2019) (Figure 4.4).

4.1.1. Identifying Health Issues Through Surveys and Data Collection

Detection of health problems in communities relies significantly on data gathering through means of surveys and other measures. Surveys are a significant method of determining quantitative and qualitative data on members' health status, needs, and perception in a community. By contacting a cross-section of people, health organizations can ideally calculate the prevalence of various health conditions, including mental health disorders, chronic illnesses, and barriers to accessing care. This process not only facilitates a broad overview of the community's health terrain but also informs directed planning and deployment of health programs.

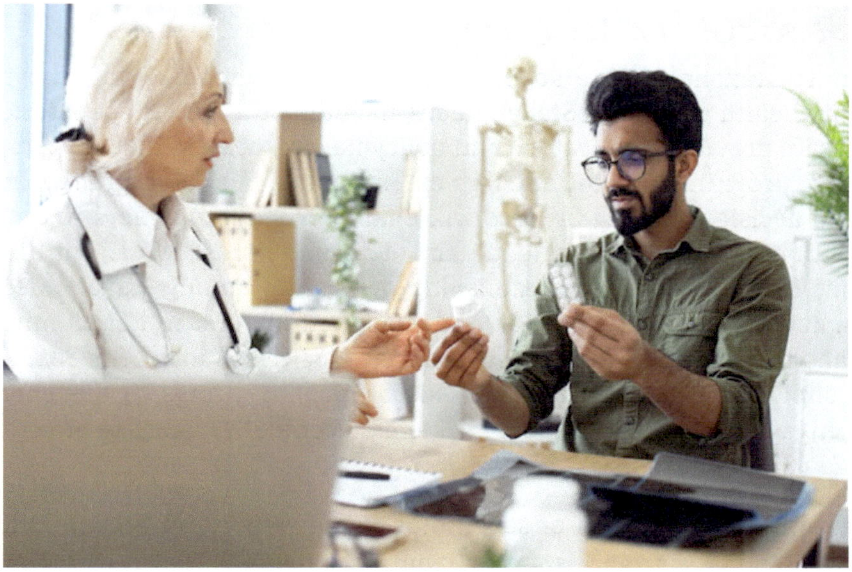

Figure 4.5. Identifying health issues through surveys and data collection.

Source: https://img.freepik.com/premium-photo/doctor-discussing-health-issues-reviewing-past-medical-data-laptop_161094-23133.jpg.

To that end, ongoing data collection has an indispensable function because it empowers stakeholders to determine new trends in health and align strategies to effectively counter change in community health needs. Evidence-based decision-making is important while creating community health programs, particularly when addressing sensitive issues like mental illness. Research indicates that teenagers in the juvenile justice system have significant mental health issues that require attention. Literature indicates that most of these individuals reside with incapacitating mental illnesses, and if left untreated, it can become a deterioration factor. Through the integration of survey results, service providers are able to view the immediate needs of vulnerable populations, such as those in the juvenile justice system, and ensure that health programs are applicable and effective. Furthermore, stakeholder feedback through community surveys leads to improved understanding of perceived barriers towards care and therefore informs efforts to achieve greater coverage and accessibility among marginalized youth populations, as indicated by the need for comprehensive health services. In community health programming, successful collaboration between the private and public sectors is essential in solving complex health issues. For instance, the Mental Health Services Act (MHSA) created a framework to fund community-based projects, and this has been evidenced by initiatives such as the Respite Partnership Collaborative (RPC) in Sacramento County. By evaluating program results methodically and gathering data through stakeholder interviews and member surveys, health organizations can rightly measure the effectiveness of partnerships. The RPC is aimed at improving respite care services for hospitalizations and local mental health, showing how the collection of data directly shapes strategic planning. Thus, community involvement in establishing the health issues not only promotes transparency but also fosters trust and ownership of the subsequent health programs generated, culminating in improved health outcomes across the community (Figure 4.5).

4.1.2. Engaging with Community Stakeholders for Input

Engaging community stakeholders to solicit their input is a fundamental step toward planning effective community health programs. Stakeholders, including the general population from the local community, healthcare providers, educators, and policymakers, possess diverse perspectives that can significantly enhance program planning and implementation of health programs. Incorporating such individuals into the decision-making process will enable program planners to determine accurate health needs, identify cultural environments, and determine trust levels within the community. Involvement of this kind is critical to establishing ownership among stakeholders, which can be converted into higher levels of participation and sustained interest in health initiatives. In recent evaluations, stakeholder-inclusive models such as the Positive Adolescent Sexual Health (PASH) Conference have shown that involving stakeholders not only brings to life educational content but also actively engages youth and support systems, eventually boosting effectiveness in health promotion at large (Crocker et al., 2019).

Furthermore, active participation of stakeholders allows program planners to utilize already established networks, and this is of great worth in outreach plans as well as distribution of resources. For instance, the participation of parents as well as community leaders in health programs has profound dividends, as witnessed by advisory groups for early childhood development. Information obtained can inform the design and presentation of programs so that they fit the community's real needs instead of imposing externally defined goals. This participation also identifies areas of shortfalls in existing health care services and suggests changes, thus providing a responsive health planning system. The partnership model, as evidenced from initiatives across various regions, showcases how strategic collaboration can build community capacity to create an active space in which stakeholders have a vested interest in health outcomes (N/A, 2015). In the end, involving stakeholders in planning community health programs represents a paradigm shift towards a democratic and inclusive process. With an emphasis on communication and collaboration among stakeholders, the integrity of health interventions is improved, as well as the possibility of innovative solutions for complex community issues. Flexible thinking is stimulated with the active exchange of ideas, and programs are thus adaptive to emerging trends in health. Successful model activities such as the PASH Conference point out the worth of such interaction, usually culminating in practical recommendations that enhance existing frameworks and initiate new avenues for public health issues. By prioritizing stakeholder contribution, health planners are able to formulate tailor-made programs that are sensitive to the vision for health by the community, achieving sustainable outcomes that foster global wellness (Crocker et al., 2019) (Figure 4.6).

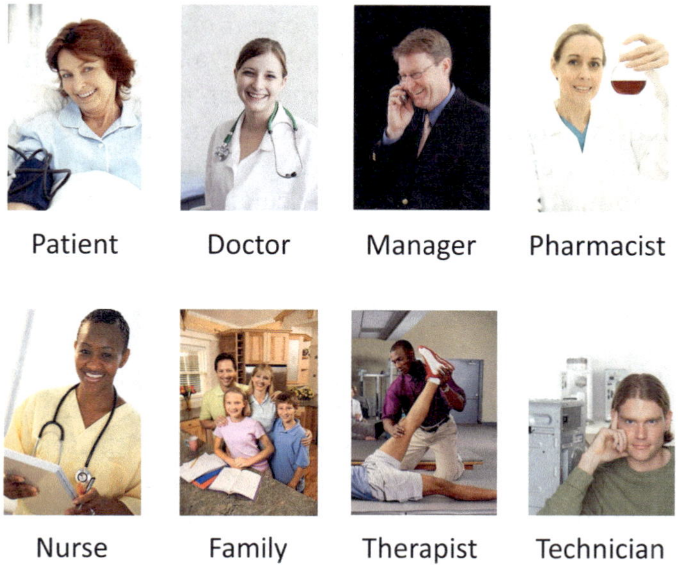

Figure 4.6. Engaging with community stakeholders for input.

Source: https://www.ssatoolkit.com/ssatoolkit/examine5identifystakeholders/stakeholderexamples.jpg.

4.1.3. Analyzing Demographic and Socioeconomic Factors

It is essential to understand the intricate relationships between demographic and socioeconomic factors in order to effectively plan community health programs. These factors bring about a dramatic effect on health outcomes in various populations. Age, gender, income level, and level of education, for instance, influence the availability of healthcare resources and personal health behavior. Detailed analysis of demographic data can highlight dramatic contrasts between access to and utilization of health care, such as with communities around the Savannah River Nuclear Weapons Site, where credibility of risk communication were influenced by local demographic characteristics (Brown et al., 2000). When analyzing how these elements interact, health planners can then design targeted interventions for the specific needs of the community, optimally maximizing the impact of health programs. Socioeconomic status remains the main factor driving health outcomes, as it is linked to access to required services and the ability to make informed health decisions. Variations in education levels are likely to translate to varying rates of health literacy, potentially affecting people's responses to health messages and consumption of health services. For example, in Nepal, socio-economic factors such as household asset indices and levels of women's education correlated with the uptake of family planning. The research demonstrated stark contrasts, where poorer ethnic women were less probable to consume contraceptives compared to those better-educated women from relatively advantageous ethnic groups like the Brahmins and Chhetries (Ghimire et al., 2025). Thus, to address the socioeconomic issues present within some populations is critical to the development of comprehensive community health policies. Incorporating demographic and socioeconomic evaluation in community health program planning will not only enhance understanding of the target population but also inform resource allocation and policy development. Evaluation of factors like ethnicity, educational attainment, and income will help in the identification of vulnerable groups that require extra support. For instance, the success of family planning programs in Nepal was based on knowing how various demographic factors influence the utilization of services (Ghimire et al., 2025). Through program designs responsive to such differences, public health authorities can ensure equitable access to healthcare and eventually achieve improved health outcomes. This advanced strategy ensures that community health programs are not only well-informed but also responsive, allowing for responsiveness to the needs of the varying populations' changing particular needs over time.

4.2. Setting Goals and Objectives

Goal setting and objectives are a core part of community health program planning, which outlines whether efforts as a whole will be successful or not. Goals provide an overall idea of what has to be done by the program, typically addressing significant health issues of the population. For instance, the goal would be on the decline in diabetes cases among the population residing within the area. Positioning these goals within a community's specific context and needs enables planners to position them according to stakeholders' interests and priorities. Setting specific objectives then turns these aspirations into tangible action. Objectives need to be SMART: Specific, Measurable, Achievable, Relevant, and Time-bound, facilitating it to track and evaluate progress. This structured process not only enhances accountability but also inspires stakeholder engagement from various sections of the community. Moreover, goal and objective-setting is a process that serves as a foundation for which strategies within a program can be developed. For instance, if the highest aim is the improvement of maternal health, some targets can be the extension of access to prenatal care or education in healthy pregnancy behaviors. Every objective serves the function of a road map which directs resources and interventions so that concerted effort reaches those who are most in need. The goal alignment and area-specific health information is also vital as it allows for the identification of priority areas that require intervention. Furthermore, using a collective process in setting these goals enhances community acceptability and ownership by residents. This collective approach also facilitates overcoming barriers, thus opening doors for improved program implementation. To reinforce the effectiveness of community health initiatives, planning processes also need to include mechanisms for feedback that gauge the relevance and efficacy of goals and objectives already set. Having the involvement of community members during the planning process not only provides input which can have a sharpening effect on objectives but also ensures cultural and socioeconomic considerations are taken into account. For example, as outlined in plans like those in Bacher et al. (2015), municipalities are encouraged to engage in inclusive strategies, supporting the involvement of citizens in projects such as solar power. The integration of learning experiences and community input into the programs assessment framework enhances resilience and flexibility. Not only are iterative alterations more apt to render programs pertinent through community input, but it also allows the initiatives to be maintained in accordance with evolving needs of the populations being served, which eventually results in long-term health benefits.

4.2.1. Establishing Clear, Measurable Goals

Formulating specific, measurable goals is a fundamental component of planning effective community health programs. These goals act as a roadmap for stakeholders, concentrating efforts towards achieving precise health outcomes. By establishing quantifiable aims, community health programs are able to measure their progress and correct for errors along the way during the process of implementing the program. This holds true for effective comprehensive community initiatives (CPIs), in which clearly specified goals have been associated with the sustainability and expandability of health gains. Also, establishing such goals harmoniously with community needs through effective participation ensures that the strategies adopted are palatable to the served population and thereby enhances commitment to the program's success (Chavis et al., 2009). Finally, goal-setting with specificity helps to ensure accountability among the team and stakeholders through the establishment of a shared vision for success.

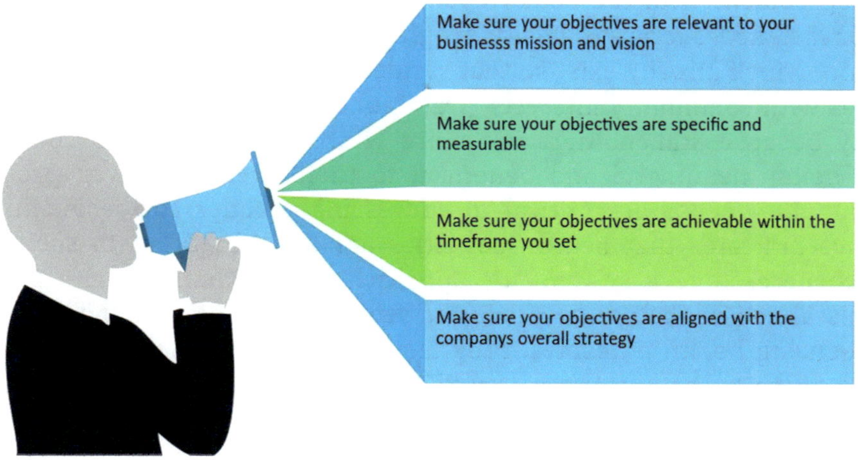

Figure 4.7. Establishing clear, measurable goals.

Source: https://fastercapital.co/i/Proven-Business-Growth-Strategies-for-Startups--Establishing-Clear-Goals-and-Objectives.webp.

Also, specifying and quantifying goals gives program planners the power to apply data effectively to assess and enhance strategy. The application of metrics for measuring progress enables stakeholders to establish trends, evaluate the impact of interventions, and make decisions on resources allocation. In the context of large-scale, multi-site projects—such as those focused on substance abuse—goal-setting becomes paramount, as demonstrated by the challenge in evaluating such programs. Stakeholders will evaluate the effectiveness and program design based on their perceptions of goal congruence and success rates (Sherwood, 2005). Therefore, having measurable goals not only provides the platform for evaluation but also encourages the spirit of collaboration whereby comments can inform ongoing improvement, thereby improving the overall efficiency of community health programs. Apart from being pragmatic, having clear, measurable goals encourages higher levels of ownership among members of the community involved in health programs. When members are seriously engaged in the goal-setting process, they become invested in the outcomes of the program. That investment can lead to increased motivation and a sense of responsibility for the achievement of the set goals. Successful CCIs have demonstrated that genuine community engagement—blended with structured goal-setting—propels momentum and endorsement behind health programs (Chavis et al., 2009). As these goals are repeatedly revisited and assessed, members of the community can observe their contributions to quantifiable improvements in health, further making the importance of collaboration evident. This process not only strengthens community trust in health programs but also with the protection of sustainability and the potential to modify, providing the potential for lasting benefits to the health of the community (Figure 4.7).

4.2.2. Aligning Objectives with Community Needs

Planning community health programs requires a sharp critique of the needs and priorities of the populations to be served. Knowing that each community is unique and possesses unique challenges, health program planners must engage in a reflective dialogue with community members to better understand their perspectives. This engagement ensures that the objectives set by health programs are in agreement with the actual needs of the community and not imposing from an external party. For instance, successful health programs always leverage on strengths and abilities within a community which already exist so that residents own and take responsibility. By aligning program objectives with community interests, practitioners achieve optimal program effectiveness and sustainability because stakeholders are more willing to engage and commit to activities they perceive as being meaningful and beneficial to their lives. Moreover, program objectives aligned with community needs are critical to addressing broader socioeconomic determinants of health. Evidence indicates that health inequities are often inherent in social and economic inequalities, which necessitate a systemwide approach to community health programming. For example, programs aimed at increasing economic security have been found to hold tremendous potential for influencing health outcomes. Programs that integrate health services with work to dismantle poverty—such as those at the center of The Urban Institute's data—provide mechanisms for individuals to build lasting financial security, and that security, in turn, maintains enhanced health (N/A, 2014). Acknowledgment and reaction to such interdependencies enable planners to create intricate programs that are not only health-focused but also successful at solving core issues that afflict communities. Lastly, successful community health programs often combine lessons from previous experiences, further harmonizing the objective-community need fit. Successful keeping of qualified health providers, as indicated in a number of case studies, is one demonstration of the importance of learning from successful methods and optimal practices (N/A, 2009). By learning from past successes and failures, health program planners can refine their approach to suit the unique contexts of the communities they are working with. Continuous monitoring and feedback systems can ensure that programs remain responsive to shifting community dynamics. This circular process not only strengthens the relationship between health providers and community residents but also makes sure that health programs are relevant, effective, and capable of inducing concrete change in the health environment.

4.2.3. Prioritizing Health Issues Based on Urgency And Impact

Effective community health programs need a careful strategy to prioritize health issues based on urgency as well as their likely impact on populations. Through the assessment of various health ailments, program planners are in a better position to make efficient use of available resources. In this aspect, priority health needs usually cover infectious diseases, maternal health, and nutrition disorders, which disproportionately impact groups that are vulnerable. The model of prioritization not only benefits short-term health crises but also takes into consideration long-term impacts, including the psychological and social dimensions of health. For instance, the fusion of urgent care and prevention decreases future health expenditures by addressing root causes. Understanding the urgency of some medical issues allows the community to craft targeted interventions appealing to the specific needs of the community and ultimately strengthening equity and outcomes in health. According to the principle of urgency, the potential effect of health issues also operates in the context of prioritizing health programs in communities. Problems that, if not solved, potentially have long-term effects on the health of communities become the focus of health planners. For example, where climate conditions are being more and more influenced by climate change, health and climate adaptation become the priority area of convergence. There is almost universal appreciation of the role of population issues in climate change adaptation policy as per a review of National Adaptation Programmes of Action (Mutunga et al., 2009). The implication for interventions is that they must contain not only direct impacts on health but also sustainability over the long term. By concentrating on health issues that are closely connected with social influences, community health programs can construct a healthier future, complementing initiatives that have the potential to change. In addition to finding solutions to immediate and salient issues, addressing cultural and social issues enhances the viability of health programs. Community health programs that recognize and operate in accordance with prevailing social norms can promote greater acceptance and participation by target groups. For instance, family planning and reproductive health interventions have had limited success whenever they do not engage men and relatives in dialogue regarding women's health issues (Venkatesh et al., 2016). It is vital to realize the position of customary decision-making in order to respond appropriately with health interventions that find suitability within existing environments. As borne out of research that prioritizes inclusion and education, health needs are also prioritized while demanding an acute knowledge of the social context of populations. Effective health program planning is thus a combination of urgency, reach, and cultural salience to make sure interventions are effective as well as sustainable (Figure 4.8).

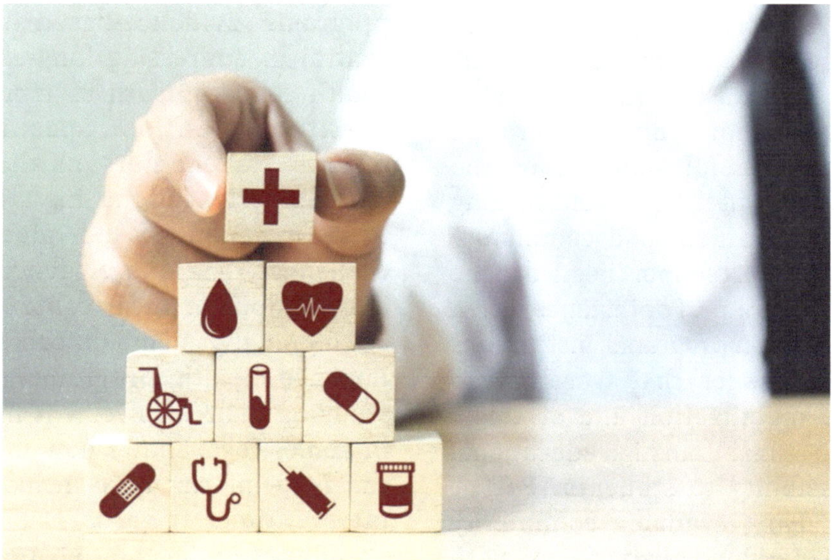

Figure 4.8. Prioritizing health issues based on urgency and impact.

Source: https://miro.medium.com/v2/resize:fit:970/1*iYrRTJCpN6pKqiAU5CJ5XQ.jpeg.

4.3. Developing Program Strategies

Program strategy development for community health programs is an organized process that considers the particular needs and challenges of the target population. The core of this process is the determination of specific health conditions that require attention, as well as the demographic and cultural setting in which these conditions exist. Utilizing data-based methods to quantify health disparities can identify areas of greatest programmatic relevance. For example, incorporating postpartum family planning services at repeated health system encounters, like antenatal care and immunization visits, has the potential to make a large difference in maternal and child health outcomes. Through developing a master plan that addresses these greater needs, community health programs can fill service gaps and make intervention available and applicable, and hence establish trust and involvement among community members, ultimately leading to successful program outcomes (Egan et al., 2014). In addition to health issues identification, the development of program strategy also includes sound review of available resources as well as potential implementation hindrances. Having infrastructure required for program operation is important to be successful. Money is just the surface of the problem, but it also means making sure there are trained staff on hand, community partnerships, and logistical support needed in the delivery of quality programs. For instance, when growing health education programs, institutions faced a number of issues that were solved through resource mobilization and strategic planning to be able to maintain high educational quality and accessibility to students (Becker et al., 2019). By using available community resources and partnership collaborations with stakeholders, program planners can be able to create a strong foundation for successful service delivery, improving the likelihood of sustainability and effects. Finally, measuring the effectiveness of program strategies is most crucial. Establishing clear, measurable outcomes helps understand whether used strategies are yielding desired results. Continuous feedback loops, encompassing qualitative and quantitative measures, help understand the programs impact as well as making the required adjustments accordingly. This assessment should be based on the original program goals and should be participatory in nature in order to reflect the actual experiences and requirements of the community. By ensuring continuous assessment, community health programs are able to become more responsive to shifting health profiles and new issues, creating an adaptable model that succeeds despite changing challenges (Egan et al., 2014).

4.3.1. Exploring Evidence-based Interventions

A foundation for effective community health programs lies in the implementation of evidence-based interventions, which are underpinned by scientifically conducted studies aimed at guiding decision-making in health-related programs. Evidence-based interventions are central in addressing long-established public health concerns such as family planning and obesity prevention. Specifically, involving diverse stakeholders in the community is most important in making a program tailored to the population's individualized needs and challenges. There is evidence to suggest that information on local contexts and attitudes of community members can significantly help improve health programs. For example, a study on male involvement in family planning in Lomé, Togo, shows how men's perspectives can help inform more inclusive and effective interventions towards the development of enabling environments for women's reproductive health choices (Bongiovanni et al., 2018). This means that the engagement of the community not only enhances the program's effectiveness but also promotes a sense of ownership by the participants. Local health departments play a key role in ensuring the implementation of evidence-based interventions that can reduce the incidence of obesity in communities. Qualitative studies of directors of state obesity prevention programs revealed that performance among local health departments is highly variable, contingent on state-level governance patterns and access to resources. Potentially significant barriers such as competing priorities and limitations in local capacity can impede the efforts of local health departments, emphasis being placed on the need for robust support systems (Khoong et al., 2014). However, those departments which can build effective communication networks, dedicated employees, and broad health screening create conditions for successful interventions. Thus, it is evident that overcoming structural barriers while building local capacity can have more significant outcomes in applying obesity prevention interventions. Further, integration of feedback and continuous scrutiny of evidence-based interventions is a requirement to maximize the effectiveness of community health programs. Engagement with the community using focus groups, questionnaires, and participatory action research can provide significant information regarding the effectiveness of existing methods and areas to be revised or enhance. For instance, LHDs' conclusions regarding obstacles met in preventing obesity support local engagement in environmental and policy changes (Khoong et al., 2014). While community health interventions are always changing, the application of a cycle of evaluation and adaptation is essential to ensuring interventions continue to be culturally adapted, relevant, and effective. A perpetual cyclical approach allows for health outcomes ultimately to be improved upon and a culture of health promotion fostered, demonstrating the dynamic character of evidence-based practice as it applies to community health planning (Figure 4.9).

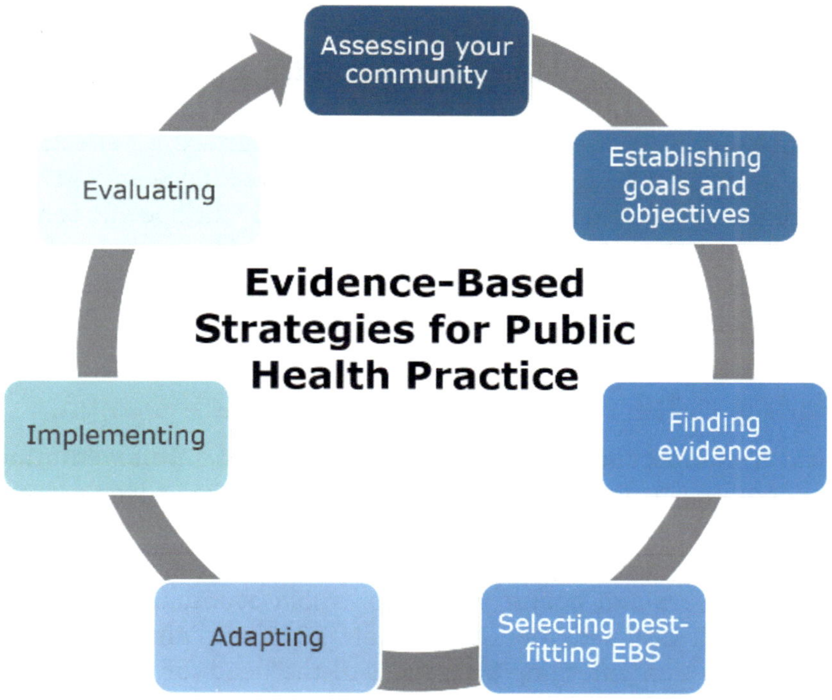

Figure 4.9. Effective community health programs lies in the implementation of evidence-based interventions.

Source: https://healthandlearning.org/wp-content/uploads/2015/02/EBS-e1435623117259.png.

4.3.2. Tailoring Strategies to Fit Community Context

The effectiveness of community health programs largely lies in the ability to adopt strategies to suit the unique contexts of different communities. Familiarity with the demographic, cultural, and socioeconomic determinants of health attitudes and behavior is essential. For instance, those communities with well-established cultural patterns will reject health measures that are incompatible with their values. Through comprehensive needs assessments and interactions with members of the community, health planners can learn from them to inform specific interventions. This helps prevent programs from being imposed but instead being co-designed with the community so that they build trust and have more chances for participation and adherence. Being aware and appreciative of the differences in every community is thus an essential starting point in the process of planning health programs that are both impactful and meaningful. Besides, active engagement from local stakeholders is key to adapting community health solutions. Local government officials, community leaders, and health activists possess extensive knowledge of the health priorities and needs of the community. Their involvement ensures that health interventions are adapted to the available resources and infrastructure in the community. This convergence can be enhanced program sustainability and flexibility in the long run, as local stakeholders will be more inclined to fight for programs addressing their community's specific health issues. Additionally, collaborative delivery fosters the sense of ownership by community members, thus leading to improved health outcomes as individuals feel empowered to be part of solutions addressing their health issues. Hence, involving local stakeholders not only localizes the programming but also builds resilience at the community level. Experience is such that effective community health programs often learn from best-case examples and the lesson of how context-specific strategies bring dramatic results. For example, the political economy of health interventions has a serious consequence on their implementation. Where political will and popular mobilization converge, as in the political economy of sanitation as exemplified in N/A (2011b), focused strategies translate to better health benefits. Failure of programs follows from ignoring local politics and culture, as effective strategies in one locale are not easily transferable. By considering such contextual elements at planning stages, community health programs can be designed most effectively for the specific context, with resources being employed in a manner that not only honors but also resists destructive tendencies in each community. Hence, an accurate awareness of local contexts is the primary determinant of effective planning and execution of community health programs.

4.3.3. Incorporating Cultural Competence in Program Design

Incorporating cultural competence into program design and implementation of community health programs is essential to foster fair health outcomes among diverse populations. Cultural competence refers to the capacity to understand and appreciate the unique experiences, beliefs, and values of different cultural populations. Such an understanding can improve communication between community members and health providers, which eventually results in increased trust and participation rates for health activities. As Yu et al. (2017) explained, early efforts at culturally responsive assessment mark an emerging awareness of the need for program alignment with the distinctive needs of various groups. By engaging community members in planning and incorporating their perspectives, health programs can better address barriers to access and adherence and thereby make them compelling for and meaningful within the cultural context of target populations. In addition, the incorporation of cultural competence promotes sustained participation and enables communities to become self-responsible for their health outcomes. Community-based agencies are pivotal in the process since they possess first-hand knowledge of the patterns of culture among their communities. With the illustration in Arifuku et al. (2003), a comprehensive study of several community-based agencies found the significance of their intervention in addressing individual needs of a given community. Through community-based agencies, trust is developed and inclusiveness is promoted through utilization of cultural knowledge, hence creating more relevant health interventions. Where program designs are being guided by the specific cultural systems of target groups, they will be more likely to return more participation rates and enhanced health outcomes, hence making the community health programs reconcile with the principles of social justice. Lastly, the importance of ongoing evaluation and adaptability in culturally responsive program design cannot be overemphasized. Continuing performance monitoring, based on quantitative as well as qualitative data, allows for continually evolving health programs that better address the ever-evolving population needs. Design must be culturally responsive and iterative, requiring participant and stakeholder feedback loops to be as relevant and effective as possible. Exhibitions of accomplishment in the community health field indicate that by having programs incorporate cultural variables into their evaluation processes, they are able to achieve significant improvement in participants' results. The commitment to culturally responsive practice, as was highlighted in Arifuku et al. (2003) and Yu et al. (2017), is not merely an ethical requirement but a practical strategy that can make the success of health interventions hinge on whether they are responsive to the character and hopes of communities with whom they are working (Figure 4.10).

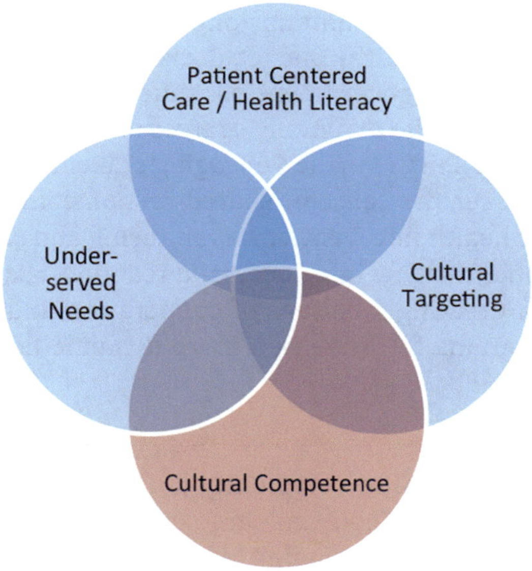

Figure 4.10. Incorporating cultural competence in program design.

Source: https://effectivehealthcare.ahrq.gov/sites/default/files/cc-fig1.png.

4.4. Resource Allocation

Effective resource allocation is a cornerstone in community health program planning since it has a direct bearing on the effectiveness and efficiency of health interventions. In situations of constrained availability of resources, the leaders in the community are forced to be cautious with spending so that resources are utilized optimally for critical health interventions. This necessitates collective efforts through the convergence of local stakeholders, including the government, non-profit organizations, and the community themselves. Through partnership, these communities can establish objective, measurable goals, analyze current funding patterns, and identify areas of potential savings or relocation. Emphasizing openness in the budgeting process is critical since it generates public confidence and encourages long-term investment in responsible health care that optimally meets local needs. Such strategic planning is thus in conformity with the Rennie Center's toolkit, which offers models of good budget analysis for the sake of facilitating leaders to make informed resource decisions (N/A, 2012). Resource allocation within community health programs continues to be made more challenging by extraneous considerations like economic trends and changing public health priorities. Deteriorating economic conditions usually compromise financing, rendering it challenging for health leaders to innovate and prioritize initiatives of maximum impact. For instance, in the event of an economic downturn, programs for addressing critical health problems such as chronic disease management or prevention services might be cut back from the budget if they are not vigorously presented with results-based data. There is evidence to indicate that pressure on performance can significantly affect resource allocation choices, and hence there is a necessity for community health planners to link financial resources to health outcomes (Demeritt et al., 2008). Through monitoring performance indicators at all times, health programs will be in a position to make adjustments and reallocate resources in real-time to meet priority health problems appropriately. In addition to strategic planning and continual assessment, community health programs also must maintain long-term sustainability of resource allocation strategy. This requires not only short-term budget decisions but also relationship building with potential sources of funding, such as government subsidies, charitable grants, and private sector partnerships. Building a diverse portfolio of funding sources allows programs to insulate against risks of budget reductions or economic shifts. Further, engaging stakeholders in open discussion on how resources are being used increases the sense of shared responsibility, and this, in turn, motivates increased investment in public health interventions. Monitoring and sharing best practices between communities can potentially offer insights into successful resource use strategies, ultimately leading to improved health outcomes. Creating a culture of cooperation and innovative efficiency will be key for community health programs to thrive in a more dynamic health landscape (N/A, 2012)

4.4.1. Identifying Funding Sources and Budget Considerations

Funding source identification is critical in community health program planning because financial resources will make the program both viable and large enough. Community health programs often rely on a diverse array of funding streams, including federal appropriations, state appropriations, and private donations. As many studies have noted, local governments often face budget constraints that make it difficult to implement or continue new programs, particularly those that address vulnerable populations, such as at-risk children or low-income families. Here, tapping into partnerships with non-profit organizations and local businesses may allow for the pooling of resources and funding for programs. By leveraging these partnerships properly, community health programs may not only secure necessary financial assistance but also create a more integrated model of health service delivery that responds to the multifaceted needs of the population they serve, hence connecting to overall health outcomes (N/A, 2011b). Other than identifying sources of financing, adequate budget consideration should be made to enable adequate utilization of resources towards advancement of the program goals. Health program planners should be data-oriented in the establishment of budgets, examining what works best as regards the utilization of resources. The use of measures such as the Early Warning Indicator Index can inform budget allocations when it comes to dropout prevention programs so that the resources are maximized to where they will be used the most effectively. The examination of per pupil expenditures associated with dropout prevention shows how effective practices can equate to increased funding for high-risk students. Besides, budgeting limitations also have to account for long-term sustainability, where there is consideration of revenues that will support periodic activities and reduce reliance on interim grants or one-time gifts (Rosales et al., 2016). Financing sustainability is paramount to sustaining long-term feasibility of community health programs, which necessitate innovative solutions to stay financially stable under evolving circumstances. Developing a blend of public and private sources of funding can establish a diversified financial base, hence mitigating risks of funding cuts. In case of threats such as budget cuts, program managers must utilize proactive strategies that involve policy advocacy for promoting sustainable levels of funding at the state and local levels. This campaigning can make resource alignment to the needs of the community simpler, particularly in underserved communities where the impact of underfunding can be significant. Finally, combining good financial planning and good community engagement can make health programs stronger, so they can change and survive in an ever-changing context (Rosales et al., 2016) (Figure 4.11).

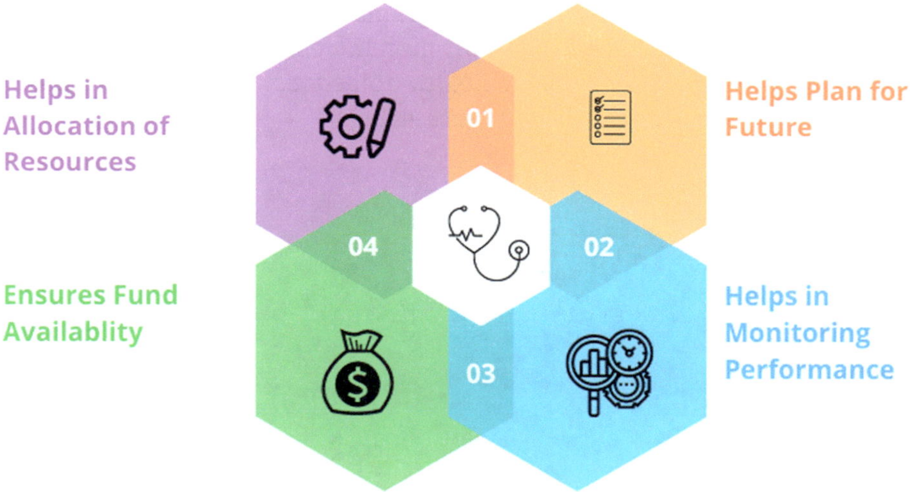

Figure 4.11. Identifying funding sources and budget considerations.

Source: https://oakbusinessconsultant.com/wp-content/uploads/2022/08/article-images-33-640x320.png.

4.4.2. Assessing Human Resources and Staffing Needs

Careful assessment of human resources and staffing needs is critical at the planning phase of community health programs. The assessment is conducted to identify individual skill sets and personnel required to effectively execute health programs for the community's precise demographics and healthcare concerns. Population numbers, disease prevalence, and community participation levels provide valuable points of data needed in the determination of staffing needs. Also, the trends within health care delivery systems nowadays often demand a more interdisciplinary process that will necessitate the coming together of other health practitioners such as public health educators, nutritionists, and mental health counselors. Effective staffing not only enhances program effectiveness but also forms trust among members of the community, a principle that is crucial in encouraging participation and compliance with health interventions. In addition to the quantitative analysis of workforce needs, qualitative factors also shape human resource assessment. The alignment of personnel with the culture and values of the community can significantly enhance program success. Recruitment strategies should look not only at competency but also at the ability of personnel to engage effectively with community members. Interventions with a high emphasis on cultural sensitivity and competence among staff are more likely to yield quality results, as they foster a culture of respect and empathy. Further, drawing upon existing resources, such as local volunteers or partnering with neighborhood organizations, can diminish staff deficits and enhance program reputation. Accordingly, establishing connections with indigenous agencies, testified by collaborative initiatives of different state agencies in the establishment of an integrated system for service delivery (N/A, 2008), is a required measure. Finally, since community health programs evolve, reassessing human resources on a continuous basis becomes imperative to adapt with shifting needs and challenges. Newness of health programs in terms of those developed from social enterprise models implies that staffing strategies must be responsive and flexible (Katz et al., 2011). The organizations would need to continually review their workforce balance and capacity in terms of turnover and employee satisfaction. By establishing ongoing training schemes focusing on skill and career development, health programs manage to retain talented staff devoted to serving communities. Lastly, sustained focus on human resource assessments guarantees that plans for staffing are coordinated with broader health objectives, ultimately resulting in improved health outcomes for the targeted population (Figure 4.12).

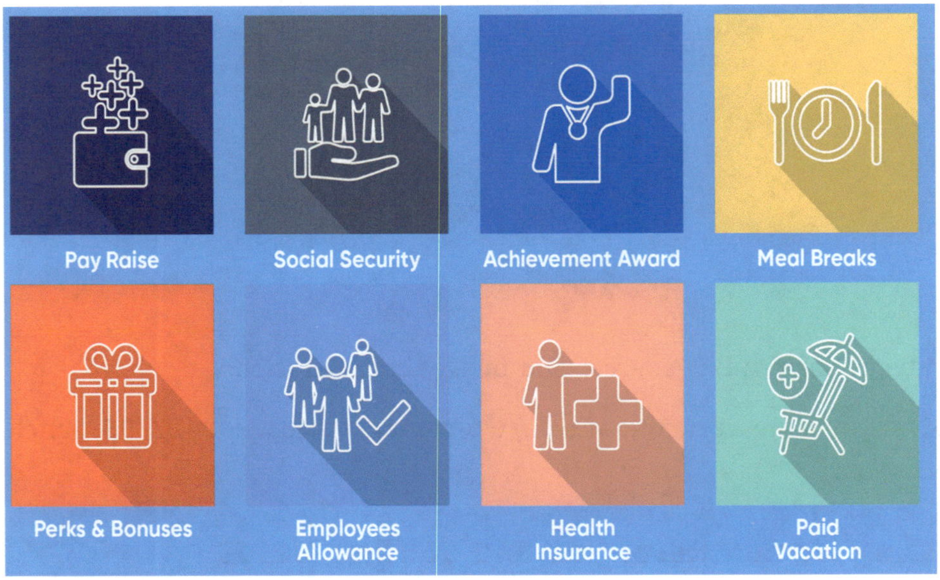

Figure 4.12. Assessing human resources and staffing needs.

Source: https://www.betterup.com/hs-fs/hubfs/Imported_Blog_Media/human%20resources%20management%20-%20employee%20benefits%201-1.png?width=4998&height=2858&name=human%20resources%20management%20-%20employee%20benefits%201-1.png.

4.4.3. Planning for Material and Logistical Support

During community health program planning, the effectiveness of logistical support can easily decide the success of interventions. A thorough assessment of material needs is essential, as it lays the groundwork for acquiring necessary resources such as medical supplies, equipment, and educational materials. This assessment should involve collaborating with community stakeholders to understand specific needs and preferences, which can enhance program acceptance and efficacy. Implementation of an organized inventory system can also provide for proper tracking and replenishment of supplies to maintain that healthcare providers will have required materials during high periods of demand. Defining organizational policies for material management can also help programs limit the opportunities for delay or shortfalls that can result in service provision disruptions and adverse impacts on community health. Logistical planning must further address the transport and distribution of materials to ensure equal access to various geographical areas of the community. Collaborating with local organizations and utilizing existing infrastructure can improve such processes while reducing operational costs. Further, the use of technology, for instance, mobile applications, can optimize routes and monitor inventory more effectively, thus making it generally more efficient. Moreover, as the example of the mFish project illustrates, innovative collaborations can deliver superior outcomes since partnerships allow leveraging on technological innovation to overcome logistical challenges in real time (N/A, 2015).

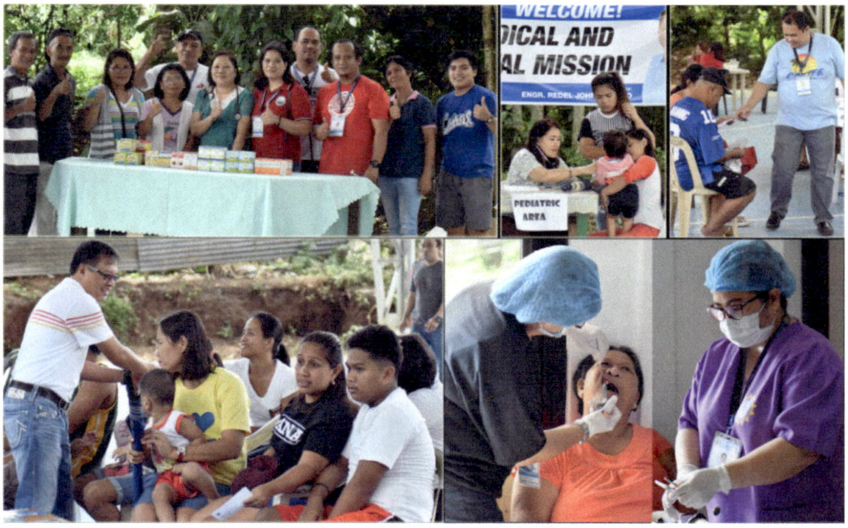

Figure 4.13. Planning for material and logistical support.

Source: https://cavite.gov.ph/home/wp-content/uploads/2018/07/PICAD2018-183-1.jpg.

Lastly, logistics support is a constantly evolving factor that needs to be continuously reviewed and adapted based on the demands of the community and on available resources. Furthermore, engaging members of the community in the planning process not only builds trust but also engenders a feeling of ownership for health initiatives. Engaging the community may provide rich details on culturally acceptable practices and local conditions that are vital for the development of effective logistical plans. Stakeholder feedback may identify probable setbacks to acquiring materials, such as transport or cultural taboos, which need to be overcome to successfully implement. As has been indicated in the review of the U.S. Department of Veterans Affairs Nursing Academy (VANA), inter-organizational collaboration can greatly enhance the capacity to effectively manage resources (Bowman et al., 2014). By prioritizing the creation of long-term collaborations that promote evidence-based practices, community health programs are able to integrate logistical necessities as a core component of their framework, which ultimately manifests as improved health outcomes for targeted populations (Figure 4.13).

4.5. Implementation of Health Programs

Successful implementation of health programmes relies on an understanding of community dynamics and community needs. Programmes among low-income and excluded groups can present unique challenges, particularly in environments where resources are limited. Pamsimas describes a community-based programme for providing clean water and sanitation, as an example, of the importance of aligning programme goals with local priorities and socio-economic context. By engaging the community in all stages of the program, from planning to implementation, Pamsimas fosters ownership and engagement, the pillars of sustainable outcomes. Involvement such as this proves that the incorporation of planning, implementation, and ongoing monitoring is the backbone of community health programs, which results in higher levels of health among the participants in the long term.

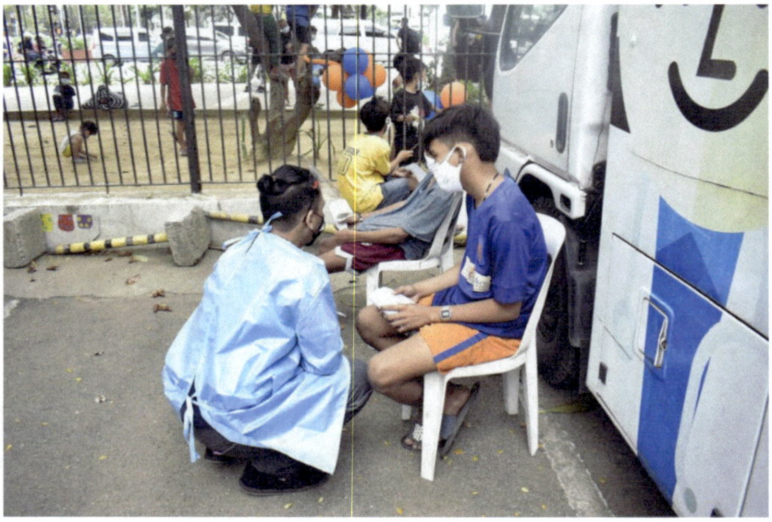

Figure 4.14. Implementation of health programs.

Source: https://childhope.org.ph/wp-content/uploads/2022/06/childhope-philippines-health-program-e1656895068613.jpg.

Ensuring that these factors are regularly evaluated can increase the program's effectiveness and responsiveness, a key to long-term success (Nofiandi et al., 2014). In addition to community outreach, the elimination of potential barriers to enrollment is required in order for successful health program implementation to occur. The results achieved from the evaluation of pharmacy staff on alcohol and drug interactions reveal considerable challenges faced by older adults in receiving health education. Within this population, illiteracy regarding health and individual attitudes may exclude participation in preventive health activities. Second, program feasibility needs to be considered carefully so that interventions are both available and possible for the targeted population. By identifying and analyzing these barriers, health program planners are able to develop interventions that promote maximized participation and minimize obstacles. This is not only an informed community but also one that encourages a working environment where people feel empowered to work on their health (Allen et al., 2018). In the end, operationalization of health programs demands a multi-faceted strategy that encompasses both education and hands-on assistance. Great messaging is necessary, as it has the power to raise awareness and achieve understanding of health problems, thus inviting community engagement. For instance, conclusions that result from comprehensive needs analyses can guide the development of targeted, relevant health programs. Additionally, multimethod dissemination strategies, such as workshops, teaching pamphlets, and doorstep delivery into communities, can enhance the coverage and effectiveness of health education programs. By engaging multiple channels of dissemination and ensuring the messaging resonates with the targeted population, health programs can be more embraced and effective. In summary, the reflective implementation of health programs with the backing of community involvement and communication tailored to needs creates the foundation for better community health outcomes (Allen et al., 2018; Nofiandi et al., 2014) (Figure 4.14).

4.5.1. Creating a Timeline for Program Rollout

Development of a master timeline for the implementation of community health programs is a significant move that ensures orderly implementation and smooth changes at various stages of the project. It must be able to accommodate various stages of the program, from planning to community outreach, deployment of resources, and evaluation. Effective time management can prevent conflicting activities to ensure that personnel, equipment, and other resources are utilized when needed. Having input from the community included in this timeline can be utilized to further enhance relevance and program effectiveness and create a feeling of ownership on the part of stakeholders. For instance, when bringing something like the Carbon Reduction Transportation Initiative (CRTI) to Northern Arizona University, preparing for meetings with the community and outreach can make projecting potential issues and more extensive community investment feasible, which is essential for gaining support and long-term sustainability (N/A, 2020). The development of particular milestones along the way also serves to track progress and holds teams accountable for various levels of program development.

The identification of key milestones along the path allows for regular checks as to whether or not the program is on course. If adjustments need to be made, stakeholders can engage in reflection to determine if or not timelines must be adjusted, keeping the initiative on course to meet its goals. These touchstones become even more critical when collaborating towards inclusivity and reaching diverse populations. For example, organizations like Microsoft and JP Morgan Chase have recognized the need for building talent pipelines among underrepresented groups by emphasizing how mapping out a timeline of well-defined goals can significantly enhance hiring from these untapped talent pools (DXC Technology, 2019). Last but not least, the final roll-out calendar should have a complete evaluation plan whereby it can be determined to measure the impact and success of the programs. Collection of data at various levels allows stakeholders to gauge the outcomes with set measures of success to ultimately enable program enhancement in the future. Organized timelines do not only simplify coordination of community health programs with strategic goals but also enhance transparency and build trust among residents of the community. By learning from previous rollouts and tailoring to specific community traits, program staff can ensure that future projects are constructed and launched more effectively. This learning loop of assessment and adjustment also serves to support the utility of a timeline as an evolving document that propels continuous improvement in community health programming.

4.5.2. Training Staff and Volunteers for Effective Delivery

Training of the staff and volunteers is an essential component of the delivery of quality community health programs. A well-organized training program equips the staff with the desired knowledge and skills to provide quality service and respond to the community in a positive manner.

The training should integrate a combination of topics, including health education, communications skills, and cultural awareness, so that all the trainees are aligned towards the goal of the programs. Through investment in large-scale training, organizations are able to build a more efficient workforce, which contributes to better health outcomes within the community. Continuous training and feedback systems can also boost staff and volunteer flexibility to changing health demands, ultimately contributing to program sustainability. With every new health problem, the abilities and skill of those charged with responding must change too, highlighting continuous professional development as a guarantee of program success. Good training policy also accepts the important contribution volunteers can make, in partnership with paid staff, towards the delivery of community health programs. Volunteers are a valuable resource, and they are likely to bring certain knowledge and connections into the communities where they work. Therefore, it is essential that organizations hold training sessions which not just familiarize volunteers with performing their responsibilities, but also give them a sense of belonging and commitment. Workshop experiences, shared training, and mentorship opportunities enable volunteers and employees to build stronger bonds. This collective environment enhances overall program efficiency by leveraging the diversified skills of both groups. Additionally, as realized through studies, organizations whose priority is strategic volunteer deployment can leverage such resources to make more of an impact, again leading to training in leveraging this vital workforce (Baker et al., 2007; N/A, 2007b). Lastly, the effectiveness of training depends on how well it is integrated into the greater planning and operation of community health programs. Training should not be conceived of as something that one does once but rather as an ongoing process that expands with the demands and developments of the programs. Ongoing review of the outcomes of training and feedback from participants can enable organizations to adapt their approaches so that employees and volunteers are sufficiently equipped to execute the demands of their position. Further, utilization of technology tools in training is also capable of reaching wider areas and offering support for multiple learning styles, which enhances participation. Effective training is, therefore, directly accountable for the effective implementation of community health programs as it makes it possible for individuals to deliver critical services with confidence and capability (N/A, 2007b) (Figure 4.15).

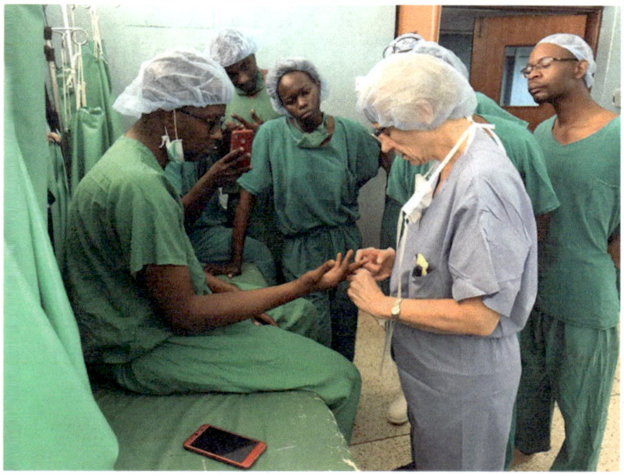

Figure 4.15. Training staff and volunteers for effective delivery.

Source: https://external-content.duckduckgo.com/iu/?u=https%3A%2F%2Fwww.ghspjournal.org%2Fcontent%2Fghsp%2F7%2F3%2F344%2FF1.large.jpg%3Fdownload%3Dtrue&f=1&nofb=1&ipt=d183ff2bf56b063c71 2fc9e44dfbe9743d41e731b90af544ea075baaec1f87e5.

4.5.3. Engaging the Community in Program Activities

Community involvement in program implementation is central to the success of community health programs. Encouraging community members to take sense of responsibility and ownership towards health programs improves their sustainability and effectiveness. Successful community participation starts with the identification of the unique strengths of the community, such as local knowledge, cultural practices, and social networks. By tapping into these accessible resources, health programs can be tailored to meet local needs in a specific way, thereby becoming more acceptable and relevant. Active participation not only builds up individuals but also facilitates cooperation as well as collective decision-making that form the basis of reaching health targets. According to studies, civic engagement teaches young people important life skills and guarantees their academic achievement and health status as well as maintains their social and emotional well-being (Hair et al., 2002). Moreover, the efforts of local organizations towards mobilizing citizens cannot be overstressed, particularly in initiatives related to health. Non-governmental organizations (NGOs), community-based organizations (CBOs), and faith-based organizations (FBOs) account for reaching out to community assets and professionals. They tend to act as in-betweeners between the health system and the community, mediating communication and offering culturally appropriate methodologies for programme implementation. Having a long history within the community allows them to pinpoint salient health issues and involve communities that have been marginalized. The capacity of local organizations to plan and establish sustainable crisis responses, such as HIV/AIDS, has been facilitated by the support and financing of global interventions, such as the Global Fund and PEPFAR. The grassroots movement not only enhances the appropriateness of the programs but also renders the interventions community reality-based, as in the meaningful improvement in resource allocation and capacity building (Cornman et al., 2005). Moreover, community participation in health program activities has also been linked to improved health behaviors and outcomes.

Community-input and community-participation programs yield higher levels of health literacy and awareness because individuals become more informed about health threats and preventive measures. Such interaction can bring about a shift in social norms that promote healthier behavior and ultimately reduce the disease burden. Moreover, community involvement in program formulation and evaluation inspires a continuous cycle of improvement because local stakeholders tend to advocate for interventions that align with their lived realities. As civic engagement has been established to build resilience and autonomy, involvement of community assets can foster long-lasting impacts. In general, active community members' involvement is vital in planning and implementing health programs so that they are functional, culturally appropriate, and sustainable (Hair et al., 2002) (Figure 4.16).

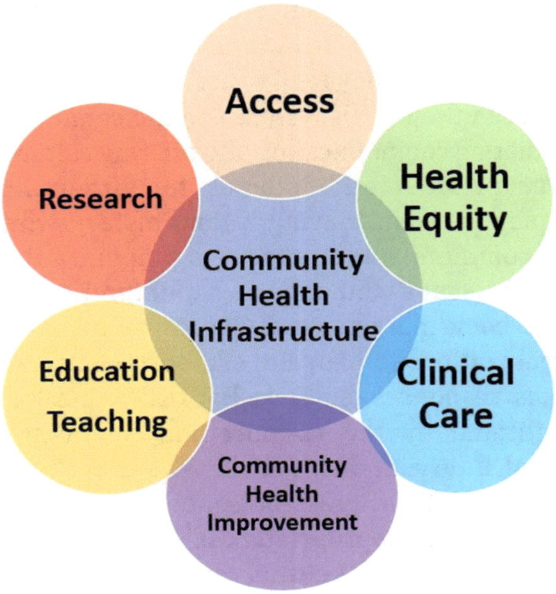

Figure 4.16. Engaging the community in program activities.

Source: https://www.massgeneral.org/assets/mgh/images/ecoch/criteria%20for%20clincal%20depts%20to%20engage%20in%20ch.jpg.

4.6. Evaluation and Feedback

Evaluation and feedback systems need to be built into community health program planning so that measures are taken to ensure activities are effective and conducive to the needs of the community. An efficient process of evaluation provides required information about program performance, and the chance to act on that basis is also there. For instance, Sacramento County's RPC Innovation Project illustrates how community-based evaluations can assist in building cooperation between stakeholders and ultimately facilitate more effective mental health services. By really involving community input when planning and implementing programs, programs can be designed to more precisely address particular needs, thus driving improved results for those served. This symbiotic interaction between evaluation and community feedback not only encourages accountability but also encourages the sustained engagement of participants, as required for long-term success in health programs. Mechanisms of feedback are crucial to refine the strategies utilized in community health programs so that they remain relevant and effective in the long run. Continuous feedback allows program administrators to assess intervention effects, track fidelity to the programmed protocols, and adapt approaches as needed to maximize effectiveness. For example, in CHARM intervention in rural India, surveys and qualitative in-depth interviews provided rich qualitative data on programs implementation and its effect on male participation in family planning. These qualitative evaluations assist in explaining the successes and challenges participants have had, and future program iterations can be informed by this. Through systematic gathering and examination of comments from all concerned parties, community health programs may change to align with shifting social forces and improve responses to the complex health needs of their populations. The worth of assessment and feedback in community health interventions extends far beyond the improvement of short-term programs; it also enhances the practice of public health as a whole by creating evidence-based interventions. By means of systematic evaluation processes, good interventions can be recorded, benchmarked, and replicated across various settings, therefore increasing their reach and impact. The RPC Innovation Project is a prime example, where its findings can inform mental health best practices in different communities. Additionally, broadcasting lessons learned from successes and failures, programs in health can build the body of knowledge that drives innovation and inclusion in public health programs. Thus, meaningful evaluation and feedback do not only strengthen programs but also expedite community health improvement by creating a learning culture and development.

4.6.1. Establishing Metrics for Program Success

Establishing program success indicators is part of community health program planning because such indicators provide a foundation upon which to assess the effectiveness and impact of various initiatives. Such indicators can be quantitative or qualitative, allowing stakeholders to track advancements relative to predetermined goals. For instance, tallying the number of individuals served or tracking gains in health outcomes, such as a fall in rates of preventable disease, will identify the quantitative improvements in community health interventions. Similarly, incorporating participant feedback enhances the quality of measurement of program effectiveness so that it is still responsive to community needs. Through the systematic examination of performance data, program managers are able to identify effective strategies, see where there's room for improvement, and make evidence-based decisions that improve upon future health programs, thereby creating a culture of ongoing improvement and accountability within community health programs. When taking on the challenge of setting metrics, it is important to combine learning from research and case studies to identify best practices. A research that considers measurement performance activity in a variety of livability programs underscores the relevance of comparing various approaches to determine good practice in measurement (Fabish et al., 2013). By considering an analysis of the factors that contributed to the success of these programs, health planners at community levels can apply relevant measurement tools appropriate to their environment. Continuing insight into the opinions of stakeholders regarding the success or failure of programs further goes to validate the relevance of chosen measures. This cycle of learning from past experience combined with feedback from the community ensures that the measures not only reflect program objectives but also are relevant to the communities being targeted, ultimately improving the programs' sustainability. Interagency coordination among various stakeholders, including government agencies, healthcare providers, and community groups, can further improve the process of creating meaningful measures. For instance, questions initiated by legislative actions, such as the proposals set by the Single Point of Entry Long-Term Living Resources System Team, illustrate the necessity of multi-agency coordination for setting sound measurement systems (N/A, 2008). Collaboration ensures that multiple perspectives are addressed, leading to a more comprehensive general feeling of community health needs. By creating partnerships among such organizations, planners can tap into collective resources, information, and expertise and therefore enhance the mechanisms utilized to measure program success. Joint efforts not only contribute to increasing the data completeness obtained but also create trust and acceptance from the community, which are critical determinants of health program success and sustainability.

4.6.2. Collecting Data for Ongoing Assessment

In community health program planning, data gathering for ongoing evaluation is a cornerstone to ensuring effectiveness and responsiveness in programs. Obtaining precise and valid data allows health planners to evaluate the impact of interventions and alter strategies through tangible findings.

Through cautious methods of data collection, such as surveys, focus groups, and public health data, planners are well-equipped to analyze quantitative and qualitative programmatic elements of health. Through ongoing assessment as well, a culture of constant improvement is facilitated whereby stakeholders can respond continuously to evolving needs in the community that they serve. As uncovered in health partnership assessments, regular monitoring can inform decision-making processes, resulting in improved community health measures and additional resource distribution where it is needed the most (Keller et al., 2012). Perhaps the most important benefit of conducting data collection for regular assessment is that it helps to inform evidence-based interventions and policies. The use of information gathered in program planning and assessment provides greater understanding of health concerns in the community, therefore informed prioritization when utilizing resources. For instance, through the Western Australian Sexual Health and Blood-borne Virus Applied Research and Evaluation Network (SiREN), qualitative community comments were collected to demonstrate that consideration of evaluation upfront in planning programs enhanced their worth for data collection purposes (Bastian et al., 2018). This forward-thinking strategy enables the identification of likely barriers and opportunities in advance and ensures programs build from actual-time data rather than gazing into the rearview mirror and examining what has transpired. In the end, continuous data collecting and analyzing helps to move towards evidence-based practices that inform improved public health outcomes. In addition, collaboration among public health researchers, service agencies, and policymakers guarantees that efforts at data collection are pushed to optimal levels. Close collaborations intensify the data collection process through varied contributions and expertise in a bid to assess needs and effectiveness more comprehensively within a community. This collaboration, as shown in the SiREN model, emphasizes resource sharing in effective data gathering and evaluation (Bastian et al., 2018). The stakeholders in such collaborations can also be the faces to advocate for the sustainability of ongoing monitoring as key tools for accountability and transparency in public health initiatives. Through the creation of a culture where shared values and goals guide assessment, community health programs can draw on collective intelligence, ensuring responsiveness to emerging health trends within their territories (Figure 4.17).

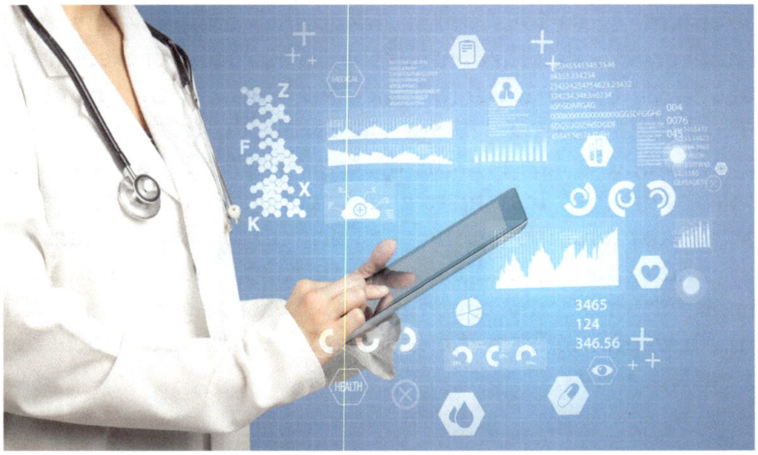

Figure 4.17. Collecting data for ongoing assessment.

Source: https://www.smartdatacollective.com/wp-content/uploads/2022/01/shutterstock_571935643.jpg.

4.6.3. Utilizing Feedback for Program Improvement

Effective program improvement in community health programs largely relies on the reflective application of feedback from various stakeholders. Such feedback may come from participants, healthcare professionals, and community members themselves, each providing valuable insights that may help characterize strengths and weaknesses in a program. Systematically gathering and reviewing such feedback allows health program planners to make sense of what changes and improvements are required. For example, feedback systems like surveys, focus groups, and individual interviews can offer qualitative and quantitative information capturing the perception of how services are understood and their effectiveness as a whole. Setting this information as a priority allows program coordinators to foster a responsive learning setting that promotes continued improvement in accord with the changing health needs of the community. Finally, the inclusion of feedback can be a force multiplier for innovation that keeps health programs adapting and thriving progressively in a constantly changing world. Informed decision-making based on thorough analysis necessitates not only the gathering of feedback but also the establishment of systematic processes for analyzing and acting on it. Enabling stakeholders to critically share their experiences with community health programs may reveal areas for improvement. For instance, clinicians and participants can identify inconsistencies in service provision or access barriers. As per Crump et al. (2015), participant feedback integration in programs, such as the Louisiana Sex Offender Treatment Program, was identified as of immense significance in therapeutic results, validating the central role of participant feedback. Furthermore, it enlightens on the significance of rigorous evaluation processes to validate whether feedback adaptations are associated with improved outcomes. Developing such a culture of evaluation enhances accountability and helps maintain ongoing discussion between all the stakeholders so that the program remains relevant and efficient in addressing community health issues. Moreover, strategic application of feedback not only enhances the efficacy of the program but also a more effective organizational framework that can support community health programs. Detailed case studies of the healthcare sector indicate that companies with high ability to institute feedback mechanisms also have the capability of keeping their talented employees and developing a good workplace culture. As is evident from N/A (2009), best practices for uses of employee feedback have proven to increase the morale of employees as well as client satisfaction, hence creating an improvement and retention cycle. By attaching a great priority to a culture of feedback, community health programs can better align their services to community expectations, thereby recording greater operational success. Alignment not only improves health outcomes but also trust and credibility, which are essential ingredients in mobilizing community members to participate in health activities. Thus, an effective creation of a feedback loop is necessary for ensuring the sustainability and effectiveness of community health programs.

SUMMARY

In planning community health programs, an integral conclusion consists of lessons learned, challenges faced, and the direct paths to follow for upcoming projects. As unveiled by the evidence of findings of the Teen Pregnancy Prevention Initiative, long-term evaluation of the health programs is crucial in revealing their effectiveness and the capability to be adjusted in real-world settings (N/A, 2007b). The program not only emphasized the targeted interventions role but also stressed the sustainability factor. When programs have grown up, it becomes very important to include feedback loops so that ongoing learning and improvement can be achieved. A well-stated conclusion must consider these and stress the need for ongoing adjustments based on the needs of the community so that the health programs remain relevant and useful. Moreover, successful community health programs must be careful in planning that is responsive to local situations and unforeseen challenges. The histories of the Merck Vaccine Network in Africa demonstrate how crucial it is to have sharp needs assessment in order to implement and integrate programs into existing health systems (Rinderle et al., 2012). Planning in this manner makes for a solid foundation that sustains long-term impact beyond the term of initial funding. The lessons learned in the program support the importance of meticulous planning that extends beyond content provision to include community engagement, partnership, and local leadership development. In short, the conclusion should look at how these strategies can be integrated into future planning in order to improve the sustainability and effectiveness of health interventions. Last but not least, the climax of community health program planning must be action-concluding in priority of stakeholder points of collaboration and empirical evidence integration. It is an appreciation of the fact that community health programs operate in complex social, economic, and political settings that demands a holistic approach responsive to diverse perspectives and life experiences. By developing collaboration among government agencies, NGOs, and community representatives, programs can be made more responsive to specific local health demands. Cooperative strategies with ongoing evaluation, adaptability, and sustainability planning are fundamental to the success of these efforts. Thus, the conclusion must contain a vision for a future of collaboration in public health, elevating the voices of served communities and driving action through shared commitment and responsibility.

The role of planning in community health programs cannot be overstated, as it acts as the template for effective health interventions. An orderly planning process enables health practitioners to identify targeted needs among a population, assess available resources, and distribute such resources optimally. Through data-driven approaches, planners can more effectively understand the specific issues that exist among different populations. Such proactive intervention not only assists in the development of special health programs but also facilitates the likelihood of achieving long-term outcomes. For instance, the implementation of successful programs, for instance, those initiated by Head Start, has been found to make a significant contribution to the knowledge base and practices of the participants, emphasizing the importance of well-crafted plans in addressing health disparities among low-income families (Chung et al., 2013). In addition, strategic planning aligns community health programs with overall public health priorities, which promotes inter-stakeholder collaboration. Effective initiatives tend to be collaborative endeavors among health organizations, local governments, and community constituents. Interagency collaboration is fundamental in addressing social determinants of health comprehensively, which have immense impacts on health outcomes. The Rhode Island Department of Health plan is a case in point, as it combined community-based approaches and data-driven assessments to establish geographically bounded Health Equity Zones (Alexander-Scott et al., 2017). By investing in local collaboratives that work on specific health issues, the program illustrates how planning can uncover unmet health needs as well as meet them. On this basis, addressing the needs of different populations is a sequential process, ultimately resulting in the enhancement of the overall effectiveness of the health system. Moreover, an effective planning process also encourages continuous monitoring and adaptation of community health programs. With ever-evolving changing health needs and emerging challenges, effective planning has feedback and reevaluation mechanisms to ensure that programs remain effective and beneficial. This iterative process is critical in fostering resilience within community health initiatives, as it allows for adjustments based on emerging data and community input. By prioritizing ongoing assessment, organizations can build on successful strategies while revising those that may not yield desired outcomes. The scalability and sustainability in health intervention, as a long-term impact of interventions such as the Health Care Institutes training program, demonstrates the interconnectedness of planning and successful health promotion activity (Chung et al., 2013).

KEY TERMS FROM THIS CHAPTER

- Civic engagement
- Community-based organizations
- Community involvement
- Cultural competence
- Drug addiction
- Ethnicity
- Family planning programs
- Flexible thinking
- Health Equity Zones
- Human resources
- Local engagement
- Non-profit organizations
- Obesity
- Community-based agencies
- Community dynamics
- Community resources
- Demographic data
- Educational attainment
- Evidence-based interventions
- Feedback mechanisms
- Goal setting
- Holistic approach
- Infectious disease epidemics
- Logistics
- Nutrition
- Participation

CLOSER LOOK

POSITIVE ADOLESCENT SEXUAL HEALTH (PASH)

Positive Adolescent Sexual Health (PASH) is a comprehensive and strengths-based approach that promotes healthy, respectful, and informed sexual development among young people. Unlike traditional sex education, which often focuses solely on risk prevention—such as avoiding unplanned pregnancies and sexually transmitted infections (STIs)—PASH takes a broader, more positive view of sexuality as a natural part of human development. It emphasizes open communication, consent, mutual respect, emotional intelligence, and the development of personal values and boundaries. By providing accurate, age-appropriate information and fostering supportive environments, PASH empowers adolescents to make informed and responsible decisions regarding their sexual health. This approach involves not just young people but also families, schools, health services, and the wider community in creating a culture of trust and respect. PASH programs often include peer-led education, workshops, and inclusive discussions that reflect the diverse identities and experiences of youth, including topics like sexual orientation, gender identity, body image, and mental well-being. By shifting the focus from fear and shame to empowerment and knowledge, PASH builds confidence and resilience in young people. Research has shown that such positive approaches do not encourage early sexual activity; rather, they support adolescents in understanding their values and making choices aligned with their well-being. Through PASH, young people learn to navigate relationships with care and respect, helping to reduce stigma, promote safer behaviors, and foster long-term sexual wellness. Ultimately, Positive Adolescent Sexual Health is about more than avoiding negative outcomes—it is about guiding adolescents through a critical stage of life with compassion, education, and support. It acknowledges that when youth are treated with respect and provided with the right tools, they are capable of making decisions that benefit their health, relationships, and future well-being.

REFERENCES

1. Alexander-Scott, N., Ankoma, A., et al. (2017). Rhode Island's Health Equity Zones: Addressing local problems with local solutions. https://digitalscholarship.unlv.edu/cgi/viewcontent.cgi?article=1643&context=jhdrp (accessed on 26th June 2025).
2. Allen, H., Antimisiaris, D., Clayton, R., Martin, M., et al. (2018). Pharmacy staff perspectives on alcohol and medication interaction prevention among older rural adults. https://core.ac.uk/download/232207281.pdf (accessed on 26th June 2025).
3. Arifuku, I., Lai, M., Nunez, M., & Morris, M. W. (2003). Culture counts: How five community-based organizations serve Asian and Pacific Islander youth. https://core.ac.uk/download/71341514.pdf (accessed on 26th June 2025).
4. Arreola, S., Ayala, G., Chong, S., Greenall, M., et al. (2014). DRAFT Report: Community systems strengthening toward a research agenda. https://core.ac.uk/download/pdf/19765254.pdf (accessed on 26th June 2025).
5. Assell, R. A. (1995). Students and service-learning: Planning programs with communities. https://core.ac.uk/download/232750622.pdf (accessed on 26th June 2025).
6. Bacher, J. A., Nolon, J. R., & Zezula, T. (2015). Land use planning for solar energy: Resource guide. https://core.ac.uk/download/80295087.pdf (accessed on 26th June 2025).
7. Baker, C., Collins, J. M., & Gorey, R. (2007). Financial coaching: A new approach for asset building? https://core.ac.uk/download/71346598.pdf (accessed on 26th June 2025).
8. Bastian, L., Brennan, S., Comfort, J., Crawford, G., et al. (2018). A research and evaluation capacity building model in Western Australia. https://core.ac.uk/download/213607723.pdf (accessed on 26th June 2025).
9. Becker, B. J., Cochran, T., Meyer, K., Norman, L., et al. (2019). Multi-campus DPT programmatic development in a public university: Leadership considerations. https://core.ac.uk/download/268253107.pdf (accessed on 26th June 2025).
10. Birnbaum, N., Masterson, E., & Schoomaker, H. (2011). State of Health Equity Movement, 2011 update Part C: Compendium of recommendations. *DRA Project Report No. 11–03*. https://core.ac.uk/download/pdf/18491812.pdf (accessed on 26th June 2025).
11. Bongiovanni, A., Emina, J., Koffi, T., Mensah, M., et al. (2018). Engaging men in family planning: Perspectives from married men in Lomé, Togo. https://core.ac.uk/download/323082130.pdf (accessed on 26th June 2025).
12. Bowman, C. C., Dobalian, A., Dougherty, M. B., Needleman, J., et al. (2014). The critical elements of effective academic-practice partnerships: A framework derived from the Department of Veterans Affairs Nursing Academy. https://core.ac.uk/download/323077324.pdf (accessed on 26th June 2025).
13. Brown, S., Greenberg, M., Vallei, A., Williams, C., et al. (2000). Frequency of use and perceived credibility of information sources and variations by socioeconomic factors among Savannah River stakeholders. https://core.ac.uk/download/72056488.pdf (accessed on 26th June 2025).
14. Carlson, N. F. (2003). Trusting in change. https://core.ac.uk/download/71355453.pdf (accessed on 26th June 2025).
15. Chavis, D. M., & Trent, T. R. (2009). Scope, scale, and sustainability: What it takes to create

lasting community change. https://core.ac.uk/download/10688026.pdf (accessed on 26th June 2025).

16. Chung, P. J., Herman, A., Nelson, B. B., Teutsch, S., et al. (2013). A structured management approach to implementation of health promotion interventions in Head Start. https://core.ac.uk/download/323079890.pdf (accessed on 26th June 2025).
17. Clymer, C., & Wyckoff, L. (2003). Employment retention essentials. https://core.ac.uk/download/71359613.pdf (accessed on 26th June 2025).
18. Cornman, H., Grimm, C. D., & Rana, S. (2005). Engaging local non-governmental organizations (NGOs) in the response to HIV/AIDS. https://core.ac.uk/download/72048685.pdf (accessed on 26th June 2025).
19. Crocker, B., Hansen, V., John-Leader, F., Pit, S., et al. (2019). A positive approach to adolescent sexual health promotion: A qualitative evaluation of key stakeholder perceptions of the Australian Positive Adolescent Sexual Health (PASH) Conference. https://core.ac.uk/download/222985547.pdf (accessed on 26th June 2025).
20. Crump, Y., Dailey, F. L. L., Merino, C., Underwood, M., et al. (2015). Preliminary results of the Louisiana Sex Offender Treatment Program. https://core.ac.uk/download/215482789.pdf (accessed on 26th June 2025).
21. Demeritt, A., Adams, J. E., Jr., Bowen, M., & De Wys, S. (2008). Performance pressure and resource allocation in Washington. https://core.ac.uk/download/71353769.pdf (accessed on 26th June 2025).
22. Derr, M. (2011). SAVI Community Information System. https://core.ac.uk/download/4696441-.pdf (accessed on 26th June 2025).
23. DeWitt John, E., Hollander, E., & Hansell, W. (2009). Putting community first: A promising approach to federal collaboration for environmental improvement: An evaluation of the Community Action for a Renewed Environment (CARE) Demonstration Program. https://core.ac.uk/download/71345950.pdf (accessed on 26th June 2025).
24. Donta, B., Battala, M., Dasgupta, A., Ghule, M., et al. (2016). CHARM, a gender equity and family planning intervention for men and couples in rural India: Protocol for the cluster randomized controlled trial evaluation. https://core.ac.uk/download/323065021.pdf (accessed on 26th June 2025).
25. DXC Technology. (2019). Organization change plan: Getting started. https://core.ac.uk/download/219376950.pdf (accessed on 26th June 2025).
26. Egan, S., Gaffield, M. E., & Temmerman, M. (2014). It's about time: WHO and partners release programming strategies for postpartum family planning. https://core.ac.uk/download/55769937.pdf (accessed on 26th June 2025).
27. Fabish, L., & Haas, P. J. (2013). Measuring the performance of livability programs, *MTI Report 12–06*. https://core.ac.uk/download/70410209.pdf (accessed on 26th June 2025).
28. Farrar, B., Gilmore, D., Lumby, E., Wang, G., Manson, K., Koester, L., & Mathew, R. (201-). Respite Partnership Collaborative (RPC) Innovation Project Evaluation: Report 1. https://core.ac.uk/download/80511005.pdf (accessed on 26th June 2025).
29. Gaddi, A. V. (2010). Alcuni abstract di articoli che trattano argomenti relativi all'eHealth. https://core.ac.uk/download/11175501.pdf (accessed on 26th June 2025).

30. Ghimire, D. R., Pratap, N., & Sharma, S. K. (2025). Ethnic differentials of the impact of family planning program on contraceptive use in Nepal. https://core.ac.uk/download/pdf/6423680.pdf (accessed on 26th June 2025).

31. Hair, E. C., Michelsen, E., & Zaff, J. F. (2002). Civic engagement programs and youth development: A synthesis. https://core.ac.uk/download/71347373.pdf (accessed on 26th June 2025).

32. Kaopua, L. S., Sy, A., Terada, T., Tofaeono, T., et al. (2019). "Making do, as best as we can" cancer in American Samoa: Qualitative methods and results. https://digitalscholarship.unlv.edu/cgi/viewcontent.cgi?article=2013&context=jhdrp (accessed on 26th June 2025).

33. Katz, E., & Kauder, R. (2011). Social enterprise businesses: A strategy for creating good jobs for people with disabilities. https://core.ac.uk/download/71345748.pdf (accessed on 26th June 2025).

34. Keller, A., Armijo, C., Bartsch, D., & Chung, P. (2012). Improving access to health through collaboration: Lessons learned from The Colorado Trust's Partnerships for Health Initiative evaluation. https://core.ac.uk/download/71360570.pdf (accessed on 26th June 2025).

35. Khoong, E. C., Lasee, C., Lewis, M., Stamatakis, K., et al. (2014). State practitioner insights into local public health challenges and opportunities in obesity prevention: A qualitative study. https://core.ac.uk/download/323079532.pdf (accessed on 26th June 2025).

36. Leibbrandt, L. (1997). Community participation in health care decisions. https://core.ac.uk/download/41234395.pdf (accessed on 26th June 2025).

37. Mutunga, C., & Hardee, K. (2009). Population and reproductive health in National Adaptation Programs of Action. https://core.ac.uk/download/71342633.pdf (accessed on 26th June 2025).

38. N/A. (2001). National blueprint: Increasing physical activity among adults age 50 and older. https://core.ac.uk/download/71346800.pdf (accessed on 26th June 2025).

39. N/A. (2007). Evaluation findings from the California Wellness Foundation's Teen Pregnancy Prevention Initiative. https://core.ac.uk/download/71351154.pdf (accessed on 26th June 2025).

40. N/A. (2007). Volunteering reinvented: Human capital solutions for the nonprofit sector. https://core.ac.uk/download/71340048.pdf (accessed on 26th June 2025).

41. N/A. (2008). Single point of entry long-term living resource system team report. https://core.ac.uk/download/11356924.pdf (accessed on 26th June 2025).

42. N/A. (2009). Wisdom at work: Retaining experienced RNs and their knowledge: Case studies of top performing organizations. https://core.ac.uk/download/71355878.pdf (accessed on 26th June 2025).

43. N/A. (2010). Healthy Returns Initiative: Strengthening mental health services in the juvenile justice system. https://core.ac.uk/download/71344788.pdf (accessed on 26th June 2025).

44. N/A. (2011). Meeting the challenge: Fiscal implications of dropout prevention in Massachusetts. https://core.ac.uk/download/71345592.pdf (accessed on 26th June 2025).

45. N/A. (2011). The political economy of sanitation: How can we increase investment and improve service for the poor? https://core.ac.uk/download/75783152.pdf (accessed on 26th June 2025).

46. N/A. (2012). Smart school budgeting: Resources for districts. https://core.ac.uk/download/71360023.pdf (accessed on 26th June 2025).

47. N/A. (2014). Disrupting poverty: Coming together to build financial security for individuals and communities. https://core.ac.uk/download/71365156.pdf (accessed on 26th June 2025)

48. N/A. (2015). Family at the center. https://core.ac.uk/download/86445003.pdf (accessed on 26th June 2025).

49. N/A. (2015). mFish Alpha Pilot: Building a roadmap for effective mobile technology to sustain fisheries and improve fisher livelihoods. https://core.ac.uk/download/80510800.pdf (accessed on 26th June 2025).

50. N/A. (2020). The Carbon Reduction Transportation Initiative at Northern Arizona University. https://core.ac.uk/download/322838318.pdf (accessed on 26th June 2025).

51. N/A. (2025). *J Public Health Manag Pract*. https://core.ac.uk/download/577754834.pdf (accessed on 26th June 2025).

52. Nofiandi, H. (Hardiles), Taufik, A. (Achmad), & Widayati, W. (Wiwik). (2014). Peran masyarakat dalam melaksanakan program Pamsimas di Desa Banjarsari Kecamatan Gajah Kabupaten Demak. https://media.neliti.com/media/publications/107730-ID-peran-masyarakat-dalam-melaksanakan-prog.pdf (accessed on 26th June 2025).

53. Poon, A., Gilmore, D., Lumby, E., Wang, G., & Koester, L. (2016). Respite Partnership Collaborative (RPC) Innovation Project Evaluation: Final report. https://core.ac.uk/download/80511006.pdf (accessed on 26th June 2025).

54. Rinderle, A., Hills, G., & Fiske, L. (2012). Boosting the immunization workforce: Lessons from the Merck Vaccine Network–Africa. https://core.ac.uk/download/71360220.pdf (accessed on 26th June 2025).

55. Rosales, L. M. (2016). An exploratory analysis of best practices for community resource coordination groups of Texas. https://core.ac.uk/download/211387225.pdf (accessed on 26th June 2025).

56. Sherwood, K. E. (2005). Evaluation of the Fighting Back Initiative. https://core.ac.uk/download/71359624.pdf (accessed on 26th June 2025).

57. Venkatesh, M. (2016). Improving women's reproductive health in India by educating men and families. https://open.bu.edu/bitstream/2144/22739/1/IIBVenkatesh.pdf (accessed on 26th June 2025).

58. Yu, H. C., Lewis-Charp, H., & Inouye, T. E. (2017). Advancing culturally responsive evaluations for boys and men of color. https://core.ac.uk/download/84911902.pdf (accessed on 26th June 2025).

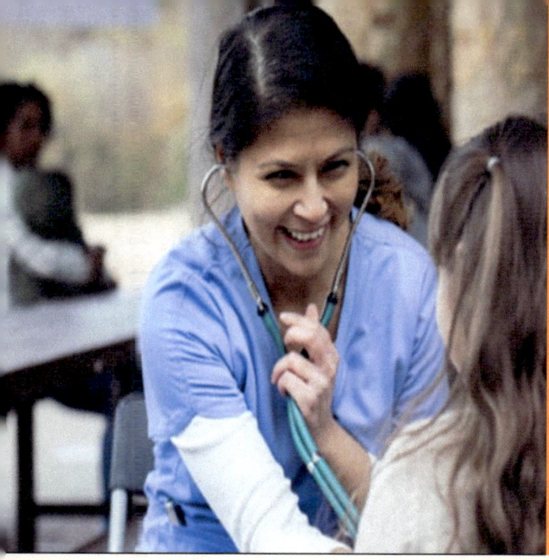

Chapter 5

COMMUNITY HEALTH IMPLEMENTATION STRATEGIES

Contents

Introduction

In current public health, implementation strategies within community health are important for developing strategies to bridge the gap between practice and evidence-based research in community settings. Since health disparities still exist, policymakers and practitioners are forced more and more to rely on effective implementation strategies in order to apply health interventions. That is where systematic analysis of implementation science—systematically analyzing how effectively health interventions are implemented within systems—enters the picture. By using a framework such as the Consolidated Framework for Implementation Research (CFIR), researchers can systematically analyze determinants of effectiveness of such interventions. This odyssey leads the way to discovering how the diverse strategies are applied in enhancing intervention effectiveness in community health, and in the process, enhancing health outcomes among diverse populations. Community health implementation strategies also encompass locating and dismantling the obstacles to the use of evidence-based practice. It will require a multi-faceted strategy in tackling such an issue by concentrating on training the workforce, activating the community resources, and encouraging leadership, among others. For instance, the CMS Accountable Health Communities (AHC) Model illustrates the manner in which collaborative activities will strengthen interventions in community health. Even with challenges revealed in qualitative assessment—e.g., inadequate staff training and resource limitation—barriers are induced by challenges like. Different organizations can find successfully prevailing facilitators that facilitate the implementation process amidst these challenges. The finding of such facilitators and barriers, particularly with qualitative assessment, informs current strategies, which are pivotal to improving health delivery systems in communities (Aarons et al., 2016). Finally, effective implementation of community health approaches demands collaborative effort among stakeholders, such as policymakers, health care providers, and community organizations. There must be context-specific evaluation of implemented strategies in which the participation of various stakeholders is promoted and in which there is a critical review of strategies against the context. Engaging community members on workgroups and advisory boards not only enhances the quality of interventions used but also ensures that interventions become more culturally appropriate and address particular needs of targeted populations. These general strategies have the ability to enable health interventions to be maintained and, through that, advance more significant public health goals to eliminate disparities and promote optimum overall community health (Aarons et al., 2016) (Figure 5.1).

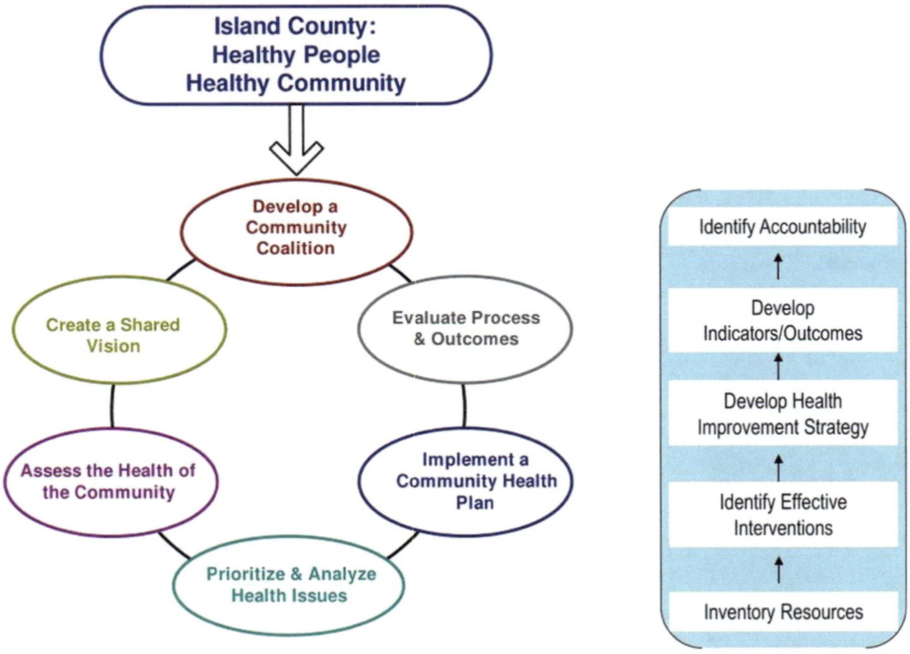

Figure 5.1. Community health implementation strategies.

Source: https://image3.slideserve.com/5933680/community-health-process-model-l.jpg.

Definition of Community Health

An interprofessional approach to the health of a population residing in an area is the definition of community health. It celebrates the general physical, emotional, and social health of people, concentrating on the relationship among various health determinants such as the environment, lifestyle, and support systems. Community health aims at ending disparities in health by ensuring that all people are treated with equal access to health care. Thus, it is an empowerment agent that stimulates the involvement of the local communities in health interventions and policies, pushing the residents to act as active players for improved health status. The active engagement translates into more responsible health education that takes into account community needs, linking the timely health interventions to long-term well-being goals.

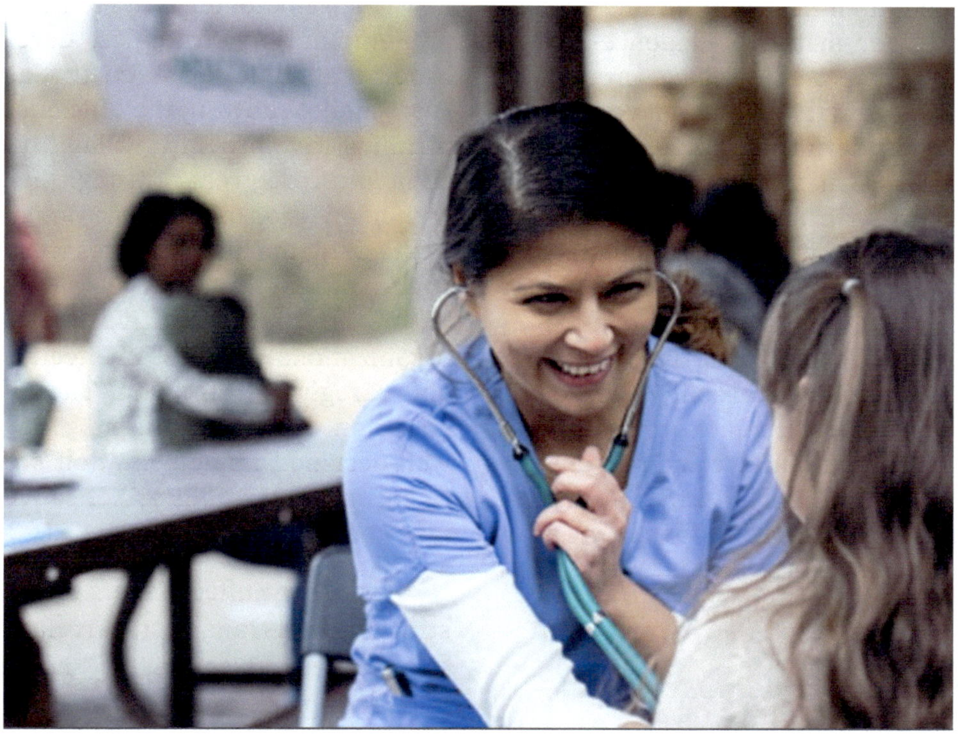

Figure 5.2. Community health.

Source: https://res.cloudinary.com/grand-canyon-university/image/fetch/w_750,h_564,c_fill,g_faces,q_auto/https://www.gcu.edu/sites/default/files/media/images/Blog/nursing-health-care/community%20health%20worker.jpg.

Community health information thus entails comprehending the link between individuals' behaviors that affect health and overall social structures, and through educational structures that affect health information at the community level (Ahmed et al., 2006). Besides ensuring individual health outcomes, community health also ensures creating and implementing effective health education programs for populations. These programs are crucial in bridging the theory-practice gap, as they allow communities to get to know their health problems and the interventions needed to correct them. Understanding that education is a necessary tool towards achieving quality health outcomes, community health practitioners can make well-being culture that spreads across the whole society. This strategy involves taking health education to various aspects of community life, beginning from schools and culminating in community organizations to ultimately an overarching focus on health in the community. Effective health education weaves in-school and out-of-school learning together to engage community resources for the extent of their importance in building long-term health literacy and resilience, as identified by the Health Action Schools project (Ahmed et al., 2006). Implementation of community health interventions typically encompasses a critical review of various innovative practices that enhance and maintain health programs across various groups. For instance, Evidence-Based Practice (EBP) Project states have created a classification system that identifies and classifies effective means of performing evidence-based health interventions. These implementations not only cater to short-term health requirements but also provide for establishing an environment for sustained improvement in health. In relation to state infrastructure, stakeholder buy-in, and routes of finance, community health programs can be initiated from the sustainability viewpoint. These aligned approaches create opportunities for replicative quality assurance and responsive service provision, which ultimately make interventions in health become pertinent and efficient in the community's constantly changing context of possible need (Figure 5.2).

Importance of Implementation Strategies

The contribution of implementation strategies towards community health cannot be overemphasized because they form the working basis on which theoretical models to practice are bridged. In efforts at improving the delivery of care, particularly among vulnerable populations, team models have been implemented variably in various practice sites. The co-integration of Medical Assistants (MAs) and Community Health Workers (CHWs), for instance, has yielded divergent results by local context, indicating the need for implementation tailoring. The findings document the heterogeneity and complexity of implementation processes and confirm that active leadership and positive team climates are enablers of MAs and CHWs' performance in their duties. Consequently, effective implementation strategies enhance not just service provision but also the professional skills of healthcare members of staff, thus contributing to improved diabetes care as well as other health outcomes in community care (Ayanian et al., 2014). In addition, the integration of technology solutions to community health is leading towards the new change potential that results from effective implementation strategies. CareNav, a web-based statewide resource in California, is a great model showing the efficiency of strategic planning in improving availability of resources to family caregivers. Through evidence-based implementation, by adopting an approach such as the CFIR, the different sites were successfully rolled out by community agencies. Results of the strategic initiative show remarkable organizational progress in effectiveness, equity, and caregiver well-being. The 18-month full adoption report highlights the importance well-designed implementation strategies have to ensure innovations are effectively instituted into current systems (Bell et al., 2024).

Finally, the effectiveness of implementation strategies has a direct correlation with the effectiveness of community health programs. Strategic gaps can lead to uneven practice and missed opportunities for increased health outcomes. As seen through the diverse experiences of employing CHWs and MAs, rigid fidelity to implementation models is perhaps not feasible in a given set of needs and settings of various healthcare organizations. A responsive and agile culture will better be able to hurdle the challenges against community health providers. Thus, utmost significance must be placed in setting, piloting, and refining evidence-based and context-specific implementation plans. Not only does it enhance the provision of care but also allows the patients to be more involved in managing their health conditions, with attendant population benefits to population outcomes of health (Ayanian et al., 2014; Bell et al., 2024).

5.1. Assessment of Community Health Needs

Community health needs assessment is a central process that guides healthcare policy and strategic decision-making at a community level. Systematic evaluation is scheduled to gather data to ascertain the health needs, resources, and service deficits relevant to a population. They are founded on tools such as surveys, focus groups, and community engagement, which enable health professionals to obtain detailed information about local determinants of health. In addition, such a knowledge base provides a basis for prioritizing in resource allocation as well as special intervention design. Additionally, tailoring these assessments to include socio-cultural environments, particularly in mixed populations, encourages the use of more culturally sensitive measures of health. Conducting community health needs assessment is vital in driving accessible health as well as improved health outcomes, particularly among vulnerable groups. The incorporation of lay people's views through participatory research facilitates a nuance of understanding barriers to care, thereby enhancing the applicability of evidence-based interventions. For example, incorporation of lay health workers can increase parental engagement in behavioral parent training programs considerably, as seen in description of their capacity to engage excluded groups more effectively (Barnett et al., 2019). These in-place residents already have valuable information to tap into regarding the identification of culturally specific barriers. Thus, these tailored strategies developed based on these assessments can be helpful contributions towards program participation and success. Additionally, this assessment process is for need determination purposes but is also for inclusion of measurement of present resources and facilities within community environments. It assists communities in optimizing the use and application of evidence-based practices that are attuned to their own settings. The utilization of models such as Implementation Mapping makes it possible to map facilitators and barriers in healthcare delivery systems (Chenier et al., 2022). As such, the evaluation produces an integrated image that, in addition to depicting health deficits, utilizes existing capacities in a manner that holds the potential for greater health dividends. By focusing on strengthening integration among services as well as widening access to interventions, community health needs assessments become central to the continuous process of expanding public health.

5.1.1. Identifying Health Disparities

Determination of health disparities is an important step in formulating responsive community health implementation strategies. Health disparities refer to health differences and access to care that are linked to social, economic, and environmental disadvantage. These disparities can be enormously significant in the case of vulnerable populations, including racial and ethnic minorities, low-income populations, and rural residents. In response to the specific health concerns and issues of these groups, public health practitioners may design professional interventions that address the underlying causes, including insufficient access to quality care, dietary problems, and inadequate health literacy. Analysis of these disparities entails multi-dimensional intervention, both the collection of health information and understanding of social determinants of health, in a situation where overall handling of disparities is crucial (Thalia, 2025). Data-driven decision-making (DDDM) plays a crucial role in identifying and intervening on health disparities among populations. By such a process, there can be systematic collection and analysis of various categories of data, i.e., epidemiologic data, demographic data, and social determinants of health data. Based on these categories of data, public health professionals can identify targeted needs at the community level and intervene to meet such needs. The issues of availability of data and ethics will obstruct the application of DDDM, but the worth of the smart investment of resources and the accuracy of intervention design which it can provide is invaluable. Health disparities must be addressed through developing policy guidelines based on identified needs as reflected by DDDM so that it not only becomes evidence-based but also fair, and effective in health promotion among vulnerable people (Thalia, 2025). Community participation is also a vital component of identification of health disparities. Interventions such as community advisory boards (CABs) have proved effective in helping to bridge the communication gap between health organizations and the communities that they represent. Health centers, for instance, in the COVID-19 pandemic, utilized CABs to decide on what community needs were and expand testing outreach to communities with high health disparities. Research indicates that engaging the local stakeholders helps to create a sense of trust and respect, thus leading to better implementation of interventions. Additionally, learning gained through the community can be utilized in developing realistic toolkits facilitating evidence-based decision-making. Through an active engagement of the community partners in program planning and health screenings, public health interventions can be designed to be more responsive to the unique challenges faced by underrepresented groups and eventually lead to more effective closure of health disparities (Figure 5.3).

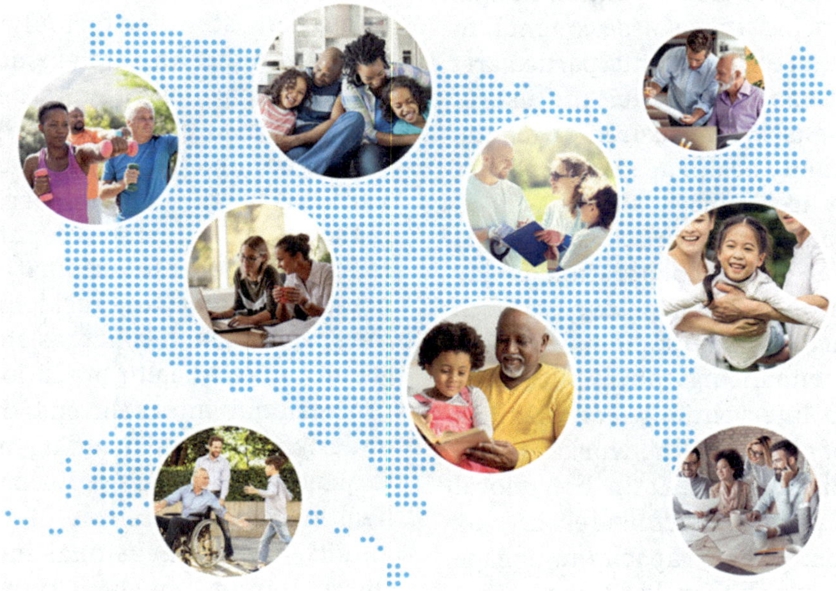

Figure 5.3. Identifying health disparities.

Source: https://eadn-wc03-8290287.nxedge.io/wp-content/uploads/2023/05/HealthEquityGuide01_thumb5.png.

5.1.2. Utilizing Community Surveys and Data

The integration of community surveys and data-collecting mechanisms is a crucial building block in the development of effective community health implementation strategies. By leveraging the richness of data available from surveys, public health leaders and managers can recognize the specific health issues, likes, and dislikes of their target populations. For instance, the onset of Big Data, characterized by its immense volume, variety, and velocity, has transformed the landscape of health research. The use of sophisticated analytic tools enables stakeholders to construct meaning from complicated data sets, thereby creating evidence that can be used for programmatic intervention and policy development (Usher et al., 2015). Such extensive engagement with community data enables the establishment of ownership and participation among residents, hence culminating in a participatory health promotion and disease prevention approach. Besides, community surveys also help determine inequalities in health outcomes and access to services among vulnerable groups. With the application of systematic data collection methods, health organizations can ascertain key issues such as environmental risks, chronic diseases prevalence, and healthcare availability. For example, the National Dialogue on Green and Healthy Homes demonstrates the potential for engaging multiple stakeholders in online discussion to yield actionable lessons contributing to low- and moderate-income families' health and safety. Through this program, the participants generated over 100 ideas and produced actionable recommendations that were effective in response to their community's particular needs (Reeder et al., 2011). These participatory strategies of information collection are essential in designing responsive health policies that translate the unique problems of different population segments. Applying the findings of community surveys in the formulation of health policies not only makes them more pertinent but also facilitates accountability and transparency in health programs. Utilizing evidence-based strategies allows for constant evaluation and improvement of programs through real-life community inputs. In addition, as stakeholders interact with each other to examine and make meaning of these data, they create a shared consensus around health determinants and interventions. This joint dynamic strengthens alliances among sectors and disciplines, ultimately leading to a more holistic approach to combating public health concerns. The successful implementation of community health strategies depends on the synergy among survey data, community involvement, and a responsive response to emergent health patterns—conditions intrinsic to healthier communities.

5.1.3. Engaging Stakeholders in the Assessment Process

Effective stakeholder engagement in the assessment process is crucial for the successful implementation of community health strategies. By engaging a multi-group stakeholder group—e.g., health professionals, community leaders, and residents—communities are able to contribute valuable information that enhances both the validity and applicability of assessments. This participation develops a stakeholder ownership that is crucial for ensuring that the health initiatives are tailored to meet the specific needs and wants of the community. Evidence indicates that actively engaging stakeholders facilitates more representative appraisals which lead to improved health outcomes and increased community trust within health systems. Engaging multiple voices not only results in richer data collected but also facilitates the identification of systematic barriers that could hamper progress for community health endeavors, reaffirming the necessity of a collaborative approach to assessment (Dary et al., 2013). Furthermore, stakeholder involvement in the evaluation process ensures that adopted strategies are aligned with the health priorities, values, and goals of the community. This agreement is essential in addressing challenges such as care access and health equity, which are more likely to be influenced by social determinants of health. For instance, when the stakeholders identify their specific needs and concerns, more effective interventions are delivered that have the potential to close the health disparities for the community's people. Additionally, the process of involvement also informs stakeholders about the health issues at stake, producing a more informed citizen well-equipped to battle for their needs and collaborate on solutions. This collective effort not only reinforces the impact of community health interventions but also builds a culture of ongoing conversation and collaboration between the community and health workers (Adelman et al., 2018). Last, sustainability of the implementation process for community health also relies on ongoing participation and feedback from stakeholders throughout the assessment process. Regular stakeholder consultation ensures accountability and promotes adaptive management, enabling health programs to adapt to changing community patterns and new health trends. Further, through open communication channels, stakeholders are able to exchange their expertise and experience, from which future assessment and interventions may be informed. This recursive process not only enhances the quality of data collected but also promotes community resilience through developing strong networks that support health initiatives in the long run. In general, putting a focus on stakeholders' involvement in planning reviews is essential to the long-term effectiveness and sustainability of community health strategies, thereby ensuring the efforts initiate desired changes in all the parties involved (Adelman et al., 2018; Dary et al., 2013) (Figure 5.4).

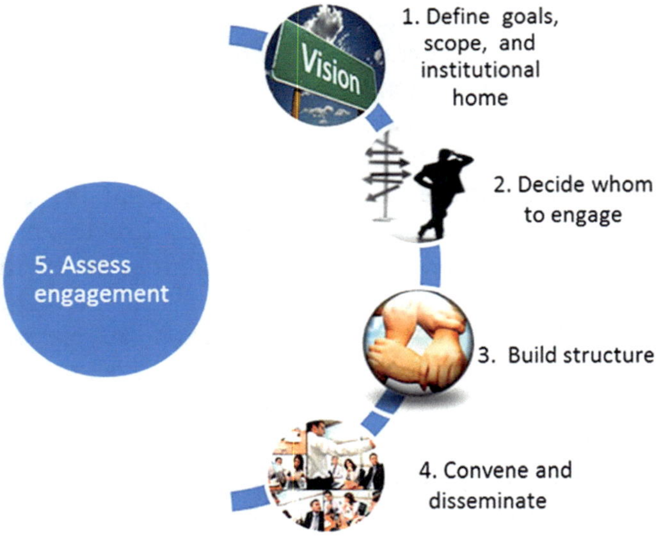

Figure 5.4. Engaging stakeholders in the assessment process.

Source: https://www.ahrq.gov/sites/default/files/wysiwyg/policymakers/chipra/demoeval/what-we-learned/implementation-guides/implementation-guide1/impguide1fig1.jpg.

5.2. Development of Health Programs

Health program development is predicated upon the diverse health needs and situations of the target communities. Effective health programs must be focused on identifying the unique health concerns of the members of the community, which can vary significantly in line with demographic, socioeconomic, and environmental factors. For instance, conducting a comprehensive health assessment can identify key elements such as availability of health foods and recreational facilities, which directly impact the formulation of targeted interventions. In line with this style of reasoning, the Eastlake-Garfield health assessment exemplifies the usefulness of community strengths and barriers to health assessment, thereby forming a solid foundation for program development. These custom approaches are capable of using existing community resources and forging alliances between various actors, creating a better and more sustainable health program that effectively improves community well-being. Key to the success of health programs is having evidence-based practices, which incorporate the latest research and community knowledge. This two-pronged approach guarantees that not only do health programs make scientific sense but also that they are fitting to the culture and acceptable to the community. Implementation of interventions in faith community nursing is one such example, proving how spiritual and holistic health can be seamlessly incorporated into public health programs.

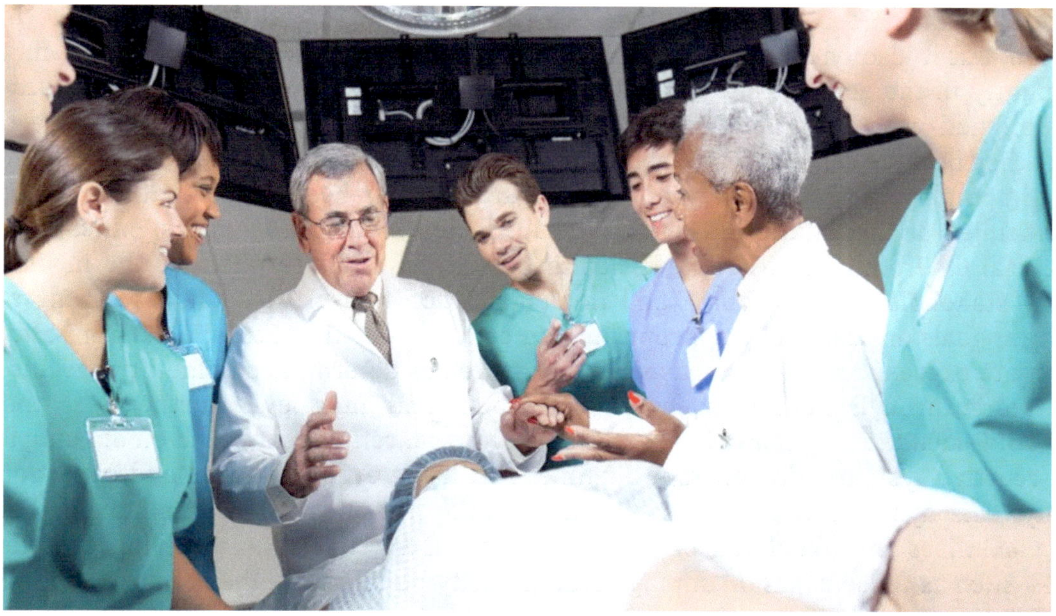

Figure 5.5. Development of health programs.

Source: https://tinehealth.com/wp-content/uploads/2017/05/Tine-Website-Photos-Articles-12.jpg.

Through support of self-efficacy and identification of health-promoting behaviors, such interventions demonstrate that health programs are able to create tangible changes in community health results. Assessments in studies reported by Callaghan found participants experienced greater adoption of healthy behaviors, particularly with nursing students and elderly groups. This achievement shows the critical role that context-sensitive strategies play in the development of successful health programs that respond to the lived experiences of community members (Callaghan et al., 2016). Finally, the sustainability of health programs is dependent on whether or not they can adapt and respond to evolving community needs and contexts. Ongoing evaluation is essential in determining the success of interventions and where there needs to be a change. Health programs must include mechanisms for participants' feedback so that their suggestions are incorporated in order to guide subsequent iterations of the program. An example of strategies developed for the Eastlake-Garfield community emphasizes continuous community involvement in planning and evaluation (N/A, 2013). In addition to increasing community ownership, this participatory planning fosters trust, which is key to long-term success. Furthermore, current partnerships with the local stakeholders and organizations maximize dynamic guideline for addressing health disparities and maximize resource mobilization. Lastly, continuous development and refinement of health programs must take an iterative process that prioritizes collaboration, responsiveness to community health needs, and sustainability (Figure 5.5).

5.2.1. Setting Clear Health Objectives

Clear health objectives are necessary in the effectiveness of implementation strategies for community health. By establishing some, measurable, achievable, relevant, and time-bound (SMART) goals, health programs are able to aim for tangible outcomes that address the unique needs of a given community. Not only does this allow for more facilitation in regard to assessing the impact of intervention, but it also encourages stakeholders to be held accountable. Engaging members from the community in the goal-setting process is necessary, as their contribution guarantees that the goals are aligned with the immediate area. Thus, the health programs become more than just initiatives; they become collective endeavors aimed at significant change, thereby making the people in the community part of what they do with regard to their health[insert citation]. Application of the principles of Community-Based Participatory Research (CBPR) can significantly improve organizational environment of definable health objectives. CBPR emphasizes the involvement of community stakeholders at planning and implementation phases of health programs to ensure that program goals are culturally appropriate and context-sensitive. Stakeholders are afforded the opportunity to express concerns and aspirations, as well as determine community-specific barriers and facilitators, through methods such as focus groups and interviews. Furthermore, the cyclical nature of CBPR facilitates an iterative process of health goal refinement based on ongoing feedback, so that a reactive system is in constant alignment with the evolving needs and conditions of the community. This dynamic approach to objective-setting not only encourages stakeholder uptake but also maximizes the likelihood of health success[insert citation]. In solving complex health disparities, such as those common among rural minority populations, the setting of defined health targets becomes increasingly significant. For instance, evidence has shown that effective application of evidence-based interventions (EBIs) hinges on detailed goals that are directly formulated for specific populations, such as African American populations with a high incidence of cardiovascular conditions. By employing a systematic method like intervention mapping with CBPR, communities can articulate goals that target determinants of individual, interpersonal, and environmental health. This multi-layered method not only enables comprehensive behavior goal assessments but also ensures that interventions are meaningful and stimulating to the target population, maximizing the impact of community health interventions[insert citation].

5.2.2. Designing Culturally Competent Interventions

In planning implementation strategies of community health, intervention design for culturally sensitive interventions is of greatest significance in dealing with pertinent and timely health issues like obesity among target populations. African-American communities, for example, have the highest incidence of obesity, an issue that causes most chronic diseases like cardiovascular diseases and diabetes. Health promotion interventions can be generated from faith-based groups considering the influential role that these groups play in African-American society. To ensure the best possible effectiveness of such interventions, it is essential that their design considers the sociocultural environment of the community. Incorporating church leaders and congregation in the design ensures not only ownership but also ensures that programs appeal effectively to the community's values and beliefs, thus ensuring higher participation and success at behavior changes towards reducing obesity in such settings (Mbe and Kougang Anne, 2017).

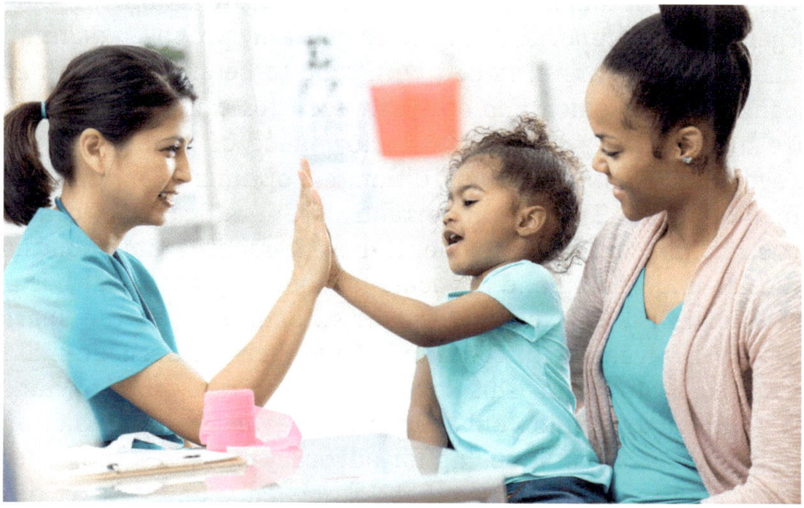

Figure 5.6. Designing culturally competent interventions.

Source: https://minoritynurse.com/wp-content/uploads/2024/05/promoting-cultural-competence-humility-in-nursing-web.png.

In addition, culturally competent intervention as a concept extends beyond reacting to health behaviors; it necessitates a profound appreciation of the cultural expectations and norms of the target population. Interaction of health educators with insight into these cultural factors enables the construction of a tailored approach that respects local tradition and practice. It has been found that interventions that recognize and draw upon the cultural strengths of communities are more effective. For instance, holistic intervention-based health interventions, which consider spiritual and cultural factors along with physical well-being, have been promising for achieving lasting behavioral changes among participants (Mbe and Kougang Anne, 2017).

Effective integration of local community leaders' viewpoints often results in higher community involvement, thus the possibility of achieving long-term health impacts. Of particular interest is the practice of culturally responsive evaluations as well, namely when applied to vulnerable populations such as boys and men of color (BMOC). BMOC programs, as initiated through efforts like the My Brothers Keeper Task Force, all point to the need for particular strategies that act upon the challenges of this population directly. However, current efforts are in their beginning stages, so there appears to be a pressing demand for robust evaluations that have the power to inform best practices. A focus on culturally responsive evaluation will enable stakeholders to ensure interventions are not only effective, but also equitable, bridging opportunity gaps that continue to leave behind BMOC. This commitment to culturally competent design not only reinforces community health strategy, but also aligns with broader public health goals aimed at health equity (Figure 5.6).

5.2.3. Incorporating Evidence-based Practices (EBPs)

Incorporating EBPs is essential in advancing community health implementation strategies, particularly as public health agencies strive to reduce disease burden and improve overall population health. Implementing EBPs enhances a rigorous approach to integrating the latest research evidence into public health interventions, enabling organizations to address present health challenges effectively. Leadership support is critical in this integration, as the necessity of having leaders to guide EBPH processes in their organizations supports. Giving priority to why proposed plans are being considered and ensuring that staff members are provided with time to be engaged with associated evidence are a few of the means through which public health agencies can ensure that EBPs flourish. This supportive structure ultimately optimizes the performance of health interventions and makes them responsive to evolving community needs, ultimately optimizing improved health outcomes in populations (Friedman et al., 2012). More importantly, the significance of community involvement cannot be overemphasized in incorporating evidence-based practices into public health interventions. Involving communities to understand and advocate for their rights to health is a direct connection to successful adoption of EBPs. This empowerment extends beyond the sharing of information to encompass the active involvement of community members in decision-making processes that guide health interventions. By following this participatory process, public health organizations are able to draw on local knowledge which enhances the relevance and uptake of health initiatives. Additionally, involving civil society in lobbying for advocacy increases the collective voices, which in turn pushes legislative and policy changes that acknowledge and respect the right to health as a right-based norm.

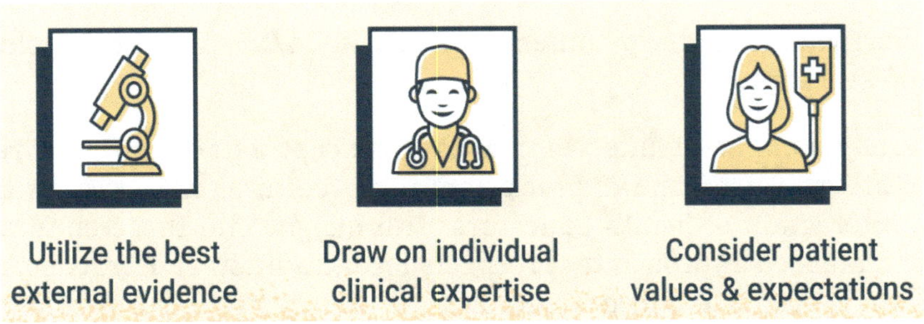

Figure 5.7. Incorporating evidence-based practices.

Source: https://www.prowritings.com/wp-content/uploads/2022/11/Evidence-Based-Practice-nursing-papers.png.

This multi-pronged strategy tackles inequalities in health while solidifying the reaffirmation of evidence-based approaches to implementation in community health (Friedman et al., 2012). For the realization of the optimal utilization of evidence-based practices as a component of community health initiatives, strong organizational systems that will support evidence-based practices need to be developed. This includes creating enabling structures which can facilitate continuous training and technical assistance to public health professionals to enhance their capacity to utilize evidence. Leadership commitment to facilitating integration between program areas is critical to the dismantling of barriers such as funding uncertainty and political resistance. Through embracing an organizational culture that is centered around EBPs, health departments can better equip their staff members to overcome challenges and to implement effective health solutions. Lastly, the successful implementation of evidence-based practices depends on a model of teamwork that brings together strategic investments, leadership, and community engagement and aligns them with one another as the drivers of effective health implementation strategies (Allen et al., 2018) (Figure 5.7).

5.3. Resource Allocation and Funding

Effective funding and resource allocation are critical elements in the implementation of community health strategies because they directly influence the capacity to act on health disparities. Local health systems are very likely to highly rely on the presence of available financial resources for ensuring accessibility and availability of services. For instance, efficient funding arrangements can facilitate the creation of health infrastructure, workforce expansions, and improved service delivery at a local community level. Through calculated investments in community health initiatives, policymakers can achieve vast long-term returns because improved access to resources directly correlates with improved health outcomes. With the rising complexity of the public health issues at the community level, this correlation is more relevant. Increased investment eventually creates a platform that not only allows for direct health interventions but also supports open-ended practice that establishes community resilience and empowers people to become active participants in their own health. Decentralization of decision-making when it comes to the provision of resources can also lead to more effective community health approaches. Where local authorities have greater autonomy in finance, they can develop interventions according to the specific needs of their populations. Localized design helps in addressing challenges such as transport, cultural specificity, and access barriers that vary across communities. Furthermore, decentralization, as seen in Mozambique's health system, aligns resources with service beneficiaries and allows for the empowerment of district-level administration (Pio et al., 2013). District capacity building ensures that the funds are utilized in an efficient manner and that community health plans consider the unique requirements of each area. Ultimately, the complementarity between resource allocation and decentralized management can stimulate improved health service delivery, increasing the aggregate quality and efficiency of community health programs. Furthermore, the application of evidence-based methods in resource allocation ensures maximum impact of spending on community health outcomes. Data-driven strategies enable health managers to track and quantify the impact of various interventions. For instance, Mozambiques Population Health Implementation and Training (PHIT) Partnership identifies the use of routine data and capacity in management as key to informing the improvement in the health system (Pio et al., 2013). With robust data, policymakers can invest in interventions that have been shown to yield beneficial health outcomes. This emphasis on data not only promotes accountability but also fosters a culture of continuous improvement in health services provision. As communities operate under limited resources, the use of data-informed strategies in the decision to fund ensures that resources are efficiently and effectively utilized, which leads to a more resilient and responsive health system that caters to different populations.

5.3.1. Identifying Potential Funding Sources

Within the scope of community health implementation strategies, identification of the possible sources of funding is critical in order to maintain programs and projects. Organizations must be able to carefully walk through the complex landscape of funding opportunities such as federal grants, state appropriations, private foundations, and corporate sponsorships. Carrying out vast research to map out available sources of funding not only allows organizations to spend monetary funds in an efficient way but also allows them to match available sources of finance to their respective missions and programmatic needs. The advanced awareness of available sources can significantly increase the chances of financing, rendering community health programs effectively funded and able to address the needs of underprivileged groups.

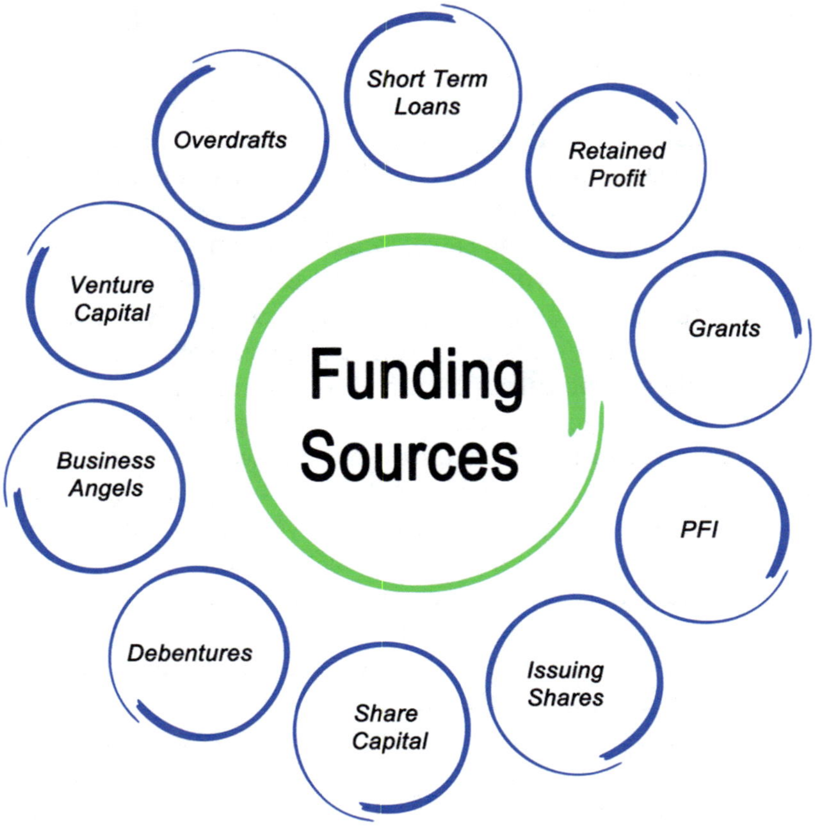

Figure 5.8. Identifying potential funding sources.

Source: https://thumbs.dreamstime.com/b/funding-sources-diagram-important-94363896.jpg.

Moreover, intermediary organizations have also emerged as key players in bridging the gap between funders and health providers at community levels. Intermediary organizations possess the expertise of enhancing service delivery by serving as conduits for funds, creating partnerships among stakeholders, and ensuring quality assurance standards compliance. Through connecting health initiatives to right sources of funds, intermediaries can significantly enhance the effectiveness of community health strategies. As defined through recent findings, these organizations help organizations navigate funding complexities while promoting broad networks of services that foster collaboration and innovation in the industry (Trends et al., 2012). Their involvement is critical for ensuring community health interventions are not only funded but also sustainable and effective. Moreover, reviewing successful case studies, i.e., those establishing mental health identification and intervention systems for youth, further supports the importance of well-systematized funding approaches. This initiative is about building systematic mechanisms in states like Colorado and Massachusetts, highlighting inclusive partnerships that create momentum and enhance service delivery (Lyman et al., 2010). Through an analysis of accomplishments and failures in such projects, organizations can gain knowledge on effective funding strategies and establish strong frameworks of partnerships to go after collective opportunities for funding. Ultimately, gaining knowledge of the intricacies of funding spaces and partnership dynamics can significantly enhance implementation strategies for community health, leading to improved health outcomes among target populations (Figure 5.8).

5.3.2. Budgeting for Community Health Initiatives

Effective budgeting for community health programs is a fundamental component of the implementation of sound health strategy. Properly formulated budget not only allocates necessary funds but also allocates priorities based on the healthcare needs of the community. By taking into account comprehensive prospective costs varying from personnel, supplies, outreach, and program maintenance, health agencies can develop financial strategies that are sustainable. Moreover, citizen participation in the budgeting process can result in greater transparency and accountability, which can be utilized to foster trust and sustainable partnerships. The participatory process is one where expenditures are a reflection of the population's needs and priorities, ensuring that there is cooperation for effective health results, thus the importance of co-participation in health projects, as reported by previous studies (Chan et al., 2025).

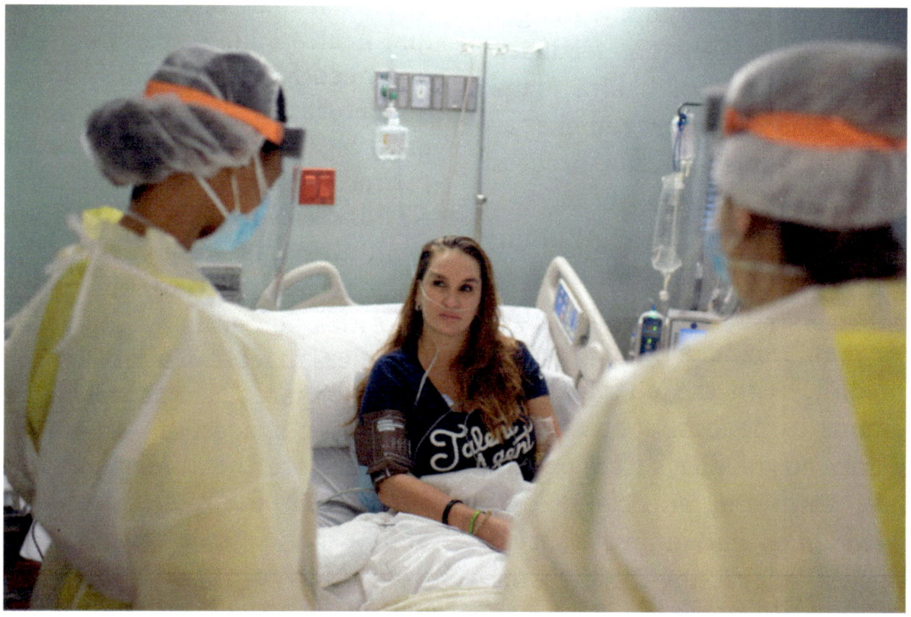

Figure 5.9. Budgeting for community health initiatives.

Source: https://www.commonwealthfund.org/sites/default/files/Murray_Global_Hospital_Budget.png.

Also, the budgeting cycle of community health programs must include financing sources which appeal to a wide range of potential stakeholders, including government agencies, nongovernmental organizations, and private sector nongovernmental partners. By securing different sources of funding, such as donations, grants, and public-private collaborations, organizations minimize the financial risk in implementing health programs. Securing stable sources of funding generally depends on demonstrating the potential benefit to health outcomes that the program will have, which can be supported by evidence-based indicators and previous successes. The MovEMENTs checklist offers models for improved implementation of health programs that emphasize the importance of resource mobilization and network development as entities are encouraged to incorporate different voices in consideration while budgeting in a bid to foster sustainability (Chan et al., 2025). Lastly, constant review of the success of the budget will help ensure that community health programs remain responsive and relevant to the needs of the community today. Budget reviews have to include stakeholder feedback in assessing the cost impact of health plans and ascertaining areas of improvement or adjustment. This constant evaluation process also dictates whether the spending is aligned with participatory methods strengthening community involvement in decision-making processes regarding health, underscoring the relationship between financial management and equity in health. With the alignment of the funding methods to fit local contexts and incorporating continuous feedback from people in the community, health programs can deliver more efficient outcomes and improve fiscal sustainability, thereby addressing the pressing challenges facing health systems worldwide (Traub et al., 2025) (Figure 5.9).

5.3.3. Ensuring Sustainable Resource Management

Sustainable management of resources is key to enhancing community health, especially in the context of scarce resources such as water land, and energy. Corrective measures should promote equilibrium between consumption and conservation while being cognizant of the fact that unrestricted exploitation of resources may have adverse public health implications. For instance, inefficient water management results in water-borne diseases while inefficient land management results in food insecurity, and both are more impactful on the poor. Community-based initiatives to promote agricultural production, water stewardship, and renewable energy utilization can play a significant role in enhancing the well-being and health of people. These initiatives also empower community members, supporting local governance and participation, thus supporting ownership. The need for strategies that align to sustainable development principles, as outlined in the UN Development Assistance Framework, cannot be overstated since they offer a framework to holistic environmental and health administration (N/A, 2014). There is a need for communities, local governments, and international organizations to collaborate in ensuring effective implementation of sustainable resource management measures. The United Nations Development Assistance Framework facilitates this cooperation by ensuring that all efforts conform to local needs and national priorities. Conformity to these allows community members to feel a sense of agency through their ability to participate actively in decision-making processes concerning resource management. Furthermore, the development of human capital through the education of people on sustainability and health fosters a culture of stewardship and awareness. As communities acquire knowledge and skills in managing resources sustainably, they are empowered to effectively deal with public health issues. The focus on participatory mechanisms provides a conducive atmosphere that leads to the creation of specific strategies that accommodate the distinct conditions in every community, thereby contributing to the general enhancement of public health and resilience (N/A, 2014). USAID's Water and Development Strategy 2013–2018 delivers critical information regarding how water management can be used to promote health. By engagement with local water sectors and operating unit coordination, the strategy focuses on having a joint framework for resource management. This guarantees that there are aligned efforts for health and water, allowing for more effective and efficient interventions to manage community health issues. Good water management practices enhance sanitation, prevent disease spread, and promote nutrition, and this is, in turn, responsible for total improvement in health. Periodic refining of such measures is evidence of the evolving nature of changing needs in communities and the evolving situation of resource management and so strategies become context-pertinent and effective. Through the integration of sustainable methods into community health planning, an opportunity is created not only for present-day health achievements but also for future sustainability of the environment.

5.4. Community Engagement and Participation

Involvement and participation of communities are pillars to the success of community health implementation plans. By engaging actively through members of the communities, programs are made relevant, responsive, and sustainable. The mutual process empowers stakeholders, ranging from health workers to those residing in neighborhoods, to provide input and expertise, which can lead to specialized health solutions addressing distinct local needs. For instance, evidence from maternal and child health initiatives research through stakeholder engagement shows a high positive relationship between stakeholder involvement and the successful achievement of community health objectives, with a reported correlation coefficient of 0.983.

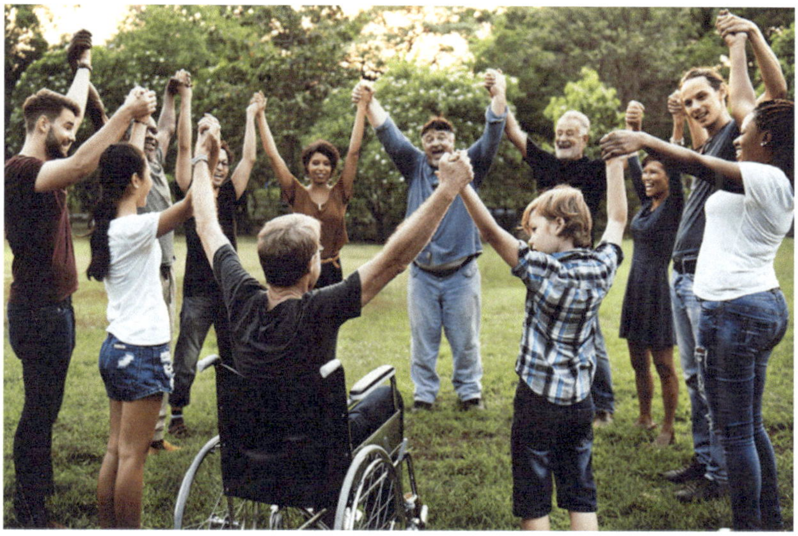

Figure 5.10. Community engagement and participation.

Source: https://rehmatsandhufoundation.com.au/wp-content/uploads/2019/11/Mar2019-community1200x630.png.

This evidence proves the fact that if community stakeholders are involved in health decision-making, there are high chances of achieving intended health outcomes, which enhance overall community health dynamics (Muasya et al., 2023). Moreover, the issue of historical distrust among certain groups calls for innovative and specifically focused work with communities. In groups such as Gypsy/Travelers who are marginalized, deep-rooted structural and cultural barriers often hinder access to health services. A multi-method study for building trust between Gypsy/Travelers and mainstream healthcare showcases the worth of methodologically diverse methods for building engagement. Through systematic reviews and case studies, the study identifies effective mechanisms of community engagement that speak to the needs of these populations. By understanding the unique health needs and attitudes in these communities, healthcare providers can implement mechanisms that enhance participation and build trust, reducing health inequalities and promoting service use (Coulter et al., 2016). Overall, promoting community involvement and participation is not merely an addendum to public health interventions; it is a requirement. Successful health interventions rely on incorporating local views and understanding community dynamics. In order to promote overall health outcomes, interventions must prioritize dialogue, collaborative decision-making, and the building of trust. As attested by the correlation between stakeholder engagement and project success, using participatory methods in community health intervention leads to better and more sustainable results. Further, studies in marginalized communities point out the inevitable necessity of tailored engagement strategies that identify and overcome current obstacles, thus facilitating an improved state of health for all communities (Figure 5.10).

5.4.1. Building Trust Within the Community

Establishing trust between people within a community is a critical component of successful implementation strategies of community health. Trust enables open communication, leads to increased collaboration in health programs, and fosters coordination among stakeholders. When members within a community feel that their health needs are genuinely valued, they will greatly cooperate with health programs seeking to improve their health. For instance, initiatives such as The Colorado Trust's strategy of Early Childhood Council Health Integration not only touched on the delivery of health services but also focused on building trust through local partnerships. This allowed for enhanced coordination of resources, ultimately leading to improved health outcomes for children and families in the community, as grantees learned how to build systems focusing on integrated care as opposed to single interventions (Bruner et al., 2011). In addition, communication is critical in the building of trust between the community.

Free discussion of health programs, practices, and policies encourages the participation of the community in the airing of their concerns and needs, which are utilized in creating relevant health services. Use of participatory methods such as focus groups and community forums can serve as channels for stakeholders to provide inputs, further enriching their ownership of health programs. Evaluations of the TICB model demonstrated that boosting community involvement not only fashioned trust but also outlined important facilitators and barriers to successful program implementation in health. Through participatory engagement, organizations can make their initiatives harmonious with what the community desires in a manner such that programs are made responsive and accessible, thus finally facilitating trust and participation by community members (Gordon et al., 2015). Finally, health organizations must have ongoing interaction and dedication to build trust within a community. Building trust is only the first step; having it followed through on continuously is what is needed to sustain it. Organizing local leaders and local voices to act as trusted middlemen can make a very large difference in how health initiatives are viewed by individuals within a community. The continued commitment provided by The Colorado Trust's programs is the ultimate example of the benefit of investing in relationships and processes that allow for long-term growth. Through requiring long-term partnership and showing a commitment to reacting to the needs of residents of communities, health organizations can create a setting in which trust can grow. This practice ultimately leads to improved health results and a healthier community, supporting the importance of trust in community health implementation strategies (Bruner et al., 2011) (Figure 5.11).

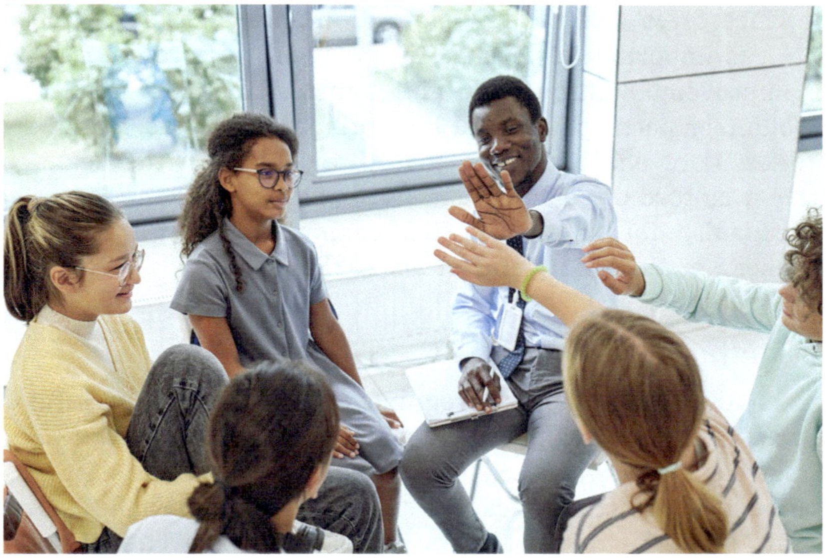

Figure 5.11. Building trust within the community.

Source: https://blog.searchinstitute.org/hubfs/blog/Key-Strategies-for-Building-Trust-in-the-Classroom.jpg.

5.4.2. Encouraging Volunteerism and Local Involvement

The importance of volunteerism in community health implementation strategies cannot be disregarded as it encourages ownership by the residents and collective action towards better public health results. Volunteers, who usually come from the communities they work in, provide important local expertise and experience with particular health issues, improving the efficiency of health interventions. Civil society organizations have a key role to play in unlocking this potential through community outreach, awareness activities, and health service provision. The World Health Organization observes that building local civil society can potentially enhance their contributions towards addressing public health emergencies like the COVID-19 pandemic. Volunteering mobilizes not only community resilience but also creates support systems important to the long-term maintenance of health interventions, making the health interventions worthwhile for the particular needs of different segments of the community (Teräs et al., 2023). Besides, the local mobilization of people through institutionalized community health programs taps into the residents' own intrinsic motivation to improve their own health. CHVs and CHMCs are important in bridging the gap between healthcare professionals and communities. These volunteer organizations enhance the efficiency of resource mobilization and offer means of simple communication that make health messages possible in a manner that makes them locally appealing. Evidence indicates that CHVs and CHMCs are not only crucial for bringing about health activities but also champions of community interests within the health system. Their processes of selection, while varied, have a tendency of taking from community involvement in order to have representatives who are well-respected and high-motivated individuals, thus rooting a system that listens and incorporates community input and participation (Sakeah et al., 2021). Last but not least, volunteerism for community health sustainability relies on the proper integration of volunteerism into broader health systems and appreciation of volunteers' efforts. Incentives, either financial or non-monetary, can significantly enhance CHVs' and CHMCs' motivation and retention. With the evolving public health environment, it is important to legalize the roles of these volunteers in health programs and continue their improvement through training and assistance for resources. By opening up clear channels for volunteer participation and rewarding their efforts, health authorities are able to engage communities more effectively and the sustainability of the health program ensured. Ultimately, cultivating a culture of volunteerism not only improves the local health environment but is an effective mechanism for building resilient communities with the capability to face future health challenges (Sakeah et al., 2021; Teräs et al., 2023).

5.4.3. Utilizing Community Leaders as Advocates

Community leaders as advocates in health programs are central to successful community health implementation strategies. They often possess a wealth of local knowledge and the trust of their locals, something that can prove vital when introducing health-related programs. Through the utilization of their influence, community leaders can effectively disseminate information, mobilize citizens, and stimulate greater participation in health programs. Their knowledge of the local culture and norms enables them to tailor health messages to suit the values of the society such that receptiveness and active acceptance are enhanced. Successful examples of this are activities that are targeting Medicaid and Children's Health Insurance Plan registration, which highlight community involvement in simplifying processes and offering accessibility to poor families (N/A, 2010). In addition, community leaders can act as a liaison between public health officials and the public, enabling the dialogue necessary to meet the unique needs and concerns of the community. Through direct participation in policy debates and voicing their constituents' opinions, these leaders contribute towards making more equitable and community-representative health policies. Their advocacy can also stand for resources that fill the gaps in health care service and address social determinants of health. One such example of lessons from programs like the California Endowments Healthy Eating, Active Communities program illustrates how community leaders are able to influence local policies to promote healthier eating among children in schools (N/A, 2008). A review of such programs indicates the strength of community advocacy to affect effective change in public health. Engaging local leaders in health activism also fosters empowerment and ownership among citizens. When citizens see their community leaders fighting for healthy programs, it builds confidence in the importance and effectiveness of such efforts. Such empowerment is sure to trigger from-the-ground activism to curb health disparities and promote wellness at the grassroots level. In addition, relying on the expertise of community leaders can also be used to mobilize volunteers and other resources that can sustain health programs in the long term. Lastly, the involvement of community advocates is a strategic approach not only to enhance program participation but to develop strong health systems responsive to the population being served.

5.5. Implementation of Health Strategies

Effective deployment of health strategies is a crucial component in enhancing community health results, particularly with respect to conditions such as dengue fever. With dengue emerging as a preeminent public health concern globally, development and implementation of vaccination programs and their integration into routine immunization platforms is the need of the hour. Currently, there are only two approved vaccines—Dengvaxia and TAK-003—yet their rollout remains hindered in areas of high burden. An extensive vaccine deployment strategy embracing tactics like school-based immunization and community engagement is required to promote greatest reach and coverage. While developing plans for introducing these vaccines, recommendations from National Immunization Technical Advisory Groups (NITAG) and local epidemiological data will be key for developing effective policies that utilize available vaccines to neutralize dengue's public health impact. The addition of these vaccines to health programs must be done cautiously to receive not only acceptance, but also effectiveness in reducing morbidity. Alongside vaccination activities, acceptability and feasibility learnings on various implementation strategies are vital to enhancing the application of EBPs within community health settings.

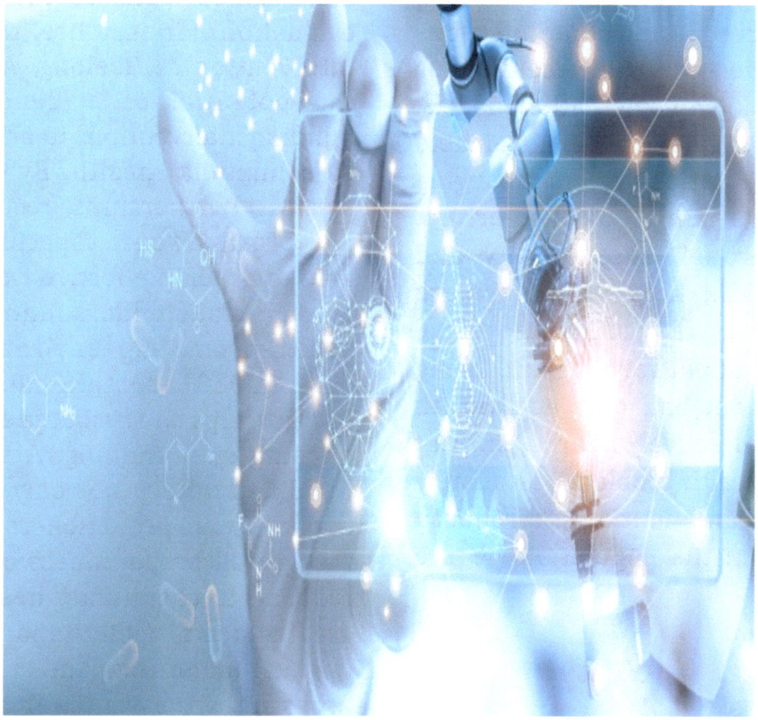

Figure 5.12. Implementation of health strategies.

Source: https://www.itconvergence.com/wp-content/uploads/2024/03/Implementing-RPA-in-Healthcare-Strategies-for-Success-blog.jpg.

Recent studies have shown that capacity-building strategies are most likely to be rated as acceptable by public agency and community organization practitioners. Capacity-building strategies are directed towards training and empowering practitioners so they can successfully implement

EBPs. Dissemination strategies are also extremely plausible and may be disseminated promptly, thereby allowing dissemination of significant health information on a broad scale. By marrying the strengths of capacity-building and dissemination strategies, policymakers can formulate effective frameworks that not only promote the adoption of EBPs but also ensure integration of those practices into community health services, thereby maximizing public health gains. The success of subsequent implementation strategies for community health hangs in the balance of the capacity to improve and adapt existing practices through ongoing evaluation and research evidence. With emerging health challenges continuing to occur, such as the threat of dengue and other infectious diseases, there is ever-growing necessity for effective and adaptable implementation models. Policymakers must strive to create sustainable approaches to be in a position to match changing health contexts while being evidence-driven. Lesson learning through acceptability and feasibility analysis can help promote more advanced policymaking. By combining these results with a commitment towards enhancing community engagement and outreach, health agencies are able to effectively address current as well as emerging health problems, ultimately leading to healthier communities and reduced disease burden within the population (Figure 5.12).

5.5.1. Training and Capacity Building for Staff

Efficient training and capacity development for staff are essential aspects of successful community health implementation strategies. These interventions target enhancing the capabilities, knowledge, and skills of health workers to help them effectively address complex health matters. One commendable approach involves the provision of specialized training programs, for instance, joint Masters in Public Health (MPH) degrees in health workforce development. This kind of capacity building program not only develops staff ability but also promotes system-wide improvement in health care provision. For example, university partnerships facilitate an environment where new teaching materials and approaches can be exchanged, ultimately contributing to an improved public health workforce. Amde et al. (2014) underscores the imperative of leadership development capacities in health ministries as part of instilling robust human resource management and public health practice. Furthermore, community health capacity building is guided by strategic frameworks that define key areas of organizational growth. A mixed methods evaluation, for instance, the Romp & Chomp intervention at Geelong, Australia, illustrates the potential of evidence-based capacity-building interventions to bring tangible benefits to community health. By addressing aspects such as partnerships, resource management, and organizational capacity, interventions are able to develop effective working relationships among stakeholders and create long-term health-promoting environments. Sanigorski et al. (2010) identifies the need to establish partnerships and resource allocation to support ongoing staff training. A successful capacity-building strategy not only builds the capacity of individual practitioners but also enhances the overall preparedness of health systems to respond to community needs, thus promoting greater health equity and accessibility. Lastly, ongoing monitoring and refinement of training programs are essential in addressing evolving needs of healthcare workers and communities. As demonstrated in the MPH program debates and the Romp & Chomp intervention debates, good capacity building is a commitment to long-term engagement and investment. Concerns such as limited finance, turnover of staff, and shifting governance arrangements must be managed strategically in order to produce sustainable results. What is gained from the assessments can be applied to future interventions so that necessary shifts in training approaches and resource allocation can be made. Consequently, constant learning and adaptation not just improve the health intervention effectiveness but also build resilience within healthcare systems. With capacity building at the staff training level, community health programs will be able to make significant advances in health outcomes and system performance as a whole.

5.5.2. Establishing Timelines and Milestones

Timeline and milestone setup is a significant component of community health implementation strategy since it helps ensure that projects advance in an organized manner. By creating well-established timelines, organizations are able to efficiently manage resources, set realistic short-term and long-term objectives, and hold stakeholders accountable. For example, having a strong review of policy can be the first step towards communities that wish to achieve priority outcomes, particularly for marginalized populations. This action should involve a systematic plan for gathering and analyzing relevant data with benchmarks to track the review process. Following this, actionable recommendations can be prepared, which results in a well-integrated plan of action that outlines the following implementation phases, thereby ensuring the pillars of long-term community health improvement (Brown et al., 2015). Milestones are milestones that allow organizations to mark their progress and make the necessary changes while working on the health programs. Having such milestones maximizes transparency and ensures a shared accountability culture among stakeholders. In community health, all stakeholders—be it academic institutions, healthcare providers, or members of the community—need to be engaged in the process. The School Accountability and Improvement Framework accomplishes this with an interlink between self-reflection and ongoing improvement planning, so all stakeholders engaged in the community health approach are all well aware of short-term successes and areas where additional effort is required. Finally, continuous tracking against established milestones not only directs future action but also serves to promote a sense of collective achievement, which is critical in engaging long-term participation (N/A, 2025). Apart from tracking progress, establishing timelines and milestones also involves significant self-evaluation at each juncture of the implementation plan. This enables alterations according to routine appraisals and feedback from the community. Effective time management is imperative; hence, health organizations need to allocate timeframes to each phase of the project, from initial assessment to end-project evaluation. Moreover, if these timeframes align with community activities or local health observance, involvement and visibility would be increased. If milestones are made clearly related to higher-order community health goals, such as disease prevention rates or consumption of healthcare services, then they become front and center and emergent in the local conversation. Therefore, a clearly documented timeline not only facilitates the implementation of a project but also assists in energizing community support and interest during the implementation process.

5.5.3. Monitoring and Adapting Strategies in Real-Time

Good community health implementation strategies are founded on the ability to monitor and modify interventions in real-time so that they can continue to be effective and relevant. As the various programs are executed by the community health workers, functioning on real-time data enables them to spot issues and opportunities that come up in real-time. The data obtained from monitoring indicators like participation rate, health effects, and feedback from the interventions offers invaluable information regarding the efficacy of the pursued strategies. For example, adaptive interventions enable one to be flexible in modifying the intervention based on continuous assessment without compromising the initial aim of the intervention. This flexibility is very important in environments that are dynamic in nature and where the determinants of health change at high speeds, thus requiring a flexible approach in programming. Highlighting flexibility underscores the thin line between staying true to intervention design and practical adaptability. Fidelity requires a program to be loyal to its fundamental features that make the program work, but changes have to be yielded to support local environments or participant demand. As is being discussed through the examination of the fidelity-adaptation continuum, certain adaptations have the potential to optimize program effect by matching strategies to the particular context of the population being served. Hence, creating a process of systematically describing the changes made—implemented as designed, changed, or added—is key in maintaining ongoing effectiveness while building resilience in implementation strategies (Castro et al., 2016). Moreover, technological application in monitoring allows for greater capacity for adaptation in real time. Technology that is founded on the application of data gathering and analytics, such as community feedback mechanisms and mobile health apps, guarantees real-time program quality monitoring. Such technology adheres to the ideals of participatory governance in that it facilitates stakeholders' participation in adaptation. As the Guidebook for climate change adaptation technology demands, involving multiple stakeholders in society enhances decision-making capacity, adding to the aggregate body of knowledge and ensuring localized solutions to health issues (Clements et al., 2011). Lastly, incorporating real-time monitoring and adaptive dynamics ensures that interventions in community health are sustainable and effective when confronted with evolving public health dynamics (Figure 5.13).

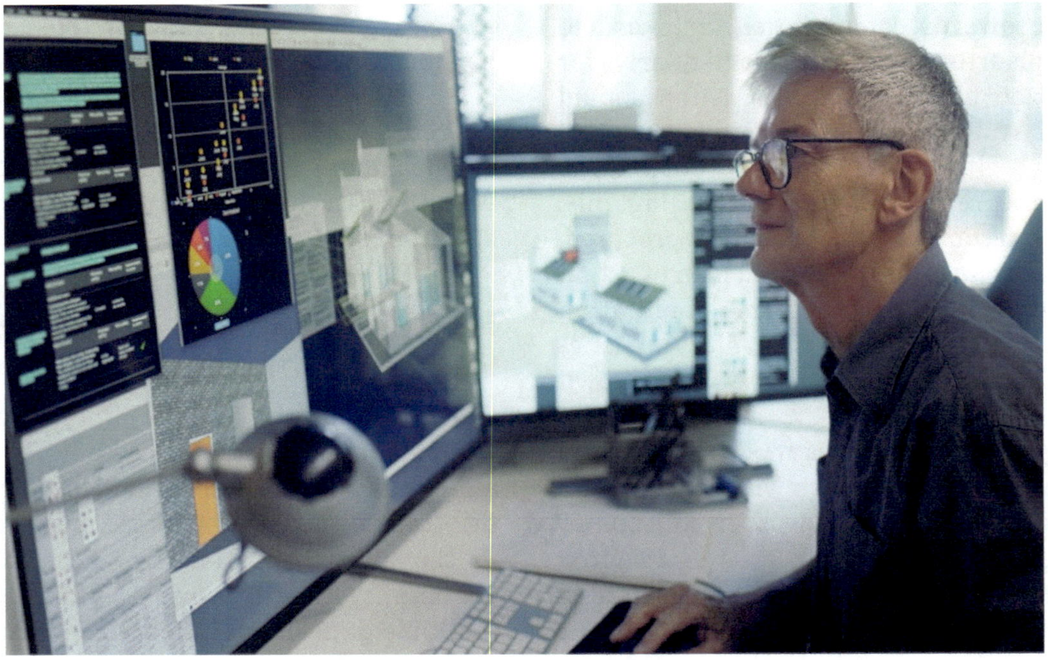

Figure 5.13. Monitoring and adapting strategies in real-time.

Source: https://www.trueprojectinsight.com/sites/default/files/inline-images/Real-Time%20 Monitoring.jpg.

5.6. Evaluation and Impact Assessment

Successful assessment and impact assessment are key components in the delivery of community health interventions, especially in addressing stigma with regard to mental health. The research presented in Ayele et al. (2024) highlights the multi-component awareness-raising intervention, Indigo-Local, in addressing stigma and increasing referrals to mental health care in low- and middle-income countries (LMICs). With the use of the mixed-methods strategy, whereby both quantitative and qualitative measures are used, the assessment is aimed at measurement of changes in attitudes, knowledge, and behavior towards mental health. Through this combined methodology, several aspects of stigma and discrimination are covered, and better insight into the effectiveness of the intervention in multiple cultural contexts is gained. Therefore, assessment not only brings to light short-term effects but also informs wider public health policy, charting the course for larger-scale application. Incorporation of varied evaluation within interventions in community health, as argued in Symons et al. (2009), is essential in guaranteeing equitable health care practices. Education plan developed for medical students with an aim of constructing their perception of disability is a wonderful example of how curriculum approaches can influence service delivery. Six-step systematic curriculum design process illustrates the importance of combining knowledge and attitude in health professions education. By employing controlled designs in educational surveys, it is possible to methodically assess the efficacy of educational interventions, demonstrating that they can influence health care practice. Such longitudinal evaluation not only adds to the training of potential health professionals but also provides a template for other studies with the same purpose that seek to improve the care of vulnerable patient groups. Therefore, systematic evaluation and measurement of the effect are important in order to make sure community health interventions produce intended results in health. Last but not least, robust evaluation systems can help community health programs learn and sustain themselves with evidence-based knowledge. According to Ayele et al. (2024) and Symons et al. (2009), collective wisdom of multiple health improvement efforts highlights the significance of feedback in a continuous loop and circular learning processes. Having this mindset, stakeholders can reinforce interventions to meet community-specific needs, hence catalyzing larger impacts. The settings given illustrate the importance of stakeholder and user participation in evaluation efforts, providing ownership that can guarantee sustainability. Thus, commitment to meticulous assessment and rigorous impact analysis not only raises standards of community health planning but also ensures that care will be provided in a fair and balanced way to various populations, ultimately leading to improved public health outcomes.

5.6.1. Defining Success Metrics

In implementation strategy for community health, success measures are a critical component to ensure that intended impacts are generated in health programs. Success indicators are typically quantitative and qualitative indicators that allow the stakeholders to gauge the efficacy, effectiveness, and consequence of the health program. Quantitative and qualitative indicators that are measurable and true allow for measuring not only short-term intervention effect—e.g., people reached—but also long-term effect, e.g., improvement of health indicators. By associating such interventions with the specific goals of community health programs, for example, reducing morbidity rates or enhancing patient satisfaction, organizations can obtain relevant lessons that will inform future interventions, enhance resource utilization, and hold stakeholders accountable who implement programs. In addition, evidence-based implementation of health programs is dependent on effective processes for data collection and analysis. For instance, developing efficient frameworks that prioritize ongoing monitoring allows organizations to contrast actual outcomes with established norms, thus initiating necessary strategy changes if and when required. Similarly, proof via research identifies inefficiencies in coordination among regional bodies as constraining successful development programs, reflecting the need for integrated measurement strategy (Nasution et al., 2025). Community involvement is also demonstrated to be a critical factor in the development of success indicators, since stakeholders' involvement is likely to ensure a sense of responsibility and ownership. Stakeholders' involvement enables the measures to be informed by and responsive to the needs and priorities of the community, thus ensuring greater satisfaction and effectiveness in the implemented strategies. Moreover, contextual drivers in the definition and measurement of success indicators, especially for varied implementation settings, are also crucial to comprehend. Problematic factors such as resource scarcity, high turnover rates among staff, and infrastructure limitations may tend to influence the development of effective metrics. The Ethiopian eCHIS program experience suggests that context constraints and enablers must be understood to develop suitable metrics that resonate with stakeholders (Hailemariam et al., 2023).

Moreover, the holding of space for engaging volunteers and community leaders in data collection ensures not only enhanced measurement of accomplishment, but strengthening of community ties as well. Taken collectively, these considerations establish the importance of a broad and evolving method of establishing measures of success for community health implementation plans, for long-term and concrete measures of health outcomes.

5.6.2. Collecting and Analyzing Data

In the context of community health implementation plans, data collection and analysis are critical to determination of program success, as well as the planning of resource allocation. The call for clear and specific data is even greater when considering public health emergencies, the HIV/AIDS pandemic being a case in point. Developing nations have come to realize in greater frequency that effective health reform initiatives are based on a systematic process in order to manage the cost of health programs. As Huff-Rousselle et al. (2001) explain, the majority of governments nowadays are working towards maximizing the use of resources in tackling the epidemic by making investments in prevention, treatment, and care programs. Policymakers can establish the cost of programs through systematic data collection methods and thus make informed decisions that prioritize essential health services in the targeted communities. Co-ordination among stakeholders is one of the most important aspects of data collection in community health programs, and through co-ordination, credibility and usability of collected data are increased. As a matter of that, government and foundation-funded programs are encouraging co-ordination to ensure collaborative work towards service delivery. Farley et al. (2012) argues that interagency collaboration puts significant importance on establishing referral and screening systems for maximum effectiveness. The programs are based on the aggregate capacity of the participating agencies to gather suitable data and employ it in informing continuous program improvement. Through synergism, these organizations not only expand the volume of data but also embed the extended community health system, ultimately resulting in improved client outcomes through evidence-informed decision-making. Data analysis is also essential in determining trends and gaps in performance that can be used to inform prospective interventions. Systematic data analysis enables stakeholders to measure the effect of strategies implemented and make necessary adjustments based on facts. For instance, the complex costing models constructed in Huff-Rousselle et al. (2001) provide valuable information on actual HIV/AIDS program expenditures, made guaranteed to be transparent and accountable. These leaders are better positioned to identify efficiency traps in resources and direct funds differently with awareness of such budget considerations. Besides, use of rigorous analytical methods produces evidence-based practice culture that engenders programs to adopt adaptive programming that is responsive to emerging needs of the populations served. This data collection/analysis/responding cycle lies at the core of long-term achievement of community health implementation plans (Figure 5.14).

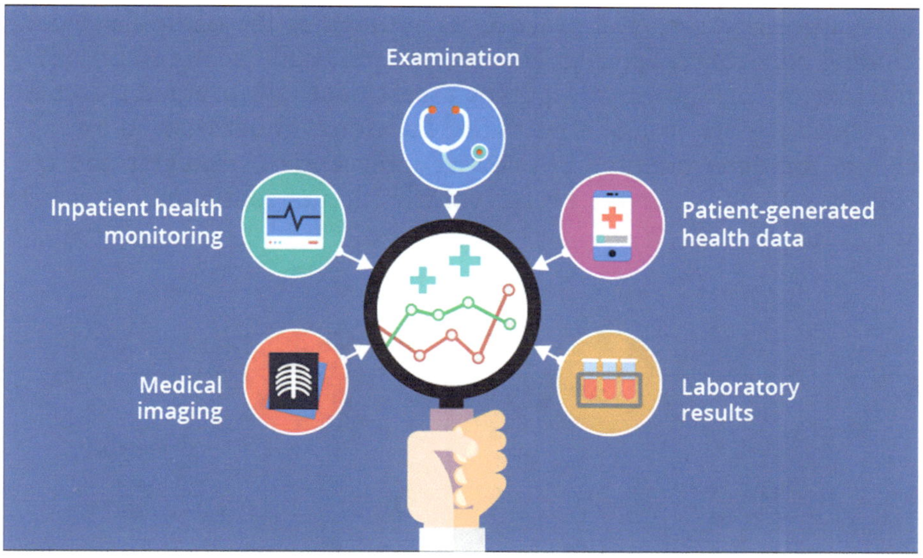

Figure 5.14. Collecting and analyzing data.

Source: https://www.scnsoft.com/blog-pictures/healthcare/health_data_analysis-01_1.png https://www.scnsoft.com/blog-pictures/healthcare/health_data_analysis-01_1.png.

5.6.3. Reporting Findings to Stakeholders

Reporting results to stakeholders is also a critical component in the implementation of community health interventions. Stakeholders like policymakers, clinicians, and the general public influence and guide health efforts. Thus, reporting research results in a manner that is appealing to such various stakeholders is central to fostering participation and stakeholder support. The use of tailored messaging can enhance stakeholders' comprehension and can be delivered through town hall meetings, presentations, and reports. Specific, brief, and clear information is essential, predominantly the good practice characteristics of interventions that can be learned from exhaustive examination like in the systematic review of the DEDPIAC Knowledge Hub. Outcome and action-oriented findings ensure research results are not only usable but also channel stakeholders into participatory processes of health improvement (Brug et al., 2015). Additionally, sharing research results should encompass process feedback that provides stakeholders and researchers with an instrument for ongoing interaction. The interactive process not only enhances understanding but also fosters stakeholder commitment, which is the essence of health program sustainability.

By cultivating a culture of collaboration, stakeholders could reap reward through a share in the development and enhancement of health practice and policy. An example thereof is the Disease Surveillance Networks (DSN) Initiative dedicated to collaboration and sharing of best practice across already operational networks aimed at enhancing the capacity of local institutions and experts (Ekirapa et al., 2011). Through. framing communication in participatory mode enabling stakeholder involvement., efforts can be placed to harness community needs and ultimately achieve enhanced health outcomes. Lastly, monitoring and evaluation procedures should be embedded within the reporting framework to enlighten stakeholders on an integrated understanding of intervention effects. By providing both monitoring findings as well as key conclusions, stakeholders are better positioned to comprehend multiplicity of community health interventions. The systematic categorization of characteristics of best practice, as outlined by the umbrella review, identifies the main issues including participant engagement, sustainability, and achievability (Brug et al., 2015). Such sophisticated reporting allows transparent assessment and promotes accountability, which ultimately allows stakeholders to make informed decisions. In addition, the reporting of trends in data can facilitate the determination of effective intervention strategies and the replication of such efforts in other settings, hence the overall contribution of community health implementation strategies (Figure 5.15).

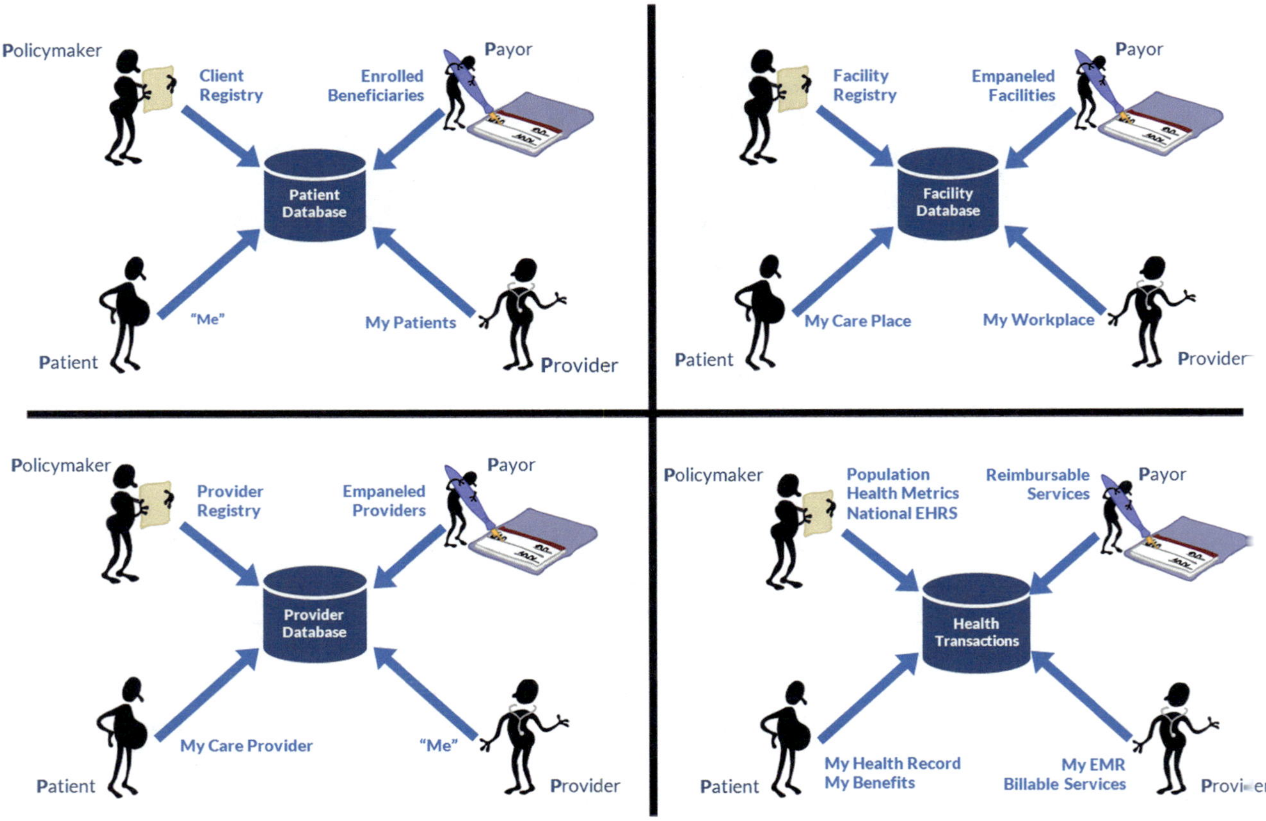

Figure 5.15. Reporting findings to stakeholders.

Source: https://www.publichealth.com.ng/wp-content/uploads/2021/01/stakeholders-in-healthcare-3.png.

SUMMARY

In summary to the previous community health implementation strategies, it is certain that proper supervision of CHWs is necessary in order to build the overall effect of health programs. Literature review shows that the quality and type of supervision has the potential to impact CHW performance, motivation, as well as retention rates. In evidence, there is suggestion that simply upping supervision frequency to placing fully supportive supervision packages can lead to improved outcomes. Not only does this method consider coverage and performance standards but also quality assurance and problem solving, showing that more intensive supervision quality is of most concern to maximizing community health programs (Benton et al., 2014). Lastly, by combining supervisory approaches with the precise requirements of health programs, stakeholders are able to generate more optimal beneficial effects for community health. Moreover, the implementation of implementation science fundamentals such as in the MyGoals rehabilitation system helps demonstrate the importance of community strategies tailored to meet the individual needs of the community. By using participatory research approaches in communities, the MyGoals intervention dissemination was informed by face-to-face interactions with target implementers and clients. Stakeholder ownership as a key to achieving successful implementation integration of health interventions is facilitated by participation. The strategies developed through this process illustrate the way determinants and action mechanisms can practically inform implementation activities, hence filling existing practice-research gaps (Foster et al., 2022). It thus follows that the incorporation of such specially crafted strategies has the potential to facilitate the effective implementation of evidence-based interventions that optimize community health outcomes. Through borrowing from such perspectives, the future adoption of community health is contingent on interaction of good supervision and proper measures. Overcoming challenges for CHWs by means of good supervision not only develops their ability but also ensures stronger and more responsive community health programs to local demands. Meanwhile, application of implementation science to context-adapted strategies provides a means of bridging the persistent disconnects between evidence and practice. In the future, policymakers and health administrators will need to prioritize these challenges in planning and implementing health programs. Through overall collaboration on the improvement of supervision strategies and the expansion of the application of matched implementation strategies, potential for achieving sustainable health gains within populations is greatly improved.

Implementation plans of community health are cross-cutting, whereby various elements work towards making their contributions to wellness and health of populations. Among significant points is the necessity to have effective partnership among stakeholders in order to have effective deployment of actions towards improving community health. The development and sustenance of partnerships demand cooperation between service providers, academic institutions, and members of society. Such collaborations are designed to facilitate integration among sectors, such as academic improvement, young people's development, and health care, in a healthy manner to address the needs of the community. Through the establishment of collaborative settings, such programs not only solve short-term health problems but also establish the basis for long-term community building (Melaville et al., 2012). Lastly, partnerships development is a force of sweeping change that can provide solutions to serious health issues prevalent in multi-group populations. Strategic interventions aimed at solving urgent health issues such as substance abuse are a second critical component of implementation plans for community health. Initiatives over the past few years like the Grand Challenge: Responding to the Addictions Crisis show the imperative of the use of an interdisciplinary model to solve intricate health issues. This interprofessional initiative aims to bring together leaders from across a multitude of disciplines to explore novel legal and policy solutions required to address the epidemic of opioid use disorder effectively. The evidence-based strategy recognizes a key aspect of public health—there exists an embrace of demand for innovative solutions that traverse criminal justice, public health, and treatment (Beukema et al., 2018). By convening experts to exchange such interventions, communities learn from successful practice that has the ability to counter the adverse effects of substance abuse and improve overall public health outcomes. Furthermore, community engagement in health implementation strategy cannot be overemphasized. Engaging communities in planning and executing interventions generates ownership and accountability, factors that are fundamental to achieving lasting effectiveness. Good communication strategies are required to ensure that everyone in the community participates and is informed and thus generate more trust among the stakeholders. Community empowerment strategies that engage the community to become active in their health program are likely to generate more sustainable outcomes. By integrating local input and knowledge in program design, the health intervention is localized and more appropriate to the needs of the target population. It is crucial for knowledge of community contributions and facilitation of collaborative health interventions in ensuring effective implementation plans in community health initiatives (Melaville et al., 2012)

KEY TERMS FROM THIS CHAPTER

- Accountable Health Communities (AHC) Model
- Civil society organizations
- Community Health Workers (CHWs)
- Community knowledge
- Curriculum
- Decentralization
- Disease Surveillance Networks (DSN)
- Evidence-based interventions
- Feedback mechanisms
- Health care
- Health decision-making
- Health program development
- Infectious diseases
- Cardiovascular conditions
- Community dynamics
- Community involvement
- Community organizations
- Data-driven decision-making
- Discrimination
- Epidemiologic data
- Evidence-Based Practice (EBP)
- Health activism
- Healthcare services
- Health disparities
- HIV/AIDS pandemic
- Local health systems

CLOSER LOOK

INTERVENTION AND POLICY DEVELOPMENT

A closer look at intervention and policy development reveals a dynamic, iterative process that bridges evidence with action to address complex societal challenges. Effective intervention begins with a clear problem definition and needs assessment, drawing on robust data and stakeholder input to identify underlying causes and target populations. From there, theory-informed strategies are co-designed with those affected—engaging community members, practitioners, experts, and policymakers—to ensure relevance, acceptability, and cultural fit. Policy development translates these interventions into institutional frameworks by articulating goals, defining roles and responsibilities, allocating resources, and establishing incentives or regulations to support desired behaviors or outcomes. Central to both processes is a commitment to evidence: systematic reviews, pilot studies, and implementation science help refine approaches before wider rollout. Equity must be embedded throughout, with deliberate attention to how interventions and policies affect marginalized groups, mitigating unintended consequences and avoiding the amplification of disparities. Monitoring and evaluation create feedback loops; real-time data and qualitative insights inform adjustments, scale decisions, and sustainability planning. Effective policies also include clear mechanisms for accountability, transparency, and public communication, fostering trust and legitimacy. Cross-sector collaboration—linking health, education, justice, and economic systems—amplifies impact, while capacity building ensures that implementers have the skills and infrastructure to carry interventions forward. Finally, policy development is not a one-time event but a living process: regular review, incorporation of new evidence, and participatory reassessment keep interventions responsive to changing contexts and emerging needs. When intervention design and policy development are integrated thoughtfully, they create resilient systems capable of producing lasting, equitable change.

REFERENCES

1. Aarons, G. A., Arch, J. J., Barnett, M., Best, L. A., et al. (2016). Proceedings of the 3rd Biennial Conference of the Society for Implementation Research Collaboration (SIRC) 2015: Advancing efficient methodologies through community partnerships and team science: Seattle, WA, USA. 24–26 September 2015. https://core.ac.uk/download/286729096.pdf (accessed on 26th June 2025).

2. Adelman, H. S., & Taylor, L. L. (2018). Addressing barriers to learning: In the classroom and schoolwide. https://core.ac.uk/download/286362370.pdf (accessed on 26th June 2025).

3. Ahmed, S. (2006). Health curriculum and school quality: AKU-IED's. https://core.ac.uk/download/47255876.pdf (accessed on 26th June 2025).

4. Allen, P., Bass, K., Best, L. A., Brownson, R. C., et al. (2018). Lessons learned in promoting evidence-based public health: Perspectives from managers in state public health departments. https://core.ac.uk/download/287887998.pdf (accessed on 26th June 2025).

5. Amde, W. K., Lehmann, U., & Sanders, D. (2014). Building capacity to develop an African teaching platform on health workforce development: A collaborative initiative of universities from four sub-Saharan countries. https://core.ac.uk/download/62635506.pdf (accessed on 26th June 2025).

6. Ayanian, J. Z., Friedberg, M. W., Guzman, E. A., Rodriguez, H. P., et al. (2014). Comparing the implementation of team approaches for improving diabetes care in community health centers. https://core.ac.uk/download/28952472.pdf (accessed on 26th June 2025).

7. Ayele, B., Bakolis, I., Bhattarai, K., Brohan, E., et al. (2024). Reducing stigma and improving access to care for people with mental health conditions in the community: Protocol for a multi-site feasibility intervention study (Indigo-Local). https://core.ac.uk/download/624327606.pdf (accessed on 26th June 2025).

8. Barnett, M., Kia-Keating, M., Landsverk, J., Lau, A. S., et al. (2019). Developing and evaluating a lay health worker delivered implementation intervention to decrease engagement disparities in behavioral parent training: A mixed methods study protocol. https://core.ac.uk/download/323062727.pdf (accessed on 26th June 2025).

9. Bell, J., Famula, J., Kelly, K., Mongoven, A., et al. (2024). The implementation outcomes and population impact of a statewide IT deployment for family caregivers: Mixed methods study. https://core.ac.uk/download/635940175.pdf (accessed on 26th June 2025).

10. Benton, L., Dumbaugh, M., Hill, Z., Kirkwood, B., et al. (2014). Supervising community health workers in low-income countries–a review of impact and implementation issues. https://core.ac.uk/download/42631763.pdf (accessed on 26th June 2025).

11. Bess, K. D., Cene, C. W., Corbie-Smith, G., Dave, G., et al. (2019). Adaptation of an evidence-based cardiovascular health intervention for rural African Americans in the Southeast. https://core.ac.uk/download/286537358.pdf (accessed on 26th June 2025).

12. Beukema, E., Hoss, A., Silverman, R. D., Terry, S., et al. (2018). Innovations in opioid law and policy interventions workshop: Summary of proceedings. https://core.ac.uk/download/160755315.pdf (accessed on 26th June 2025).

13. Brown, L., Philpart, M., & Masoud, S. (2015). Building place-based initiatives for boys and men of color and vulnerable populations: A community planning guide. https://core.ac.uk/

download/75782836.pdf (accessed on 26th June 2025).

14. Brug, J., De Bourdeaudhuij, I., Hendriksen, M., Horodyska, K., et al. (2015). Good practice characteristics of diet and physical activity interventions and policies: An umbrella review. https://core.ac.uk/download/55847520.pdf (accessed on 26th June 2025).

15. Bruner, E., & Schroeder, J. (2011). Early childhood councils: Effective planning processes for health systems integration. https://core.ac.uk/download/71345847.pdf (accessed on 26th June 2025).

16. Callaghan, D. M. (2016). Implementing faith community nursing interventions to promote healthy behaviors in adults. https://core.ac.uk/download/43651447.pdf (accessed on 26th June 2025).

17. Castro, M., Lefevre, P., Pérez Chacón, D., Van Der Stuyft, P., et al. (2016). A modified theoretical framework to assess implementation fidelity of adaptive public health interventions. https://core.ac.uk/download/84044522.pdf (accessed on 26th June 2025).

18. Chan, F. J. H., Chan, A. Y., Wen, Z. X., Rajendram, P., Quek, J. J. H., Tan, W. M., Yong, Y. L., et al. (2025). Classifying strategies for building community health movements: A guide for implementers. *BMC Public Health, 25.* https://www.semanticscholar.org/paper/1021da069964561cc87d318d9cbd34c744149636 (accessed on 26th June 2025).

19. Chenier, R., Fernandez, M. E., Garza, E. R., Heredia, N., et al. (2022). Using implementation mapping for the adoption and implementation of Target:BP in community health centers. https://core.ac.uk/download/604668825.pdf (accessed on 26th June 2025).

20. Child Trends, Walker, K. E., & Delale-O'Connor, L. (2012). Rising to the challenge: The strategies of social service intermediaries. https://core.ac.uk/download/71359901.pdf (accessed on 26th June 2025).

21. Clements, R., Haggar, J., Quezada, A., Torres, J., et al. (2011). Technologies for climate change adaptation: Agricultural sector. https://core.ac.uk/download/316337.pdf (accessed on 26th June 2025).

22. Coulter, A., Maduma-Butshe, A., Morgan, A., O'Cathain, A., Ryder, A., Wilkin, A., McFadden, A., et al. (2016). Community engagement to enhance trust between Gypsy/Travelers, and maternity, early years and child dental health services: Protocol for a multimethod exploratory study. https://core.ac.uk/download/74233682.pdf (accessed on 26th June 2025).

23. Dary, T., & Pickerel, T. (2013). School climate: Practices for implementation and sustainability. https://core.ac.uk/download/71361523.pdf (accessed on 26th June 2025).

24. Ekirapa, A., Matthys, B., Zinsstag, J., Crump, L., Yatich, N., & Ettarh, R. (2011). Disease Surveillance Networks Initiative Africa: Final evaluation. https://core.ac.uk/download/86445038.pdf (accessed on 26th June 2025).

25. Farley, C., Walker, K. E., & Polin, M. (2012). Using data in multi-agency collaborations: Guiding performance to ensure accountability and improve programs. https://core.ac.uk/download/71359978.pdf (accessed on 26th June 2025).

26. Ferguson, G. M., Highfield, L., & Holcomb, J. (2022). Barriers and facilitators to implementation of the Accountable Health Communities (AHC) model: Findings from a between-site qualitative assessment of implementation strategies. https://core.ac.uk/download/604668532.pdf (accessed on 26th June 2025).

27. Foster, E. R., & Kang, E. (2022). Use of implementation mapping with community-based participatory research: Development of implementation strategies of a new goal setting and goal management intervention system. https://core.ac.uk/download/551306903.pdf (accessed on 26th June 2025).

28. Friedman, E. A., & Gostin, L. O. (2012). Pillars for progress on the right to health: Harnessing the potential of human rights through a Framework Convention on Global Health. https://core.ac.uk/download/70374763.pdf (accessed on 26th June 2025).

29. Gordon, D., Rebanal, D., Tokunaga, J., Wolin, J., & Simon-Ortiz, S. (2015). Trauma informed community building evaluation: A formative evaluation of the TICB model and its implementation in Potrero Hill. https://core.ac.uk/download/80511020.pdf (accessed on 26th June 2025).

30. Gore, A., Alschuler, A. A., Lehman, A. F., Daniels, A. S., Young, A. S., Perrin, B., Emery, B. D., et al. (2006). Innovations in mental health services implementation: A report on state-level data from the U.S. Evidence-Based Practices Project. https://core.ac.uk/download/pdf/4043514.pdf (accessed on 26th June 2025).

31. Hailemariam, T., Atnafu, A., Gezie, L., Kaasbøll, J., Klein, J., & Tilahun, B. (2023). Individual and contextual level enablers and barriers determining electronic community health information system implementation in northwest Ethiopia. *BMC Health Services Research, 23*. https://www.semanticscholar.org/paper/da979ae48413b96e5f20024d991c20903894b6ca (accessed on 26th June 2025).

32. Huff-Rousselle, M., & Phillips, M. (2001). Resources and tools: A step-by-step methodological guide for costing HIV/AIDS activities. https://core.ac.uk/download/pdf/11306982.pdf (accessed on 26th June 2025).

33. Kougang, A. (2017). Culturally competent health education in African-Americans' faith-based communities for better health outcomes: A literature review. https://core.ac.uk/download/70427442.pdf (accessed on 26th June 2025).

34. Lee, R. M., Mallick, K., Daly, J. G., Thompson, V. S., Hoffman, E., Papadopoulos, M., & Curry, S. (2024). Community advisory boards as implementation strategies to center partner and patient voice in community health centers. *Journal of Clinical and Translational Science, 9*. https://www.semanticscholar.org/paper/98e56880de8241274956e8ef8603c67c23702a98 (accessed on 26th June 2025).

35. Lyman, D. R., Dougherty, R. H., & Holt, W. (2010). State case studies of infant and early childhood mental health systems: Strategies for change. https://core.ac.uk/download/71355034.pdf (accessed on 26th June 2025).

36. Melaville, A., Blank, M. J., & Jacobson, R. (2012). Achieving results through community school partnerships. https://core.ac.uk/download/71356859.pdf (accessed on 26th June 2025).

37. Muasya, J. N., & Nyakundi, M. B. (2023). Stakeholder involvement and the implementation of maternal and child health projects of Safaricom Public Limited Company in Siakago Sub-County, Embu County, Kenya. https://core.ac.uk/download/654958919.pdf (accessed on 26th June 2025).

38. N/A. (2008). Key lessons from California schools working to change school food environments. https://core.ac.uk/download/71352567.pdf (accessed on 26th June 2025).

39. N/A. (2010). Maximizing enrollment for kids: Results from a diagnostic assessment of enrollment and retention in eight states. https://core.ac.uk/download/71352983.pdf (accessed on 26th June 2025).

40. N/A. (2013). Eastlake-Garfield District: Health impact assessment report. https://core.ac.uk/download/97830891.pdf (accessed on 26th June 2025).

41. N/A. (2014). United Nations Development Assistance Framework for Kenya. https://core.ac.uk/download/75781829.pdf (accessed on 26th June 2025).

42. N/A. (2014). Water and development strategy: Implementation field guide. https://core.ac.uk/download/75777299.pdf (accessed on 26th June 2025).

43. N/A. (2025). Accountability and improvement framework for Victorian government schools 2012. https://core.ac.uk/download/pdf/30679017.pdf (accessed on 26th June 2025).

44. Nasution, M. A., Ginting, W. O., Revida, E., & Trimurni, F. (2025). Evaluation model of sustainable development planning in regional policy implementation and local government administration. *Journal of Eco Humanism*. https://www.semanticscholar.org/paper/4d918fe1dd3da9bbb384efab979f27742522b739 (accessed on 26th June 2025).

45. Pio, A., Michel, C., Cuembelo, F., Pfeiffer, J., Manuel, J. L., Sherr, K., Kariaganis, M., et al. (2013). Strengthening integrated primary health care in Sofala, Mozambique. https://core.ac.uk/download/71362101.pdf (accessed on 26th June 2025).

46. Purtle, J. I., Stadnick, N., Wynecoop, M., Walker, S. C., Bruns, E. J., & Aarons, G. A. (2024). Acceptability and feasibility of policy implementation strategies for taxes earmarked for behavioral health services. *Frontiers in Health Services, 4*. https://www.semanticscholar.org/paper/be225834cf753c308923b52a6bdf06ecf351f5b6 (accessed on 26th June 2025).

47. Ravichandran, N. (2025). Vision 2020: The role and scope of operations research models. https://core.ac.uk/download/pdf/6443695.pdf (accessed on 26th June 2025).

48. Reeder, F. S., Christopherson, G., Mihm, J. C., & Glendening, P. (2011). Achieving green and healthy homes and communities in America. https://core.ac.uk/download/71345918.pdf (accessed on 26th June 2025).

49. Sakeah, E., Aborigo, R., Debpuur, C., Nonterah, E., Oduro, A., & Awoonor-Williams, J. (2021). Assessing selection procedures and roles of community health volunteers and community health management committees in Ghana's community-based health planning and services program. *PLOS ONE, 16*. https://www.semanticscholar.org/paper/1845a8c32efe7048e10f4d630c1b030fad29e282 (accessed on 26th June 2025).

50. Sanigorski, A., Simmons, A., Steckler, A., Bell, A. C., de Silva-Sanigorski, A. M., Sanigorski, A. M., de Silva-Sanigorski, A. M., et al. (2010). Increasing community capacity to prevent childhood obesity: Challenges, lessons learned and results from the Romp & Chomp intervention. https://core.ac.uk/download/pdf/8453785.pdf (accessed on 26th June 2025).

51. Sharkey, S., & Sharples, A. (2008). From the beginning: Negotiation in community evaluation. https://core.ac.uk/download/76704.pdf (accessed on 26th June 2025).

52. Symons, A. B., Kern, D. E., McGuigan, D., Morrison, E. H., Akl, E. A., Martin, H. L., Thistlethwaite, J. E., et al. (2009). A curriculum to teach medical students to care for people with disabilities: Development and initial implementation. https://core.ac.uk/download/pdf/8370449.pdf (accessed on 26th June 2025).

53. Teräs, H., & Kartoglu, N. (2023). Resilience to emergencies and civil society organizations. *Bulletin of the World Health Organization, 101*, 162–162A. https://www.semanticscholar.org/paper/ba85d07bd625f5fb410d7de682832800402d6dd6 (accessed on 26th June 2025).

54. Thalia, O. P. (2025). Data-driven decision making in public health initiatives. *Research Invention Journal of Biological and Applied Sciences*. https://www.semanticscholar.org/paper/a3118146cd506bca6a5661d0e2bf766c716adfa6 (accessed on 26th June 2025).

55. Traub, C., & Kovacevic, R. (2025). Exploring co-participation in health: Strategies and initiatives towards inclusive well-being. *International Journal of Health Governance*. https://www.semanticscholar.org/paper/11f014ce88a89ab242ae136094fd955a6dc6784c (accessed on 26th June 2025).

56. Usher, A., Lampe, C., Kreuter, F., Alvarez, G., Lane, J., Japec, L., Berg, M., et al. (2015). AAPOR report on big data. https://core.ac.uk/download/75781498.pdf (accessed on 26th June 2025).

57. Wilder-Smith, A., Cherian, T., & Hombach, J. (2025). Dengue vaccine development and deployment into routine immunization. *Vaccines, 13*. https://www.semanticscholar.org/paper/a10598f5245cddff06f3ac99a046578bcf2f6537 (accessed on 26th June 2025).

58. Yu, H. C., Lewis-Charp, H., & Inouye, T. E. (2017). Advancing culturally responsive evaluations for boys and men of color. https://core.ac.uk/download/84911902.pdf (accessed on 26th June 2025).

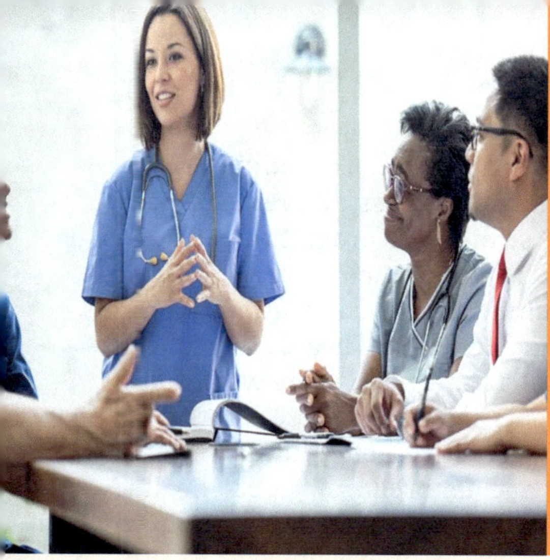

Chapter 6

HEALTH PROMOTION AND DISEASE PREVENTION

Contents

Introduction

Introduction to disease prevention and health promotion is a critical foundation of knowledge on how proactive strategies can make a significant difference in public health results. By focusing on the discovery and re-engineering of lifestyle factors, health promotion aims to enable individuals and populations to take control of their health, thus avoiding chronic disease and reducing healthcare expenses. Of specific interest, though, is that the World Health Organization (WHO) places an emphasis on strengthening capacities at the individual- and community-levels, leading to successful health improvement. Despite the recognized benefit, however, there are still issues in the deployment of effective health intervention recruitment processes, such that recent work has indicated the presence of significant variation in the rates of participation by targeted populations and representativeness. Intervention of such problems is required to facilitate the advancement of health promotion and ensure that it reaches the most vulnerable members of society (Estabrooks et al., 2025). More critical examination of recruitment practices in health promotion programs makes the necessity for a clearly defined strategy to ensure increased participation and engagement apparent. The findings of a scoping review indicated a wide variety of recruitment strategies utilized across different studies, where some interventions were capable of using more than one strategy in order to maximize reach. The current studies did not, however, provide adequate details about their methodological design, such as dose and timing of the strategies, thus often resulting in low comparability and reliability in findings. Thus, a critical component of facilitating the advancement of health promotion is developing standardized criteria upon which to evaluate recruitment strategies. Future work must not only aim for more clarity but also build the theoretical concepts informing these strategies, and as a result, more effective implementation and monitoring of health promotion interventions across a range of populations (Estabrooks et al., 2025). Under the umbrella of global health initiatives, particularly in nations like those in Latin America, equal access to healthcare promotion through community outreach is essential. Ecuador, for instance, has implemented a Ten-Year Health Plan post-COVID-19 to meet holistic improvements in health according to the different needs of its population. A role of utmost importance belongs to community involvement in establishing widespread health problems and formulating prevention programs accordingly in this situation. These local interventions have the potential to establish strong partnerships that address social determinants of health and foster sustainable development. Moreover, by emphasizing health promotion interventions aimed at building healthy behaviors, the stakeholders can contribute significantly towards narrowing gaps in health status and quality of life, thereby moving towards an equitable society (Figure 6.1).

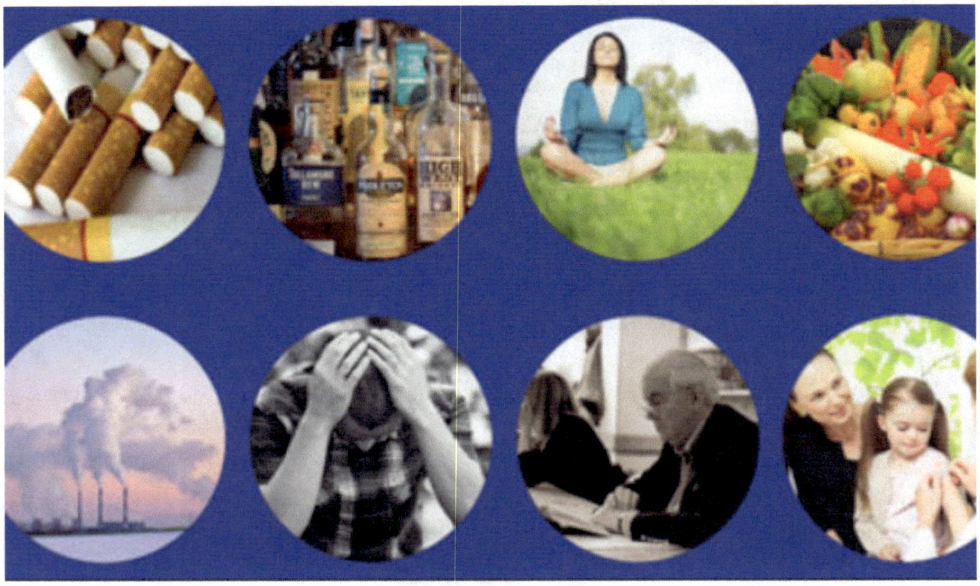

Figure 6.1. Health promotion and disease prevention.

Source: https://www.aim-mutual.org/wp-content/uploads/2017/02/position.jpg.

Definition of Health Promotion

Health promotion is a general process to enhance the physical and mental health of individuals and populations by using various strategies and interventions. It is not simply disease prevention, but it is a more integrative idea that grasps health as an evolving construction that relies on various determinants. Such determinants include but are not limited to social, economic, environmental, and behavioral determinants that have strong potentials of affecting an individual's ability for optimal health. By equipping people with information and resources, health promotion seeks to promote healthier lifestyles as well as choices that eventually lead to improved well-being in the long run. Besides, this comprehensive approach recognizes that health is a dynamic process requiring ongoing effort and social support to cope with the complex interactions between these determinants. Central to the concept of health promotion is the emphasis on modifying risk factors associated with chronic diseases, which permeate modern society. For instance, cardiovascular risk factors were recently discovered to correlate significantly with dementia and cognitive impairment, and that further reflects the significance of addressing those areas of health as part of overall health promotion. The research from the American Heart Association elaborates on ideal brain health as well as ideal health behavior and factors that may be quantified and changed to reduce chronic disease risks. These health-enhancing behaviors are such as frequent physical exercise, proper nutrition, and regulation of cholesterol and blood pressure levels. Such health-promoting activities are not only meant to cut back on the development of disease but also propagate a health-conscious culture that indirectly benefits communities and improves quality of life (Gorelick et al., 2017). The application of systems thinking to health promotion also enhances its potential for the effective prevention of disease. Systems thinking considers how all the various determinants of health interlink, understanding that individual health behavior is not independent. In Australia, for example, public health policymakers are exploring how systems thinking can revolutionize chronic disease prevention strategies by providing a holistic picture of how so many various determinants of health are interlinked. This method encourages intersectoral collaboration, integrating evidence-based methods with local practice and policy in a way that will create an efficient framework for health intervention. Although some practitioners have questioned applying systems approaches, the study describes an optimistic path toward developing effective health promotion plans that can provide sustainable improvement in health (Wutzke et al., 2016).

Importance of Disease Prevention

Successful disease prevention is crucial in enhancing the general health of populations and reducing the effects of different medical conditions. Ensuring preventive interventions takes high priority and can highly decrease the prevalence of diseases, resulting in healthier populations. For instance, the global burden of visual impairment shows the need for specific interventions. With some 1.1 billion people estimated to have distance vision impairment or uncorrected presbyopia in 2020, effective interventions, such as early access to eye care services and accessible treatment paths, can prevent preventable visual loss (Burton et al., 2021). Disease control programs of early detection and proper treatment can not only enhance individual health but also enhance economic productivity by reducing burdens of health care costs and lost labour productivity. Moreover, the approach of integrating measures of health promotion and disease prevention has been found to be high in effectiveness in control of infectious diseases. Interventions that consider human, animal, and environmental determinants—embracing the One Health concept—are critical in outbreak management and improving public health outcomes (Ellwanger et al., 2021). Critical interventions include vaccination programs, sanitation enhancement, and educational programs in the public sphere promoting personal hygiene and safe food preparation. Combining these interventions generates a more holistic health system with improved ability to handle the multicausal nature of diseases. Overall prevention of disease can significantly reduce health inequalities and promote resilience in communities, particularly relevant for poor settings where access to health resources is likely to be weak. Finally, the establishment of disease prevention on the public health agenda is central to sustainable development goals. Health promotion not only enhances the health of individuals but also has broader benefits for improving society as a whole, such as reducing poverty and education. In terms of vision health and other preventable diseases, there is clear evidence that expanded access to care has the ability to greatly improve quality of life and economic well-being for populations, particularly those in low- and middle-income environments (Burton et al., 2021). In addition, integrating disease prevention programs into national health policy ensures that arrangements for healthcare are both equitable and comprehensive, thus confirming the significance of prioritizing health programs that are not only effective but also socially fair and sustainable in the long run (Figure 6.2).

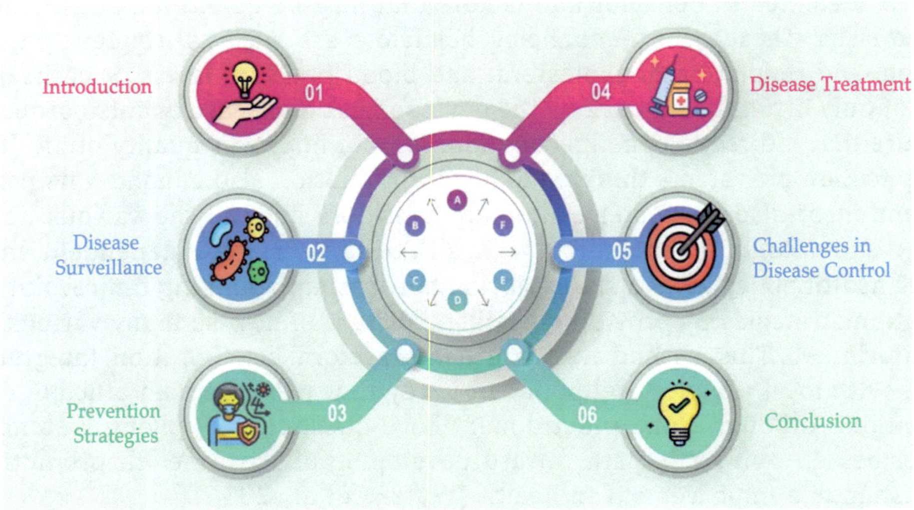

Figure 6.2. Importance of disease prevention.

Source: https://www.intakelearn.com/wp-content/uploads/2023/10/Prevention-of-Communicable-Diseases-banner-1024x655.webp.

6.1. The Role of Education in Health Promotion

Education plays an important role in health promotion since it is one of the key tools through which individuals acquire the skills and knowledge necessary to make informed choices about their health. Through the education of health literacy at an early stage, education can empower individuals to take on healthy living, mitigate the risk factors of chronic diseases, and embrace preventive measures. For instance, comprehensive health education curricula can cover several areas, including nutrition, physical fitness, and mental health, thereby equipping learners with the ability to learn about the importance of such areas in ensuring overall health. Besides that, as the contribution of health professionals like Physician Assistants (PAs) to health advocacy adequately shows, education can also extend beyond the classroom to empower practitioners to create innovative educational interventions within their communities to promote health and prevent disease (Alvarez et al., 2018). Such initiatives underscore the essential interdependence between education and successful health promotion strategies. Besides, the integration of health education into public health nursing school curricula reflects the discursive nuances of health promotion and disease prevention. Public health nurses are taught to operate at both the individual and population levels, facilitating easy transfer of knowledge essential for active management of health. Through critical analysis of the educational framework, several discourses become clear that shape the handling of health promotion in nursing education. As an example, there is a recognized tension between paternalistic and cooperative healthcare models responding to prevailing social values and the roles placed upon health professionals. This tension implies that effective health promotion depends on an understanding of not just clinical skills but also the socio-political narratives that inform them (Dahl et al., 2017). Consequently, the role of education is not merely didactic but inextricably participatory, designed to facilitate a shared context open to enhancing health. Finally, evidence of the impact of education on health outcomes demonstrates the necessity of constant innovation in pedagogy and practice. Just as public health evolves, so must the practice employed to educate populations. Population-specific interventions with particular population health issues can introduce enhanced motivation and efficiency in health promotion. An example is the application of technology and social media platforms to disseminate health messages that cater to diverse populations and thus improve accessibility and awareness. Educational approaches need to offer empowerment and self-efficacy for communities so they can take up health responsibility for themselves. As indicated in the involvement of PAs in health advocacy, education of healthcare professionals to perform the role of health promoters is crucial in bridging the knowledge-practice gap (Alvarez et al., 2018). Through this, education becomes a critical pillar within the overall plan of health promotion and disease prevention (Figure 6.3).

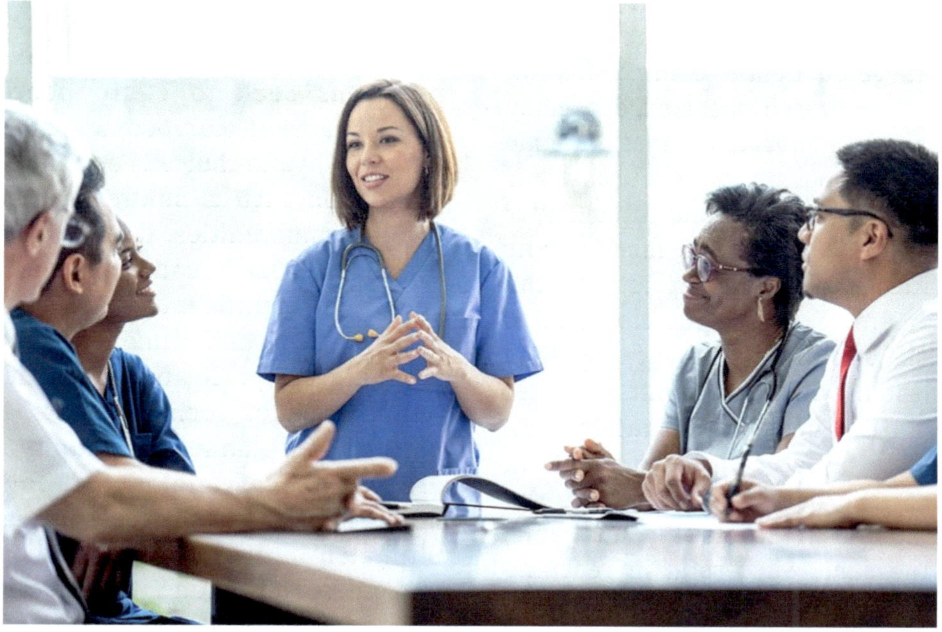

Figure 6.3. The role of education in health promotion.

Source: https://www.usa.edu/wp-content/uploads/2020/08/public-health-nurse-hero-2.jpg.

6.1.1. Health Literacy and Its Impact

Health literacy is a central determinant in the field of disease prevention and health promotion that plays a strong role in determining individuals' ability to navigate the healthcare system. Individuals with high health literacy have the ability to interpret medical language, follow treatment directions, and make health decisions independently. On the other hand, individuals with low health literacy will likely find it difficult to understand health information, resulting in worse health outcomes and higher healthcare expenditure. This gap not only amplifies prevailing health disparities but also reinforces cycle of confusion and mismanagement of chronic illnesses. Acceptance of the critical nature of health literacy is necessary to develop effective health promotion approaches that are appropriate for diverse populations so that everyone has the ability to interact with their health care in a meaningful way. Effective communication is central to improving health literacy, especially among diverse populations with specific challenges. As indicated in recent studies, the need for targeted health communication strategies cannot be overemphasized, especially in populations that are expected to face systemic barriers to access healthcare resources. For example, lesbian, gay, bisexual, and transgender (LGBT) populations are likely to face specific health disparities and misconceptions in the healthcare system. Such populations have specific health communication campaigns developed for them, which can facilitate better communication with health information that, in turn, results in better health outcomes. In such situations, it is necessary to involve the communities' people in developing the same, thus making the same successful in reaching out to the target groups (Drabble et al., 2003). By so doing, health promotion interventions are able to achieve a maximum level of health literacy and enable individuals to take control of their own health. In addition, integrating health literacy interventions into vast public health strategies shows a comprehensive approach to health promotion and disease prevention. It is also crucial to note that health literacy is not just a matter of individual capacity; it is a matter of collective responsibility to create settings that can facilitate the capacity to access clear and correct health information. As noted in the State of Health Equity Movement report, placing health equity on the forefront of policymaking is crucial to address the structural issues that lie behind low health literacy (Birnbaum et al., 2011). With community-based education programs and available health resources, public health can narrow health disparities. Thus, this multi-component intervention not only benefits individual well-being but healthier communities by way of improved health literacy and equitable access to healthcare.

6.1.2. Community Health Education Programs

Community health education programs are a fundamental component in the area of health promotion and disease prevention. These programs seek to equip people with the knowledge and competence needed to make informed health choices. Focusing on a particular population, such as children, the elderly, or low-income communities, these programs address disparate health concerns specific to each subgroup. Significantly, these programs look at how social determinants affect health and, in doing so, place individual health choices within broader social contexts. For instance, efficaciously planned community interventions are capable of minimizing poverty-related, illiteracy-related, and access to healthcare risks, ultimately promoting improved public health outcomes. The action to inform communities on health issues is one of the proactive measures needed for a successful health promotion policy and a step towards reducing health inequalities through evidence-based action. The success of community health education programs is enhanced through the application of evidence-based practices that resonate with targeted audiences. These strategies often build on appropriate cultural materials and methods, so that not just are messages being heard but also being absorbed by the participants. Collaboration with local agencies and leaders can provide a basis for trust and enhance participation and ensure a better likelihood of program success. The Centers for Disease Control and Prevention (CDC) has depicted this model by promoting programs that give priority to the most emphasis on nutrition, physical activity, and obesity prevention, highlighting the need for concerted focus in the community environment (O'Toole et al., 2022). The establishment of partnerships within communities could lead to enhanced participation rates, essential for long-term health education program sustainability. Lastly, the ability of outreach programs to respond to the needs of diverse populations is essential to the long-term effectiveness of such programs. Advances in technology and communications have also widened the reach and impact of community health education programs. The Internet and other online platforms facilitate the dissemination of health information and opportunities for interactive and interactive learning experiences readily accessible to a greater number of individuals. Aside from this, social media campaigns have proven efficient in raising awareness about public health, as they can spread vital information quickly and elicit community participation. Despite all these advancements, there remain concerns, primarily the digital divide that heavily disadvantages marginalized communities the most. Yet, integrating technology with the traditional education systems offers potential avenues for enhancing the effectiveness of community health programs. As public health becomes increasingly advanced, maintaining the emphasis on these complex educational approaches, which couple direct contact with technological innovation, will be key to establishing a healthier society and ultimately preventing disease (Jumba, 2024) (Figure 6.4).

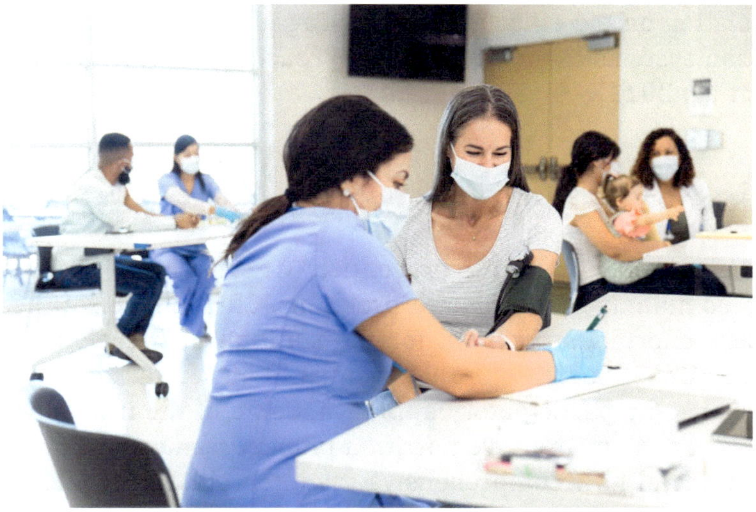

Figure 6.4. Community health education programs.

Source: https://www.usmhe.com/wp-content/uploads/2023/03/iStock-1361778800.jpg.

6.1.3. School-Based Health Education Initiatives

School-based health education efforts have been a core focus in the health promotion and disease prevention effort over the past few years. These programs aim to improve health literacy among students by including elementary health information in school curricula. Addressing issues of nutrition, physical exercise, mental health, and sanitation, these programs empower young people to make informed choices about their health and form better habits. The applicability of such programs is vindicated by global health experts that advocate for the holistic strategy to ensure health education in schools, emphasizing its impact on health outcomes on a long-term basis in various populations, particularly in middle- and low-income nations (Burton et al., 2021). Furthermore, the implementation of structured health education programs in schools is potentially likely to have a significant impact on society, particularly if directed towards vulnerable populations. Youth from disadvantaged groups will tend to experience disparities in the quality of health education, potentially with adverse health impacts. Interventions designed to correct the inequalities have the potential to bridge health literacy gaps, thereby improving health outcome equity among student populations. Increased interest in inclusive approaches aligns with global aspirations to reduce health disparities alongside attaining universal comprehensive health coverage across all citizens. Well-funded and supported programs may allow for successful involvement and create awareness among students regarding their health needs and available resources, thereby stimulating pro-active health-seeking practices (Bull et al., 2020). Additionally, collaborations between various stakeholders—educators, health personnel, families, and policymakers—are required for the effectiveness and sustainability of school-based health education programs. An effective health education program not only requires adequate funding and resources but also the inclusion of teachers who are adequately trained to carry out such curricula in a confident and competent manner. Technical assistance by state, local, and national governments can institutionalize health education in schools and render the program a permanent fixture in schools. The imperative to develop such multi-dimensioned partnerships demonstrates that health promotion is everyone's business, as collaborative strategic action can lead to improved health among students. With the evidence still accumulating on the efficacy of these programs, it becomes imperative to raise their profile within education systems as an integrated approach towards health promotion and disease prevention (Burton et al., 2021).

6.2. Behavioral Strategies for Disease Prevention

Behavioral strategies play a role in disease prevention, where they go beyond individual behavior and are interested in community-based health programs. CBHP models of health promotion have been shown to possess enormous potential for the solution of prevalent health issues, such as cardiovascular disease (CVD). Locating the determinants of health socially, the models facilitate long-term behavior change by participatory approach. Some of the interventions that are used to promote healthy physical activity, improve nutrition practices, and advocate for smoking cessation are just a few illustrations of how comprehensive the interventions are. There is robust evidence supporting the effectiveness of CBHP interventions, with statistics indicating that concerted efforts can lead to considerable public health improvements. Moreover, integrating technology solutions, such as digital health platforms, has the potential to enhance access and utilization across populations, ultimately enhancing the overall efficacy of these behavioral interventions towards disease prevention (Komi et al., 2024). Furthermore, education forms a fundamental element to enhance health promotion and disease prevention. The multiplicity of the nature of education, particularly when taking into account health practice among children and adolescents, brings into context its important role. Educational programs with a behaviorally grounded strategy, including interactive learning experiences, can facilitate young people with the knowledge and skills needed for healthier choices of living. Through the delivery of evidence-based information on nutrition, active living, and dangers of substance use, such programs instill a health literacy culture. As a result of the collaborative nature of these initiatives, the development of effective strategies for specific communities occurs, thus responding to precise health needs. Integrated educational systems are able to build successful long-term behavioral change and assist in the promotion of a long-term reduction in the incidence of preventable diseases (Khalifa et al., 2024). Overall, the implementation of disease prevention behavior programs necessitates an integrated intervention with the participation of the community, education, and policy adjustment. Successful interventions address not only individual behavior but also leverage the strength of social networks and localized support networks. Overcoming barriers to access to health care, facilitating inclusive strategies, and promoting stakeholder collaboration are critical factors that make preventive initiatives scalable and sustainable. As society struggles with numerous health issues, the integration of behavior change interventions into health promotion programs can yield improved health status and reduced disease prevalence. By continuous optimization of the same and their optimization based on emerging needs, public health programs can effectively capture the complexities of health promotion and disease prevention of the present times (Khalifa et al., 2024; Komi et al., 2024) (Figure 6.5).

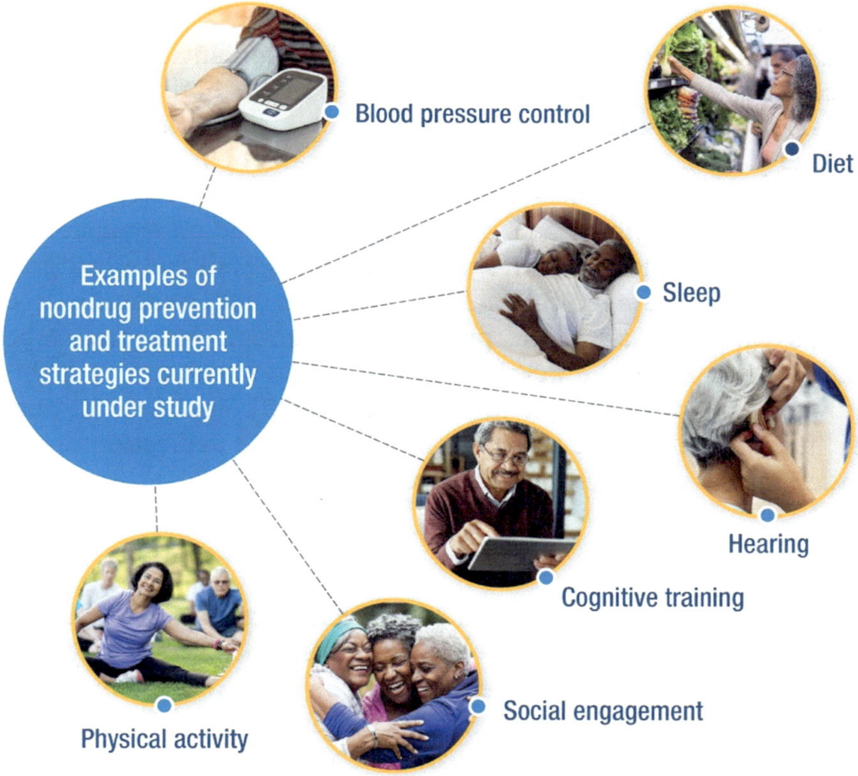

Figure 6.5. Behavioral strategies for disease prevention.

Source: https://www.nia.nih.gov/sites/default/files/styles/none/public/2020-08/NIAAD-Bypass-Budget-Layout_Figure4_1920x1080px_1.jpg .

6.2.1. Importance of Lifestyle Choices

The importance of lifestyle decisions for health promotion and disease prevention cannot be overstated. Daily decisions regarding diet, exercise, and stress control have a pivotal role in the outcome of health. For instance, dietary habits involving high intake of fruits, vegetables, and whole grains have been found to reduce the risk of chronic diseases such as heart disease, diabetes, and obesity. Regular exercise not only assists weight maintenance but also improves cardiovascular health and improves emotional well-being. Hence, promoting healthier lifestyle choices is included in controlling healthcare costs for preventable diseases, ultimately saving the people and society at large. By understanding the impact of their choices, people can take initiative in safeguarding their health and wellness, exemplifying the crucial connection between lifestyle and preventing long-term disease. Moreover, the effect of lifestyle choices goes beyond physical healthcare, having a significant impact on mental health and affecting cognitive functioning and emotional balance. Studies have indicated that regular physical exercise can reduce anxiety and depressive mood, thereby promoting healthier mental health outcomes. Proper nutrition has also been linked to better mood and intellectual function, again illustrating the mind-body connection. Mindfulness practice and stress management are equally crucial because ongoing stress has been demonstrated to exacerbate physical issues. In understanding the link between mental health and lifestyle habits, healthcare providers are better able to move patients toward holistic practices of health promotion and disease prevention. Through establishing environments that support well behaviors, society can construct a culture of wellness that benefits both the physical and the mental health of individuals. Finally, the role of healthcare and public health interventions in promoting a healthy lifestyle choice plays a crucial role in narrowing health disparities at the population level. Healthcare providers can utilize evidence-based recommendations to integrate lifestyle counseling into routine care, thus enabling patients to choose lifestyle based on their health. As highlighted in right health guidelines, e.g., the guidelines provided by the ESC, there is a great responsibility of health professionals to implement care as per complete understanding of every individual patient's setting. This planned care should prioritize prevention strategies, especially for those with higher vulnerability towards the development of chronic diseases, as highlighted in recent discussions about preventing dementia (Livingston et al., 2020). Thus, raising public awareness of the importance of lifestyle can provide a greater sense of shared dedication to disease prevention and health promotion, and a healthier and more resilient society.

6.2.2. Role of Physical Activity

Physical activity is critical in health promotion and disease prevention. Regular physical activity contributes to improved cardiovascular health, weight management, and enhanced metabolic function. Studies have proven that a healthy, active lifestyle not only keeps a person from becoming obese but also decreases the chances of developing chronic diseases such as hypertension, diabetes, and cardiovascular disease. As recommended by health agencies, exercise is important for achieving optimal health, and it should be an integral component of public health interventions to promote quality of life. Through physical activity-supportive environments, communities can make significant contributions to health outcomes, reduce health care costs, and maximize well-being in diverse populations. Evidence supporting these claims identifies a critical need for increased public education about the benefits of regular physical activity for long-term health gain and the prevention of disease. The link between physical activity and mental well-being is another significant health promotion area. Regular exercise has also been associated with fewer symptoms of depression and anxiety and a higher level of cognitive function and mental health overall. New studies have discovered that physical exercise can lead to enhanced brain health by reversing the effects of aging and fostering the risks associated with cognitive decline. As highlighted in the American Heart Association guideline, healthy behaviors like regular physical activity are most important to maintaining cognitive health among adults, therefore lowering the risk of dementia and other neurodegenerative disorders. Furthermore, physical exercise fosters social engagement and community involvement, which can reverse loneliness, an experience that is prevalent with mental illness. Therefore, by promoting physical exercise, not only do individuals ensure their physical well-being but also improve their psychological strength and emotional calmness. In presenting the integrative function of physical exercise in promoting health and preventing illness, its impact on public health initiatives needs to be taken into account. Governments and public health agencies need to support active living through policy and programs fostering access to safe recreation spaces, physical education instruction, and community health promotion activities. These strategies have been demonstrated to yield astonishing gains in population-level health outcomes and indicate that the group benefits of enhanced physical activity can lead to decreases in healthcare costs and disease incidence. With countries seeing mounting levels of obesity and associated health expenditures, prioritizing physical activity as the key to health promotion is crucial. Through focusing public health efforts on comprehending the gigantic impact of physical activity on the body and mind, we can aim for a healthier community with decreased disease rates and a better quality of life for all, according to contemporary literature on trends in global health (Bray et al., 2018; Gorelick et al., 2017) (Figure 6.6).

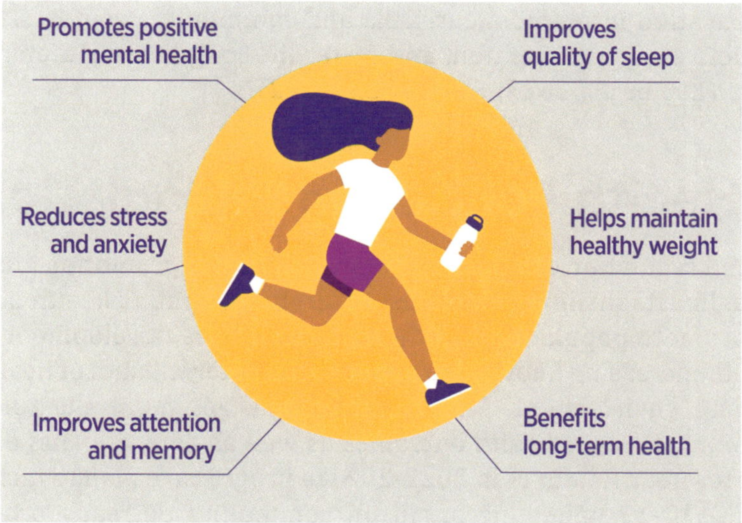

Figure 6.6. Role of physical activity.

Source: https://habs.uq.edu.au/files/52816/Instagram%20Post%20%E2%80%93%20Top%206%20benefits%20of%20PHYSICAL%20ACTIVITY.jpg.

6.2.3. Nutrition and Dietary Guidelines

Nutrition is a key to health promotion and disease prevention and the basis for the prevention of the chronic diseases of obesity, diabetes, and cardiovascular disease. Extensive dietary recommendations are needed in developing a home that will inform individuals about healthier food choices. These guidelines have been developed based on extensive literature, demonstrating the link between diet and health effects. In particular, special interventions must be created to address the unique issues of poor families that may be subject to restrictions on healthy nutrition due to limited budgets or inadequate nutrition education. Evidence shows that during the COVID-19 pandemic, the majority of families reported a negative dietary pattern shift, characterized by increased reliance on processed foods and self-reliance on nutrition program services, hence necessitating the need for new and situation-specific nutritional advice for public health interventions (Lee et al., 2023). The impact of food patterns extends beyond individuals; they impact community well-being and health. Local dietary patterns need to be known in order to construct effective guidelines that resonate with local populations. In countries like Pakistan, research has indicated that food selection is highly influenced by socioeconomics and cultural way of life. There has been a rising energy food demand with saturated fat and added sugars that has helped fuel an alarming rise in cardiometabolic disease among young people. This scenario highlights the imperative need for comprehensive national dietary recommendations that are sensitive to indigenous food habits, economic statuses, and accessibility of healthy foods so that alterations can be sustained economically at the community level (Shah et al., 2022). These dietary recommendations should also incorporate systematic behavior change strategies because advice itself might not be sufficient. There is a need for public health campaigns and education programs to improve nutrition literacy and encourage more appropriate food choices. Health promotion interventions through the use of technology, such as social media and mobile phone applications, are able to reach and effect various populations, particularly young people. In addition, collaborative efforts by healthcare providers, educators, and policymakers are needed to integrate nutrition education into school curricula and community programs. Such a multi-faceted strategy can help enable early intervention, and foster life-long healthy dietary habits and overall public health benefits (Lee et al., 2023; Shah et al., 2022).

6.3. Public Health Policies and Regulations

Public health policy and regulation are the basis on which health promotion and disease prevention activities are founded. In establishing guidelines underpinning public health activity, these policies seek to protect and promote population health. Historically, the development of such policies has gone hand-in-hand with increasing knowledge about social determinants of health, such as economic security, education, and environment. This trend emphasizes more the role of comprehensive strategies that contribute to better health outcomes as well as determinants of ill health. One such example is Ecuador's Ten-Year Health Plan 2022-2031, a progressive plan to tackle health disparities in the wake of the COVID-19 pandemic based on community outreach programs that enhance access to treatment and health literacy in marginalized groups (Zúñiga Sosa, 2025). Moreover, integration of public health policy into health systems is essential for maximizing the efficacy of health promotion efforts. As was witnessed through some of the case studies, for example, those of Ontario and Uganda, public health policy can catalyze system-wide transformations that help manage and prevent disease. Through these policies, there are linkages between health departments and community players, which means an integrated approach to health problems. Through addressing systemic issues through policy-making, public health interventions can focus on improving health outcomes and supporting sustainable health systems. Such mergers boost efficiency as well as enable communities to be actively involved in their health affairs, proving that efficient public health policy has a pivotal role to play in disease prevention as well as health promotion (Jumba, 2024). The role of public health policy extends beyond regulation; it is to facilitate healthy lifestyle in the community. Policies must be responsive to national and local health priorities to make people adopt healthier living. For instance, policies that help make communities educated about dietary habits and exercise can significantly reduce rates of chronic disease. This can be observed in many outreach programs that employ health education as a unifying component, serving to actively engage the public. Furthermore, policy interventions targeting environmental determinants can reduce barriers to health, such as access to clean water and healthy food. The success of such initiatives is a reflection of the fundamental position that properly designed public health policies occupy in creating healthier societies, leading ultimately to mortality and morbidity rates reductions (Zúñiga Sosa, 2025) (Figure 6.7).

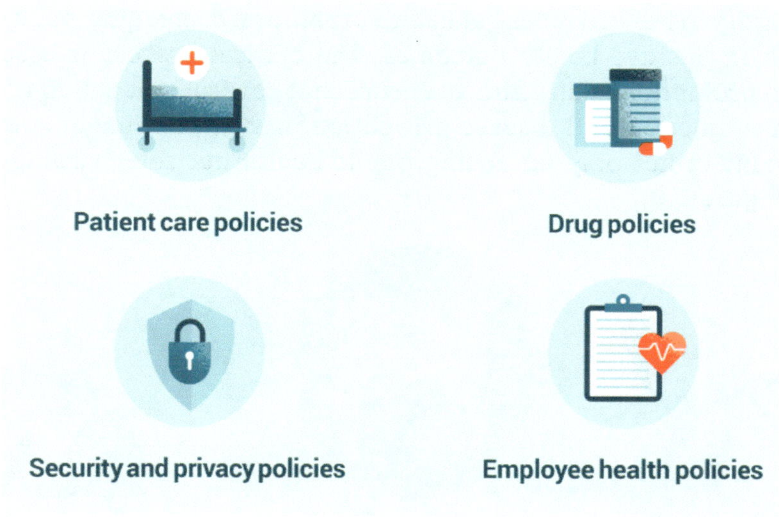

Figure 6.7. Public health policies and regulations.

Source: https://www.usa.edu/wp-content/uploads/2021/10/healthcare-policy-examples.png.

6.3.1. Government Initiatives for Health Promotion

Government health promotion initiatives are of vital importance in influencing public health outcomes by addressing the underpinning social determinants of health. Such programs tend to concentrate on developing health-supportive environments that promote healthier lifestyles while emphasizing the necessity for addressing socioeconomic determinants of the health status. For instance, as noted in Philip O'Hara (2005), a realization of the social determinants of health can pave the way for radical health care reforms. By incorporating these social determinants into policy, governments are able to enact strategies that directly address the broader context of health inequalities, ultimately working towards the goal of enhancing the overall health equity within communities. These measures not only encourage the healthiness of individuals but also work to promote the collective health of populations, supporting the sound claim that health is a collective societal responsibility. Also characteristic of effective health promotion initiatives are coalition partnerships between government and non-governmental agencies. Through partnership building, e.g., with health professionals and community leaders, and through their inclusion in the planning process, initiatives can craft programs designed specifically to address determined needs for improved local health. The Playbook for Action outlined in N/A (2008) offers a tool for leaders wishing to translate health policy ideas into operational activities. It harmonizes speech among the key stakeholders towards the implementation of evidence-based health interventions. Such collaborations enhance the chances of successful policy uptake and facilitate the exchange of best practices among different regions. Such government-sponsored initiatives can, thus, induce actual far-reaching health changes, ensuring that preventive interventions are not just initiated but sustained in the long run. In addition to social determinants and partnership models, successful health promotion also relies on continuous monitoring and program evolution to respond to emerging health concerns. Governments must remain responsive to emerging health threats, such as the incidence of chronic disease or pandemics, by examining strategies and reallocating resources accordingly. Data-driven programs can do a great deal to enhance their efficiency. By using metrics to quantify the effectiveness of health promotion campaigns, policymakers can inform decisions that result in positive health outcomes. The cyclical process is essential in enhancing approaches in health promotion in an effort to ensure that government action remains effective and applicable in health promotion and disease prevention. Lastly, such ongoing evaluations validate the role of government in not only advancing public health but safeguarding the future welfare of the population (Figure 6.8).

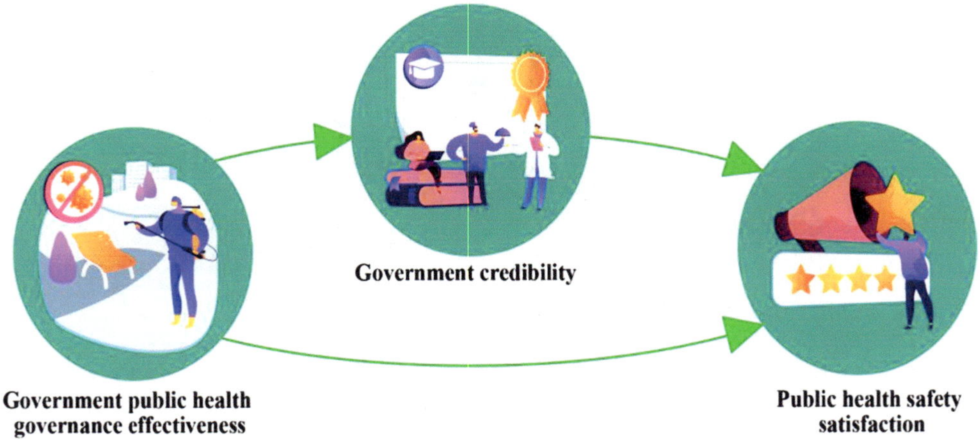

Figure 6.8. Government initiatives for health promotion.

Source: https://media.licdn.com/dms/image/v2/D4D12AQFWAESlIX-enQ/article-cover_image-shrink_720_1280/article-cover_image-shrink_720_1280/0/1692677390250?e=2147483647&v=beta&t=zNnRMO1_-iMaU21S2Y6D7BFhk8aywtWBNpNJtVKSGEs.

6.3.2. Impact of Regulations on Disease Prevention

Regulatory regimes play a critical role in the determinants of public health, especially in the context of disease prevention activities. In-depth regulations set boundaries for health practices and conduct, affecting community health habits significantly. For instance, regulations in urban planning to restrict greenhouse gas emissions have a significant impact on public health. Cities like Bologna, which strive to be climate neutral, demonstrate how targeted regulations can reduce health risks from environmental changes. The interconnection between built environments and health becomes clearer, where interventions to improve built environment and transport can lead to decreased rates of respiratory diseases and improved overall well-being within the general community, consequently fulfilling the objectives of disease prevention and health promotion (Nuvolari-Duodo et al., 2024). In oral health, preventive strategies based on fluoride emphasize the effectiveness of policy regulations in preventing dental disease. Regulatory guidelines facilitated the introduction of community-based interventions, such as water fluoridation, as inexpensive methods to prevent dental caries, the most prevalent infectious disease in the world. The implementation of fluoride in public health programs indicates the significance of aligning interventions with community needs and risks to reduce inequalities in oral health. Of importance, regulatory frameworks also control safe levels of fluoride exposure, given that there have been heightened suspicions of overexposure to systemic amounts especially in children. By having clearly demarcated standards, regulations are able to strike a balance for maximizing preventive effects of fluoride while protecting vulnerable populations from negative effects on health (Veneri et al., 2024). The impact of regulation extends beyond individual prevention of disease to extend to broader policy measures that address social determinants of health. Public participation in the development and implementation of health regulations can make them more effective, as well as more accepted by the public. Policies that seek to promote oral health literacy, access to preventive dental care, and dental product affordability can all contribute to improving health inequities. For instance, regulative programs that mandate school-based dental programs or community health outreach are best able to reach underrepresented populations and ensure preventive services are accessible to everyone. In this way, regulations can facilitate comprehensive health promotion programs that not only prevent targeted disease but also promote overall community health and robustness (Veneri et al., 2024) (Figure 6.9).

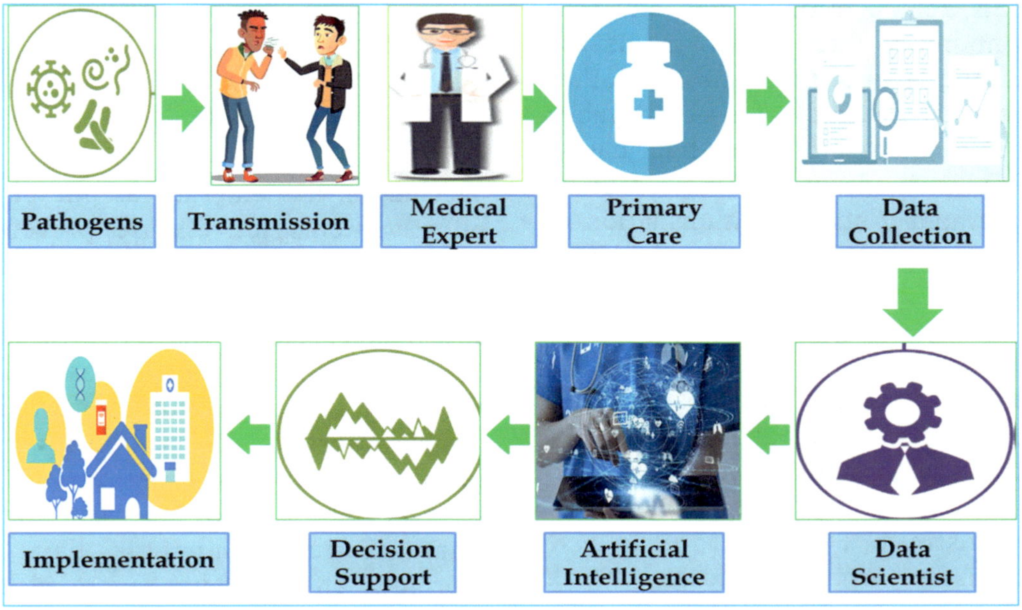

Figure 6.9. Impact of regulations on disease prevention.

Source: https://www.researchgate.net/publication/359437289/figure/fig1/AS:1147550837018626@1650608848877/nfectious-disease-prevention-principles-must-be-followed-The-series-presents-the-main.png.

6.3.3. Case Studies of Successful Public Health Policies

Public health policy has been a vital tool in the war against health challenges, with numerous successful case studies demonstrating its potential for triumph. One such example is the effective exercise of integrated tobacco control policies, best exemplified in Australia and Canada. Australia and Canada have undertaken an all-encompassing effort to combat tobacco use in the form of graphic warning labels on tobacco, bans on smoking in public areas, and a wide-ranging taxation of tobacco products. Evidence indicates that such policies have contributed to a significant decrease in smoking prevalence and related health ailments. The WHO report asserts that integration of comprehensive anti-tobacco policies has not only decreased the rates of occurrence of smoking-related diseases but also contributed to a cultural change towards improved lifestyles. This case illustrates the ability of targeted political and social interventions to effectively reverse public health threats, demonstrating the effectiveness of persistent policy intervention in disease prevention and health promotion. Another very compelling case study of effective public health policy is the case of water fluoridation programs implemented in various regions. Brazil has demonstrated a strategic fluoridation of public water supplies to significantly lower the prevalence of dental caries in populations, particularly in high-risk groups. Such prevention is supported by the WHO, as it cites that water fluoridation is one of the most cost-effective public health interventions available to us today. In low-income communities, where access to dental care is typically low, these kinds of programs constitute a first line of defense against oral disease. What is particularly worth noting is that the enactment of fluoridation is also a model public-private partnership that aggregates resources and capabilities across different sectors for enhancing community health outcomes and paving the way for follow-up policies for prevention of disease in the area of dental health. Cardiovascular health is another area where sound public health policy has been a real payoff. Various nations have had comprehensive plans encompassing dietary guidelines, exercise advice, and regulation of unhealthy products like trans fats and sodium. Decreasing rates of cardiovascular disease in nations with tight food regulation, for instance, parallel the extent of success for comparable public health efforts. The Global Burden of Disease Study reveals that such specific policies are required in an effort to address the overwhelming rise of noncommunicable diseases worldwide. Public health experts consider that increasing the profile of heart health-initiative programs has the potential to mobilize resources effectively in a bid to address this top health issue, affirming the need for ongoing investment in evidence-based public health interventions to realize long-term success in health promotion and disease prevention (Roth et al., 2020).

6.4. The Importance of Vaccination

Vaccination has emerged as one of the most effective tools for disease prevention and health promotion, and it has changed the face of public health globally. Not only does the vaccination of individuals protect the immunized individuals but also contributes to population immunity, hence protecting communities from future outbreaks. It is especially critical for populations who are unable to be vaccinated due to health problems or age-related limitations. Immunization campaigns have reduced morbidity and mortality due to such diseases as polio, measles, and influenza substantially, showcasing the important role that vaccines play in developing broader public health and well-being. The development history of vaccines illustrates the possibility of vaccine efficacy in eliminating diseases, further highlighting that prevention through vaccination is not only a moral imperative but also a viable public health strategy. Nevertheless, the dividends of immunization extend beyond immediate improvements in health; they also create significant economic payoffs to nations. A successful vaccination campaign has the potential to reduce healthcare costs associated with the treatment of diseases, epidemics, and lost productivity. Successful immunization drives also translate into fewer cases of morbidity, healthier individuals, and improved life expectancy, which are a measure of the eventual long-term economic viability of such health campaigns. While these benefits are real, public hesitation over vaccination is a significant constant challenge. Social media and cultural norms-based misinformation often creates uncertainty regarding vaccine safety and effectiveness. Strategic communication, educational efforts, and collaboration with advocacy organizations must address these concerns in an effort to maximize vaccination rates and cultivate a preventive care-focused culture. To realize the full potential of vaccination as a means of health promotion, it is essential to have inclusive public health policies that promote equal access to immunization. This entails identification and removal of systemic barriers to vaccination, especially among vulnerable groups. For instance, systemic factors such as socioeconomic disparities and unaffordable healthcare services can have a significant effect on vaccination coverage. Additionally, public discourse on vaccination on sites such as social media can counter misinformation and set the importance of vaccines. In addition to that, as recognized in current research, efforts at mobilizing the public on vaccination issues, particularly in instances like male HPV vaccination, reflect the need to confront gender norms and stereotypes (Zhou et al., 2025). Hence, a wider and composite strategy, as suggested by public health objectives, is critical in supporting the practice of immunization as a cornerstone of disease prevention policies in society (Nyiramana, 2024) (Figure 6.10).

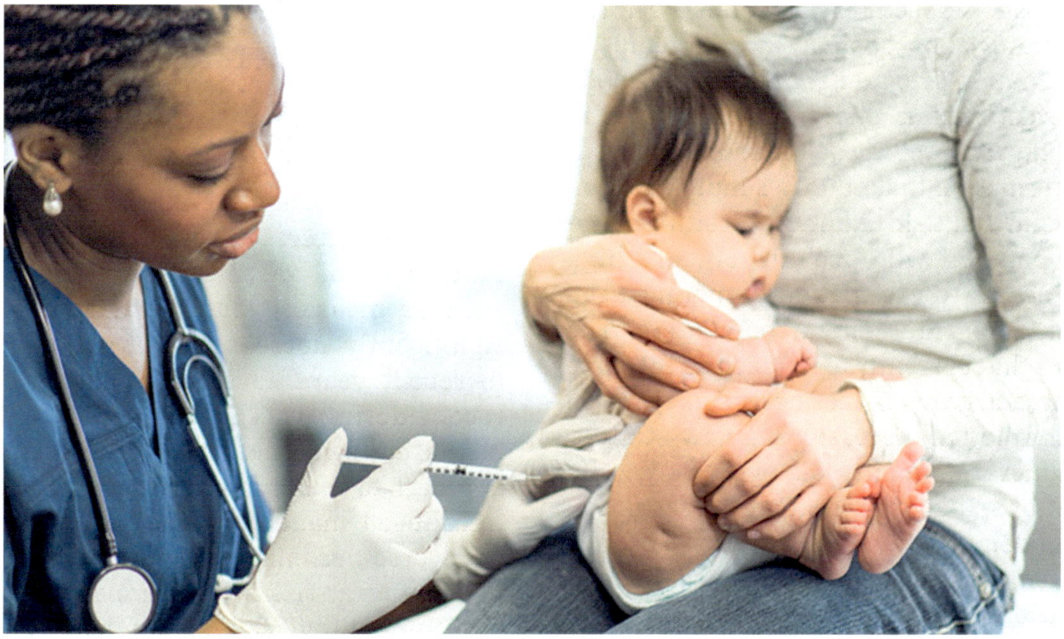

Figure 6.10. The importance of vaccination.

Source: https://images.agoramedia.com/wte3.0/gcms/The-Importance-of-Vaccines-722x406.jpg.

6.4.1. Overview of Vaccination Programs

Vaccination programs form part of public health interventions that aim to prevent disease and are a significant determinant of the health of populations. They prevent infectious diseases from becoming epidemic in populations through the creation of herd immunity. Vaccination has, in the past, led to the eradication of smallpox and a massive decline in cases of measles and polio. But implementation success relies on many factors, including social acceptability and availability of vaccines, as well as public perception. For example, HPV vaccination programs attempt to vaccinate men as well as women, but are foiled by cultural sentiments and policy delays in individual countries, most significantly in China, where public opinion reflects prevailing gender norms and widespread misinformation about health behavior. Debates are overcome by taking this step in a bid to maximize vaccine uptake and encourage healthier populations (Zhou et al., 2025). The solution requires a multi-faceted approach, such as education, policy reform, and community engagement, in an attempt to push vaccination program enhancement. Public health organizations strive to build trust in vaccines through the dissemination of broad-based information that educates individuals on benefits and risks. In addition, health equity-focused policies will provide equally high levels of access to vaccination to marginalized communities as the general population. The challenges that currently exist, such as resource constraints and growing vaccine hesitancy driven by misinformation, necessitate a new strategy that includes community dialogue. Successful interventions, like the Diabetes Prevention Program, demonstrate how effective public health interventions can be to create change and positive health outcomes, and similarly too might targeted education programs increase public immunization support (Nyiramana, 2024). For the future, the future of vaccination programs hangs in the balance depending on technology and research advancements, with doors open to increased health promotion intervention. New vaccine technology such as mRNA vaccines has turned the tide and offered hope in the battle against not only active infectious disease but future pandemics. Further, the application of social media for education in health can increase public discourse and help counter misinformation. Policy and health educators need to collaborate to counter challenges that continue to constrain effective immunization campaigns, particularly in regions with deeply entrenched bias against specific vaccines. A coordinated and holistic approach will make communities more resilient, promote evidence-based decision-making, and ultimately lead to increased immunization rates, thereby making public health interventions more effective and allowing for broader disease prevention (Nyiramana, 2024; Zhou et al., 2025).

6.4.2. Impact of Vaccines on Public Health

The impact of vaccines on public health is far-reaching and complex, serving as a keystone of global health promotion and disease prevention efforts. Vaccination has led to the significant decline in the occurrence of infectious diseases, thereby improving overall community health status. This success is evident when one realizes that cases of vaccine-preventable diseases such as measles, mumps, and rubella have significantly decreased. Outbreak responses in recent years have led to many countries reconsidering vaccination policies, with an increasing awareness of the necessity for an approach to health. Some European nations have introduced mandatory vaccination programs to reverse declining vaccine coverage, thereby protecting at-risk populations and enabling herd immunity. While the policies have been reported to improve uptake of the vaccine, the issue remains on how preventive healthcare procedures are followed in an educated way by the public, and therefore the need for ongoing health education campaigns (Odone et al., 2021). Besides, the emergence of vaccine distribution and acceptance issues, particularly in the context of the COVID-19 pandemic, has exposed public health inequities. The high-income countries have greater access to vaccines, resulting in enormous roll-out gaps compared to low- and middle-income countries. This imbalance raises critical ethical questions concerning global health responsibilities and resource allocation. Vaccine hesitancy, which has risen due to misinformation, uncertainty, and perceived risk, needs to be overcome in achieving mass vaccination coverage. For instance, findings indicate that in most African nations, COVID-19 vaccine uptake levels are critically low, which further highlights the significance of employing effective health communication strategies based on local contexts. It is important that there should be coordination between local communities, health authorities, and global agencies to build trust and increased vaccine uptake (Nachega et al., 2021). Ultimately, vaccines play a greater role than disease prevention; it is a vision for building stronger public health infrastructure and more resilience. The importance of a robust cold chain, proper storage, and distribution channels cannot be emphasized enough, particularly in environments of resource limitation that pose logistical challenges. As countries make efforts at equitable vaccine distribution, it is important to learn from past vaccination campaigns against polio and measles. Future health interventions must pay special attention to harmonized approaches addressing vaccine hesitancy and encouraging increased initiatives in community outreach. It will take an effort to break down the barriers to vaccination and establish a preventive health culture in diverse populations in order to achieve herd immunity against COVID-19 as well as against VPDs (Nachega et al., 2021) (Figure 6.11).

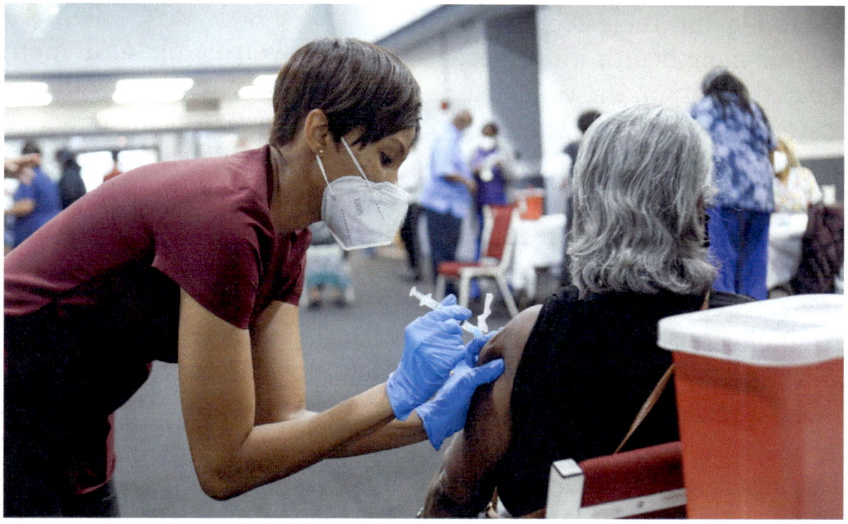

Figure 6.11. Impact of vaccines on public health.

Source: https://static01.nyt.com/images/2021/04/02/well/02WELL-NL-VACCINEFAQ3/02WELL-NL-VACCINEFAQ3-videoSixteenByNineJumbo1600-v2.jpg.

6.4.3. Addressing Vaccine Hesitancy

Vaccine hesitation is an important issue in health promotion and disease control, most commonly resulting from a multi-faceted convergence of misinformation, cultural perceptions, and discontent with health authorities. The rapid dissemination of health information—for better or worse—

has been facilitated a great deal through online media. Social media then becomes a double-edged sword; while facilitating quick dissemination of accurate health facts, it also offers avenues for the spread of misinformation. The role of Digital Opinion Leaders (DOLs), in particular, health professionals who are web participants, is critical in this regard. They have been effective in enhancing public health communication, prioritizing misconcept correction and role-playing preventive actions. Their influence can be used to fight vaccine hesitancy by educating the audience about the efficacy and safety of vaccines, as evidenced by their efforts at reducing fear of diseases like pertussis and dengue (Garbarczyk et al., 2025; Green et al., 2025). In the fight against vaccine hesitancy, strategic partnerships among DOLs and health sector stakeholders are important. The majority of the DOLs have reported working with pharmaceutical companies, government agencies, and NGOs to expand their scope and increase the efficacy of their health messages. Such partnerships can draw upon the expertise of medical professionals while harmonizing efforts in the community values to nullify such stereotypes. The success of these partnerships lies in staying on the high grounds of ethics to guarantee that the information being disseminated is medically correct and becomes rooted among the audiences. Through resource and information consolidation, health programs are better placed to articulate the importance of immunizations, leading to enhanced uptake rates ultimately. The collaborative actions also seek to enhance public engagement such that members of the community feel engaged and knowledgeable in the discourse of vaccinations and their crucial role in disease prevention (Garbarczyk et al., 2025; Green et al., 2025). To effectively combat vaccine reluctance, it is also important to discover and tackle specific demographic drivers that are drivers of the public's attitude toward vaccines. Evidence indicates that some groups express higher degrees of vaccine doubt based on previous wrongs, socioeconomic disparity, or cultural knowledge. Population-based health promotion interventions that consider such individual contexts can significantly enhance the efficacy of vaccination campaigns. Maternal immunization and promotion of booster are combined efforts to reach the high-risk groups, when herd immunity is compromised. By such priority for targeted interventions, health workers can not only promote vaccination but also restore faith in the health system. Public health communication, especially in the case of emerging health crises, must signal openness and sensitivity to public issues to establish a more informed and tolerant public attitude towards vaccinations (Garbarczyk et al., 2025; Green et al., 2025).

6.5. Mental Health and Well-being

Mental well-being and mental health form key components of overall health, which often dictates physical health outcomes as well as social productivity. World Health Organization (WHO) emphasizes that mental health transcends mere absence of mental illness, comprising a state of well-being whereby people are conscious of their potential and can cope adequately with issues of life (Gautam S et al., 2024). This broader definition emphasizes the need for active health promotion and disease prevention efforts. Through designing environments that support mental health, we can enhance community and individual coping capacity as well as resilience. Effective health promotion can only be attained through collaborative efforts among policymakers, health agencies, and stakeholders in the community to address the multifaceted determinants of mental wellbeing such as social capital and civic engagement, which are critical to enhance wellbeing alongside reducing mental health disparities. Furthermore, trauma in childhood can have huge effects on mental health as appreciated by trauma-informed care

(TIC). The TIC principles emphasize the need to recognize and respond to the impact of trauma on children and families. Research demonstrates how trauma can disrupt neurodevelopment and ultimately the trajectory of lifelong health (Duffee et al., 2021). Clinicians can create secure environments that build relational health and resilience in children in adversity using TIC in health systems. Placing emphasis on interventions in early life to reverse the effects of childhood trauma is essential in the prevention of adult-onset mental disorders. This approach allows the detection of supportive relationships that can serve as buffers to stress and facilitate resilience, demonstrating how prevention of mental disorders begins at an early age through comprehensive support systems. In the context of prevention of disease and health promotion, actively involving mental health is central to individual and general well-being. Effective coping strategies, which are based on education and social support, have been shown to enhance mental health resilience. Interventions to promote mental well-being can potentially build problem-solving capability, emotional regulation, and social connection. Research demonstrates that higher well-being is linked to lower prevalence of mental illness and improved quality of life (Gautam et al., 2024). Thus, the integration of mental health promotion within public health programs not only supports disease prevention but also leads to more successful and peaceful societies. This integrated approach requires a focus on mental health literacy, stigma prevention, and a conducive environment for well-being, ultimately producing a healthier population and cheaper care in the long term (Figure 6.12).

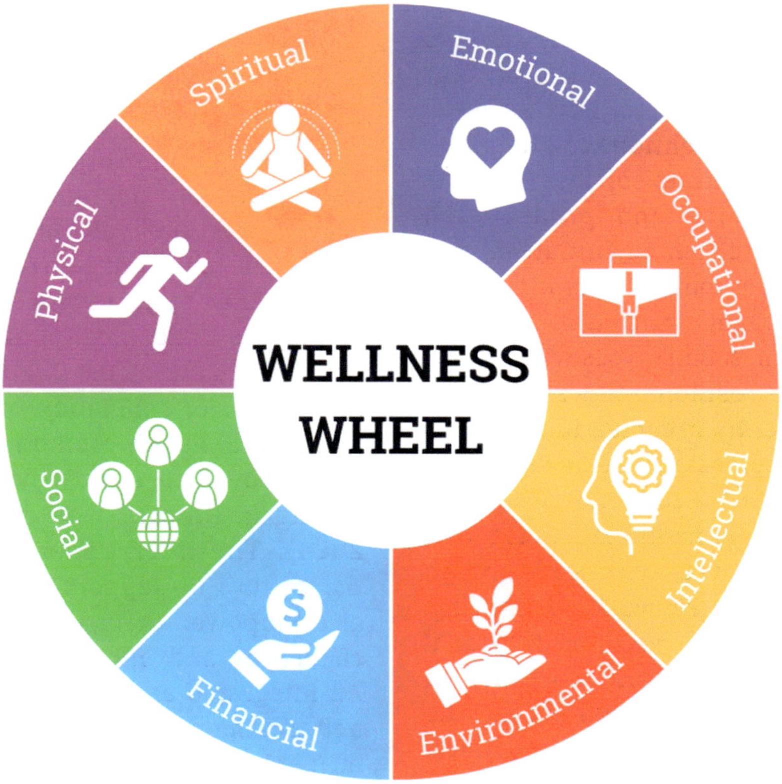

Figure 6.12. Mental health and well-being.

Source: https://tandempsychology.com/wp-content/uploads/2023/04/chart.png.

6.5.1. Connection Between Mental and Physical Health

The interlink between physical and mental health is one of the main pillars of overall health promotion and disease prevention. The evidence confirms that mental health plays an enormous role in physical health, as individuals who are experiencing stress, anxiety, or depression are more likely to develop chronic diseases such as heart disease and diabetes. This mutual relationship of symbiosis emphasizes the need for an integrated approach that addresses both body and mind. Investment in mental health care not only fosters resilience at an individual level but also subsequently enhances health outcomes, with an upward cycle creating healthier living and reduced disease prevalence. The impact of effective management of mental health means that healthcare measures must extend beyond the usual physical health markers to incorporate mental well-being as a focal point in public healthcare measures. Furthermore, effective workplace interventions can help link mental and physical health to support workers' psychological well-being and productivity. Wellness and health coaching initiatives can enable individuals to recognize the importance of self-care and stress management, as documented by multiple case studies. Employees who receive coaching are more resilient and self-aware, and this is subsequently reflected in improved physical health outcomes and decreased rates of chronic diseases. This association recognizes the importance of organizational investment in mental health initiatives, evidenced through organizations that emphasize worker well-being. This not only benefits the health of individual workers but also contributes positively to organizational performance, again stating the interdependent nature of mental and physical health in maximizing overall health promotion effectiveness (Lawson et al., 2019). Lastly, initiatives for promoting mental health are part and parcel of public health policy which is integrated in full into disease prevention. Models of public health which consider mental health and physical health might be able to minimize the social cost of stress-related disease. For instance, the Playbook for Action urges leaders to develop action plans to help strengthen both areas. By integrating mental health into physical health programs, public health programs have the capability to address root causes of chronic disease and subsequently lower long-term healthcare costs and improve quality of life. The dual strategy encourages policy-makers to realize that the promotion of mental well-being is not secondary to the promotion of physical health but a critical component of an integrated public health, facilitating resilient communities (N/A, 2008).

6.5.2. Strategies for Promoting Mental Well-Being

Evidenced-based ways of improving mental health are central to health promotion and prevention. Among these, one of the promising approaches is implementing organized interventions, particularly in high-stress professions such as nursing. The evidence indicates that organized programs can successfully build psychological resilience in employees under high-pressure conditions, as experienced during the COVID-19 pandemic. The integration of simulation-based team training and mental health promotion intervention has been proven to avoid psychosocial problems among healthcare workers (Wahyuni et al., 2024). The interventions not only enhance the culture of support among employees but also empower them with stress management capacities and enhanced overall well-being. An integrated approach combining prevention and treatment could yield long-term dividends in mental health outcomes for at-risk groups. Moreover, the promise of creative expression, and particularly the arts, has fallen into prominence as a key intervention for moving forward toward improved mental well-being. Creative endeavors could serve as a powerful tool for promoting the health of individuals and communities. Research indicates that art can promote emotional expression and social bonding, both of which are essential to enhancing mental health (Jumba, 2024). Art-integrated community health programs offer people a chance to establish bonds, create coping strategies, and manage stress. The collaborative approach in such programs promotes social cohesion, playing a critical role in enhancing collective mental health among communities. Through arts-based health interventions promotion and facilitation, public health policy can not only address short-term psychological need but also support long-term resilience and good health in diverse populations. In addition to training and aesthetic engagement, digital interventions represent an emerging frontier in promoting mental health. As technology use increases, digital spaces present new frontiers for mental health aid and support. Virtual counseling, mental health applications, and online community-based support groups have been successful as vehicles for individuals who require access and convenience in mental health treatment. These digital approaches can diminish access barriers, particularly in rural or underserved populations, in achieving access to individuals who might otherwise be reluctant to seek care (Wahyuni et al., 2024). Emphasizing the importance of integrating technology into health promotion programs reflects an understanding of contemporary society's needs. Thus, an integrative approach comprising various modalities—a continuum from face-to-face to virtual—can create a general framework for enhancing mental well-being as part of comprehensive health promotion and disease prevention.

6.5.3. Importance of Mental Health Resources

The value of mental health services cannot be highlighted enough in the context of their fundamental role in health promotion and disease prevention. Mental health services are essential tools in the early identification and treatment of many psychological diseases. According to the American Academy of Pediatrics, many adverse childhood experiences (ACEs) could have significant and enduring influences on both mental and physical health throughout one's life. By providing access to trauma-informed care (TIC) models, health practitioners can work with such early traumas effectively, promoting resilience among adolescents and youth, relational well-being, and ultimately minimizing the long-term effects of exposure to trauma. Not only does this benefit individuals but also makes families and communities stronger, making the community as a whole better (Duffee et al., 2021). The integration of mental health resources into health care systems thus becomes crucial for the provision of integrated patient care focusing on long-term outcomes. Apart from the alleviation of early-life traumas, mental health resources are vital for enabling the promotion of the well-being of populations facing various problems. The World Health Organization new guidelines emphasize physical activity for health promotion but not with the inclusion of mental health loses a little to the strategies for overall well-being (Bull et al., 2020). Physical activity is a significant aspect of mental well-being, but individuals must have access to mental health centers that foster healthy engagement in physical activities. This access generates a collaborative environment that can lead to increased self-efficacy, motivation, and overall mental health improvement. By integrating mental health services into community programs and health systems, stakeholders are in a position to create tailored initiatives that directly address the unique needs of specific populations, leading to a healthier society. Moreover, the impacts of inadequate mental health resources trickle down through society and affect not just individuals but populations' health as well. Poor mental health is also established to be a predictor for chronic diseases, which the CDC has linked to a number of risk factors, among them being social determinants of health (Duffee et al., 2021) Mental health managed by readily available resources is an effective solution to disease prevention because it can reduce health disparities brought about by largely untreated psychological disorders. Sensitizing individuals and making support groups, therapy, and counseling accessible can help public health programs eliminate the stigma of mental health disorders. Hence, this will encourage people to seek assistance and engage in preventive interventions, resulting in healthier populations and reduced disease burden in total. Expenditure on mental health resources is thus not merely an ethical necessity but a strategic public health necessity (Figure 6.13).

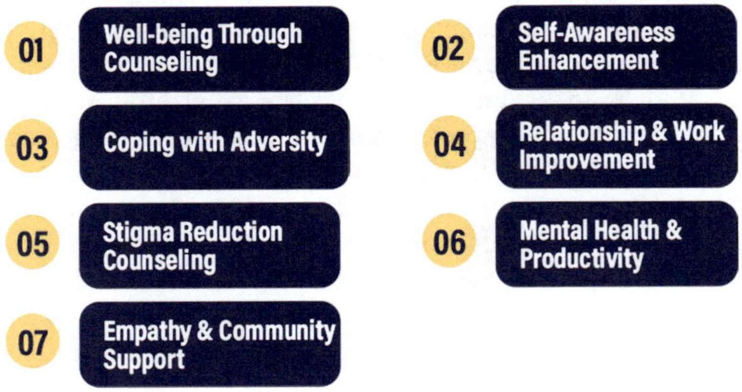

Figure 6.13. Importance of mental health resources.

Source: https://www.brightpoint-md.com/wp-content/uploads/2024/05/importance-of-mental-health-counseling.jpg.

6.6. Technology in Health Promotion

The use of technology in health promotion is a big leap for disease prevention measures. Telemedicine and mobile health apps are all types of digital health that bring health information and services closer to the reach of diverse populations. Technologies assist in delivering more personalized approach in terms of health management so that patients can monitor their own health, be given customized health advice, and become active participants in care. Through the provision of information and tools to users, technology serves to bridge disparities in access to health care, particularly for the uninsured. These technologies are required in order to decrease health disparities and formulate equitable health outcomes. As indicated in a systematic review, the application of community-led interventions with these technological tools constitutes an integrated framework for effective health promotion and disease prevention, further outlining the potential for technology to be a driving force for healthier communities (Scarpa et al., 2024). In addition to supporting the promotion of health management, technology also plays a critical role in the collection and processing of public health data. The use of big data analytics and health informatics transforms the way disease trends are understood and responded to by health workers. By pooling large datasets, officials in public health can identify trends, quantify health interventions, and adjust methods in real-time feedback. Moreover, instruments such as wearables facilitate continuous monitoring of health, with researchers being able to learn about patterns of behavior and health outcomes. This data-driven approach not only enhances the precision of public health interventions but also encourages preventive health against disease. As noted in the advancements regarding One Health initiatives, the integration between genomic data and health data can unlock significant progress in controlling zoonotic diseases and improving world health outcomes (Scarpa et al., 2024). Technological advancements also facilitate enhanced engagement with health promotion programs via innovative communications. Online learning programs and social media platforms are good tools for the dissemination of health information and mobilization of communities. These give health organizations a platform for engaging a wide population within a short time, sharing vital health tips, and stimulating open involvement in health programs. Further, application of technology in community health programs provides outreach efforts with the guarantee that contents are delivered to the community in a culturally sensitive form and at accessible levels. Such participatory practices have been seen to foster improved health literacy and stakeholder ownership of health in the community. The systematic review highlights that successful integration of technical innovations into health promotion activities has the potential to significantly affect health outcomes, accentuating the need for multi-faceted approaches that utilize these tools for a holistic approach to disease prevention (Saman et al., 2024) (Figure 6.14).

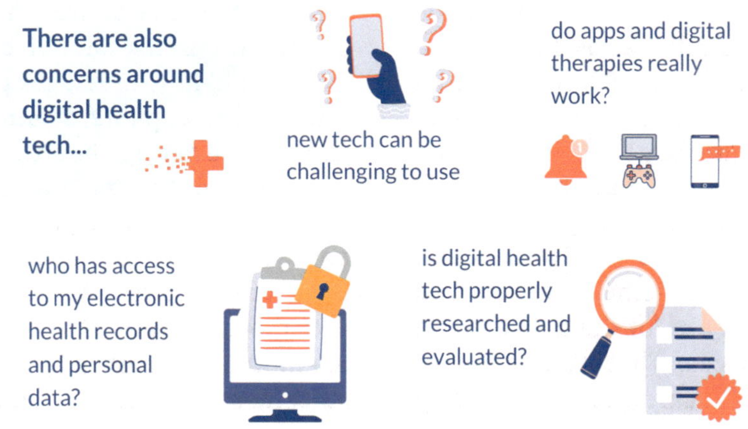

Figure 6.14. Technology in health promotion.

Source: https://evidence.nihr.ac.uk/wp-content/uploads/2022/09/2-1-1536x864.png.

6.6.1. Role of Telehealth and Digital Health Tools

The integration of digital health tools and telehealth has a transformative contribution to the promotion of health and prevention of disease, particularly as health systems adapt to address the challenges of diverse populations. Through the applications of mobile phones, teleconferencing, and wearables, healthcare professionals are able to expand services and provide support that is effective and convenient. Digital health solutions facilitate the delivery of preventive care by allowing individuals to take an active role in engaging with their health information. For instance, applications that contain patient-reported outcomes provide users with the ability to track their health behavior and receive personalized advice, engaging them more in preventive care and promoting healthier lifestyle choices. As technological advancements advance, so does their ability to improve health outcomes, particularly in underserved communities, which brings into view the imperative convergence of technology and public health interventions (Keane et al., 2025). Added to this, the infusion of civic engagement in designing digital health tools serves to further enhance their capacity to improve health promotion and disease prevention. One such example is the digital platform BIBOPP, which facilitates risk assessment of long-term conditions while allowing users to share their health data with healthcare providers. The creation of BIBOPP was preceded by co-creation workshops conducted among citizens, healthcare workers, and policymakers to ensure the tool caters to the end-users' needs and expectations. This collective process not only enhances the accessibility of the tools but also fosters a sense of ownership among the participants, contributing to improved health behavior within society. Additionally, as is highlighted in the case of BIBOPP, the involvement of various stakeholders underscores the need for comprehensive methods of integrating technology and indigenous health programs to manage disease prevention (Lambrechts et al., 2025). Lastly, the role of digital health technologies and telemedicine goes beyond convenience; it is a new era for the delivery and access to health services. These technologies have the capability to fill care gaps, particularly in rural and underserved areas, and enable personalized and preventive healthcare models. In addition, as healthcare providers struggle with the issues of equity and keeping up with increasing patient volumes, technologies such as telehealth provide creative solutions for enhanced access and participation. Digital health program success depends on continuous monitoring and uptake by both patients and providers, creating a dynamic healthcare system that can shift to meet evolving demands. In short, strategic integration of telehealth and digital health materials into health promotion efforts not only enhances individual health outcomes but is also vital in the development of strong healthcare systems that are capable of adequately addressing public health issues of the day (Keane et al., 2025).

6.6.2. Social Media as a Platform for Health Education

Social media has transformed a number of sectors, health education being one of them, such that it is now easy for health practitioners and ordinary people to freely communicate. Social media websites provide an easily accessible avenue through which health professionals can share vital health information that defines public health practice and attitude. Utilizing such websites enables health influencers to communicate to larger numbers of individuals, tailoring their messages to specified audiences. For instance, the Source Credibility Model and the Health Belief Model enable us to better understand how messages provided by credible sources are capable of altering health beliefs and encouraging health behavior changes regarding nutrition and overall health. The social media participation and engagement not only disseminate information but also form communities that prioritize health promotion and disease prevention, thereby facilitating the mutual interest in optimizing public health outcomes through peer support and evidence-based decision-making, such as the case for social medias influence on dietary habits (Ali et al., 2025). In more specific context, the function of social medias in health education is prominently highlighted within the context of specific groups, i.e., students. Various studies indicate that students, especially students in higher learning institutions, use media such as WhatsApp, Instagram, and Twitter actively to search for health information. The media are commonly employed for varied functions based on educational backgrounds, reflecting a bipartite divide between disciplines, such as pharmacy and political science. For students in pharmacy, focus will be on specific drug interaction and safety information, while political science students will more than likely be addressing more universal health concerns. This disparity in involvement is in line with the necessity for targeted health education campaigns with regard to distinct student populations' interests and concerns. Since appreciation of these differences highlights the potential of social media as an individualized platform for health education programs (Osahon et al., 2024), besides, the interactive nature of social media opens up space for responsive health messaging that could prompt immediate action among the followers. For example, health-conscious consumers are likely to report alteration to diet or lifestyle behavior based on compelling evidence attained through social media influencer who they believe in. Such immediate responsiveness is extremely conspicuous in high-risk health conditions, where information gone wrong can lead to unwanted results. Strategic utilization of credible sources and factual evidence is necessary to combat this menace to develop effective and credible health promotion campaigns. Interactive communication through social media, along with proper knowledge regarding the psychology of the target group, can bring about the change in behavior by instilling confidence in health-promoting behavior. Thus, the use of social media in health education is not just a fad, but an integral component in the creation of responsive public health interventions that extend to a variety of populations and promote informed health practices in the midst of an increasingly dynamic world (Ali et al., 2025) (Figure 6.15).

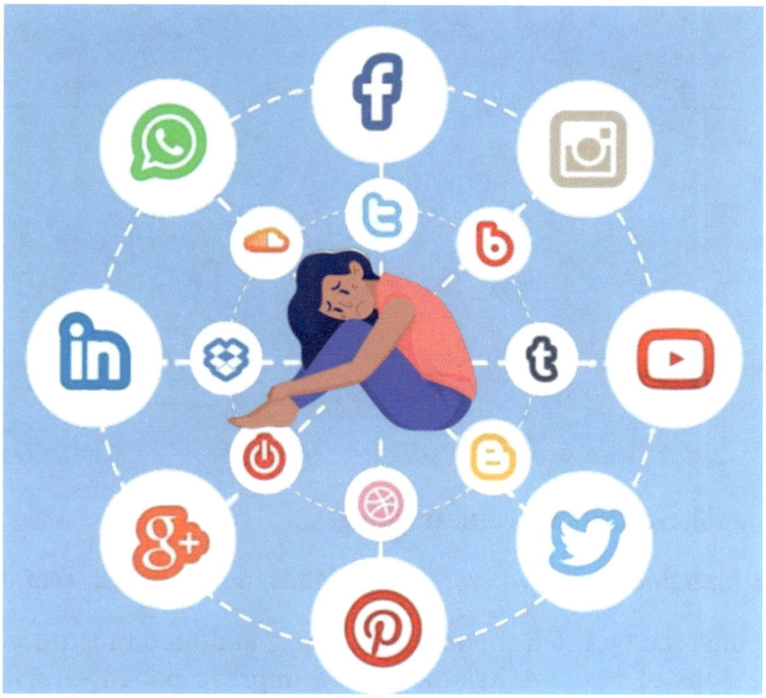

Figure 6.15. Social media as a platform for health education.

Source: https://miro.medium.com/v2/resize:fit:1148/1*0iwfW4kFj4Qwo1burd6J3Q.png.

6.6.3. Mobile Applications for Health Tracking

The use of health-monitoring mobile apps has become a pivot point in the landscape of disease prevention and health promotion. As healthcare is transforming towards a modifiable behavior approach, such applications are invaluable assets for enabling individuals to monitor and improve their health outcomes. By facilitating real-time tracking of various health parameters such as physical activity, diet consumption, and stress levels, such apps allow users to make smart decisions regarding their health. Furthermore, the use of these technologies also lightens the burden on healthcare professionals by automating repetitive processes and ongoing communication with users, thereby increasing the overall quality of care as a better experience. This is particularly crucial in environments where healthcare resources are scarce since it contributes to better health outcomes through long-term individual responsibility and motivation (Fadhil et al., 2019). In regions with poor health, such as Latin America, mobile health apps are especially convenient for addressing regional health issues. An increase in CVD death rates shows the necessity of pragmatic health interventions specifically tailored for local environments. Given the extensive use of mobile telephones in these countries, mHealth programs offer a realistic and fruitful means of reaching non-communicable diseases (NCDs).

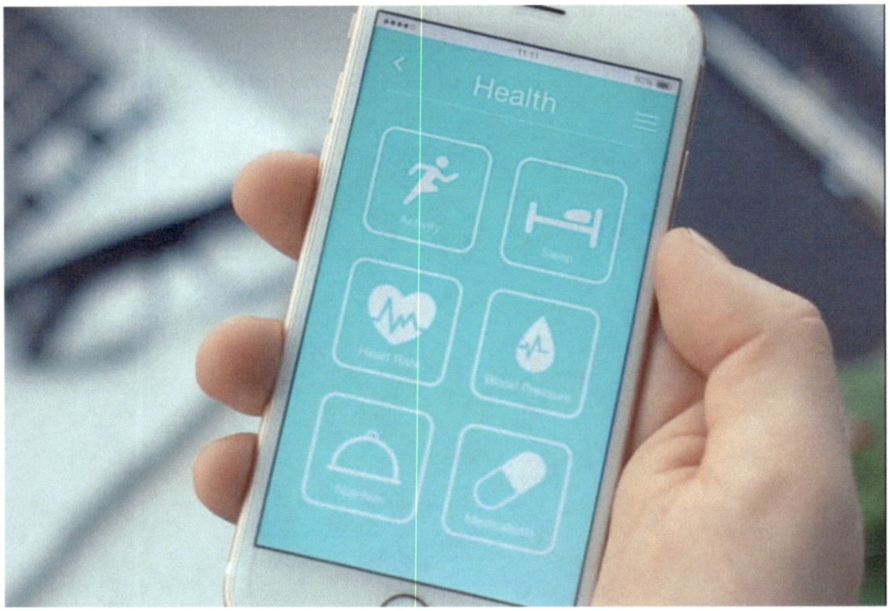

Figure 6.16. Mobile applications for health tracking.

Source: https://www.hhmglobal.com/wp-content/uploads/news/19092/remote_monitoring.jpg.

The programs sponsored by the National Heart, Lung, and Blood Institute have demonstrated the ability of mobile apps to improve health literacy, improve patient-provider communication, and deliver evidence-based interventions for particular health problems (Beratarrechea et al., 2016). These studies show how mobile technology can be used to bridge existing healthcare system gaps, ultimately enhancing public health interventions among marginalized populations. Mobile applications have more to offer than tracking; they have the ability to alter user behavior by using customized feedback and supportive interventions. Health coaching technologies, as seen within CoachAI, leverage conversational agents to initiate and maintain interaction between users and health interventions. By providing individualized advice and continuous support, such apps facilitate accountability and sustainable lifestyle change, a crucial element of disease prevention interventions. Moreover, through their ability to learn and adapt to users' needs and preferences, such technologies allow for a user-centered approach to managing health that not only supports adherence to health recommendations but also improves people's capacity to manage health issues (Fadhil et al., 2019). As mobile health monitoring technologies advance, they are a paradigm shift in the development and enactment of strategies for health promotion and disease prevention among populations (Figure 6.16).

SUMMARY

The conclusions from the analysis of health promotion and disease prevention are that successful public health programs need to be multi-component. As made apparent in the literature, creative methods that integrate community engagement, technology, and cultural relevance are powerful in their ability to impact health outcomes dramatically. For instance, community involvement interventions improve increased engagement and empower people to take control of their health, resulting in greater health literacy and behavior. This analysis reinforces the need for regular research grounded on cooperative endeavors among stakeholders in meeting the complexities of contemporary health challenges, thus complementing the contention that a holistic approach is imperative for successful health promotion initiatives. The merging of differing methods, as evidenced by the study, highlights the imperatives for addressing comprehensive health inequalities within groups (Saman et al., 2024). In considering the role of health promotion in an outbreak, anticipatory education and community-based interventions are evidently of utmost concern to promote public adherence to health intervention. Past outbreaks, as detailed in the critique, are key learning experiences in informing the creation of interventions that successfully communicate risks and enhance preventive behavior. The incorporation of community mobilization into epidemic response is witnessed not only in heightened alertness but also in changed behavior with the potential to sharply decrease transmission of disease. But limitations such as uneven levels of health literacy and resource limitations persist, with the need for adaptive solutions based on local conditions. This again supports the necessity for constant evaluation of health promotion practice so that it continues to be effective and current in the face of evolving public health issues (Katmini et al., 2024). Lastly, the results of the literature underscore the requirement of a holistic approach to health promotion and disease prevention that leverages technology and engages the community. With the changing complexion of healthcare, particularly in the context of global health crises, solutions must be innovative and responsive to population needs that are fast-changing. Future public health interventions must involve evidence-based interventions that take into account cultural, socioeconomic, and contextual determinants influencing health behavior. Ranking among them are these factors, which not only enhance disease prevention but also enhance community resilience in handling future health concerns. The conclusions derived from the review present a call for greater collaboration and strategic use of digital technologies to facilitate such processes towards an improved healthier population (Saman et al., 2024).

In the health promotion and disease prevention arena, countless evidence-based interventions have been found, yielding significant effects on the health status of children and adolescents. Over the past several decades, researchers have unraveled a range of approaches to enhancing cognitive, affective, and behavioral well-being among youngsters. These interventions not only are critical for acute health benefit but also can promote long-term wellness. However, despite numerous successful implementations, there is still much work to be undertaken to enhance such interventions further and optimize their implementation in various settings. This is particularly crucial as the potential benefits translate into population-level improvements in health outcomes when paired with effective implementation science approaches that ensure these interventions are implemented sustainably within existing health and education systems (Livingston et al., 2020). Another essential field of health promotion is in disorders such as dementia, particularly in the older patient in the facility. Recent literature addresses the importance of holistic care plans that address dementia and also attendant conditions such as delirium, affecting cognitive skills drastically. By offering appropriate sensory stimulation, hydration, and infection protection to hospital inpatients, the onset of delirium is avoided, thus improving the overall quality of care delivered to patients with dementia. It plays a pivotal role in improving not only the lived experience of individuals with dementia and their family members but also the broader social consequence of health care for older people. These prevention interventions emphasize the necessity of bridging care gaps to improve health outcomes among high-risk persons (Livingston et al., 2020). Moreover, flexibility in delivering health interventions is now a top priority. The dynamic nature of public health ensures that interventions not only must be evidence-based but also flexible enough to fit local contexts and population needs. Studies point out that classical models tend to ignore the intricacies of how interventions need to learn and adapt continuously from real-life practice. This level of adaptability increases the chances of getting optimal results since it caters to the fact that heterogeneous populations can react differently to uniform interventions. By creating an understanding culture for intervention design and delivery subtleties, health promotion strategy can be inclusive and more effective and result in positive health outcomes among all groups but particularly those most vulnerable (Chambers et al., 2016).

KEY TERMS FROM THIS CHAPTER

- Behavioral strategies
- Community health
- Curriculum
- Environmental determinants
- Health Belief Model
- Healthcare services
- Hypertension
- Integrated educational systems
- Mind-body connection
- Non-communicable diseases (NCDs)
- Public awareness
- School-based health education
- Stress management
- Civic engagement
- Community outreach programs
- Educational programs
- Health advocacy
- Healthcare expenditure
- Health literacy
- Infectious diseases
- Mental disorders
- Mindfulness practice
- Pandemics
- Sanitation enhancement
- Socioeconomic disparities
- Sustainable development

CLOSER LOOK

MIND-BODY CONNECTION

A closer look at the mind-body connection reveals the intricate and powerful relationship between our mental and physical health. Far from being separate systems, the mind and body continuously influence each other through complex networks of communication involving the nervous, endocrine, and immune systems. Thoughts, emotions, and stress levels can directly impact physical well-being, while bodily health in turn shapes mood, cognition, and behavior. For example, chronic stress can trigger hormonal responses that suppress the immune system, increase inflammation, and contribute to conditions like heart disease, digestive issues, and anxiety disorders. Conversely, practices that support mental wellness—such as mindfulness, deep breathing, regular exercise, and adequate sleep—can improve physical health by reducing stress hormones, enhancing immune function, and promoting overall balance. This bidirectional relationship is particularly evident in conditions such as depression, which often presents with physical symptoms like fatigue, pain, or sleep disturbances, and in chronic illnesses that can affect mental health due to ongoing discomfort or lifestyle limitations. Understanding the mind-body connection empowers individuals to take a more holistic approach to their health by recognizing the importance of emotional regulation, positive thinking, and self-awareness. Interventions such as yoga, meditation, cognitive-behavioral therapy (CBT), and biofeedback are increasingly used in both clinical and everyday settings to support this integrated view of health. Medical professionals are also beginning to adopt more interdisciplinary approaches that acknowledge the psychological aspects of healing and wellness. Ultimately, honoring the mind-body connection means seeing health not just as the absence of disease but as a dynamic balance between mental, emotional, and physical well-being. By nurturing both the mind and body together, individuals are better equipped to achieve resilience, prevent illness, and live more fulfilling lives. This connection underscores the importance of treating the whole person, not just isolated symptoms.s

REFERENCES

1. Abdullah Othman Khalifa, H., & Benissa, R. T. (2024). Health promotion and disease prevention in children and adolescents: An update of literature study. *Scholars Academic Journal of Pharmacy*. https://www.semanticscholar.org/paper/8d6580d1e51469507a6f13f7e3a8f83efdff24ee (accessed on 26th June 2025).
2. Alvarez, E., Dang, A. T., Elzibak, O. H., et al. (2018). Physician assistant involvement in health advocacy, health promotion and disease prevention: A scoping review. https://core.ac.uk/download/635073444.pdf (accessed on 26th June 2025).
3. Beratarrechea, A. G., Diez Canseco, F., Irazola, V., Miranda, et al. (2016). Use of m-health technology for preventive interventions to tackle cardiometabolic conditions and other non-communicable diseases in Latin America–Challenges and opportunities. https://core.ac.uk/download/159285900.pdf (accessed on 26th June 2025).
4. Birnbaum, N., Masterson, E., & Schoomaker, H. (2011). *State of Health Equity Movement, 2011 Update Part C: Compendium of Recommendations DRA Project Report No. 11–03*. https://core.ac.uk/download/pdf/18491812.pdf (accessed on 26th June 2025).
5. Bray, F., Ferlay, J., Soerjomataram, I., Siegel, R. L., Torre, L. A., & Jemal, A. (2018). Global cancer statistics 2018: GLOBOCAN estimates of incidence and mortality worldwide for 36 cancers in 185 countries. *CA: A Cancer Journal for Clinicians, 68*, 394–424. https://doi.org/10.3322/caac.21492 (accessed on 26th June 2025).
6. Bull, F., Al-Ansari, S. S., Biddle, S., Borodulin, K., Buman, M. P., Cardon, G., Carty, C., et al. (2020). World Health Organization 2020 guidelines on physical activity and sedentary behavior. *British Journal of Sports Medicine, 54*, 1451–1462. https://doi.org/10.1136/bjsports-2020-102955 (accessed on 26th June 2025).
7. Burton, M. J., Ramke, J., Marques, A. P., Bourne, R., Congdon, N., Jones, I., Ah Tong, B. A. M., et al. (2021). *The Lancet Global Health Commission on Global Eye Health: Vision beyond 2020. The Lancet Global Health, 9*, e489–e551. https://doi.org/10.1016/s2214-109x(20)30488-5 (accessed on 26th June 2025).
8. Chambers, D. A., & Norton, W. E. (2016). The Adaptome. *American Journal of Preventive Medicine, 51*, S124–S131. https://doi.org/10.1016/j.amepre.2016.05.011 (accessed on 26th June 2025).
9. Dahl, B. M. (2017). Critical discourse analysis perspective on Norwegian public health nursing curriculum in a time of transition. https://core.ac.uk/download/322430910.pdf (accessed on 26th June 2025).
10. Drabble, L. A., Keatley, J., & Marcelle, G. (2003). Progress and opportunities in lesbian, gay, bisexual and transgender health communications. https://core.ac.uk/download/70410107.pdf (accessed on 26th June 2025).
11. Duffee, J. H., Szilagyi, M., Forkey, H., & Kelly, E. T. (2021). Trauma-informed care in child health systems. *Pediatrics, 148*. https://doi.org/10.1542/peds.2021-052579 (accessed on 26th June 2025).
12. Ellwanger, J. H., da Veiga, A. B. G., Kaminski, V. de L., Valverde-Villegas, J. M., de Freitas, A. W. Q., & Chies, J. A. B. (2021). Control and prevention of infectious diseases from a One

Health perspective. *Genetics and Molecular Biology, 44*. https://doi.org/10.1590/1678-4685-gmb-2020-0256 (accessed on 26th June 2025).

13. Estabrooks, P. A., Bolyard, M. L., Casucci, T., Christensen, J. T., Gibson, B., Golden, C., Hill, J. L., et al. (2025). Identifying recruitment strategies to improve the reach of evidence-based health promotion, disease prevention, and disease self-management interventions: A scoping review. *Frontiers in Public Health, 13*. https://www.semanticscholar.org/paper/2f09bd4250f87da1e87f0b642fbf567a2695323d (accessed on 26th June 2025).
14. Fadhil, A., Schiavo, G., & Wang, Y. (2019). CoachAI: A conversational agent assisted health coaching platform. http://arxiv.org/abs/1904.11961 (accessed on 26th June 2025).
15. Garbarczyk, W., Napieralska, A., Kapla, A., Černohorská, A., Bednarczyk, D., Białeta, J., Siembab, K., et al. (2025). Systematic review of pertussis: Trends, challenges, and advances in care and prevention. *Journal of Education, Health and Sport*. https://www.semanticscholar.org/paper/8b0188b60f5ccaadae8251b17ce7c0d15832165a (accessed on 26th June 2025).
16. Gautam, S., Jain, A., Chaudhary, J., Gautam, M., Gaur, M., & Grover, S. (2024). Concept of mental health and mental well-being, its determinants and coping strategies. *Indian Journal of Psychiatry, 66*, S231–S244. https://doi.org/10.4103/indianjpsychiatry.indianjpsychiatry_707_23 (accessed on 26th June 2025).
17. Gorelick, P., Furie, K., Iadecola, C., Smith, E. E., Waddy, S. P., Lloyd-Jones, D., Bae, H., et al. (2017). Defining optimal brain health in adults: A presidential advisory from the American Heart Association/American Stroke Association. *Stroke, 48*(10), e284–e303. https://www.semanticscholar.org/paper/bdfb5e28fe77abe8675cdd7d96e851d59f91dae8 (accessed on 26th June 2025).
18. Green, A., Wu, S., Di Pasquale, A., & Pang, T. (2025). The role of digital opinion leaders in dengue prevention through health promotion and public health collaboration: Qualitative semi structured interview study. *Journal of Medical Internet Research, 27*. https://www.semanticscholar.org/paper/ff522af4696d0ad352e5cbdc237aacf407bcde7f (accessed on 26th June 2025).
19. Jain, N., Dutt, U., Radenkov, I., & Jain, S. (2023). WHO's global oral health status report 2022: Actions, discussion and implementation. *Oral Diseases, 30*, 73–79. https://doi.org/10.1111/odi.14516 (accessed on 26th June 2025).
20. Jumba, K. (2024). Exploring the role of art in community health initiatives. *Newport International Journal of Law, Communication and Languages*. https://www.semanticscholar.org/paper/fe0afead09858d3490689159f557a36c8a34e35b (accessed on 26th June 2025).
21. Katmini, K., & Nazliyah, I. (2024). Health promotion for the prevention of extraordinary events or outbreaks: A systematic review. *Journal of Applied Nursing and Health*. https://www.semanticscholar.org/paper/ddf6493ae48db06162ff4cccc2484d6f866ff0d4 (accessed on 26th June 2025).
22. Keane, D., Calbimonte, J. P., Pawłowska, E., Kassianos, A., Medina, J. C., Gregório, J., Serra-Blasco, M., et al. (2025). Protocol for an umbrella review of systematic reviews evaluating the efficacy of digital health solutions in supporting adult cancer survivorship care. *PLOS ONE, 20*. https://www.semanticscholar.org/paper/7a446ec7df6fd2d3a49fe9720bb111986b01be07 (accessed on 26th June 2025).
23. Komi, L. S., Mustapha, A. Y., Forkuo, A. Y., & Osamika, D. (2024). Community-based health

promotion models for cardiovascular disease prevention: A conceptual and evidence-based review. *International Journal of Multidisciplinary Research and Growth Evaluation*. https://www.semanticscholar.org/paper/91529b353ea18b4135a8ab0b6da6dfdeb081106a (accessed on 26th June 2025).

24. Lambrechts, N., De Clerck, C., Goesaert, E., van Schyndel, C., Van der Auwera, V., Vermeylen, S., Vandenhoudt, H., et al. (2025). A community engagement strategy for health promotion through co-created digital solutions, the BIBOPP project. *International Journal of Integrated Care*. https://www.semanticscholar.org/paper/69d39e899a443018128559009e647fd372293396 (accessed on 26th June 2025).

25. Lawson, K., Yocum, S., et al. (2019). Health coaching case report: Optimizing employee health and wellbeing in organizations. https://core.ac.uk/download/223117465.pdf (accessed on 26th June 2025)

26. Lee, H., Oldewage-Theron, W., Lyford, C., & Shine, S. (2023). Nutrition and health challenges among low-income families of young children in the post COVID-19 era: A qualitative study. *Nutrition Research and Practice, 17*, 1185–1200. https://www.semanticscholar.org/paper/48031479ec3b0187d3f1fea342706c45eef31656 (accessed on 26th June 2025).

27. Livingston, G., Huntley, J., Sommerlad, A., Ames, D., Ballard, C., Banerjee, S., Brayne, C., et al. (2020). Dementia prevention, intervention, and care: 2020 report of the Lancet Commission. *The Lancet, 396*, 413–446. https://doi.org/10.1016/s0140-6736(20)30367-6 (accessed on 26th June 2025).

28. Md Saman, K., Alias, R., Kadir, N. A., Mohd Halimi, H., Md Isa, K. A., & Ibrahim, N. (2024). Health promotion and disease prevention in health: A comprehensive systematic review. *International Journal of Education, Psychology and Counseling*. https://www.semanticscholar.org/paper/627b9eeea1815049a0f9dd796e9cfd22a338c66d (accessed on 26th June 2025).

29. Mukamurera, P. N. (2024). The impact of public health on disease prevention. *Research Invention Journal of Scientific and Experimental Sciences*. https://www.semanticscholar.org/paper/f033830171a63569a17504b6ebad8d9532ebabf4 (accessed on 26th June 2025).

30. N/A. (2008). Finding the voice of public health. https://core.ac.uk/download/71344387.pdf (accessed on 26th June 2025).

31. Nachega, J. B., Sam-Agudu, N. A., Masekela, R., van der Zalm, M. M., Nsanzimana, S., Condo, J., Ntoumi, F., et al. (2021). Addressing challenges to rolling out COVID-19 vaccines in African countries. *The Lancet Global Health, 9*, e746–e748. https://doi.org/10.1016/s2214-109x(21)00097-8 (accessed on 26th June 2025).

32. Nuvolari-Duodo, I., Dolcini, M., Buffoli, M., Rebecchi, A., Dall'O,' G., Monticelli, C., Vertua, C., et al. (2024). Integrated climate change mitigation and public health protection strategies: The case of the City of Bologna, Italy. *International Journal of Environmental Research and Public Health, 21*. https://www.semanticscholar.org/paper/6be6736fff222319cabf5ef419188c255779df3a (accessed on 26th June 2025).

33. O'Toole, T., Lavinghouze, S. R., Pejavara, A., & Petersen, R. (2022). State and local chronic disease programs adapt and pivot to address community needs during the COVID-19 pandemic: Examples from CDC funded SPAN, REACH, and HOP programs. *Health Promotion Practice, 23*, 12S–20S. https://www.semanticscholar.org/paper/76efd5171a1b05fdc44592bb47cf670b2b134a46 (accessed on 26th June 2025).

34. Odone, A., Dallagiacoma, G., Frascella, B., Signorelli, C., & Leask, J. (2021). Current understandings of the impact of mandatory vaccination laws in Europe. *Expert Review of Vaccines, 20*, 559–575. https://doi.org/10.1080/14760584.2021.1912603 (accessed on 26th June 2025).

35. O'Hara, P. (2005). Creating social and health equity: Adopting an Alberta social determinants of health framework. https://core.ac.uk/download/71343870.pdf (accessed on 26th June 2025).

36. Omar Ali, S. R., Che Noh, C. H., Mohd Said, N. S., & Mansor, F. A. (2025). Health influencers on social media: Shaping followers' beliefs and behaviors. *International Journal of Research and Innovation in Social Science*. https://www.semanticscholar.org/paper/8de120156e0882539192552c2646e03815b2d4b2 (accessed on 26th June 2025).

37. Osahon, P. T., Mote, L. A., & West, I. S. (2024). The role of social media in health promotion, disease prevention, and drug use among University of Benin students. *Journal of Basic and Social Pharmacy Research*. https://www.semanticscholar.org/paper/95d01048f4ff761eeeb886099505c4ecb612dab4 (accessed on 26th June 2025).

38. Roth, G. A., Mensah, G. A., Johnson, C. O., Addolorato, G., Ammirati, E., Baddour, L. M., Barengo, N. C., et al. (2020). Global burden of cardiovascular diseases and risk factors, 1990–2019. *Journal of the American College of Cardiology, 76*, 2982–3021. https://doi.org/10.1016/j.jacc.2020.11.010 (accessed on 26th June 2025).

39. Scarpa, F., & Casu, M. (2024). Genomics and bioinformatics in One Health: Transdisciplinary approaches for health promotion and disease prevention. *International Journal of Environmental Research and Public Health, 21*. https://www.semanticscholar.org/paper/7c04eedb475853b56ff4b4eb9bd971ed28e5d246 (accessed on 26th June 2025).

40. Shah, S., Hamid, F., Malik, J., & Jhumra, E. (2022). The need for optimum nutritional strategies for cardiovascular health in Pakistani population. *Pakistan Heart Journal*. https://www.semanticscholar.org/paper/5443e1369d0f71979e9b8bb0330250d89d4dece3 (accessed on 26th June 2025).

41. Veneri, F., Vinceti, S. R., & Filippini, T. (2024). Fluoride and caries prevention: A scoping review of public health policies. *Annali di Igiene: Medicina Preventiva E Di Comunita*. https://www.semanticscholar.org/paper/7d7ccd134b924c1bfc2a94232a5c5562ec7d3a8a (accessed on 26th June 2025).

42. Visseren, F. L. J., Mach, F., Smulders, Y. M., Carballo, D., Koskinas, K. C., Bäck, M., Bénétos, A., et al. (2021). 2021 ESC Guidelines on cardiovascular disease prevention in clinical practice. *European Heart Journal, 42*, 3227–3337. https://doi.org/10.1093/eurheartj/ehab484 (accessed on 26th June 2025).

43. Wahyuni, S. E., & Keliat, B. (2024). Interventions addressing nurses' psychological well-being during COVID-19 pandemic: A systematic review. *Acta Medica Philippina, 58*, 67–76. https://www.semanticscholar.org/paper/b23eec3bcd4fa3588e1eeb3d61796cdd101366a4 (accessed on 26th June 2025).

44. Wutzke, S., Morrice, E., Benton, M., & Wilson, A. (2016). Systems approach for chronic disease prevention: Sound logic and empirical evidence, but is this view shared outside of academia? *Public Health Research & Practice, 26*(3). https://www.semanticscholar.org/paper/50abb82e9edaaeb9b8f612fc08bc2187a05f7624 (accessed on 26th June 2025).

45. Zhou, X., Gao, H., & Wang, J. (2025). A computational framework analysis of public

attitudes toward male human papillomavirus infection and its vaccination in China: Based on Weibo data. *Healthcare, 13*. https://www.semanticscholar.org/paper/ec358aaf9dcaecb29e3906906b9d92bcb6b09226 (accessed on 26th June 2025).

26. Zúñiga Sosa, E. A. (2025). Prevention and health promotion: A strategy for linking academia with society. *AG Salud*. https://www.semanticscholar.org/paper/dec017ce8aa52c7d08df4fb42e1941936c18c645 (accessed on 26th June 2025).

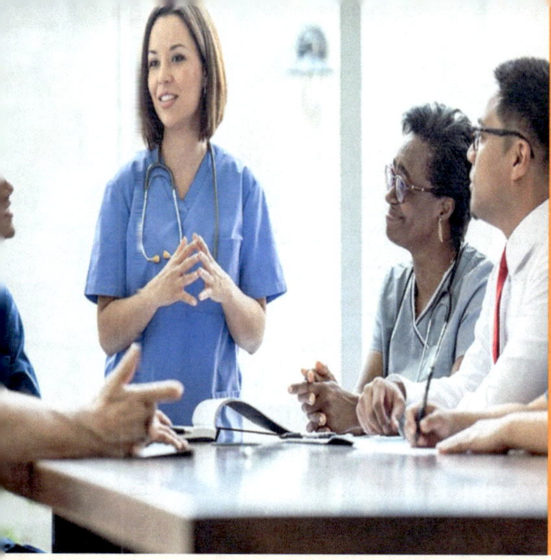

Chapter 7

EVALUATION OF COMMUNITY HEALTH PROGRAMS

Contents

Introduction

Introduction to the evaluation of community health programs is an education point to understand the intricacy of health programs aimed at fostering the health and well-being of diverse populations. Community health programs are given top priority in the case of public health issues because, apart from having direct impacts on health, they also consider social determinants of health, which contribute to overall health status to a large degree. Comparing these programs enables the stakeholders to determine best practices, what needs to be improved, and whether or not the resources are being utilized effectively to address the needs of the community. This preliminary assessment is fundamental to program development and sustenance, ultimately starting to resemble constructs of community-oriented medical education as described in the existing literature, which is centered on learning environment and in practice in health education (Khadivi et al., 2004). Second, community health program evaluation operates on a broader basis of social justice and equity, especially in the management of marginalized individuals. As identified in service research with intellectually disabled individuals, effective community health programs demand profound understanding of multicultural requirements and advocacy-oriented provision of services (Blackman et al., 2005). Program assessment not only assesses the effectiveness of programs but also examines whether programs match community desire and worth. With the aid of stakeholder and community feedback, health programs could be tailored to fit the specific requirements of each subgroup in a manner in which maximum health equity is achieved. This comprehensive needs assessment is pivotal for establishing community trust and participation, both of which are determinants of health program success. Finally, the constantly evolving health issues require an on-going evaluation process that is always sensitive to potential problems and developments in public health. The connection of continuous evaluation processes enables the ability to react to the flexibility required for program adjustments due to changing community needs and healthcare trends. In addition, the dynamic interaction of numerous variables, such as economic progress, population fluctuations, and advances in medical technology requires that evaluations are not static but rather cyclical. By following a process of assessment and revision, community health programs can remain effective and timely, ultimately resulting in better health status for everyone in the community. The evaluation process is not only utilized as a method of accountability but also as an innovator so that community health programs evolve in parallel with the societies that they are meant to serve (Figure 7.1).

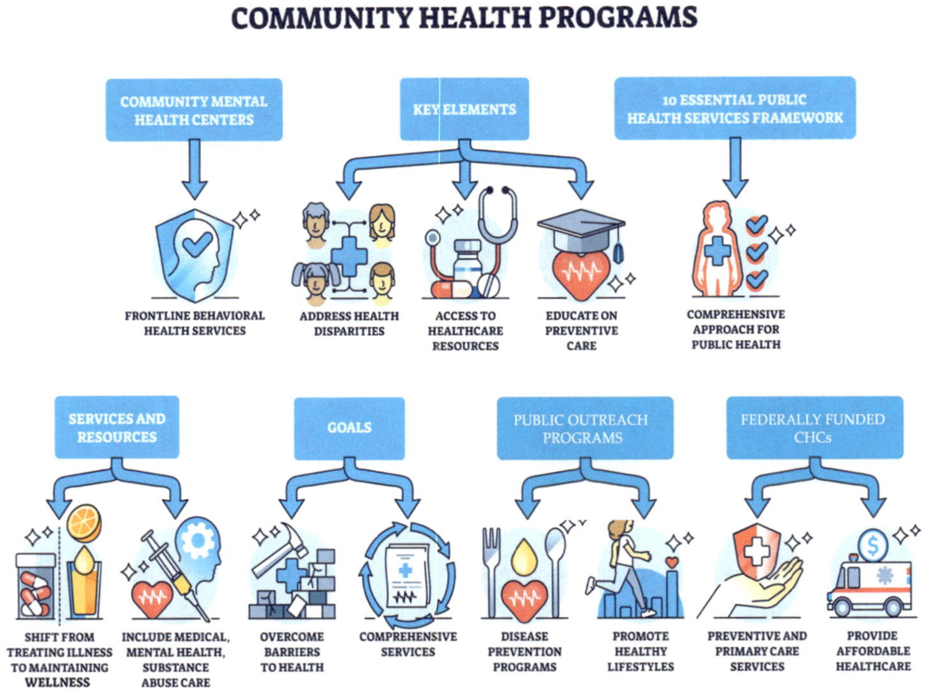

Figure 7.1. Evaluation of community health programs.

Source: https://thumbs.dreamstime.com/b/community-health-programs-society-education-treatment-outline-diagram-labeled-educational-detailed-scheme-elements-299850664.jpg.

Definition of Community Health Programs

Community health programs are coordinated activities whose aim is to improve the health status of specified populations. They encompass a variety of services, from preventive and health education to community outreach endeavors to react to problems in the local health status. The programs fundamentally are predicated upon the belief that health is shaped by a multicausal interaction of determinants, social, environmental, and economic, and this gives weight to the value of the individualized method for community health. By understanding the distinct health requirements of individual communities, such programs aim to establish equal access to healthcare and improved overall health results. Recent research has illustrated that it requires high levels of understanding of community trends in order to properly design interventions that are attractive to desired groups. This entails not just offering services, but also developing a situation where communities are actively involved in decision-making regarding their health, hence enhancing the effectiveness of the programs as well as sustainability. Evidence-based practice is one of the most essential elements of community health programs that necessitates stringent evaluation methods. Evaluation is applied to measure the impact of such interventions in quantitative terms, holding the programs accountable as well as developing evidence for the next intervention. Community health program measurement involves qualitative and quantitative data collection to measure the effectiveness of health interventions through predetermined indicators and outcomes. Indicators such as the scale capture this approach as a psychometric tool for assessing health programs across multicultural environments. A good evaluation system is not only crucial in examining program effects but also in informing resource allocation and policy development.

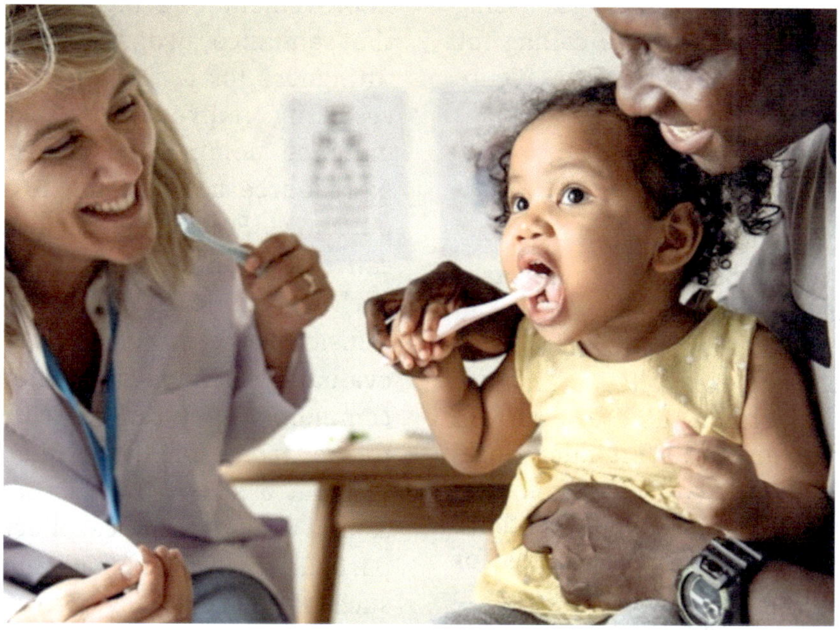

Figure 7.2. Community health programs.

Source: https://publichealth.tulane.edu/wp-content/uploads/sites/3/2020/05/blog-healthcare-provider-teachers-toddler-to-brush-teeth.jpg.

Therefore, rigorous assessment processes are of great importance to ensure program planning and overall quality of community health services and ultimately enhance enhanced health equity and outcomes for populations (Ahn et al., 2014). Community health programs also intervene primarily on common social determinants of health, being aware that poverty, education, and health service access contribute significantly to the determination of health outcomes. Interventions aimed at orphans and vulnerable children (OVC), for example, reveal this approach—recognizing the necessity of concerted effort in such targeting among health, education, and social support. Evaluation of these interventions would actually entail analysis of existing policies and the loopholes within these, and identifying the general effectiveness of interventions aimed at targeting assistance to OVCs. By obtaining data on OVC populations and reviewing programs and policies that exist, stakeholders can make evidence-based choices to strengthen health services in the long term. Therefore, community health programs play a critical function in increasing resilience and addressing the multifaceted challenges facing vulnerable populations, once more calling for overall evaluations (Beard et al., 2009) (Figure 7.2).

Importance of Evaluating Health Programs

The evaluation of health programs is important in order to ascertain their effectiveness and whether they are meeting targeted needs of the community. By utilising controlled evaluation techniques, stakeholders are able to establish if a health program meets its intended goals and objectives. This is particularly crucial in community health programs, where there are limited resources and high demands for accountability. By identifying areas of strength and weakness in program functioning, evaluators are able to make recommendations that are feasible and can guide future programs. Evaluation also promotes trust and openness among community stakeholders and funders, thereby increasing the programs credibility and chances for long-term funding. Because most community programs are dependent on sustained funding, demonstrating effectiveness through strong evaluation is essential to long-term sustainability and effectiveness. Another important role of assessing health programs is in the development of innovative intervention strategy. Ongoing evaluation makes it possible for health practitioners to understand which areas of a program are succeeding and where they are failing. For instance, a robust assessment framework can monitor to what extent advocacy and policy interventions are truly translating into concrete health outcomes, making better decisions (Gienapp et al., 2012)

In addition, knowledge of the individual settings where programs are being used, for example, socio-economic settings and public health challenges, is able to ensure enhanced understanding of their efficacy. Such cyclical analysis enables the process of reinforcing improvement for bringing about improvements that enhance program responsiveness and fittingness for a changing health terrain. The resulting improvements can subsequently enhance community health and efficiency of resource use, leading to improved health outcomes. Finally, measuring health programs can also identify issues of general interest, such as public health policy and structural transformation. As policymakers and researchers evaluate the impact of interventions in the community, they can contribute rich evidence to the debate on the public health response. Without a sound process of assessment, one cannot establish the real effect of interventions, particularly in the management of acute issues such as malnutrition (Renzaho et al., 2002). Apart from determining the short-term effect of a program, evaluation is also a platform for extensive change and innovation. This is crucial in the pursuit of evidence-based policy-making in responding to population health challenges and redistributive forces. Systematic reviews are thus a driver of ongoing development and a promoter of public health accountability.

7.1. Historical Context of Community Health Programs

Political, economic, and social history of community health programs is greatly rooted in processes of transformation in the 20th century. The history of community health programs starts with the early public health initiatives on infectious diseases, aimed to improve sanitation, nutrition, and coverage of primary medical care. As urbanization was simmering after World War II, the public health model was extended to cover more determinants of health, including socioeconomic status and the environment. Development of many government agencies brought into focus the increased appreciation that health is not only determined by biological factors, but also by social differences. This movement established the groundwork for community health programs that aimed to eliminate differences, paving the way for more holistic strategies toward the promotion of health equity and improvement in population health outcomes at a systems level. In the subsequent decades, the international health programs and civil rights movement played an important role in defining the course of community health programs. The human rights and cause of social justice became endowed in the health policies, with the outcome of community participation in implementing and planning for health. There had been interventions set up during this period to remove the adverse effects of the socioeconomic disparities, concentrating on community engagement among marginalized groups. The participatory philosophy acknowledged that people have an understanding of their health requirements in a setting, which resulted in culturally-tailored programs to address particular groups. The evolution of these guidelines represented a paradigm shift in public health theory, prioritizing locally-initiated interventions and coming to realize the central role that empowering the community must play in fostering wellness and disease prevention. De-implementation has also gained traction in community health programs, as a strategy for dealing with the problem of managing undesirable outcomes of interventions that do not yield intended results. As programs expanded, there was a need to decide which of such programs to halt and substitute with improved strategies. Building on recent research, certain conditions under which de-implementation would be warranted have been suggested, such as whether an intervention is not working or even harmful, whether more effective options exist, or in changing community needs. This more subtle reaction has prompted re-evaluation of past intervention and enabled ongoing improvement in community health programming. Through the focus on responsiveness and responsiveness to context at the community level, these paradigmatic changes in public health over time purportedly work towards improving the efficacy and appropriateness of community health programs, developing healthier populations in an evolving world.

7.1.1. Evolution of Public Health Initiatives

Public health program evolution is an evolving process between new health issues and societal efforts to address them. Over time, the efforts themselves have also seen dramatic shifts from intervention for sole diseases in individuals to models of joined efforts to tackle general determinants of health. For instance, 19th-century public health interventions were primarily focused on sanitation and the prevention of infectious diseases, largely reactive to epidemics such as cholera. This reactive function had yielded to more proactive measures, emphasizing disease prevention and health promotion during the latter part of the 20th century. The growing interest in social determinants of health has led public health programs to integrate economic stability, education, and access to health services, such that a multi-dimensional community health program evaluation became a necessary mandate. When assessing community health projects, it is informative to look at how work in public health has evolved to address new populations and novel health inequities. Perhaps the most important part of this evolution has been broadening focus on inclusion, especially of marginalized groups. Contemporary best practices for youth, specifically boys and young men of color (BYMOC), attest to this shift. With awareness of the unique needs of such populations, public health programs have not only sought to enhance the quality of service delivery but also to mobilize these communities. The programs have come to rely more on community participation, with the belief that change is a bottom-up process through grassroots activism and mobilization. As highlighted by current literature, experts are more and more engaged in defining what works in practice via the use of collective mechanisms and evidence-based information, consequently shaping the course of public health interventions (Gilgoff et al., 2015). Moreover, analysis of data and technological advancements have transformed the creation of public health interventions. These technologies have improved better community health need appraisal such that programmed interventions can be aimed specifically and applicable. More advanced communication systems have also had a significant contribution in the dissemination of health news, which has resulted in improved overall public awareness and engagement. Social media-driven health campaigns, for instance, have reached diverse populations, but most significantly, generations at a younger age. As public health interventions in communities become complex, it becomes necessary that evaluators observe the implications of such drivers of technology on health outcomes. Experience lessons documented in TCWFs grant reflections also provide valuable lessons on evaluation that necessitate rethinking legacy models to adaptive and iterative models that are more appropriate in addressing the multifaceted health issues of the day (Brousseau, 2004) (Figure 7.3).

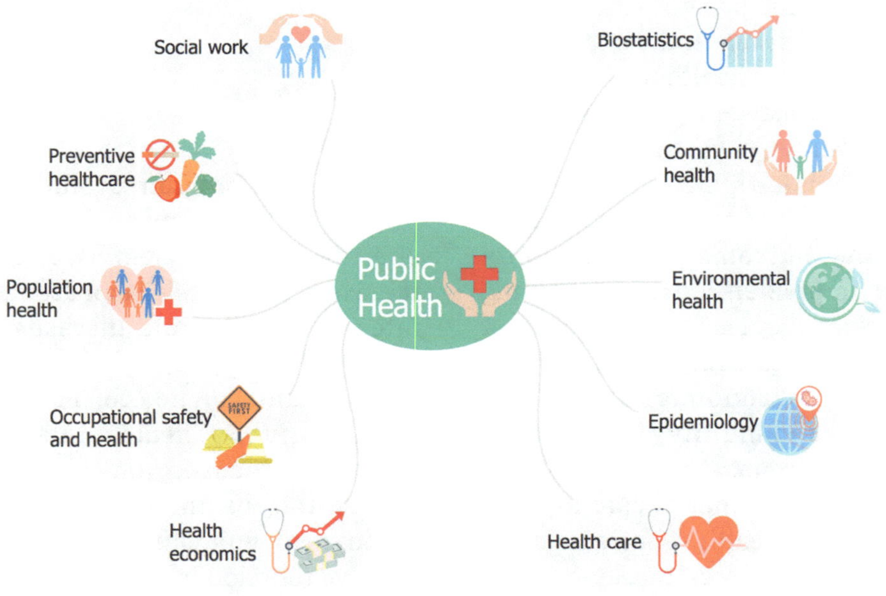

Figure 7.3. Evolution of public health initiatives.

Source: https://www.conceptdraw.com/How-To-Guide/picture/Health-Sciences-Public-Health.png.

7.1.2. Key Milestones in Community Health Development

The evolution of community health has been marked by many historic landmarks that have greatly shaped public health policy and practice. Some of the landmarks include the establishment of the World Health Organization (WHO) in 1948, when universal health was forcibly recognized as a shared responsibility. This was an evolution from single-nation health interventions to concerted action at decreasing health disparities across borders. The work of the WHO provided room for an international regime of administration of health, with nations meeting to discuss numerous public health matters. Apart from this, this global vantage provided space for infectious disease and health education interventions, thereby paving the way for general well-being community health interventions. As countries adopted the WHO's guiding principles, stress on preventive practice and community participation became key to successful health systems. In the latter half of the 20th century, the primary healthcare movement was another landmark in community health development. The 1978 Alma-Ata Declaration laid emphasis on universal access to essential health care for all, which revolutionized the strategy of community health from being only clinical to socially based. It was an inclusive outlook that valued the aspect that health is not a personal issue but a public concern encompassing education, environment, and economic development. Primary care focus led to the opening of health centers that address local concerns in an integrated fashion. Greater participation and utilization of the local resources, these health centers attempt to create long-term solutions to healthcare. The Alma-Ata Declaration thus not only shaped health systems around the world but gave individuals a sense of belonging to their health needs. The role of technology in developing community health over the last few years has been a turning point factor, as it has led to a change in the assessment of health programs. Development in telehealth and health informatics has made access to healthcare services within the broader community easier, especially for marginalized groups. Health care providers have been able to provide care from a distance using such technological innovations, thus bridging geographical and enhancing health outcomes. Information gathered by health informatics also assist health organizations in tracking indicators and outcomes of community health to facilitate effective decision-making and allocation of resources. Use of technology in community health programs again emphasizes that there have to be dynamic mechanisms to address new arising health issues. To these trends, community health programs are forced to evolve continuously in a bid to assume new tools and techniques (N/A, 2010), all under the paradigm of the fundamental principles expounded by research and policies aimed at health as found in Bozeman et al., (2009).

7.1.3. Impact of Historical Events on Current Programs

Historical viewpoints of community health programs significantly contribute to their evolution and existing programs. Past histories of flooding have been central to shaping health program design and priority. For example, repeated instances of flood occurrence observed in places such as Galena, Alaska, have guided prevention efforts in community health preparedness. An assessment of flood management programs identifies how past difficulties and interventions can be applied as templates for more sustainable health programs. Methods applied following past floods, observed from comparative studies, center on gaining insight from policy through learned history and the community-based approach. Through learning from such events, it is easier to develop well-coordinated disaster preparedness actions and, in the long run, reduce vulnerabilities in future situations and public health resilience in general (Kontar et al., 2017). The interaction of history with socioeconomic also plays an important role in determining community health programs today. Disaster preparedness for older persons varies by income and race/ethnicity based on history of injustice. Lower-income older persons, for instance, particularly Hispanics and poor Black older persons, have lower rates of preparedness compared with Whites. The trend, therefore, shows that past trends in inequality continue to influence present health outcomes and preparedness activities. These results are helpful when designing specific interventions to fight such inequalities so that vulnerable groups have access to suitable intervention at the time of disaster. They learn from the history of marginalization, and as a result, community health programs are well-positioned to modify their strategies to suit different populations (Cox et al., 2017). Studying the past episodes that have shaped community health programs offers some lessons to be applied in future programs. The interplay of the history of flooding and public health response exhibits a tendency of integrating people's participation into program planning. Moreover, definition of populations at risk in various socio-economic settings emphasizes the need for allocation of balanced resources. Historical analysis, like comparative study of flood risk management in Galena and Edeytsy, makes it possible to better comprehend effective communication and coordination among agencies. Use of these lessons in practice today is contingent upon ongoing evaluation and adaptation of programs following historical experience. Lastly, appreciation of the history helps in improving the efficiency and completeness of community health programs, which is important in addressing issues of the present health (Kontar et al., 2017).

7.2. Types of Community Health Programs

Community health programs are extremely valuable resources by which many varieties of health disparities are dealt with and well-being is improved at the community level. Stress-reduction programs are among the most prevalent types that are increasingly becoming well-recognized to improve mental health. RELAX: Alternatives to Anger and Stress Less with Mindfulness, among others, is structured to enable individuals to learn to manage their emotions and remove stress through systematic educational processes.

Apart from providing the much-needed coping skills, the courses also promote a sense of community engagement. As observed through partnership between West Virginia University Extension and Michigan State University, mutual curriculum sharing as well as mutual application of assessment measures ensures programme effectiveness and responsiveness while inter-organizational collaboration becomes critical in advancing community health programmes (Jones et al., 2021). Community health programmes may also address specific health issues, such as oral inequities among vulnerable people. One rich example is the Alaska Dental Health Aide (DHA) program that was established in order to turn around tooth decay trends among American Indian and Alaska Native children. It offered a new model of learning by empowering individuals to provide necessary dental services within a federally sanctioned setting. The DHA program includes a broad array of provider types from Primary Dental Health Aides to Dental Health Aide Therapists, each uniquely designed to meet local demands for the provision of culturally appropriate care. Through embracing such strategy, the program not only increases access to preventive and restorative oral health care but also emphasizes the significance of culturally specific care in the achievement of enhanced health outcomes (Bolin et al., 2013). The multiplicity of community health programs manifests the multi-dimensional methods essential for effective public health governance. Addressing the mental and physical health demands through focused programs allows communities to create integrated health plans to improve overall health. Evaluation of the programs is also required to ascertain their effects as well as where they can be optimized. Proper evaluation can offer information regarding satisfaction by participants, development of skills, and health outcomes, thereby allowing for decision-making informed by evidence to support long-term program planning. Lastly, ongoing assessment and revision of community health programs are required to make them useful and effective in addressing evolving health needs among various populations (Figure 7.4).

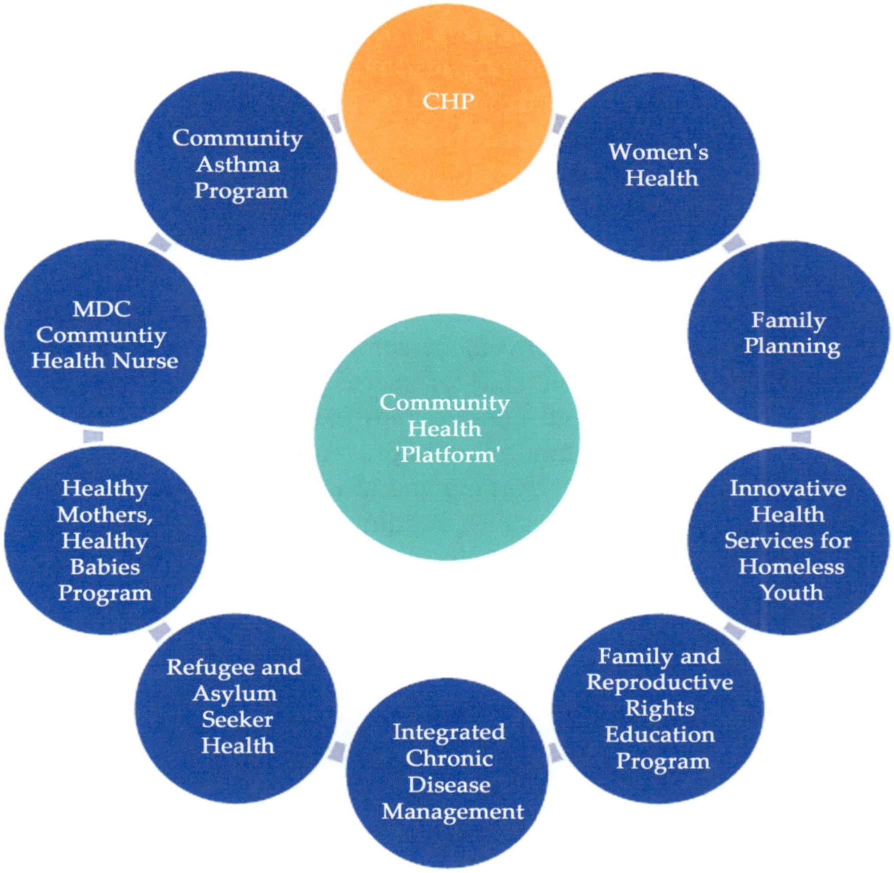

Figure 7.4. Types of community health programs.

Source: https://www.audit.vic.gov.au/sites/default/files/2018-06/Community-Health-Services/1c.PNG.

7.2.1. Preventive Health Services

Preventive health services are a crucial component of community health programs in that they attain a proactive approach to disease prevention and the sustenance of well-being. They encompass a sequence of interventions from immunization and screening to interventions in lifestyle for health. They aim to avoid disease before it occurs and not merely the management of illness and thus improve population health outcomes as well as reduce chronic disease expenses. Also, preventive health care services work extremely well when integrated into general community systems, for example, schools and primary care centers, as they enable better provision of health information and resources in an integrated fashion. Such integration is equally important in accessing deprived groups, who are discouraged from going to main-stream healthcare facilities, thus enhancing health equity among the population. In addition, the significance of certain preventive health services is brought about through dealing with certain demographic needs for health. Strategies to reach children have been challenged to consider certain needs in child development, and as a result new advances in preventive oral health have ensued. New programs have had promise to increase access to basic care by bringing dental care into primary health centers or community programs such as WIC and Early Head Start. Such programs emphasize the significance of reaching beyond socioeconomic, cultural, and geographic boundaries that generally limit access to preventive care. For instance, the inclusion of dental health facilitates greater comprehension and management of a child's overall well-being, not merely addressing mouth-related problems but encouraging health as a whole. These extended programs indicate a thoughtful approach towards meeting the specific needs of poor families through preventive care to those most in need (Krol et al., 2013). Evaluation of community health programs delivering preventive health care stresses the importance of innovative solutions to existing barriers to care. Offering new models of care delivery is integral, particularly in areas where healthcare provision has been low in the past. Enlarging the dental provider workforce, taking services to convenient community settings, and designing culturally sensitive outreach efforts are highly promising for success. Not only do they increase access, but also they seek to bring communities and families into partnership with one another in making health priorities, and to foster shared commitment to preventive care. Within comparison of various community health programs, it is evident that big and innovative approaches actually enhance the effectiveness of preventive health care services, building a more promising future with improved well-being among vulnerable populations (Krol et al., 2013) (Figure 7.5).

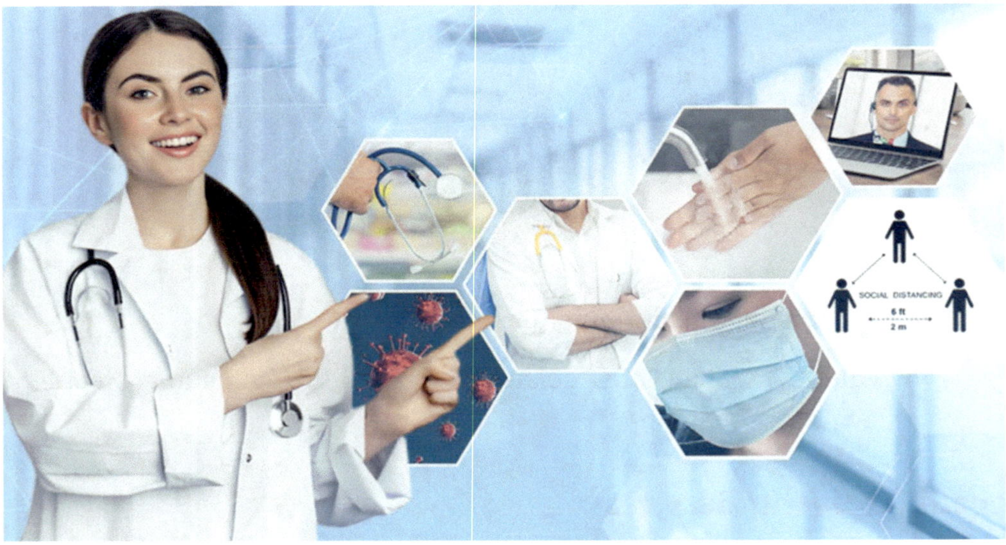

Figure 7.5. Preventive health services.

Source: https://healthgroovy.com/wp-content/uploads/2023/10/preventative-health-services-prevent-disease.webp.

7.2.2. Health Education and Promotion

Health education and promotion are central to community health programs policy since they serve as momentum towards modifying the public's health behavior and outcomes. Essentially, the programs aim at creating awareness of the health risks and making people adopt better lifestyle options. By taking advantage of the utilization of advanced methods such as online media, interactive training, and local events, health educators are best suited to convey significant information that is relevant to various populations. Technology interventions such as health education video and interactive nutrition tools, for example, have been found to be effective in augmenting involvement among populations and supporting lasting behavior change. The significance of responding to specific community needs cannot be overemphasized since adapting health messages to cultural contexts enhances understanding and adherence to health behavior, finally enhancing the general health condition of the community (Harwanto et al., 2024).

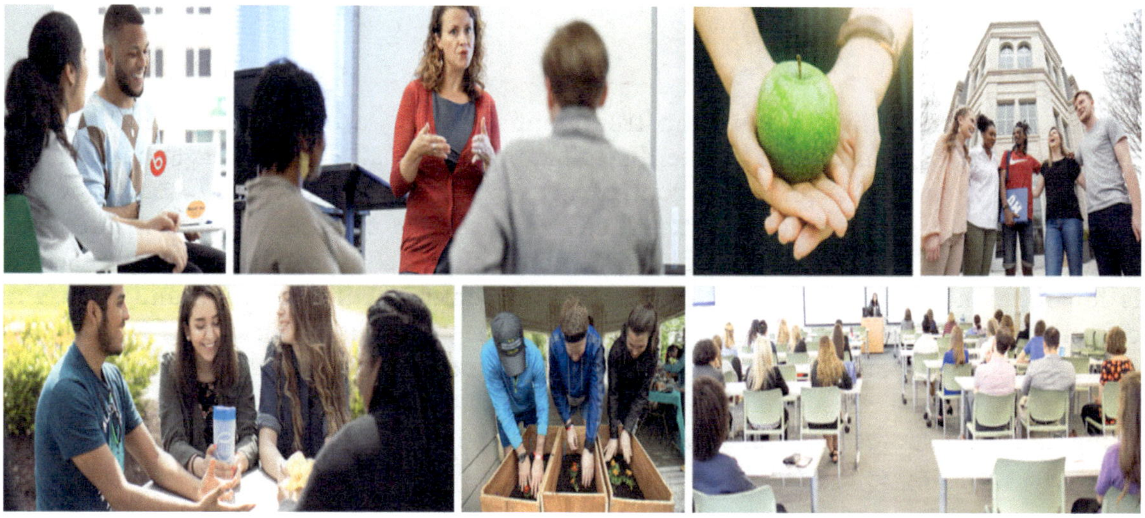

Figure 7.6. Health education and promotion.

Source: https://external-content.duckduckgo.com/iu/?u=https%3A%2F%2Fmarymount.edu%2Facademics%2Fwp-content%2Fuploads%2Fsites%2F3%2F2022%2F03%2FM.S.-in-Public-Health-Education-Promotion_Header.jpg&f=1&nofb=1&ipt=819c6767db1505d2949b7a9c07e91aa437a853c48b8a3155d4a6692cd6f8992f.

In the context of specific health conditions, the requirement for specialized learning becomes increasingly evident. Diabetes, for instance, is now a focal public health issue in most of the globe, as well as in the Philippines, with exponential growths in prevalence (Barcial et al., 2022). In response to this pressing demand, diabetes education-based health promotion programs not only educate the population regarding the risk caused by the diseases but also provide proper prevention and management advice. Among the successful strategies is the implementation of interactive sessions that give participants information in terms of nutrition, exercise, and lifestyle change in an effort to engage participants actively in their health process. Through the utilization of systematic channels of feedback after program implementation, these programs have the ability to gauge participant understanding and adjust their methodology with the goal of enhancing follow-up interventions. It is a process of continuous evaluation and revisions bringing programs up-to-date and responsive to emerging community needs. Participant outcomes and effects on the community are primarily used to assess the effectiveness of health education and promotion programs. Successful interventions will most likely generate meaningful, quantifiable change in behavior, attitude, and knowledge among participants in the intervention. A good example includes the diabetes education project carried out in Barangay Lalakhan, which recorded high success rates, high levels of satisfaction among the learners, and improved health habits among young adults (Barcial et al., 2022). The impact says a lot about the indispensable role of active community participation in health education, as involvement ensures a sense of ownership and responsibility. Additionally, the responsibility cycle and continuous feedback maintain a culture of learning under which health promotion programs can flourish. By assets at the community level and multi-sector collaborations' emphasis, such programs can drive enduring improvements to health and result in higher overall effectiveness of community health programs (Figure 7.6).

7.2.3. Disease Management and Treatment Programs

Interventions for controlling disease and treatment need to be integrated with objectives for community health programs in case an interdisciplinary public health program is to be implemented. Not only are these programs aimed at controlling already existing chronic diseases but also at instituting preventive interventions that reduce the incidence of such diseases in the long run. Through change in lifestyle and knowledge, the community health programs are able to establish a basis for better health. For instance, combined interventions with nutrition and counseling on physical activity have been promising in addressing obesity, which is important given that there has been a rising issue with obesity being a leading risk factor for chronic diseases. The collaborative approaches seen in projects such as the CPRC and the NICHQ Childhood Obesity Action Network help to highlight the success of collaborative approaches in responding to system issues of health in populations (Murphy et al., 2008).

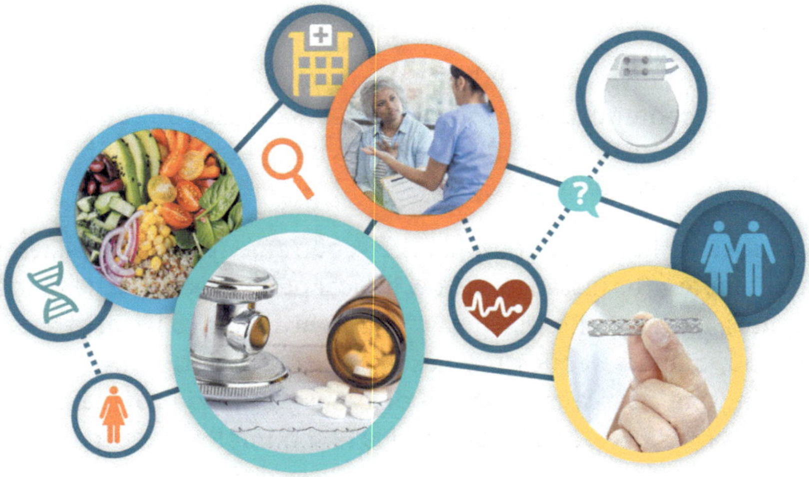

Figure 7.7. Disease management and treatment programs.

Source: https://domf5oio6qrcr.cloudfront.net/media/content/images/cr/ab327e1d-2014-43ff-ba[illegible]-d2fbf0b2dee8.jpg.

The application of the medical home model has also significantly transformed the disease care landscape, particularly for Medicaid and Children's Health Insurance Programs. In encouraging care coordination and overall care, such new models particularly emphasize the need for family-based deliveries of care. More significantly, in addition to trying to enhance the degree of care quality, these models also try to rein in the cost of care, which is a huge in today's financially strained settings. The models that also emphasize respectful communication among healthcare professionals, clients, and their families show more capacity to improve health outcomes in an orderly manner. Every state's experience in creating such models is instructive, being reproducible, transferable, and also applicable in guaranteeing effectiveness of community health initiatives towards managing chronic disease (Takach et al., 2009). Lastly, evaluation of the programs in disease control and treatment is crucial in verifying their effectiveness and overall effect on the population's health. Continuous evaluation helps in easier understanding of the common strengths and weaknesses associated with such health interventions, which helps in evidence-based refinement and improvement. Collection of information on health outcomes, patient satisfaction, and accessibility allows decision-makers to know where to make a change, thus the optimum use of resources. Secondly, engagement of members of the population in the assessment process makes them own the process and feel responsible, thus increased commitment towards health interventions. As one goes through the programs, there is a need to share documented best practices and methods, which can potentially inform the design of future community health programs for disease treatment and management, resulting in healthier lives and less healthcare inequality (Figure 7.7).

7.3. Evaluation Criteria for Community Health Programs

Determining the success of community health programs depends on a good grasp of some standards in order to ascertain whether they can work and last. One basic framework is assessing each program's viability, which focuses on obvious, overall goals and projected activities and results. According to January 2006 discussions, successful evaluation depends on establishing those definite goals in the attempt to have a point of reference for measuring program performance against. Without this grassroots level of knowledge, program stakeholders will be in the dark to align their efforts, leading to fractured results. Along with this, this knowledge can not only guide operational deployment but also increase the participation of participants, anchoring community investment and commitment in health programs. As an element of community health program evaluation, feasibility testing is also critical. Feasibility involves real-world considerations of putting a program in place, including resource availability and stakeholder involvement. The program itself needs to be robust but still flexible, capable of being inserted into community circumstances. As described in newer policy guidelines, the inclusion of a behavioral risk management framework is one illustration of a double focus on systematic intervention strategies without sacrificing responsiveness to patterns in unique communities. This reconciliation enables a modified response with the potential to achieve health hazards, such as the spread of AIDS, effectively by taking into consideration locally suitable conditions during planning of programs. This is why strong feasibility analysis not only directs implementation but also ensures optimal likely effectivity of health intervention. Finally, good standards of assessment must engage in a careful process and ensure outcome measurement.

Community health programs are effective not only for short-term health but also for long-term sustainability of the programs. Programs that demonstrate dramatic changes not only lead to short-term health but also lead to long-term behavior change within communities. The emphasis on behavior knowledge, as evident from the design of flexible intervention programs, implies the necessity of mechanisms for ongoing assessment like ongoing feedback loops. These enable programs to adapt in line with effectiveness in the real world, hence leading to higher community-level participation and improved public health outcomes. A multiperspective evaluation is therefore essential in ensuring community health programs have holistic, sustainable outcomes (Figure 7.8).

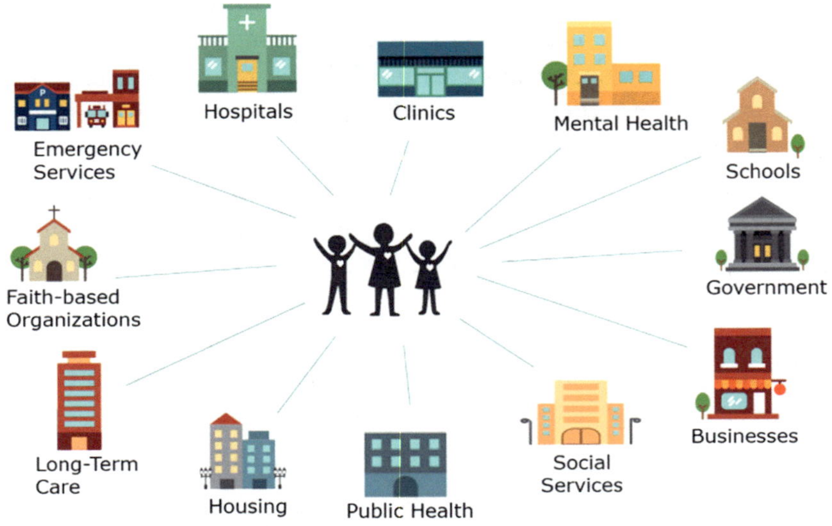

Figure 7.8. Evaluation criteria for community health programs.

Source: https://www.ruralhealthinfo.org/assets/1493-6245/1019-rhi-behavioral-health-integration-model-fullsize.jpg .

7.3.1. Effectiveness and Outcomes Measurement

Effectiveness and outcomes measurement of community health programs is crucial to determine the effectiveness of interventions and guide subsequent strategies. The measurements allow health practitioners to look at the various aspects of health programs, including general improvement of community well-being and diverse health outcomes. Through the use of a balanced framework for assessment, stakeholders are able to ascertain what is effective and what is not within a particular program. Successful measurement contributes to the determination of areas for development, the proper use of resources, and the enhancement of positive impacts. A solid foundation for effectiveness measurement can also contribute to accountability by program officials while increasing public confidence in community health programs. One of the key aspects of outcome measurement is understanding how civic participation creates improved health outcomes in communities. Engaging youth and other community members in health interventions not only enhances the effectiveness of interventions but also provides a sense of ownership and responsibility to local health issues. Youth citizens participating in civic engagement develop strong capacities that drive improved health outcomes, academic achievement, and social well-being. By prioritizing civic engagement as a key component, programs can be better designed to target youth populations, ultimately leading to healthier outcomes for the population overall, as has been determined about the impact of civic engagement on improving health and self-sufficiency (Hair et al., 2002). Finally, the ever-growing creation of models to evaluate must take into account collaborative approaches to measuring effectiveness. This collaboration among stakeholders—e.g., health care providers, community organizations, and the target groups themselves—is more comprehensive elucidation of program impacts. Expansion of the frame of reference to multiple-component evaluations as well as short-term health outcomes captures not only the acute effects of health but also long-term effects involving social equity and community resilience. Also, research initiatives led by institutions like the World Bank emphasize the importance of evaluating youth civic engagements impacts and how it can drive holistic community development (Campbell-Patton et al., 2009). As community health programs continue to expand, issues of inclusiveness and equity will be crucial to adapt to make them relevant and effective in addressing health disparities in society.

7.3.2. Accessibility and Equity Considerations

Accessibility and equity are fundamental in the evaluation of community health programs since they have a direct impact on the effectiveness and coverage of health interventions. Vulnerable populations are typically faced with systemic barriers that limit access to health services, resulting in differential health outcomes. For example, ethnic minorities and low-income households typically reside in areas with substandard housing that not only increase their utility costs but also result in health hazards. Both of these groups have disproportionately high levels of exposure to environmental pollutants, which contributes to the inherent health disparities.

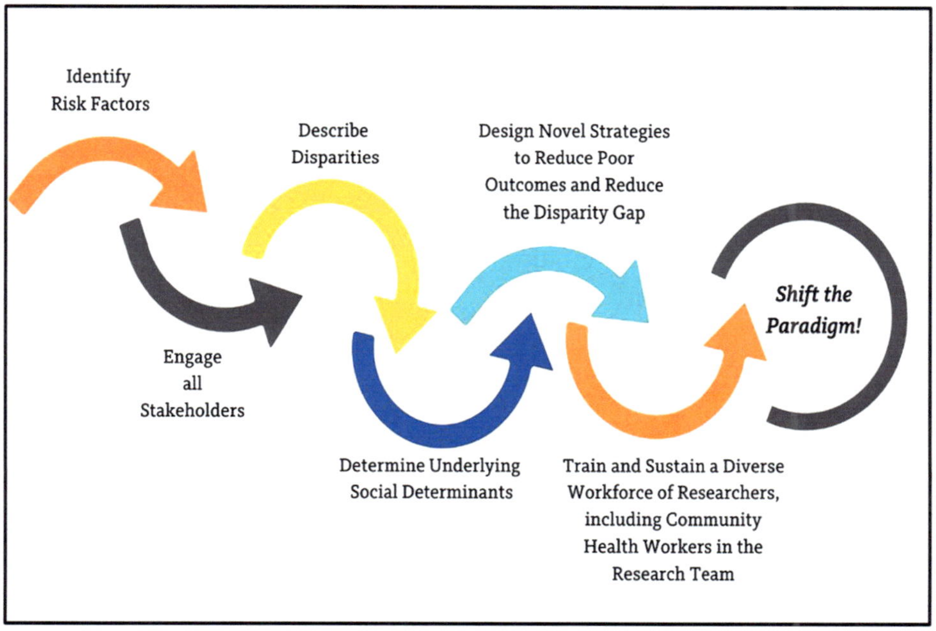

Figure 7.9. Accessibility and equity considerations.

Source: https://www.ahajournals.org/cms/asset/e22d3bca-a7e0-4a93-8641-dc5e2afb6efe/strokeaha.124.046958.fig04.jpg.

Striving for community health programs to address these inequities straight on can lead to more equitable outcomes in health, as well as increase the general performance of programs aimed at ensuring community wellness, stressing the importance of targeted interventions that consider the specific challenges of distinct parts of the population (Boston University Institute for Sustainable Energy et al., 2019). Equity also in community health programming calls for intentional design and implementation. For instance, public transportation access is central to making health service access a reality, but too many communities, and in particular those with high populations of people of color, are suffering from the absence of good public transportation. By prioritizing transportation access in program planning, communities can advance equity in health and ensure that everyone has an equal opportunity to seek needed care. In addition, evaluation of community health programs must involve the voices of marginalized populations to identify barriers and enhance services accordingly. As evidenced by the majority of livability programs, the integration of stakeholders' perspectives into practices of performance measurement can result in more responsive and more effective health strategies aligned with multicultural members' needs (Fabish et al., 2013). Finally, preserving an inclusive viewpoint in the process of building and implementing health programs is essential to achieving long-term equity goals. Health intervention development must incorporate a social justice approach that actively seeks to address past inequities and allow all parties to be heard in decision-making. Community participation and collaboration with local organizations could not only make programs more responsive but also allow marginalized groups to advocate for their health needs. In doing so within a collaborative context, health programs can create supportive environments that address root determinants of health disparities, thus moving further towards greater social and economic justice. Ultimately by integrating accessibility and equity concepts into community health efforts, stakeholders are able to build healthier, stronger communities (Boston University Institute for Sustainable Energy et al., 2019) (Figure 7.9).

7.3.3. Cost-Effectiveness Analysis (CEA)

CEA is a valuable method to measure community health programs by offering an organized approach to compare the relative cost and impact of different interventions. This method allows policymakers and health administrators to decide the optimal use of limited resources, particularly in settings where health budgets are tight. Measuring health outcomes against cost, CEA can guide program decision making for as varied as prevention and chronic disease management. The application of CEA helps in revealing the worth of health interventions, making the argument for cost-effective practice that yields a substantial return in the form of public health benefits without exacting overly high costs on health care systems. In international health programs, the application of cost-effectiveness analysis is even more essential with the range of different health problems vying for restricted funds. For example, studies have pointed out how the economic effectiveness of cessation programs can considerably influence public health outcomes. By presenting the costs of smoking-related illnesses against the cost of introducing cessation procedures, stakeholders are able to determine whether financial prudence is served by investing in prevention programs. Studies have indicated that effective cessation of smoking produces not only short-term health benefits but also huge economic returns in the way of lower healthcare expenditure and enhanced productivity, warranting the application of CEA in measuring health interventions (Brown et al.,

2025). Moreover, the growing emphasis on evidence-based practice further increases the relevance of CEA in planning effective community health interventions. By utilizing a systematic review of economic evaluations best recognizes the importance of good methodologies in evaluations of programs for community health. This practice development guarantees that future appraisals not only are comprehensive but also based on a framework that supports health equity as well as enhancement of population health. Accordingly, research like that in Bangladesh demonstrates a significant disparity between the use of CEA systematically and the requirement for increased methodological robustness in analyzing health programs (Gazi et al., 2011). Through closure of this disparity, health decision-makers will be able to develop a better-informed view of the effects of their interventions, thus towards improving the health outcomes of populations (Figure 7.10).

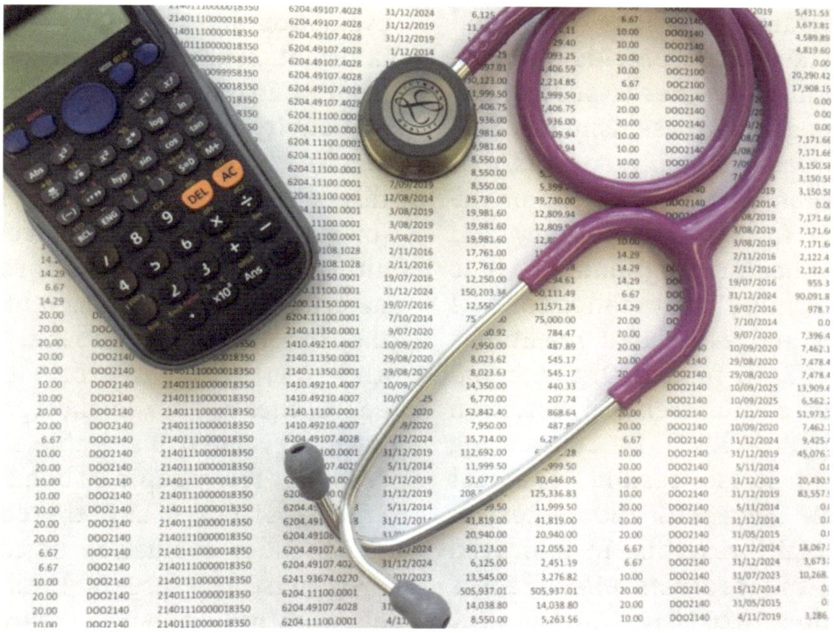

Figure 7.10. Cost-effectiveness analysis (CEA).

Source: https://s3-ap-southeast-2.amazonaws.com/os-data/aithm-jcu-edu-au/images/pageattached/392/blogskale_big_img_3570.jpg.

7.4. Methodologies for Evaluating Health Programs

The evaluation of community health programs necessitates a multi-modal methodology that includes both quantitative and qualitative approaches. Quantitative methods are likely to use the application of formal tools such as surveys and statistical analysis in quantifying health outcomes. These methods provide for a numerical basis that may be helpful in comparison among different groups of demography. For instance, understanding the condition's prevalence prior to and subsequent to program initiation may be significant in impact measurement. Alternatively, qualitative techniques attempt to achieve intensive understanding utilizing interviews and focus groups, where individual experiences and contextual concerns that cannot be measured can be explored. Therefore, the blending of these methods results in a robust mechanism for evaluating health programs since it is capable of including empirical data alongside the multifaceted realities confronting community members. The inclusion of stakeholder perceptions into the evaluation process is another fundamental methodological component. Community member, healthcare provider, and policymaker consultation can render health program evaluations more valid and applicable. Stakeholders provide opinions that might represent difficulties or success not readily observed in standard assessments. This participatory approach not only ensures that assessment is responsive to the needs of the community, but it fosters transparency and accountability for health programming. It is necessary to determine the implications of existing programs and associated results, as evidenced in the USAID-funded Orphans and Vulnerable Children Comprehensive Action Research Project (OVC-CARE). By considering these perspectives, it is possible to adjust programs to better align with the context of the community, finally resulting in improved health outcomes and program effectiveness (OVC-CARE project, 2010). Lastly, new technologies and methods are transforming how health program evaluations are conducted in contemporary settings. Digital technologies such as data analytics platforms and mobile health apps are also being used to gather and analyze health information in more efficient and real-time manners. This significantly enhances the possibility of adaptive management, with programs being modified based on real-time feedback and emerging data. In addition, awareness of the necessity to address epistemic loss within evaluation practices is growing due to its link with protecting and blending local knowledge systems. In a participatory culture of evaluation where indigenous knowledge is valued together with recent innovations, health programs can be made more suitable to tackle the unique challenges of climate change and other community issues of the time (Werkheiser et al., 2017).

7.4.1. Qualitative vs. Quantitative Evaluation Methods

The evaluation of community health programs often necessitates integrating qualitative and quantitative strategies, each contributing in its own way to the evaluation strategy. Quantitative evaluation most often makes use of numerical information and statistical methods to measure health outcomes and provide definiteness and objectivity. For instance, an evaluation may quantify behavioral change or enhanced health through surveys and clinical records, allowing for generalizable inferences. Nevertheless, although quantitative approaches thrive in determining correlations and assessing effec , they can neglect people's individual experiences and contextual factors that qualitative approaches can tap. By incorporating qualitative means, evaluators are able to understand the reasons for people's behaviors, attitudes, and experiences and thereby add depth to the broader evaluation of community health programs. The use of both qualitative and quantitative evaluations through the mixed-methods approach has increasingly been applied in measuring community health programs. t allows for effective analysis of program efficacy by situating quantitative information within the context of actual participant narratives. For example, an assessment of a French national health promotion program in primary school children utilized a mixed-method design where information developed from qualitative approaches was a secondary validation to a more quantitative rigorous examination. This conjoining enabled researchers to construct a more detailed picture of how health promotion affected children's physical and emotional health in the school setting, illustrating that it is important to capture not just statistical outcomes but also the lived experience that creates these outcomes (Guével et al., 2010). Whether or not to employ qualitative or quantitative approaches can also have an immense impact on implications of findings and policy implications. For instance, evaluations of Eastern European mine closures showed how the consideration of community impacts included quantitative findings and individual accounts from those affected. Employing qualitative interviews alongside quantitative questionnaire results, researchers not only determined economic effects of mine closure but also the broader social impacts on entire communities, which tended to include insecurity and a loss of community identity. These evaluations highlight how combining approaches can render findings more relevant and useable, finally leading to soundly well-rounded policy recommendations for highly single-industry-dependent communities (Haney et al., 2025) (Figure 7.11).

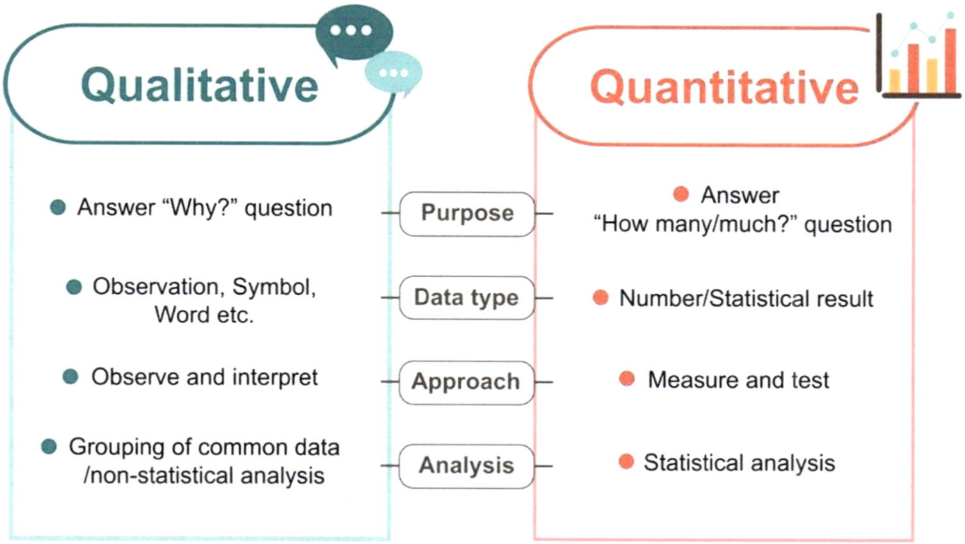

Figure 7.11. Qualitative vs. quantitative evaluation methods.

Source: https://www.bachelorprint.co.uk/wp-content/uploads/2023/07/qualitative-vs-quantitative-data-analysis-1.jpg.

7.4.2. Use of Surveys and Interviews

Surveys and interviews are essential tools to apply to the evaluation of community health programs, yielding rich descriptions of participant experience and program achievement. The official structure of questionnaires allows for quantitative measurement of numerous factors, such as participant satisfaction, demographic information, and health outcomes. Interviews, on the other hand, allow a deeper understanding of individual attitudes through the respondents' ability to explain their own feelings, ideas, and worries in their own words. Qualitative data of this kind is invaluable, revealing issues that would go unnoticed were generic questionnaires used. Employing both approaches, evaluators are able to triangulate results, enhancing validity of the findings and giving a more comprehensive view of program effect in communities. For the Respite Partnership Collaborative (RPC) Innovation Project, combining surveys with interviews from stakeholders was critical in assessing collaborative work between public and private sectors. The American Institutes for Research (AIR) assessors gathered questionnaires among the RPC members to gauge perceptions of how effective the projects are in improving respite services. Stakeholder interviews were also utilized to provide qualitative data on collaboration dynamics and community-led action of the initiative. This twofold strategy not only brought out the strengths and weaknesses in providing services but also highlighted how the community could be involved in shaping mental health resources within Sacramento County, with a particular emphasis on stakeholder engagement in the evaluation process (Poon et al., 2016). Similarly, survey and interview use are emphasized in the CHARM intervention study in rural India, where both assessed the impact of the programs on men's participation in family planning. Both quantitative survey data were used to give baseline and follow-up measurements for contraceptive use and reproductive health outcomes among couples. Meanwhile, qualitative, in-depth interviews with purposively sampled couples uncovered the prevailing beliefs and limitations influencing family planning decisions, giving essential background to the quantitative findings. Collectively, these methods enable program implementers to shift approaches as a response to feedback, fostering an open space satisfying the particular demands of rural populations. Thus, this methodological consistency not only enhances program evaluation but also assists in constructing culture-sensitive health interventions so that community health programs are efficient and responsive to local contexts (Balaiah et al., 2016).

7.4.3. Data Analysis Techniques

Data analysis techniques play an essential role in evaluating community health programs because they provide a paradigm for integrating complex data on health outcomes, behavior, and program effectiveness. Employing a combination of qualitative and quantitative methods, researchers can track patterns of health in data that inform decision-making. For instance, qualitative methods such as interviews and focus groups can yield rich contextual information on the community's perceptions of health programs, whereas quantitative methods can statistically analyze health indicators to establish the effect of a program. The union of both approaches enhances findings strength, allowing inclusive assessment that considers numbers and stories and hence best serving the overall aim of community health programs. In assessing community health programs, one has to use systematic data analysis techniques that allow rigorous policy evaluation and outcomes. These techniques have a tendency to encompass data reduction, presentation, and interpretation as discussed in a number of studies. For example, the assessment of youth-friendly community programs could show this strategy; the investigators may utilize interviews and observation techniques to gather qualitative information, which is subsequently triangulated with quantitative assessments of program impact. The strategy can complement blueprints such as the District/City Worthy of Children strategy, which is centered around bringing together government and community resources to fulfill children's rights. Using such thorough analytical methods ensures that evaluations accurately reflect the extent to which community health programs are reaching their objectives and addressing the needs of the population in question, directly informing policy implementation.

The circular process of data analysis in assessing community health programs is key in ensuring continued improvement and accountability. As reported in other studies, as well as findings resulting from forums for dialogue with experts internationally, the assessment process should be flexible and responsive to the emerging data as well as community demands. This flexibility is crucial in making sure that programs are not just implemented successfully but are continually sharpened through participatory feedback. A key aspect of this analysis is the quantification of youth engagement in civic activity, which has been linked to broader developmental impacts. Engaging the community in the analysis promotes transparency and stimulates a feeling of ownership of health initiatives, reaffirming the interconnectedness among data analysis, community participation, and quality health outcomes. So, a firm dedication to applying multiple data analysis methods helps enhance the integrity and effectiveness of community health program assessments (Figure 7.12).

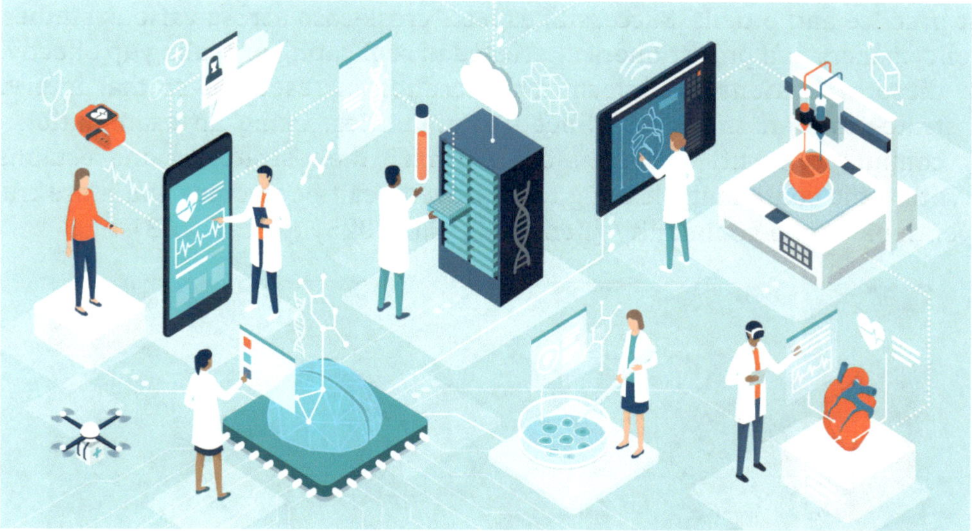

Figure 7.12. Data analysis techniques.

Source: https://blog.decos.com/hubfs/Hero%20blog%20data%20analytics.png#keepProtocol.

7.5. Case Studies of Successful Community Health Programs

Successful case studies are often implemented by community health programs during their planning and evaluation. A successful example can be found in various nutrition programs that were implemented across Africa. In-depth analysis of the projects revealed that seven key factors were largely responsible for the success of the programs, i.e., community involvement, program flexibility, and institutional setting. These were conditions in which stakeholders were interested in the outcomes, and therefore the overall effectiveness of the programs was increased. Furthermore, the emphasis on holistic activities and highly qualified staff allowed such programs to be sensitive to the specific demands within different populations. Through an emphasis on local knowledge and abilities, health programs could be sustainable and effective, and there was an argument for such measures to be replicated in subsequent programs (Kennedy et al., 2025). Apart from nutrition-specific programs, case studies with planetary health practice integrated in community health education have also yielded promising outcomes. Employing a six-stage design-based education research strategy, various countries, including Australia and the United States, have managed to implement the Planetary Health Education Framework effectively in health professional courses. All of these courses emphasize community engagement, cultural competence, and interprofessionalism, which are essential in developing curricula for diverse groups. The final case studies illustrate the ways in which integrating Indigenous perspectives into health education embeds holistic well-being strategies. Importantly, the case studies can serve as an educator's toolkit if one is to take up and implement similar projects, thereby broadening the debate on health education and encouraging an holistic approach to public health (Luebke et al., 2024). Moreover, effective community health programs need to be scrutinized for their impact on outcomes in health and participation in the community. Not only are programs tested, but they are also utilized to guide future programs by defining best practice and pitfalls. Successful aspects cross-case across various studies that are of interest to policymakers and practitioners interested in replicating or scaling up effective programs. Besides that, these evaluations can inform the allocation of resources so that interventions can be targeted strategically at the most in-need communities. Using an examination of effective case studies, community health programs can optimize their strategies and establish stronger connections within the community, leading to improved health outcomes and more trust in public health interventions by the community (Kennedy et al., 2025) (Figure 7.13).

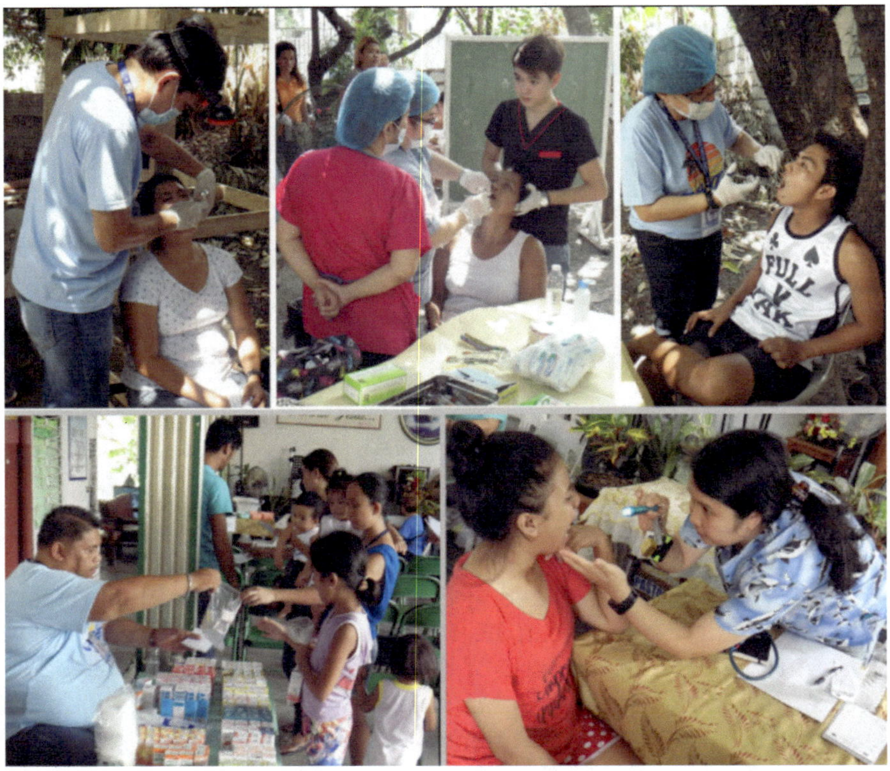

Figure 7.13. Case studies of successful community health programs.

Source: https://cavite.gov.ph/home/wp-content/uploads/2018/06/MD-Mission-in-Bayan-Luma-5.jpg.

7.5.1. Overview of Notable Programs

Programs in community health are multifaceted programs that seek to address specific health issues in diverse populations. A good example is various mental health consultation programs that have proved to be effective due to the systematic approach and competent professionals. One of the primary explanations for the effectiveness of such programs is the extensive infrastructure behind them, making it possible to implement targeted interventions. Organizations that have highly educated consultants working for them and provide quality support services are found to make considerable mental health outcome gains. In prioritizing precision when measuring targeted outcomes, such initiatives not only enhance individual mental health but also help community wellness at large through early intervention and ongoing support (Anthony et al., 2009). Very significant among the exemplary programs of community health engagement is that of the Center for Service and Learning at IUPUI. The program integrates effectively academic resources and community engagement, opening doors to the involvement of faculty and staff in community-engaged activities. A study of the IUPUI faculty and staff who were found to have positive attitudes towards the role that CSL programs play in reinforcing service learning and community engagement. The findings emphasized the experience of respondents in converting academic ability to real-life problem-solving, stressing the need for institution cooperation with their immediate surrounding communities. Such programs are key in establishing participants' sense of civic participation as well as enhanced health and educational access (Hahn et al., 2019). Additionally, extensive evaluation of community health programs is important to ensure constant improvement and functionality. By soliciting feedback from stakeholders and participants, such appraisals enable programs to adjust and revise their strategies in line with empirical evidence. For instance, information that is acquired from surveys and evaluations provides a clearer picture of the health needs of the community as well as the gaps existing within the health services. This cycle process not only aids in improving existing programs but also in preparing new programs that are sensitive to the dynamic shifts of community health. Constant evaluation thus forms a foundation for successful program planning, ensuring the interventions remain appropriate, effective, and reactive to the needs of the population.

7.5.2. Key Factors Contributing to Their Success

The effectiveness of community health programs is based on a variety of critical factors brought together to enhance their effectiveness and sustainability. The focus on social and economic determinants of health, particularly among vulnerable populations, is one of the critical aspects. Programs that directly address greater educational access, housing stability, and economic opportunities have been linked with better health outcomes. Through interventions on these determinants, programs will be making long-term changes, as evidenced in efforts to close the life expectancy gap between Indigenous and non-Indigenous Australians. Recognizing that most interventions target individual determinants rather than proximal health outcomes is critical in understanding the multifaceted nature of public health benefits (Baum et al., 2013). This inclusive strategy not only enhances the immediate effect of health programs but also contributes to long-term community resilience. Effective community engagement emerges as a consequence as another major reason for the success of health programs. If communities are engaged in planning, implementation, and evaluation of such interventions, ownership and commitment are highly increased. Successful programs are most commonly incorporated with local stakeholders along the way so interventions are culturally relevant and tailored to the particular needs of the served community. Such participation is useful for the establishment of trust and partnership, essential elements to the addressing of health improvement challenges. Successful leadership and staff who are well informed in the health arena and also aware of the community environment can perhaps enable more quality implementation strategies. This type of leadership contributes greatly to resource mobilization and momentum maintenance in the program, and in turn, enhances its effectiveness (Chavis et al., 2009). Finally, strategic, cross-level relationships are needed to scale and uphold community health programs. Systems that collaborate resources and interventions from sectors like healthcare, education, and social services can provide comprehensive solutions to health problems. Successful programs often benefit from a single broker or organization to coordinate these activities, with a common vision that aligns multiple groups of stakeholders to collective health objectives. Clearly defined roles within the partnerships also reduce conflict and foster cooperation, required to generate larger community-level effects. Additionally, the application of data to inform decisions and track progress can establish the program's impact and responsiveness over the long term. Programs that recognize these relational dynamics are more likely to create long-term change in their communities (Chavis et al., 2009) (Figure 7.14).

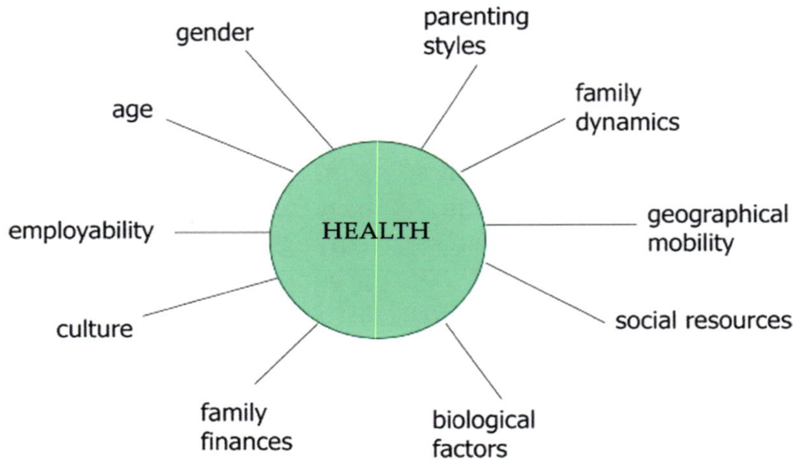

Figure 7.14. Key factors contributing to their success.

Source: https://image.slideserve.com/1083821/factors-affecting-health-n.jpg.

7.5.3. Lessons Learned from These Case Studies

Lessons below, taken from various community health program case studies, are useful in understanding the success of capacity-building initiatives. The following main finding highlights the emphasis on the participation of the community in all phases of program implementation. Community members' participation builds trust and confidence that interventions applied are impactful and relevant to the local context. As is evident in the evaluation of the Cancer Prevention and Control Research Network (CPCRN), community members' participation helps in enhancing capacity to select and apply evidence-based interventions appropriate to specific population health concerns. This participatory approach is essential in facilitating long-term sustainability and community adoption of health interventions and calling for future efforts to be directed towards involving strategies that involve the voices and perspectives of the communities at the planning and implementation stages of health interventions (Escoffery et al., 2023). Of importance too is the need to develop and sustain partnerships among various stakeholders involved in community health projects. The evaluation of Partnerships in Health Initiative winners placed importance on the fact that collaborative processes were capable of influencing communities' access to health resources in a productive manner. Successful partnerships leverage diverse strengths and resources bases, leading to an interdependent problem-solving approach. Not only does this interconnectedness enhance the coverage of health initiatives, but it also fosters ownership among partners, leading to greater community health impacts. The findings indicate that actively developing and cultivating such relationships and supporting collaborative efforts can overcome adversity and promote resilience in combating health issues (Keller et al., 2012). Furthermore, co-learning is a significant component in the paradigm of the community health program. The experience gained through CPCRN offers evidence that co-learning among community organizations, researchers, and practitioners can lead to improved implementation processes and better health outcomes. When different stakeholders get together to share knowledge, experience, and best practices, there is a better understanding of complex health issues. This not only fosters a culture of development but also empowers local organizations to adapt evidence-based practice according to their local contexts. The emphasis on co-learning means that subsequent evaluations of community health programs must consider processes for ongoing knowledge exchange and adaptive learning to enhance program effectiveness and long-term sustainability (Escoffery et al., 2023).

7.6. Challenges in Evaluating Community Health Programs

Evaluating community health programs is very challenging since program models and the settings for their implementation are heterogeneous. Implementation strategies, target populations, and types of health problems addressed contribute to complexity. For instance, the current pattern of ICT-delivered health programs has added more levels of complexity to evaluation as observed in studies with findings revealing broad variations in program design, methodology, and outcomes across studies. From the literature as examples, it is observable that only a small proportion of programs identified persistently had strong methodologies, and thus it becomes hard to ascertain best practices and generalizability of study findings. The combination of program attributes with heterogeneity means that evaluators must adopt elastic frameworks that can accommodate heterogeneity, but these tend to be non-specific, which leads to inconclusive evidence on program efficacy (Alston et al., 2022). Second, the protocols for the use of RCTs as the gold standard evaluation method pose significant constraints, particularly for complex community health interventions. RCTs, while helpful in a broad variety of contexts, are deficient when assessing the everyday realities that accompany programs that treat issues of domestic violence. The nature of such programs necessitates an assessment process that will incorporate qualitative methods that can capture the lived experiences of participants and the uncertain character of intervention effects. Critics argue that following RCTs rigidly constrains our understanding of community health program efficacy since it ignores the abundance of qualitative data that can be utilized in informing program refinement and adaptation (Epstein et al., 2017). Examining a broader array of evaluation strategies might thus be more insightful regarding the realities of community health initiatives. And finally, stakeholder participation is also a critical problem hindering the proper evaluation of community health programs. Successful programs are based on active input from local people and organizations, but their input into the evaluation process remains subpar. Such low co-design has the impact of not only reducing the value of evaluation indicators but also program acceptability in target communities. For instance, evaluations can overlook culturally modified needs or fail to account for the inclusion of genuine program beneficiaries' input, and in doing so, produce skewed outcomes that do not reflect the actual effect of the programs. Closing the gaps entails a conscious intent towards participative evaluation approaches that empower community voice to ensure that evaluations not only quantify outcomes but also ensure continuous improvement and sustainability in the community health sector (Alston et al., 2022).

7.6.1. Data Collection and Reliability Issues

Ensuring data collection integrity is of utmost concern when evaluating community health programs, as this directly influences the reliability of outcomes and subsequent health interventions. Effective data collection procedures ensure that the data obtained is accurate and relevant, hence supporting informed decision-making.

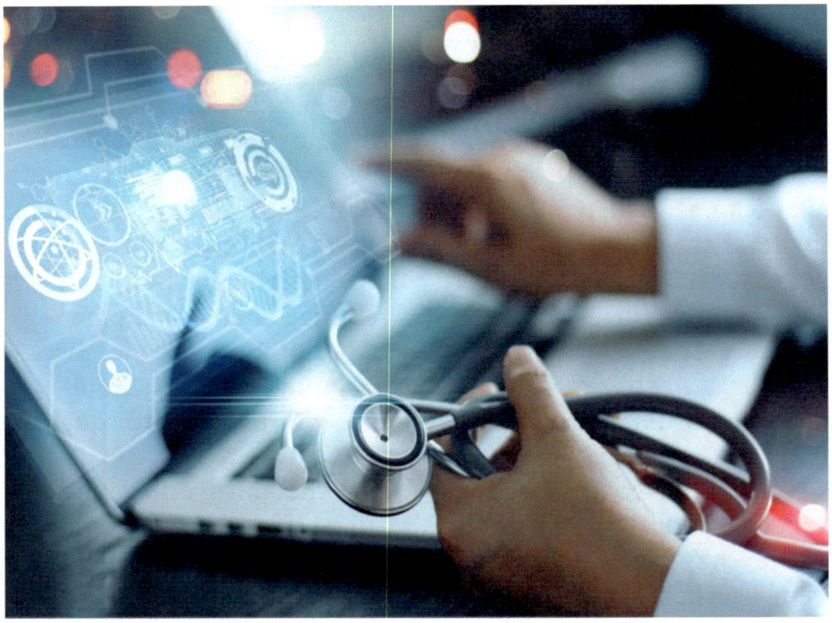

Figure 7.15. Data collection and reliability issues.

Source: https://prognocis.com/wp-content/uploads/2022/09/Data-collection-in-healthcare.jpeg

The issues typically manifest in the form of sampling bias, data entry mistakes, and substandard measurement tools. Such variables can significantly skew findings, leading to inaccurate strategies that will fail to address actual community health needs. For instance, misreporting due to unrepresentative samples can decrease the perceived effectiveness of a healthcare program, denying communities precious resources. Ensuring data collection procedures are reliable is central to the capacity of delivering credible evaluation that may inform the future community health plans sufficiently, as noted by Klima et al. (2013) when considering evaluating the health programs. Moreover, evaluation of the community health programs entails not only collection of data but also analysis of the same, which may identify crucial information or unveil basic gaps in knowledge regarding processes of community health. As noted by Colburn et al. (2011), the need for frequent reporting and monitoring progress is crucial in ascertaining the success of such programs. After systematic collection, data can be analyzed for patterns and trends, enabling the determination of the successful elements and those that need strengthening. Periodic monitoring of community progress improves health objectives and develops new strategic plans. But when there is not good data or bad data, then it compromises the entire evaluation process, and there are unmet healthcare issues. Strong practices of data collection are required to generate high-quality evaluations that are not only responsible but also actionable. Moreover, data reliability in the evaluation of community health programs is also complicated by other external considerations like socioeconomic conditions and health behavior and outcome-cultural environments. Such issues necessitate all-round data collection that captures the intricacies of public health. For example, an assessment of health program performance could be substantially different in various demographic communities due to variations in access to resources or variations in views regarding health among people within a community. Thus, program evaluators need to consider both qualitative and quantitative data to form an overall picture of community health needs. Through the gathering of various forms of data, evaluators can provide higher reliability and context in analysis that leads to more useful health intervention. Lastly, highlighting data reliability not only facilitates appropriate evaluation but also helps formulate particular programs that resonate with the needs and values of the community (Figure 7.15).

7.6.2. Stakeholder Engagement and Participation

Effective stakeholder participation plays a key role in the evaluation of community health programs, as it provides partnership relations that ensure maximum program relevance and sustainability. Having a wide variety of stakeholders on board—local residents, policymakers, etc.—protects the concept that the programs will be developed in order to meet the specific preferences and needs of the populations being targeted. Engaging stakeholders at the evaluation's front end can earn one a deeper understanding of the local health issues and the capacity to create interventions that are culturally and contextually relevant. This involvement not only creates a sense of ownership among participants but also allows them to contribute inputs in planning and implementation of health programs, thereby having more prospects of program success and social solidarity. By tapping into such collaborative efforts, community health programs can bank on local wisdom, thus gaining more effective strategies and outcomes. Partnerships play an essential part in stakeholder engagement, particularly in public health evaluations. Partnerships, as articulated by collaborative frameworks such as Western Australia's SiREN, demonstrate how strategic alliances between researchers, service providers, and policymakers can bridge evaluation knowledge and capacity needs. These partnerships allow for immediate stakeholder engagement in evaluation processes, improving valuing and understanding of the evaluation process by policymakers and service providers. Above all, such partnerships can be employed to enhance local evidence generation, which is an utmost requirement for community-level health issues. By engaging stakeholders through coordinated partnerships, not only is the development of actionable results promoted, but the translation of these into policy and practice is also guaranteed. It is this interaction that ultimately makes the entire group of community health initiatives more efficient and even fosters a culture of improvement. However, effectiveness in stakeholder involvement continues to be challenged in communication and role understanding within collaborative arrangements. University Social Responsibility (USR) implementation requires a clear communication factor in engaging various stakeholders. Without the common understanding of objectives and expectations, stakeholders could be hindered in their participation, which restricts the desired advantages from collaborative efforts. As implied from evidence regarding USR, there can be a hindrance to integrating strategic plans with inadequate communication within communities. This could deny valuable participatory chances. To address such challenges, inclusive communication strategies need to be developed by community health programs that facilitate participatory involvement and foster trust among the stakeholders. By prioritizing these efforts, community health assessments can not only promote greater stakeholder engagement but also lead to more impactful and enduring health outcomes for the targeted groups.

7.6.3. Funding and Resource Limitations

In terms of community health programs, funding and resource limitations are significant hindrances to effective provision and sustainability. Government and private fundings are the sources of most of the programs and are susceptible to diverse political, economic, and social changes. For instance, a program may get initial funding but struggle to maintain financial support as grant cycles close or policy priorities change.

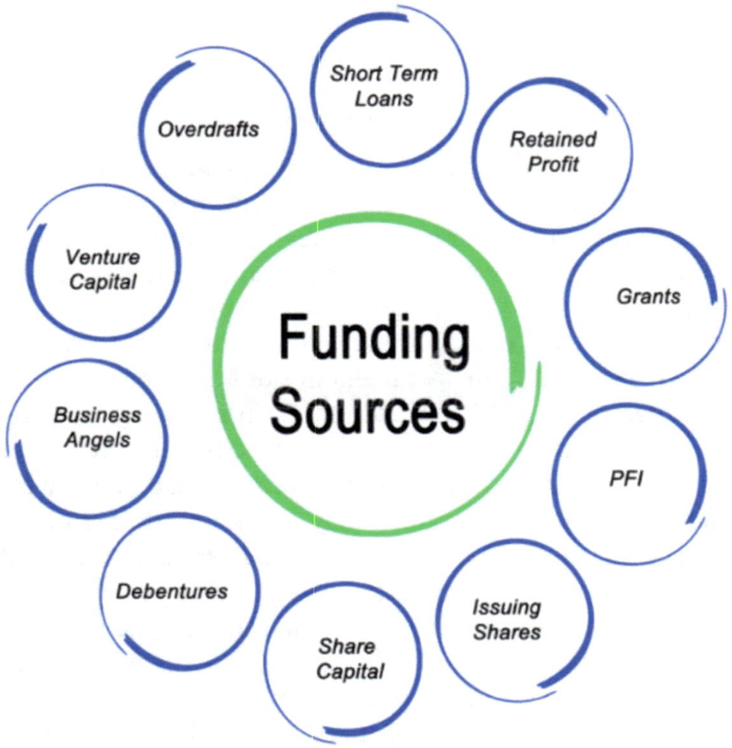

Figure 7.16. Funding and resource limitations.

Source: https://thumbs.dreamstime.com/b/funding-sources-diagram-important-94363896.jpg.

Such unpredictability in funding usually discourages the adequacy of services or even program expansion to meet community needs. As a result, equitable access and health gains that such programs aim to create are significantly diluted. Also, without a specified program data collection and evaluation budget, the majority of programs lack the appropriate feedback systems to accurately assess their impact and improve strategies. In addition, the shortage of resources is not just monetary; it also involves human resources, infrastructure, and technology. Community health initiatives typically have a challenge in obtaining and keeping good individuals, particularly in poor neighborhoods where financial gain might be less attractive than in urban centers. A successful program will fail if it does not have talented professionals to carry out its vision, illustrating the interdependence of human resources and funding. Infrastructure limitations, such as inadequate buildings or access to technology, also limit the potential of community health efforts. As highlighted by the Rhode Island Department of Health (RIDOH), adequate investment in local programs like Health Equity Zones can be capable of reducing such barriers and facilitating enhanced health outcomes through collective action and targeted resource allocation (Alexander-Scott et al., 2017). Furthermore, results in evaluating collaborative action in health programs emphasize the strategic use of funds toward realizing maximized impact. Reports of evaluation identify that collaborative partnerships between organizations increase the sharing of resources, resulting in better access and health equity, as noted in the results of the Partnerships in Health Initiative (Keller et al., 2012). Such collaborations allow communities to pool sources of funding and expertise and target the constraints presented by single organizations working in isolation. But their effectiveness is contingent upon achieving stable funding and open communication among stakeholders. Thus, overcoming funding and resource limitations is critical to making community health programs effective in their ability to serve populations and react to emergent health disparities in a changing setting (Figure 7.16).

SUMMARY

In evaluating community health programs, the discovery emphasizes the need for reflective critique in order to achieve their intricate impacts. These evaluations gain significantly in molding existing frameworks as well as guiding future implementations. Experiential engagement-oriented medical education in the context of community-based medical education is evidenced to indicate stakeholder satisfaction and the success of the program. The point here is the understanding that satisfaction among students and health professionals not only reflects the immediate quality of education but also provides the foundation for better community health. With over 80% of Clerkship students satisfied with their training, there is a clear link between good education and enhanced practice in managing health that calls for the replication of courses in community medicine in medical curricula globally, as hypothesized by the need for them to be revised (Khadivi et al., 2004). Another critical point coming out of the evaluation concerns accountability and strategic planning in realizing effective implementation of health programs. Statistics of maternal and child health programs indicate a failure in reducing the most critical indicators for health, such as the reduction in mortality rates and the eradication of malnutrition. The findings from the research of the local government indicate that there is an absence of correlation between allocations and tangible health outcomes, as unveiled through fluctuating maternal and infant mortality rates (Astuti et al., 2014). This highlights the importance of enhanced monitoring and accountability mechanisms within community health programs to ensure resources are utilized effectively in order to make meaningful progress in public health programs. Secondly, identification of gaps in local action plans reflects the importance of strategic systems of governance that enable community engagement and quality provision of health services. Lastly, the implications of the community health program assessment provide actionable advice that has the potential to significantly improve health results. The recommendations underscore the importance of education interventions that are specific to community needs and sound, evidence-based program implementation and funding strategies. Adopting a paradigm of community health that insists on cooperation between stakeholders ensures that investments are channeled into regions of maximum impact, with resulting responsiveness to local health priorities. Inasmuch as these assessments call for continuous improvement and adjustment of health programs, they also make clear the paramount requirement for policy improvements that create a strong system of monitoring and assistance. This comprehensive vision of community health not only pushes the agenda of disease prevention and health promotion forward but also enables communities to seize control of their own health futures.

The assessment of community health programs demonstrates a number of important findings that highlight the role of community involvement and community-based health initiatives. A major inference is that CBPHC is a central driver of improved maternal, neonatal, and child health. The inferences made by an Expert Panel are that investing in CBPHC is critical in order to build healthier systems, accelerate progress towards universal health coverage, and eliminate avoidable maternal and child deaths. The assessment included comprehensive examination of reports that highlighted partnership between health systems and communities. It is through collaboration with communities and their health systems that partnerships can really harness evidence-based interventions and ensure that interventions reach the most vulnerable communities in every society in order to meet global health goals established by agencies like the World Health Organization (Arole et al., 2017). Another key finding is concerning the Mental Health Services Act (MHSA) and how it is affecting community-based mental health programs. The RPC Innovation Project funded by MHSA, is just one example of how public-private partnerships can successfully facilitate localized mental health care. The American Institutes for Research assessment found that the RPC significantly improved interagency collaboration and community organization collaboration and demonstrated the effectiveness of a community-based approach to handling mental health crises. The assessment, founded on stakeholder interviews and surveys, underscored that increased local mental health respite services can be strong hospitalization alternatives. This finding confirms that community-centered methods enhance mental health care quality and accessibility, in accordance with overall objectives of promoting mental well-being and treatment access (Poon et al., 2016). Finally, a persistent theme emerging in the evaluations is the necessity for ongoing research and data collection to optimize community health program impact. The findings suggest extensive operations research and continuous assessment, both of which are important for maximizing intervention strategies and informing policy-making. Systematic assessment of programs like CBPHC and the RPC Innovation Project enables stakeholders to identify best practices and points of improvement. Above all, these findings are an eldorado for creating future health initiatives that are evidence-driven and tailored to responding to specific needs of communities. Finally, incorporating people's feedback and evidence-based methods is crucial to accomplishing the envisioned health outcomes and promoting sustainable health systems that empower.

KEY TERMS FROM THIS CHAPTER

- Accessibility
- Advocacy
- Civic engagement
- Community member
- Community resources
- Cost-Effectiveness Analysis (CEA)
- Dental Health Aide (DHA) program
- Economic stability
- Ethnic minorities
- Flood management
- Flood risk management
- Healthcare expenditure
- Healthcare provider
- Healthcare services
- Health Equity Zones
- Holistic approach
- Housing stability
- Human resources
- Human rights
- Malnutrition
- Marginalization
- Orphans and vulnerable children (OVC)
- Outcome measurement
- Policymaker consultation
- Preventive health services
- Public awareness

CLOSER LOOK

PEACE EVALUATION ACROSS CULTURES AND ENVIRONMENTS (PEACE)

A Peace Evaluation Across Cultures and Environments (PEACE) is a framework designed to assess and understand peace from a holistic, inclusive, and culturally sensitive perspective. Rather than viewing peace solely as the absence of conflict or violence, the PEACE model recognizes that true peace encompasses social justice, environmental sustainability, human rights, and individual well-being. It emphasizes that peace must be evaluated within specific cultural and environmental contexts, acknowledging that communities define and experience peace in diverse ways. The framework seeks to include voices from marginalized groups and indigenous populations, ensuring that local knowledge, traditions, and values inform the understanding and measurement of peace. PEACE uses both qualitative and quantitative tools to assess factors such as access to resources, equity, governance, cultural harmony, ecological balance, and personal safety. It encourages collaboration between community members, researchers, and policymakers to identify strengths and challenges, and to co-create strategies that promote sustainable and inclusive peace. By addressing structural inequalities, historical injustices, and environmental degradation, the PEACE framework highlights the interconnectedness of global and local peace efforts. It also supports ongoing monitoring and adaptation, recognizing that peace is a dynamic process requiring continuous engagement, dialogue, and healing. Ultimately, PEACE moves beyond simplistic or one-size-fits-all solutions, advocating for a nuanced approach that respects the complexity of human societies and ecosystems. It provides a valuable tool for guiding peacebuilding efforts, promoting intercultural understanding, and ensuring that peace is meaningful, measurable, and sustainable across all communities and environments.

REFERENCES

1. Ahn, R., Blais, M., Burke, T. F., Nelson, B., et al. (2014). Development of a scale to measure individuals' ratings of peace. https://core.ac.uk/download/28951886.pdf (accessed on 26th June 2025).
2. Alexander-Scott, N., Ankoma, N., et al. (2017). Rhode Island's Health Equity Zones: Addressing local problems with local solutions. https://digitalscholarship.unlv.edu/cgi/viewcontent.cgi?article=1643&context=jhdrp (accessed on 26th June 2025).
3. Alston, L., Beks, H., Clapham, R., Glenister, H., et al. (2022). Community health programs delivered through information and communications technology in high-income countries: Scoping review. https://core.ac.uk/download/587393688.pdf (accessed on 26th June 2025).
4. Anthony, B., Perry, D., Duran, F., Hepburn, K., Irvine, M., Horen, N., & Kaufmann, R. (2009). What works? A study of effective early childhood mental health consultation programs. https://core.ac.uk/download/71355788.pdf (accessed on 26th June 2025).
5. Arole, S., Bang, A., Bhutta, Z. A., Black, R., et al. (2017). Comprehensive review of the evidence regarding the effectiveness of community-based primary health care in improving maternal, neonatal and child health: 8. Summary and recommendations of the expert panel. https://core.ac.uk/download/212879387.pdf (accessed on 26th June 2025).
6. Astuti, W. D., Laksono, A. D., Oktarina, O., Pratiwi, D., et al. (2014). A policy review on the distribution of health operational aid funds in achieving maternal and child health program (MDGs 4, 5) in three districts/cities of East Java Province. https://media.neliti.com/media/publications/20919-ID-a-policy-review-on-the-distribution-of-health-operational-aid-funds-in-achieving.pdf (accessed on 26th June 2025).
7. Barcial, K. R. B. (2022). Simple steps in preventing diabetes: A healthier diet and active lifestyle promotion for the young adults aged 20 to 39 in Barangay Lalakhan, Sta. Maria, Bulacan. https://core.ac.uk/download/599598021.pdf (accessed on 26th June 2025).
8. Barrena Martínez, J., Llinàs Audet, F. J., & Ramos-Monge, E. (2019). Drivers and barriers of university social responsibility: Integration into strategic plans. https://core.ac.uk/download/157810895.pdf (accessed on 26th June 2025).
9. Bastian, L., Brennan, S., Comfort, J., Crawford, G., et al. (2018). A research and evaluation capacity building model in Western Australia. https://core.ac.uk/download/213607723.pdf (accessed on 26th June 2025).
10. Baum, F., Osborne, K., & Brown, L. (2013). What works? A review of actions addressing the social and economic determinants of Indigenous health. https://core.ac.uk/download/pdf/30675270.pdf (accessed on 26th June 2025).
11. Beard, J., Biemba, G., Brooks, B., Costello, J., et al. (2009). Kenya research situation analysis on orphans and other vulnerable children. https://open.bu.edu/bitstream/2144/26989/1/Kenya-Research-Situation-Analysis-Country-Brief.pdf (accessed on 26th June 2025).
12. Blackman, D. H. (2005). Current developments in services for people with intellectual disabilities. https://core.ac.uk/download/5124575.pdf (accessed on 26th June 2025).
13. Bolin, K. A., Indian Health Service (IHS), Jones, C. M., Nash, D. A., & Trueblood, G. (2013). Alaska Dental Health Aide Program. https://core.ac.uk/download/pdf/26744475.pdf (accessed on 26th June 2025).

14. Boston University Institute for Sustainable Energy, Castigliego, J., Cleveland, C., Fortune D., et al. (2019). *Carbon Free Boston: Social equity report 2019*. https://open.bu.edu/bitstream/2144/39229/1/CFB_Social_Equity_Report_053119.pdf (accessed on 26th June 2025).

15. Bozeman, B., Purdy, C., Williams, C. L., Garrison, D. F., Comfort, L. K., & Hillsman, S. T. (2009). Department of Homeland Security Science and Technology Directorate: Developing technology to protect America. https://core.ac.uk/download/71345935.pdf (accessed on 26th June 2025).

16. Brousseau, R. T. (2004). Reflections on evaluating our grants. https://core.ac.uk/download/71354307.pdf (accessed on 26th June 2025).

17. Brown, A. K., & Ekpu, V. U. (2025). The economic impact of smoking and of reducing smoking prevalence: Review of evidence. https://core.ac.uk/download/30650105.pdf (accessed on 26th June 2025).

18. Brownson, R. C., McKay, V. R., Morshed, A. B., Proctor, E., et al. (2018). Letting go: Conceptualizing intervention de-implementation in public health and social service settings. https://core.ac.uk/download/287888057.pdf (accessed on 26th June 2025).

19. Campbell-Patton, C., & Mattero, M. (2009). Measuring the impact of youth voluntary service programs. https://core.ac.uk/download/71342437.pdf (accessed on 26th June 2025).

20. Chavis, D. M., & Trent, T. R. (2009). Scope, scale, and sustainability: What it takes to create lasting community change. https://core.ac.uk/download/10688026.pdf (accessed on 26th June 2025).

21. Colburn, K., Cole, C., Hazel, D., McClarnon, T., et al. (2011). Assessing community progress on the Blueprint to End Homelessness. https://core.ac.uk/download/84885740.pdf (accessed on 26th June 2025).

22. Cole, G. E., Holtgrave, D. R., & Rios, N. M. (1993). Systematic development of trans-theoretically based behavioral risk management programs. https://core.ac.uk/download/72056919.pdf (accessed on 26th June 2025).

23. Cox, K. M. (2017). Race and income disparities in disaster preparedness in old age. https://core.ac.uk/download/215521387.pdf (accessed on 26th June 2025).

24. Donta, B., Battala, M., Dasgupta, A., Ghule, M., et al. (2016). CHARM, a gender equity and family planning intervention for men and couples in rural India: Protocol for the cluster randomized controlled trial evaluation. https://core.ac.uk/download/323065021.pdf (accessed on 26th June 2025).

25. Epstein, D., Goodman, L. A., & Sullivan, C. M. (2017). Beyond the RCT: Integrating rigor and relevance to evaluate the outcomes of domestic violence programs. https://core.ac.uk/download/213035189.pdf (accessed on 26th June 2025).

26. Escoffery, C., Fernandez, M. E., Friedman, D. B., Hannon, P., et al. (2023). Twenty years of capacity building across the Cancer Prevention and Control Research Network. https://core.ac.uk/download/604668621.pdf (accessed on 26th June 2025).

27. Fabish, L., & Haas, P. J. (2013). Measuring the performance of livability programs, MTI Report 12–06. https://core.ac.uk/download/70410209.pdf (accessed on 26th June 2025).

28. Gazi, R., Hoque, M. E., Hossain, S. S. A., Khan, M. A., et al. (2011). A systematic review of

economic evaluations of health and health-related interventions in Bangladesh. https://core.ac.uk/download/pdf/8608044.pdf (accessed on 26th June 2025).

29. Gienapp, A., Reisman, J., & Stachowiak, S. (2012). *A Handbook of Data Collection Tools: Companion to "A Guide to Measuring Advocacy and Policy."* https://core.ac.uk/download/84911833.pdf (accessed on 26th June 2025).

30. Gilgoff, J., & Ginwright, S. (2015). Toward more equitable outcomes: A research synthesis on out-of-school time work with boys and young men of color. https://core.ac.uk/download/75786240.pdf (accessed on 26th June 2025).

31. Guével, M. R., Jourdan, D., & Pommier, J. (2010). Evaluation of health promotion in schools: A realistic evaluation approach using mixed methods. https://core.ac.uk/download/49282375.pdf (accessed on 26th June 2025).

32. Hahn, T., Makki Alamdari, S., Price, M. F., Studer, J., et al. (2019). Perceptions of IUPUI faculty and staff regarding the Center for Service and Learning faculty/staff development programs. https://core.ac.uk/download/228066320.pdf (accessed on 26th June 2025).

33. Hair, E. C., Michelsen, E., & Zaff, J. F. (2002). Civic engagement programs and youth development: A synthesis. https://core.ac.uk/download/71347373.pdf (accessed on 26th June 2025).

34. Haney, M., & Shkaratan, M. (2025). Mine closure and its impact on the community: Five years after mine closure in Romania, Russia and Ukraine. https://core.ac.uk/download/pdf/6521952.pdf (accessed on 26th June 2025).

35. Harwanto, F., Saci, M. A., & Yuliana, I. (2024). Innovation in nutrition promotion: Literature analysis to increase community awareness and healthy practices. https://core.ac.uk/download/617989014.pdf (accessed on 26th June 2025).

36. Jones, C., Eschbach, C., Nichols, A., Riffe, H., et al. (2021). Lessons from two states with extension programs for managing stress. https://core.ac.uk/download/492914788.pdf (accessed on 26th June 2025).

37. Keller, A., Armijo, C., Bartsch, D., & Chung, P. (2012). Improving access to health through collaboration: Lessons learned from The Colorado Trust's Partnerships for Health Initiative Evaluation. https://core.ac.uk/download/71360570.pdf (accessed on 26th June 2025).

38. Kennedy, E. (2025). Successful nutrition programs in Africa: What makes them work? https://core.ac.uk/download/pdf/6616189.pdf (accessed on 26th June 2025).

39. Khadivi, R., & Khosravi, Sh. (2004). The viewpoints of interns and clerkship students about community medicine course. https://core.ac.uk/download/143845060.pdf (accessed on 26th June 2025).

40. Klima, N., O'Duill, B., Vanhauwaert, R., Wijckmans, J., et al. (2013). Evaluation of crime prevention initiatives. https://core.ac.uk/download/55812547.pdf (accessed on 26th June 2025).

41. Kontar, Y. Y., & Контарь, E. E. (2017). Comparative analysis of spring flood risk reduction measures in Alaska, United States and the Sakha Republic, Russia. https://core.ac.uk/download/286607717.pdf (accessed on 26th June 2025).

42. Krol, D., Cheung, K., Cruz, K., Carver, L., & Revels, M. (2013). Providing preventive oral health care to infants and young children in Women, Infants, and Children (WIC), Early Head Start,

and primary care settings. https://core.ac.uk/download/71362896.pdf (accessed on 26th June 2025).

43. Krol, D., Jacobs, E., Cheung, K., Carver, L., Revels, M., & Dawkins-Lyn, N. (2013). Dental professionals in non-dental settings. https://core.ac.uk/download/71362887.pdf (accessed on 26th June 2025).

44. Luebke, J., LeClair, J., Patz, J. A., Leder, K., Barbour, L., Flynn, M., et al. (2024). Integrating planetary health education into tertiary curricula: A practical toolbox for implementation. https://core.ac.uk/download/631417023.pdf (accessed on 26th June 2025).

45. Murphy, C. G., Alendy, C., Cooper, J., & Simpson, L. (2008). Childhood obesity: The role of health policy. https://core.ac.uk/download/71342400.pdf (accessed on 26th June 2025).

46. N/A. (2007). Early assessment of environmental interventions to prevent childhood obesity. https://core.ac.uk/download/71346543.pdf (accessed on 26th June 2025).

47. N/A. (2010). A guide to actionable measurement. https://core.ac.uk/download/71351649.pdf (accessed on 26th June 2025).

48. OVC-CARE Project. (2010). OVC costing technical consultation meeting report. https://open.bu.edu/bitstream/2144/26995/1/OVC-Costing-Technical-Consultation-Final-Report.pdf (accessed on 26th June 2025).

49. Poon, A., Gilmore, D., Lumby, E., Wang, G., & Koester, L. (2016). Respite Partnership Collaborative (RPC) Innovation Project Evaluation: Final report. https://core.ac.uk/download/80511006.pdf (accessed on 26th June 2025).

50. Purnomo, E., & Yohana, N. (2017). Strategi komunikasi Badan Pemberdayaan Perempuan, Perlindungan Anak dan Keluarga Berencana dalam mewujudkan program Kabupaten Layak Anak di Kabupaten Siak. https://media.neliti.com/media/publications/200320-strategi-komunikasi-badan-pemberdayaan-p.pdf (accessed on 26th June 2025).

51. Renzaho, A. (2002). Selective feeding centers in refugee settings: Evaluation framework protocol. http://hdl.handle.net/10536/DRO/DU:30004292 (accessed on 26th June 2025).

52. Takach, M., & Kaye, N. (2009). Building medical homes in State Medicaid and CHIP programs. https://core.ac.uk/download/71349689.pdf (accessed on 26th June 2025).

53. Unnithan, M. (2015). What constitutes evidence in human rights-based approaches to health? Learning from lived experiences of maternal and sexual reproductive health. https://core.ac.uk/download/30614934.pdf (accessed on 26th June 2025).

54. Werkheiser, I. (2017). Loss of epistemic self-determination in the Anthropocene. https://core.ac.uk/download/131213868.pdf (accessed on 26th June 2025).

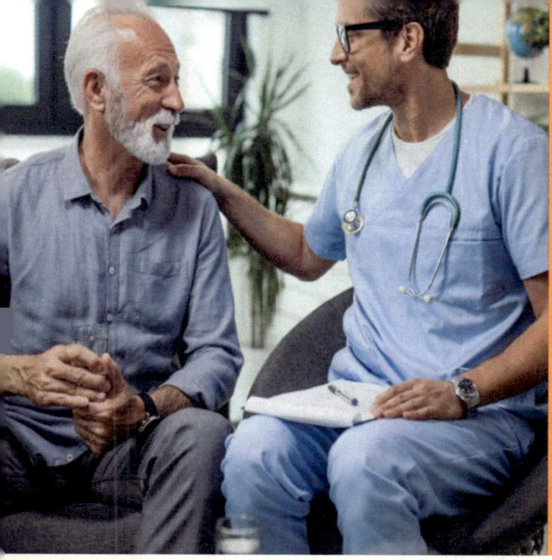

Chapter 8

HEALTH COMMUNICATION AND SOCIAL MARKETING

Contents

Introduction

Health communication and social marketing are two significant disciplines in contemporary society that contribute to influencing public health efforts and behavior change. The intersection of the two disciplines provides a unifying principle for effectively communicating health messages and engaging diverse communities in healthy behaviors. As new media begin to emerge, communicators are able to leverage innovative methods for influencing target populations and enhancing the impact of health messages. This multidisciplinary approach not only conveys vital information about health risks and prevention methods but also addresses the socio-cultural determinants of health behavior. As health problems grow in complexity, the understanding of the theories of health communication and social marketing is essential for practitioners in attempts to establish healthier communities. A more critical examination of health communication recognizes its central role in generating awareness and understanding of health matters. Effective communication strategies are not just about the transmission of information but also presenting messages to resonate with intended audiences. Secondly, using social marketing principles ensures that health campaigns are designed such a way that they inspire people towards health-positive behaviors. As confirmed by various studies, effective communication has the capability to alter perceptions and behavior and thus lead to improved health outcomes. For instance, Marseille et al. (2008) directs towards the need for specially tailored intervention strategies which address at-risk populations, emphasizing the importance of refining the dissemination of health messages within the most vulnerable. Practitioners thus need to utilize the synergy of vast knowledge bases in both social marketing and health communication to bridge gaps in knowledge and create a lasting legacy. Furthermore, social marketing dynamics are a perceptive type of behavior change theories in the context of promoting health. Social marketing, following the traditional marketing principles, utilizes commercial marketing practices for social good, with the aim to alter behaviors that are in the best interest of people and society at large. Successful implementation of social marketing campaigns relies on an understanding of the forces driving consumers' behavior and addressing barriers to change. For example, Basurto et al. (2018) illustrates the way in which well-planned health interventions are capable of mobilizing the community during periods of low activity, by presenting innovative solutions which address the audience's requirements. If professionals implement an integrated approach which integrates health communication and social marketing ideas, they are able to develop comprehensive methods which do not only inform but empower people towards healthier lifestyles. Later on, the constant development of these fields is crucial in navigating the intricacies of public health in the midst of a rapidly changing world (Figure 8.1).

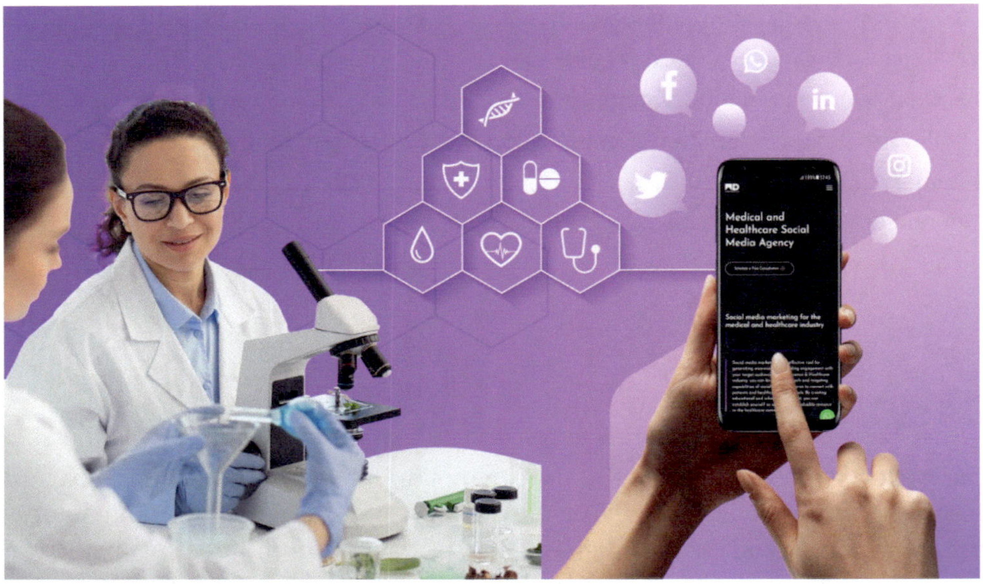

Figure 8.1. Health communication and social marketing.

Source: https://medicaldigitals.com/blogs/wp-content/uploads/2024/01/3advantages-of-social-media-in-healthcare.webp.

Definition of Health Communication

Health communication entails the process of conveying information on matters of health with the purpose of educating, inspiring, and influencing people and communities towards transforming to healthier behavior. It encompasses several formats, including public service announcements, educational programming, and web campaigns, all aimed at addressing health issues effectively. A critical component of health communication is understanding the target population's values, beliefs, and motivations because this builds more effective messages that are grounded in their experience and needs. As highlighted in the synthesis commissioned by the National Co-ordinating Centre for Public Engagement (NCCPE) and the Economic and Social Research Council (ESRC), successful engagement relies on identification of public opinion on health matters, which means audience segmentation tools play an important role in guiding effective health communication strategies (Barnett et al., 2011). Secondly, implementing health communication strategies will need coalition-building in many sectors, including healthcare providers, policymakers, and community organizations. Such coalitions will help health communicators tap into diverse resources and expertise to amplify their messages and outreach efforts. Public will campaigns also illustrate the utility of convergent strategies in creating momentum for community involvement on health issues. These agenda-building and social movement theory models provide handy frameworks for measuring the impact of health communication efforts. With concrete evaluation criteria, communicators can modify their strategies to be most effective, demonstrating the value of adaptability in health communication models (Salmon et al., 2003). In addition to strategic planning, ethical issues are of the highest priority in health communication practice. These ethics encompass the responsibility to provide evidence-based, honest information in a manner that is sensitive to the autonomy and culture of the target audience. This ethical construct is particularly significant in applying audience segmentation since there is risk of leaving some groups behind based on perceived assumptions or stereotypes. Thoughtful application of segmentation strategies has the capability of enhancing participation, but it also calls for inclusiveness to be a top priority so diverse perspectives have a voice. Thus, health communication is not only a tool for information dissemination but also a vital means of promoting equitable health outcomes among diverse populations and underscoring the broader social effects of effective health messaging (Barnett et al., 2011) (Figure 8.2).

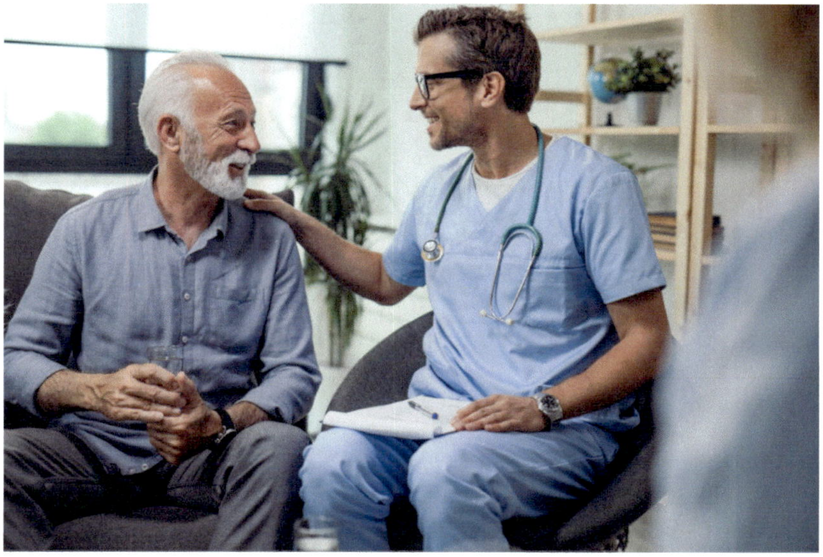

Figure 8.2. Health communication.

Source: https://www.goodx.healthcare/wp-content/uploads/2023/04/patient-communication.jpg.

Importance of Social Marketing in Health

Social marketing is an important tool in public health utilized to promote behavior that leads to individual and community health. As opposed to conventional marketing that targets profit-making, social marketing aims to influence health behavior through emphasizing the gains that come with adopting new habits. For instance, communications focused on specific medical conditions, such as giving up smoking or healthy diets, use strategic messaging in a bid to reach people with information about something that pertains to them. Such programs are vital as they not only raise awareness but also mobilize the entire community, hence creating a healthy environment where healthy choices can thrive. One notable aspect of such campaigns is their reliance on evidence-based methods and research, which enhance their effectiveness in reaching various populations and addressing particular health issues (Salmon et al., 2003). Moreover, successful social marketing campaigns depict the intersection of various strategies with an eye to applying long-term behavior modification. Interventions for urgent health concerns have a tendency to draw upon public will in an effort to address more societal problems, using formats that include media advocacy and social capital building. The example of the collective campaign in Vietnam towards improving handwashing of the populace illustrates how understanding of local customs can be used in intervention strategies. By observing how individuals actually act and not the ideal, health communicators can craft messages with a touch of personalization. Such campaigns like in Indonesia also reflect this, where private-public partnerships achieve the widest coverage and public health communications sustain momentum (N/A, 2011).

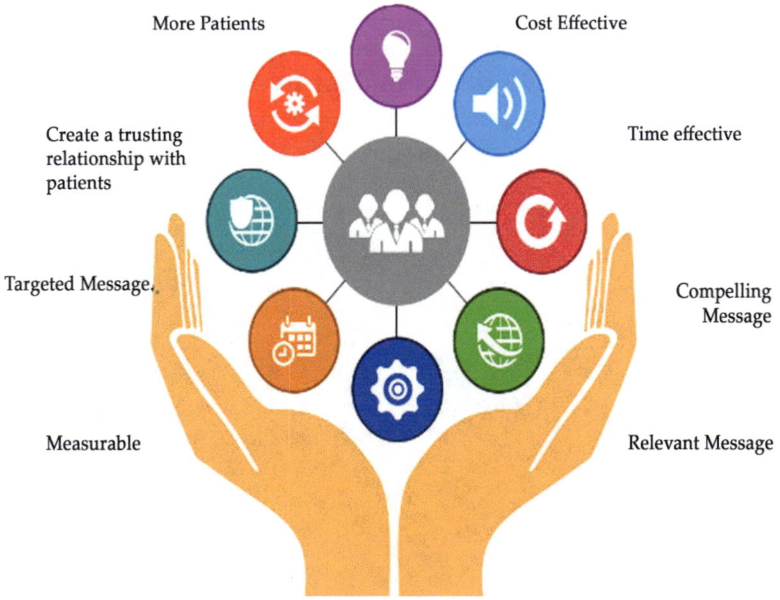

Figure 8.3. Importance of social marketing in health.

Source: https://media.licdn.com/dms/image/C4E12AQEZGpAY5WH67Q/article-cover_image-shrink_600_2000/0/1520064698830?e=2147483647&v=beta&t=WUIMnSCWmBLTzcG_Rnz-frvj1sD9-gi9yqRFzc9_MNI.

This multi-pronged intervention captures the dynamic nature of social marketing in addressing health inequities. Monitoring and assessment of social marketing campaigns are key pillars establishing their long-term contribution to public health. Researchers and practitioners set the standards for measuring progress through various stages of a health issue life cycle in an effort to measure campaign success. Evaluation not only involves direct measurement of short-term outcomes, such as behavior change, but also seeks to the broader reaches of shifts in community norms and values regarding health. The abundance of case studies documented in the literature at hand assists in laying out an orderly plan for measuring success in public will campaigns. Based on these observations, communicators of health can refine their strategies so that subsequent interventions continue to engage and impact. The ongoing debate on the social marketing practice and their evaluation promotes the culture of learning that can enhance the health outcomes among different populations significantly (Salmon et al., 2003) (Figure 8.3).

8.1. The Role of Health Communication

Successful health communication is a critical instrument for delivering information influencing public knowledge and conduct regarding health. It is therefore a pivotal role in both population and individual health impacts. Health communication is not merely the presentation of health-related information, but also the engagement of the audience that generates an urge to understand and prompt action. For example, successful campaigns tend to customize messages so that they appeal to certain groups of people, making it possible for them to identify with the content provided. Through the use of multiple channels, such as social media, public service announcements, and community outreach programs, health communication strategies have the potential to raise awareness and create behavioral changes that result in healthier lifestyles and decision-making, thus closing gaps between knowledge and action within public health initiatives. Besides that, health communication may also play an important role in promoting the success of social marketing programs, where they aim to promote public health activities through the strategic application of marketing practices. Such programs have a tendency to apply convincing messages to affect behavior change by engaging in areas of social norms, perceived risk, and reward in adopting healthier behaviors. Through the addition of emotional and psychological aspects of decision-making, health communication becomes more profound interaction with target populations and more engagement. Therefore, programs on matters such as vaccination campaigns or smoking cessation programs may become more successful, as evident in targeted communications that relate more profoundly to specific groups. Thus, through the integration of health communication and social marketing, there is more impact and facilitation of sustained change within communities. In addition, the health communication concerns extend beyond mere message dissemination; they involve trust and transparency between the public and the health authorities. Credibility building by way of guaranteed and trusted messaging is crucial in shaping people perceptions on health tips and policy advice.

For instance, health organizations must guarantee accuracy, timeliness, and relevance of information, which raises the level of public confidence in preventive interventions and services. Failure to sustain such trust will lead to suspicion and hesitance to adopt health practices, such as during health crises when rumors of wrong information go around. Second, response to health literacy is at the center of effective health communication since creation of awareness among individuals will help them make informed health decisions. Collaborative practice among health communicators and organizational stakeholders can significantly enhance overall health outcomes, where safety, efficacy, and community well-being are given high priority to public health interventions (Basurto et al., 2018; Sharma et al., 2018).

8.1.1. Facilitating Patient-Provider Interactions

Effective patient-provider interactions are the foundation for delivering good quality health care and enhancing the quality of patients' outcomes. The ability of health professionals to communicate openly and empathetically with their patients is critical in the process of establishing trust and the development of a cooperative climate for decision-making. Such communication is more crucial in marginalized populations, like the LGBT, where health disparities have typically emerged due to prior neglect and discrimination in healthcare settings. Studies have shown that culturally focused health communication strategies that address specific needs and issues of these groups can enhance participation and health literacy, finally reducing barriers to care (Drabble et al., 2003).

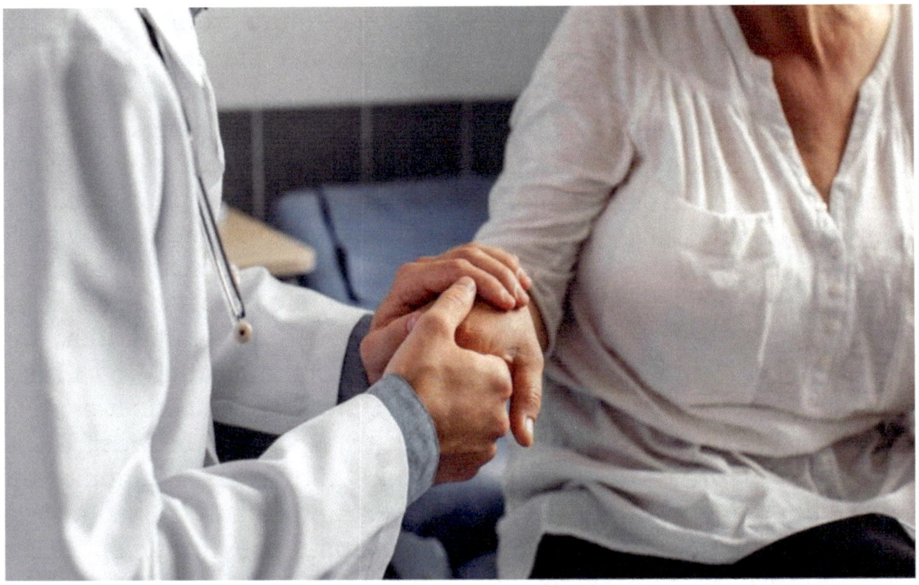

Figure 8.4. Facilitating patient-provider interactions.

Source: https://mayflax.com/wp-content/uploads/2021/06/How-To-Improve-Your-Doctor-Patient-Relationship-1024x576.jpg.

Through engaging with culturally skilled communication strategies, caregivers are not only able to address immediate health concerns of patients but also promote a heightened sense of being accepted and belonging in healthcare environments. Aside from cultural competence, provider attitudes and professional traits impact the quality of patient-provider interactions. Negative attitudes of providers toward certain patient groups, i.e., drug users, have been found to significantly impair effective interactions and reduce the overall effectiveness of care provision. Evidence obtained from Chinese methadone maintenance treatment clinics indicates that clinicians who have negative attitudes toward their patients tend to communicate less and for less time, which further exacerbates issues with treatment adherence and satisfaction (Cao et al., 2016). This supports the importance of correcting underlying biases and promoting positive attitudes through training and education. These programs can empower health care providers to communicate more effectively with diverse patient populations and establish enhanced interactions that are critical to successful treatment outcomes. In the end, causing powerful patient-provider interactions necessitates a multi-pronged approach that involves training, sensitivity, and appropriate health communication strategies. One effective way of enhancing such interactions is through embedding feedback mechanisms in which patients can provide feedback about their experiences and preferences. Engaging the patients in their care processes not only increases their satisfaction levels but also rewards providers with valuable feedback on the diversity of their clients' needs. Health communications in the future must focus more on collaborative processes between healthcare providers and patients such that all stakeholders in the system are heard and valued. By communicating the complexity of patient-provider relationships and encouraging inclusive patterns of communication, health systems can work towards minimizing health disparities and ensuring equitable care to every individual (Cao et al., 2016; Drabble et al., 2003) (Figure 8.4).

8.1.2. Enhancing Public Health Campaigns

Public health campaigns have the potential to influence population behaviors and promote community health outcomes in a meaningful way. To make them more effective, the campaigns need to adopt an inclusive approach that incorporates community engagement, audience segmentation, and tailored messaging. Engaging community members in campaign development can assist public health programs in ensuring that the content can reach various populations, including marginalized groups such as the LGBT community. Such participatory approach facilitates a greater understanding of health needs and preferences, ultimately contributing to more effective health promotion interventions. Based on evidence, individualized evidence-based communication to specific groups is required in order to assist in diminishing health disparities as well as facilitate increased community participation (Drabble et al., 2003). Public health campaigns therefore require not just innovative messages but also consideration of inclusion and representation during the process of health communication. Audience segmentation is a critical component of effective health communication programs, allowing for a more nuanced understanding of varied public attitudes and motivations. The application of segmentation methods allows public health campaigns to tailor messages to specific demographic, psychographic, and behavioral segments of target populations. Strategic planning can assist in the creation of outreach efforts, forging productive connections between health agencies and the populations they desire to reach. However, it should be noted that segmentation by itself is not enough; its power lies in the overall organizational desire to make use of the insights gained. Engaging the target audience in a thought-provoking manner can discern some barriers and myths that need to be addressed to develop better public health outcomes (Barnett et al., 2011). Therefore, the integration of audience segmentation with overall campaign strategies is important to achieve the maximum reach and effect of health communication campaigns. Furthermore, the ethical considerations of public health campaigns must be addressed in designing and conducting the campaigns. Specifically, the use of segmentation involves concerns about representation and potential discrimination against marginalized groups. Designers of campaigns ought to place main emphasis on ethical involvement to make sure that all demographic populations are represented in an equitable way and interventions do not have the effect of encouraging existing disparities inadvertently. Through ethical emphasis on segmentation, public health campaigns have fewer reputational risks associated with messaging that alienates the targeted group. It is essential that public health workers remain open and gain the trust of communities by demonstrating their dedication to being inclusive and equitable in promoting health. Essentially, putting ethical values first in public health communication strengthens community relations and maximizes the overall impact of health campaigns, ultimately leading to healthier populations (Figure 8.5).

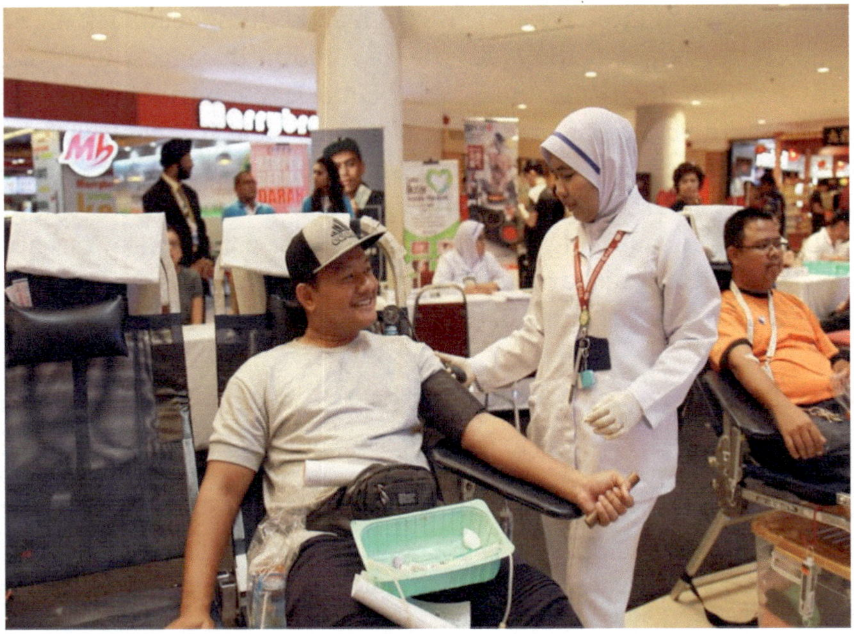

Figure 8.5. Enhancing public health campaigns.

Source: https://qiu.edu.my/wp-content/uploads/2018/09/Public-Health-Campaign-2018-3.jpg.

8.1.3. Promoting Health Literacy

Promoting health literacy is a key component of effective social marketing and health communication campaigns. Health literacy is the ability of an individual to access, process, and understand basic health information, which in turn influences his/her decision-making capacity in matters related to health. In the increasing dominance of healthcare on the Internet, web-based Customer Relationship Management (CRM) programs can enhance health literacy among various groups. By using Social CRM and mix-marketing, healthcare organizations are able to provide significant interactions to enable patients to receive and comprehend health information more effectively. Empowerment through mix-marketing is essential, as it enables people to take active roles in their health and navigate the insurance system complexities, leading to improved health outcomes (Almunawar et al., 2012). Effective health communication also needs to address the unique needs of various populations, including marginalized communities. It has been found by research that multidimensional approaches are warranted in targeting interventions on both the macro and micro levels. For instance, specially targeted health campaigns to lesbian, gay, bisexual, and transgender (LGBT) communities identify the necessity of responsive messaging to specific populations. Not only do these efforts diminish disparities, but they also enhance overall health literacy since they promote participation and familiarity. By involving members of the community in formulating targeted health communication strategies, health professionals can ensure that the content is apt, accessible, and relevant to the population (Drabble et al., 2003). This practice is critical in establishing trust and improving health status among different populations. Moreover, education is second to none in improving the level of health literacy. Health education programs that aim at improving media literacy prepare the general population with the ability to decode health information. With misinformation spreading across many platforms, such programs become critical to the extent that individuals will be able to recognize the credible sources of health information and distinguish them from untrustworthy sources. Additionally, medical professionals need proper training to present health information clearly and compassionately, especially for patients who may not speak the same language. By improving communication competency, health care providers can improve patients' comprehension, facilitating patients' authority to engage with and control their health care experiences successfully. This integrated approach to improving health literacy is vital in forming an informed public that can make sense of their own health decisions (Figure 8.6).

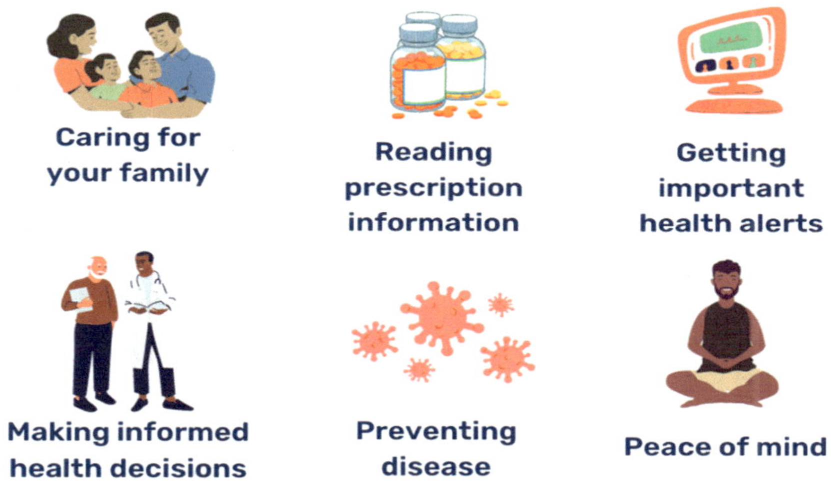

Figure 8.6. Promoting health literacy.

Source: https://www3.erie.gov/health/sites/www3.erie.gov.health/files/2022-10/healthliteracybarriers.png.

8.2. Principles of Social Marketing

Social marketing principles play a major role in health behavior promotion and promoting well-being in the community. The audience segmentation is a critical principle of these social marketing principles that allows the marketer to develop messages appealing to different population segments. Having knowledge about certain audiences depending on their values, beliefs, and needs, the health communicators are able to develop targeted campaigns responding to particular health issues effectively. This is an interesting concept supported by research that indicates segmentation strategies enhance citizen engagement by revealing complex interests and attitudes towards health. For instance, health campaigns applied through these strategies have managed to reach vulnerable groups effectively, ensuring the campaigns are inclusive and responsive to their unique problems. Subsequently, effective segmentation not only generates more interaction but also increases success in general health outcomes in broader public health campaigns (Barnett et al., 2011). In addition, the marketing mix involving the traditional 4Ps—product, price, place, and promotion—extended with additional components such as partnership and policy also plays an integral part in developing successful health communication strategies. Social marketing programs must not only seek to provide helpful health information but also provide accessible support and resources for behavior change. The mention of partnership in the marketing mix highlights the importance of collaboration among stakeholders, including healthcare professionals, non-profit organizations, and community leaders, in an effort to expand outreach efforts. Besides, using a policy framework in social marketing ensures that structural changes can facilitate healthier choices in communities where individuals live, work, and play. By embedding health campaigns within the broader agenda of social marketing, organizations are able to use their resources most effectively and induce long-term transformation of public health (Rosidah et al., 2012). Finally, ethical dilemmas have a significant role in utilizing social marketing principles. Given that campaigns are formulated with target groups in mind, there is a call for marketers to be sensitive to the stigmatization or unintended consequences arising from their marketing campaigns. The ethical dimensions of audience segmentation, for example, demand an openness and sensitivity in group definition and targeting. In addition, the reputation of health-promoting organizations can be harmed when their message fails to align with community values or fails to establish trust. Social marketers need to incorporate reflective practices and maintain the wellbeing and dignity of target publics in a manner that will have their institutions seeking not only to inform but to empower individuals to make healthier choices. Adhering to these ethical guidelines strengthens the credibility of health communication campaigns and ultimately serves their purpose in promoting public health (Barnett et al., 2011).

8.2.1. Understanding Target Audiences

Knowledge about target audiences is at the core of successful health communication and social marketing interventions. Obtaining complete information on audience demographics, motivations, and behaviors is the basis for developing communications that genuinely connect and captivate. Segmentation methods can also amplify this information by segmenting audiences into specific groups based on shared characteristics such as age, socioeconomic status, and health beliefs. Not only does this enhance communication strategy to better align with the audience's expectation but also caters to the different interests and perspectives other segments hold regarding health. As stated in existent literature, utilization of segmentation tools can increase participation by revealing concealed values and incentives, which generates a better, well-informed, and empathetic health messaging strategy (Barnett et al., 2011). Beyond foundational segmentation, understanding audiences involves an ongoing dialogue between stakeholders and communicators. Health communication is the most effective when organizations engage in active listening and responsive action. This entails incorporating target group opinions and adapting messages according to their shifting issues and interests. Utilizing new media channels contributes even more to such a responsive communications environment, facilitating organizations to respond interactively to the audience. This framework has the case studies analyzing documentary films demonstrate how multimedia can act as a vehicle for community building and outreach, specifically within the context of social media (Barrett et al., 2008). Through careful assessment of these mediums' impacts, health communicators can optimize awareness and attain sustained engagement. Last but not least, ethical implications of segmenting specific audience segments in health communication should not be overlooked. As segmentation yields strategic advantages, it unavoidably suffers from perpetuating inequalities if certain segments are excluded or stereotyped. Practitioners will therefore need to undertake audience segmentation from a social responsibility standpoint, with caution to ensure their efforts are balanced and inclusive. Addressing these ethical issues not only mitigates reputational risk for health organizations but also enables sustained dedication to public trust and community well-being. Findings presented through segmentation research can be utilized for planning strategy and to deliver health messages in a relevant manner without reaching exclusions among underserved populations, thus constituting an integrated model for successful social marketing of health (Barnett et al., 2011).

8.2.2. Creating Effective Messaging

Creating effective messaging in health communication involves a close understanding of the target audience and their individual concerns and behaviors. It is all about crafting messages in ways that address specific demographic segments, particularly for social marketing efforts where the aim is to promote health behaviors and awareness. Research has identified that messaging strategies should consider the social and cultural contexts of various populations, especially such vulnerable populations such as racial minorities and mentally ill populations. For instance, research has indicated that the tobacco industry designs its advertising campaigns particularly to match various groups of people, which is essential for public health campaigns to reach.

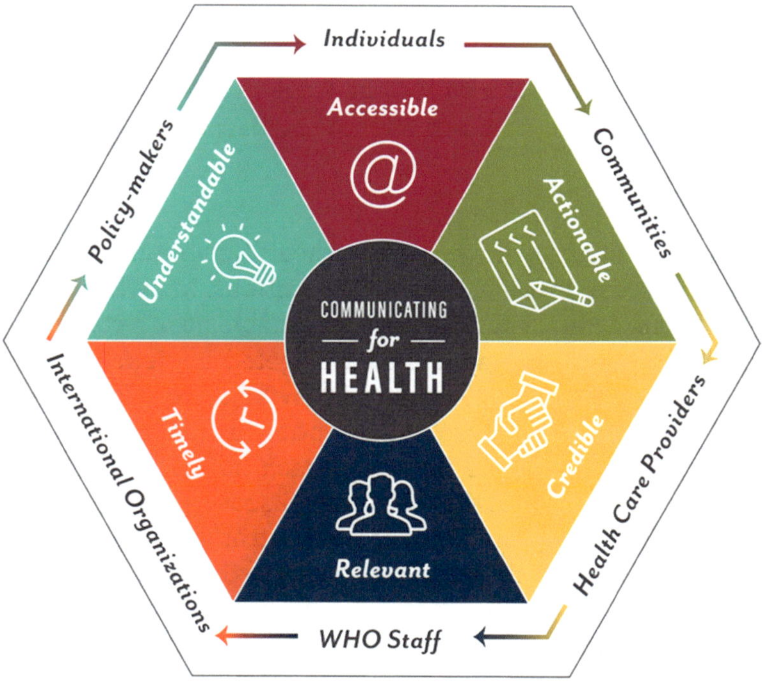

Figure 8.7. Creating effective messaging in health communication.

Source: https://www.who.int/images/default-source/communicating-for-health/principle-infographic-630.tmb-1920v.png?sfvrsn=2d4ca839_1.

By examining literature on anti-tobacco campaigns and pro-tobacco advertisements, Baezconde-Garbanati et al. (2019) emphasizes the importance of crafting messages to reach these wide-ranging groups directly, consequently reducing health disparities and augmenting the influence of public education programs. The means of disseminating health messages also play a critical role in determining communication efforts' success. Internet websites have become pivotal mediums in reaching young individuals, who are more likely to be subjected to health information through social media, video games, and videos. When these websites are paired with health communication, it has the potential to make it more effective and promote behavioral changes. Alongside this is an enormous ethical issue, particularly regarding food and beverage companies' influence on children through advertising. It has been recommended that government regulations be put on the exploitation of youths and children from exploitative advertising practices, as quoted in N/A (2007). Establishing messages that can move through such channels and also meet ethical requirements is fundamental to developing a sustainable and effective health communication campaign. Besides that, ongoing evaluation and adaptation of messaging tactics are required to monitor and be effective in health communication. The constantly changing universe of public health risks requires continuous research to uncover areas of discrepancy in current strategies and new emerging health issues. For example, the literature on anti-tobacco campaigns today has revealed notable gaps in the reach of such campaigns to specific populations, such as Asian Americans and LGBTQ+, that could mean these groups are not represented sufficiently within health stories. These gaps will be filled, expanding the scope of health campaigns but also enacting marginalized communities as stronger, with a more inclusive platform to deliver public health messaging. Being responsive to the ever-evolving nature of health communication, message makers are in a position to create improved health outcomes and promote a culture of prevention and awareness that finds common ground among various audiences, as noted in Baezconde-Garbanati et al. (2019) (Figure 8.7).

8.2.3. Utilizing Behavioral Change Theories

The use of behavioral change theories in the field of health communication and social marketing platforms can enhance the success of public health interventions. Knowledge of the psychological and sociocultural factors that affect individual behaviors can enable health communication professionals to create messages that are tailored to appeal to a targeted audience. The use of theories such as the Health Belief Model or Theory of Planned Behavior allows for an advanced examination of perceived benefits, risks, and barriers to the adoption of healthier behaviors. These models promote an integrative strategy that does not only teach but also prompts individuals to learn behaviors that make them healthier. Further, creating disease prevention and health promotion awareness becomes stronger if communicators ground strategies on these established theories, leading to long-term behavior change in the population. Further, working with the public through social marketing campaigns provides a practical pathway to implementing these theories of behavior change. Using knowledge of consumer behavior and decision-making habits, health campaigns can develop messages that are not only informative but also persuasive. For instance, social marketing-based campaigns can replicate successful public will campaigns aimed at building community support on health issues. As introduced in the discussion of public will campaigns, the use of models of agenda building and social movements can propel health communications from information dissemination to something more. Such strategic framing allows campaigns to successfully mobilize action within communities, fostering a healthy climate for health change.

Accordingly, the use of behavioral change theories acts to anchor social marketing initiatives in a strong theoretical foundation, which increases their combined impact on public health. Additionally, the place of environmental education in public health highlights that having initiatives aimed according to behavioral change theories is crucial. Public health-oriented organizations involved in educating the general public on health matters tend to focus on increasing awareness. However, as research integrates psychosocial determinants of behavior change, knowledge alone cannot suffice in bringing about significant behavior change. Bolt et al. (2017) advance that pragmatic examples elucidate the means through which application of behavior theory can inform understanding for why people are convinced to adopt pro-health behavior. Such details enable health communicators to assess prevailing practice and adapt effective strategies. By applying these theories to both communications and education efforts, health marketing can better take on complex social and environmental determinants that influence health decisions, ultimately contributing to healthier communities and improved public health results.

8.3. Strategies in Health Communication

Effective strategies of health communication are crucial in changing public behavior, especially preventive health behavior. Social marketing strategies, which borrow from conventional marketing, provide useful paradigms for selling health-related goods, such as condoms. As effective as condoms are in preventing HIV, a concerning gap in utilization is being faced in risky sexual acts.

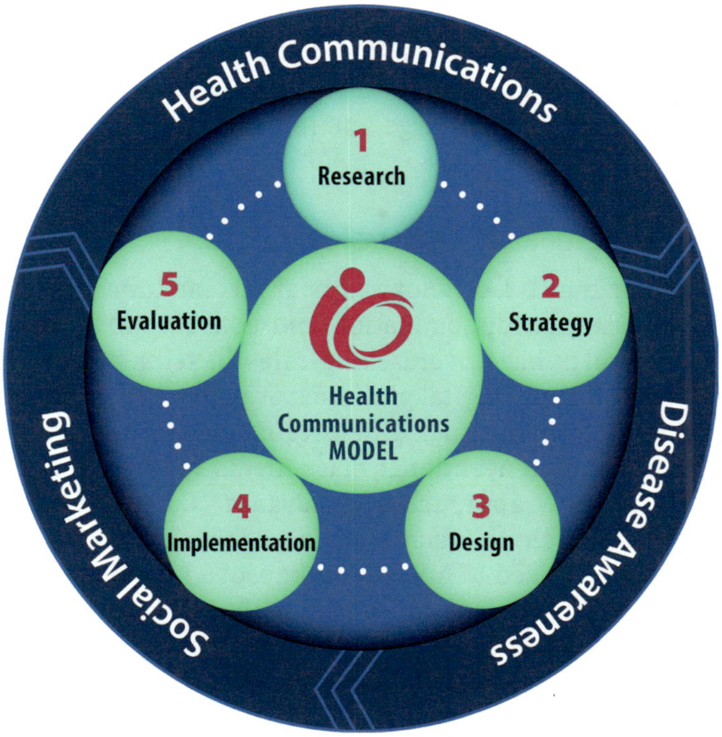

Figure 8.8. Strategies in health communication.

Source: https://i.pinimg.com/originals/fc/33/96/fc3396596c4904fa7699dbd449c39f98.jpg.

A study of 52 countries shows that marketing considerations, including prices and promotional strategies, are significant in influencing the demand for female and male condoms. Notably, female condoms show greater price elasticity, which highlights the need for strategic product- and population-specific decisions. By optimizing the utilization of marketing resources in health communication, public health programs can better tackle condom availability and acceptability barriers to achieve better prevention outcomes (Terris-Prestholt et al., 2016). Beyond product promotion, health communication programs must be grounded in the diverse experiences of specific demographic groups such as the LGBT communities. Historically marginalized from health promotion campaigns, LGBT communities face unique acute health disparities that need to be addressed through responsive communication strategies. Multidimensional theories promoting interventions at both macro- and micro-levels have shown potential to address these needs. Studies suggest that health campaigns often fail to engage LGBT communities, leading to the inability to create culturally adapted communication strategies. To bridge this gap, future health communication interventions need to involve these communities in campaign planning and material development and, therefore, foster an inclusive dialogue and amplify the impact of health messages (Drabble et al., 2003). Further, the integration of media literacy and health education among LGBT can allow them to critically receive health communication. This becomes increasingly critical as both consumers and health practitioners are confronted with the complexities of multiple health issues, including sexual health and mental health. Training health care providers on how to increase their communication capacity can enhance interaction with LGBT patients and enhance health outcomes. Continued research for health communication tailored to LGBT will inform best practices so that practitioners can effectively modify their interventions. By highlighting inclusion and understanding the unique characteristics of the targeted populations, health communication can become increasingly able to meet the needs of several communities at large and increase public health engagement in general (Drabble et al., 2003) (Figure 8.8).

8.3.1. Use of Digital Media and Technology

The application of digital media and technology in health communication and social marketing is a revolutionary shift in information dissemination and consumption. For contemporary society blogs, social media, and podcasts have overarching roles in telling public health narratives and determining consumer behavior. These digital platforms provide un-previous reach for organizations to engage with their publics directly, messaging that resonates particularly with specific audiences. As witnessed, the effectiveness of conventional mass media keeps deteriorating at a rapid pace, necessitating the use of these new approaches in advance (Constantinides et al., 2008). Digital consumer interaction not only extends reach but also offers interactive dialogue, which creates avenues for real-time feedback utilized to adjust and improve marketing campaigns. Furthermore, the strategic use of digital media provides a more personalized approach in health communication. Active professionals utilizing online social media platforms have a superior understanding of their audience, which enhances the effectiveness of health campaigns. In accordance with research, professionals with high usage of social media platforms value social media sites more, since they are familiar with their influence on internal and external stakeholders (Moreno et al., 2014). This sensitivity points to an important dynamic: that between online engagement of individuals and broader implications for public health initiatives. Technology empowers health communicators to create personalized content on chosen health matters, and thereby render their messages more relevant and compelling. In addition, emergence of digital media has yielded innovative strategies to maximize levels of engagement and retention in health communication. The shift from passive consumption of information to active participation is critical towards creating a healthier, better-literate citizenry. Programs that encourage user-generated content, i.e., testimonies, shared experiences, and testimonials, enhance credibility and connectivity. In this context, the strength of community-based programs can be utilized by health institutions to drive the agenda of healthy living and behavior change. By adopting Web 2.0 tools and focusing on user interaction, such institutions can effectively address the complexities of modern health communication, whereby their messages are not only heard but obeyed, eventually leading to improved health outcomes for people and populations (Constantinides et al., 2008) (Figure 8.9).

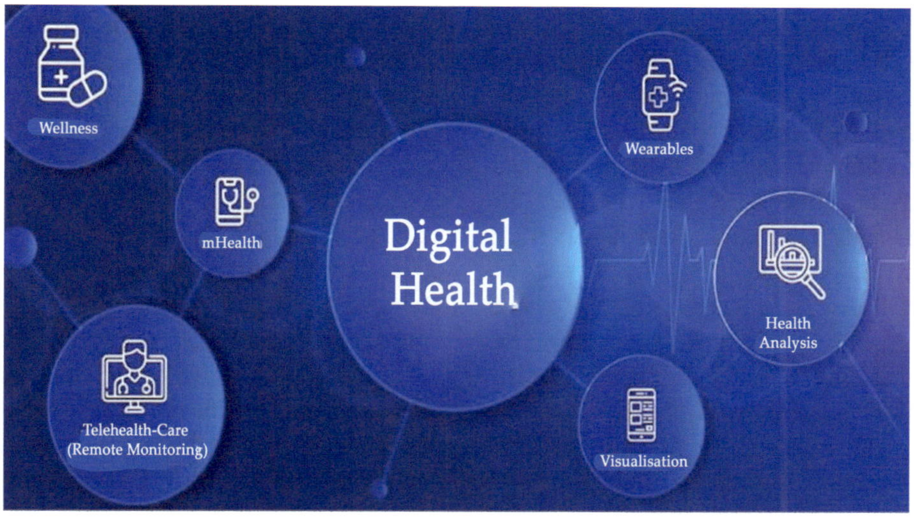

Figure 8.9. Use of digital media and technology.

Source: https://www.tigahealth.com/wp-content/uploads/2021/06/digital-health.jpg.

8.3.2. Community Engagement and Outreach

Effective community outreach and participation are integral components of social marketing and health communication. Active involvement of the community in health programs can strengthen awareness and foster ownership of health concerns. In a scenario where false information can spread via social media and other channels at the speed of lightning, an approach of participatory practice is that much more vital. As seen through the recent evaluations, the utilization of creative media, such as documentary films, can prove to be an effective outreach instrument that optimizes community participation. The films not only communicate vital health information but also stimulate dialogue among the members in the community, enabling them to share their experiences and perspectives. This leads to a more informed population, which is in the best position to address its health challenges in an effort to contribute to a greater social movement, which pressurizes for alteration at the system level (Barrett et al., 2008). Community health programs, to a large extent, depend upon the ability to build trust and rapport between communities and their respective health agencies. This relationship-building relies on ongoing communication and dialogue so that the programs are targeted to the needs and desires of the target group. One example is the North

Lanarkshire Choose Life program, which employs social marketing strategies to raise awareness about mental health services. Evaluation of such social marketing efforts provides valuable insights into the level at which they reach out to the population and de-stigmatize illness. In understanding the specific social and cultural forces at play in the community, health communication campaigns can be designed to overcome barriers to participation while creating an enabling environment that encourages individuals to engage and attend programs (Braybrook et al., 2012). Moreover, getting community members on board as co-creators of outreach activities can lead to more sustainable health communication practices. When community members are involved in planning and delivering health messages, they become advocates of the change that they desire to occur. This can lead to ownership and investment in health impacts, thus promoting a likelihood of sustained involvement. Health programs that leverage this co-creation model can potentially draw upon local information and resources, producing a cyclical process that continually feeds and refines health communication. By incorporating information derived from co-creation, public health campaigns become more focused and effective, eventually leading to healthier populations through public cooperation and shared responsibility for well-being (Barrett et al., 2008; Braybrook et al., 2012).

8.3.3. Tailoring Messages for Diverse Populations

Successful health communication strategies demand an understanding of the different population groups in a society. Messages should be adapted to engage different cultural, socioeconomic, and linguistic groups meaningfully. This entails not merely translating but adapting messages to consider cultural values, norms, and beliefs that might influence health behaviors. Organizations can gain knowledge about which specific needs and preferences belong to which segments through user profiling insights. These personalized messages can potentially promote the efficacy of health campaigns because they address the target population, thereby making them more vulnerable to health interventions (Dijk et al., 2005). The value of such diversity in user profiles not only enhances communication but also acts as an enabler of inclusivity and eradication of health inequities between populations. Furthermore, culturally competent communication is a fundamental component of adapting health messages across populations. Culturally competent messaging is aimed at addressing unique barriers confronted by unique populations, e.g., language competence and cultural myths about health behavior. Cultural competent practice adoption contributes to building successful interactions between receivers and providers of health care and therefore contributes to eliminating health disparities. Evidence has shown that when doctors or other medical personnel engage their patients in a culturally appropriate manner, they enhance patient trust and facilitate collaboration in healthcare decision-making (Keys et al., 2012). Hence, companies targeting individuals from various backgrounds must incorporate culturally proficient communication tactics into their overall efforts to promote health so that the messages are rendered understandable and available to every section of society. In order to transcend cultural competence, employing multiple communicative strategies is necessary to fit messages appropriately into various populations. Utilizing more than a single platform, for instance, social media, workshop settings, and conventional printed media, guarantees that health messages reach individuals from various population segments. Visual aids, storytelling, and mobile health technology may also be utilized to make messages understandable and engaging, particularly for lower literacy populations. Use of innovative techniques such as local narratives or peer educators who belong to the community can enhance bridging of communication gaps and provide a true sense of connect with the audience. The multi-faceted strategies of message adaptation, thus, not only enhance chances for behavioral change but also facilitate the overall goal of inclusive health communication for every member of a community (Dijk et al., 2005).

8.4. Case Studies in Health Communication

Effective health communication is an important part of public health programs that impact behavior and health outcomes. Case studies in health communication highlight the methods of communicating health messages to different groups of people. Excellent case studies illustrate the methods through which health authorities utilize segmentation methods for tailoring messages to attract given groups. For instance, awareness of specific values, beliefs, and motivations of target groups enhances the effectiveness of public engagement activities. Segmentation not only aids in producing adequate content but also in strategic planning and participation activities within healthcare systems, thereby resulting in improved health literacy.

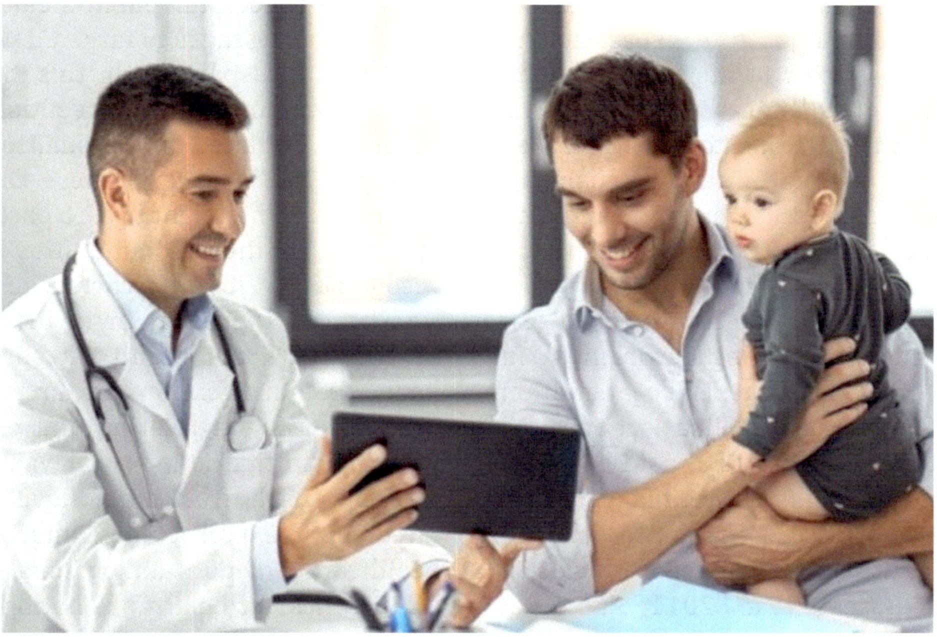

Figure 8.10. Case studies in health communication.

Source: https://healthcare-communications.com/wp-content/uploads/2024/04/Maximising-the-Benefits-of-Waiting-List-Validation_AdobeStock-777x437-1-600x400.jpeg.

By way of critical examination of various models of audience segmentation, it is feasible for practitioners and researchers to rationalize their approach toward health communication and ensure that resources are being utilized maximally to have a broader impact (Barnett et al., 2011). Social marketing approach to health communication accentuates the role of audience in promoting healthy behavior. Public will campaigns case studies demonstrate the ways in which the integration of theoretical models—such as social problem construction and media advocacy—

can guide effective strategies. These activities seek to attempt to build public support for health problems, creating a climate supportive of behavioral change. Case studies reveal that well-designed and well-implemented campaigns are able to actually impact awareness and shift public opinion regarding health issues. Besides, comparing the campaigns with criteria helps ensure continuous improvement and adaptability to changing social contexts. This cyclical method is significant in health communication because it ensures the use of the best methods in addressing various health concerns (Salmon et al., 2003). Incorporating analysis from effective case studies in health communication helps to better understand the complexities involved in public health communication. Lessons from previous campaigns find expression in the development of new strategy, particularly in the presence of constantly shifting media landscapes. Health communicators will be tasked with working across platforms and channels, adapting their messages to be preferred and befitting the audience's behavior and preference. The immediacy of response through social media, for instance, may be leveraged to test interest and mold messaging accordingly. In addition, the moral challenges of segmentation and audience interaction remain a part of health communication practice. Care should be taken to ensure that campaigns do not inadvertently reinforce stigma or discrimination in order to make public health approaches more inclusive and equitable (Barnett et al., 2011; Salmon et al., 2003) (Figure 8.10).

8.4.1. Successful Public Health Campaigns

Successful public health campaigns employ a combination of strategic communication techniques and social marketing strategies to attain their objectives of influencing public behavior and improving health outcomes. Public health campaigns increase health awareness, mobilize public opinion, and encourage individuals towards a healthier lifestyle. For instance, government campaigns employing models of agenda building and media advocacy have succeeded in putting major health concerns at the forefront of discussion, which allow for a more effective public discourse regarding social concerns. Through an assessment of successes in public health, we better understand how the convergence of these communication strategies and community action leads to substantial improvements in public health. Most importantly, evaluation of such campaigns provides valuable insights regarding their long-term impact and efficacy, ultimately helping in future health promotion (Salmon et al., 2003). Another significant aspect of successful public health campaigns is tailoring messages to targeted populations to limit health disparities. In this, the success of health communication intervention can be seen in initiatives aimed at marginalized groups, for example, LGBT groups. These campaigns are successful in highlighting the particular health concerns for these communities because they recognize that it is not correct to apply a one-size-fits-all approach. In involving members of the LGBT community in producing the health communication resources, campaigns are successful in relating and establishing a relationship that is more relevant. This multi-level approach, from macro-level strategies to imperceptible interpersonal interactions among healthcare providers and persons, optimizes the effectiveness of health promotion activities as well as makes them accessible and meaningful for diverse groups (Drabble et al., 2003). Moreover, the success of successful public health interventions relies significantly on continuous evaluation and improvement based on available emerging evidence. Employing criteria to analyze these campaigns at various levels of development, organizations can identify not only what works but where they must improve. Implementing feedback loops allows immediate improvements for the greatest overall impact of health programs. Additionally, encouraging intersectoral collaboration among healthcare sectors, community-based organizations, and media can maximize the reach and impact of health messages. Finally, successful public health campaigns do not only seek to alter individual behavior but also seek to build an enabling environment that fosters sustained health changes in communities (Salmon et al., 2003) (Figure 8.11).

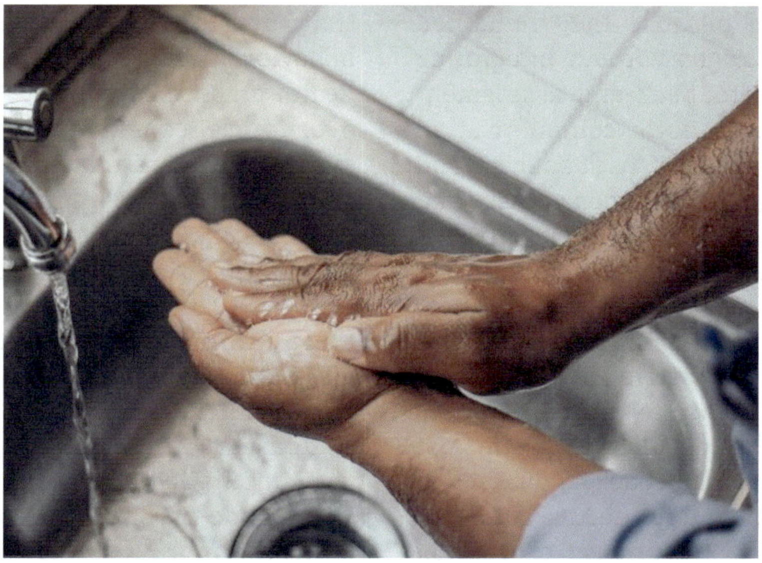

Figure 8.11. Successful public health campaigns.

Source: https://www.betteryou.ai/wp-content/uploads/2020/10/successful-public-health-campaigns.jpeg.

8.4.2. Lessons from Failed Health Initiatives

Lessons learned from failed health initiatives give invaluable insights into the intricacies of health communication and social marketing. One of the leading things that tend to detract from the success of these activities is the failure of stakeholders to develop successful partnerships. Upon examining several programs, such as those aimed at creating mental health identification systems for children in states of Colorado and Massachusetts, weaknesses such as a lack of collaboration between health organizations and community providers have been seen. These failed efforts confirm the necessity of alliance development that leverages mixed expertise and resources. Therefore, the establishment of effective partnerships can facilitate an integrated practice of health communication and improve opportunities for positive outcomes and prevention against future failure (Lyman et al., 2010). Another lesson learned from unsuccessful health initiatives relates to familiarization with the needs and cultural contexts of the target communities. Most health campaigns have failed due to ignorance of the very particular perspectives and realities of communities. For example, neighborhood revitalization projects have traditionally failed when they are not informed by local input and participation, resulting in a mismatch between program objectives and community aspirations. These imbalances typically translate to low rates of participation and decreased confidence in health programs. In contrast, effective programs engage community members in the planning and delivery processes, ensuring that health messages are locally relevant on a personal scale. By putting cultural competence and community engagement on the front burner, health communication is greatly improved, establishing credibility and efficacy in addressing public health concerns (N/A, 2004). Lastly, the scenario of continuous monitoring and adaptability comes as a valuable learning experience from previous health programs. Few of them have failed because they remained too rigid to initial designs without integrating changes relative to feedback and assessment in real time. Effective health communication requires an iterative process, with analysis and data informing change to strengthen strategy and implementation. As an example, incorporating feedback loops can allow health communicators and marketers to identify new opportunities and barriers in advance, such that initiatives can stay salient and effective. By embracing flexibility and adaptability to program design, stakeholders are able to pick up from past errors and refine their approaches, which will eventually translate into more effective outcomes for health promotion and disease prevention programs. Being able to make shifts in health communication strategy will be paramount in the ever-changing environment of public health (Lyman et al., 2010).

8.4.3. Impact of Social Media on Health Messaging

The evolution of social media networks has significantly redefined health messaging, offering opportunities for greater interactivity and information sharing. As opposed to traditional media of health communication, social media offers a platform for direct interactivity between publics and health institutions, allowing instant propagation of health-related information. Through this real-time flow of information, vital messages on health can be efficiently disseminated with immediacy, particularly during emergency situations of public health, when rapid communication can affect health behavior among large segments of the population. However, the effectiveness of such communications is dependent on their ability to resonate across different groups, a call that health communicators need to modify content that recognizes the unique facilitators and inhibitions within specific groups. It is from such an understanding, as observed (Musekiwa et al., 2017), that one can plan for health campaigns that possess the potential to encourage behavioral change and drive compliance with health practice. Moreover, social media is also a peer-to-peer communication platform on which individuals share individual health experience and results. This grass-roots participation can potentially raise the credibility of health information since individuals are more likely to follow their peers' recommendations than those from authority figures. These unofficial discussions are capable of significantly affecting health habits, as in the case of anti-smoking campaigns, where tailored messaging to at-risk populations has proved to be effective (Baezconde-Garbanati et al., 2019). Social media is, furthermore, an interactive platform, and health agencies can measure public sentiment and adjust messaging strategies accordingly, thereby making campaigns more attuned to target communities' sentiments and needs. Hence, the deployment of social media as part of health messaging not only optimizes coverage but also creates a community-oriented model of health promotion. Despite all the advantages of social media in health communication, there is no risk-free aspect. The velocity of the spread of misinformation is a key risk, for that erroneous health message will mislead individuals and destabilize public health programs. This is particularly concerning in the situation of novel health risks when crosscutting stories overwhelm the public and lead to less than ideal health decisions. Therefore, health agencies must adopt proactive strategies in countering misinformation, including monitoring online discourse and engaging directly with users. Furthermore, because social media websites continue to evolve, health communicators must continually update themselves on new trends and technologies in order to remain effective and relevant. Lastly, while social media provides many avenues for health messaging promotion, careful attention to its nuances must be given in order to assure that health communication campaigns are accurate, effective, and evidence-based (Musekiwa et al., 2017) (Figure 8.12).

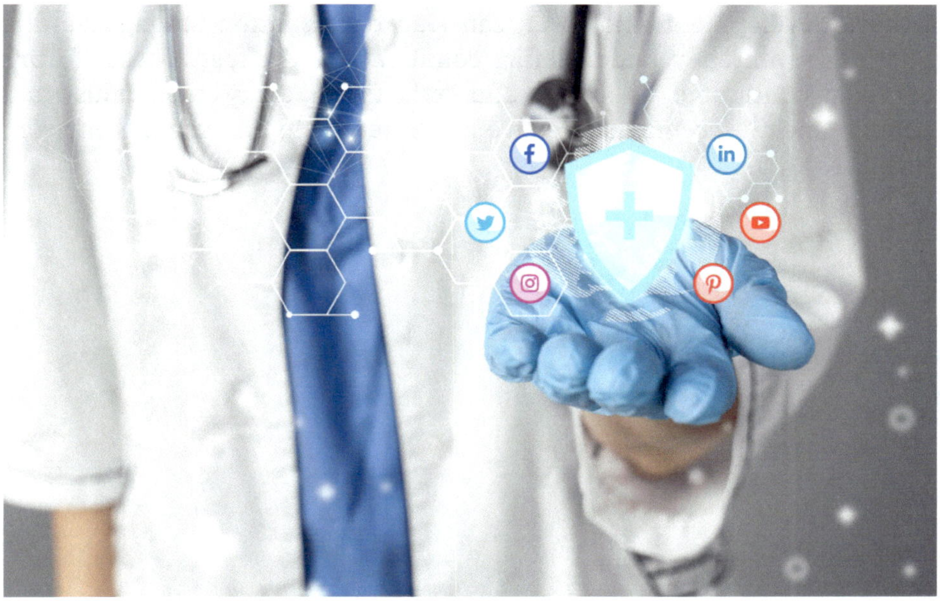

Figure 8.12. Impact of social media on health messaging.

Source: https://www.socialpilot.co/wp-content/uploads/2023/05/Social-Media-in-Healthcare.jpg.

8.5. Challenges in Health Communication

Health communication is faced with numerous serious difficulties that can adversely affect the process of effective information provision and public understanding of health issues. The most critical difficulty is perhaps the survival of misinformation, particularly in the current digital era where social media is a dominant source of information for many individuals. This trend was particularly dominant in the COVID-19 pandemic, with fast-spreading misinformation and unverified information about the virus, which complicated health marketing strategies. As noted, the pandemic triggered a shift in consumer behavior, with increased use of digital media for passing health information. Such is the dual burden on health communication practitioners to combat misinformation and effectively target an audience that is inherently more cynical of traditional health messaging (Micah et al., 2023). Cultural competence for healthcare practitioners is also an important issue that needs to be addressed for health communication. Populations' multicultural backgrounds and experiences call for tailored communications that resonate with diverse demographic groups. Strong communication regarding health must take into account language, level of health literacy, and varying cultural beliefs regarding health and well-being. Occupational therapy graduates, for instance, have been said to benefit from effective communication skills as part of their professional arsenal (Bell et al., 2025). These skills are essential to enable that health messages are conveyed inclusively in modes that encourage understanding and cause affirmative health behaviors in various groups. On top of that, the evolving healthcare policy and practice environment presents its own set of challenges. As seen through the reorganization of health and social care required under the Health & Social Care Act (2012), the practice of health communication has to be agile in reacting to legislative developments and service delivery models. Such ongoing change requires health communicators to continually adjust their messages and methods based on new regulations and social needs. Missing out on the rhythm of these developments, however, can lead to alienation among health organizations and their populations, eventually undermining confidence and effectiveness. To bridge this gap, conscious attempts at continuous education and stakeholder engagement must take precedence so that health communication remains effective and relevant in an evolving environment (Bell et al., 2025) (Figure 8.13).

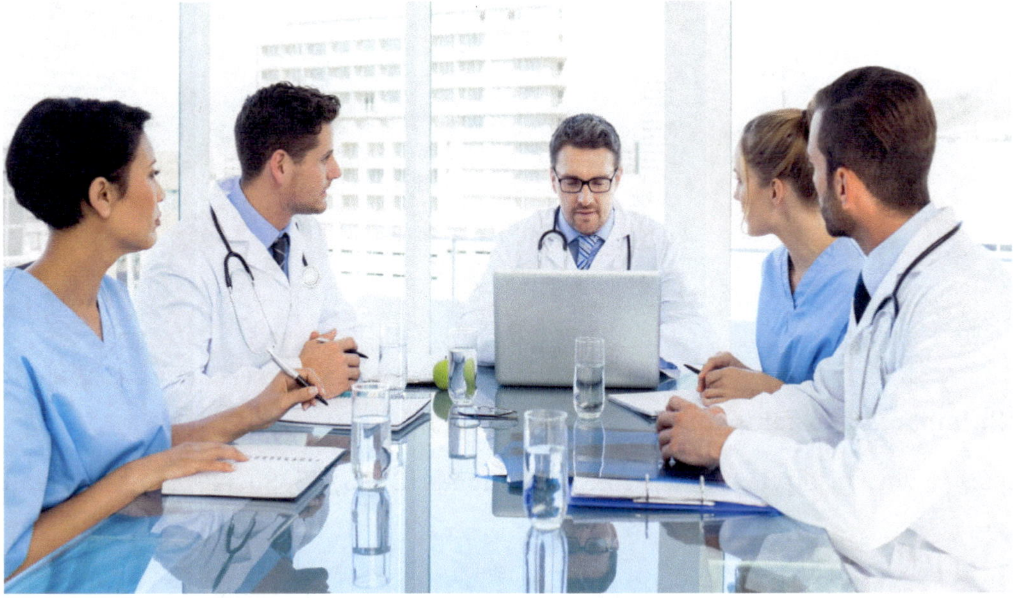

Figure 8.13. Challenges in health communication.

Source: https://www.sermo.com/wp-content/uploads/2023/02/effective-communication-img6-min.jpg.

8.5.1. Misinformation and Disinformation

The dissemination of misinformation and disinformation represents significant challenges for social marketing and health communication. It is essential to define these terms since misinformation refers to the spread of inaccurate or false information, while disinformation has been deliberately crafted with the intention of misleading. During health emergencies such as the COVID-19 crisis, misinformation about vaccines had already extensively circulated through social media in a matter of days, shaping public views and behaviors. This is a factor that brings out the work of health marketers and communicators to not only disperse accurate information but also to effectively counteract misinformation. As has been demonstrated through studies, the persuasive power of misinformation actually has the ability to significantly influence people's beliefs and actions regarding health interventions, pointing to the significance of strategic intervention in dispelling public misconceptions regarding health issues (Mahoney et al., 2021). In addition, the impact of disinformation and misinformation extends beyond individuals' health behaviors to span communities and public health programs. The spread of fallacies can chip away at trust in health systems and practitioners, thus placing obstacles in vaccine uptake, for instance. The virtual environment has also optimized the virality of disinformation, which complicates audiences to discern between credible sources. In order to defeat a force like that, health communicators must adopt proactive strategies that not just present understandable, evidence-based facts but also neutralize the underlying assumptions and hotspots of emotion that make such facts attractive. By understanding and stipulating the type of misinformation that occurs in health conversation, practitioners can shape their strategies to become immune to that sort of information (Taraghi and Nima, 2023). Finally, to counteract the effects of misinformation, efforts must be two-fold and include both communications tactics and community engagement. Target groups can be reached through social marketing techniques that promote critical thinking and build the publics ability to manage health information. Media literacy educational campaigns that emphasize questioning the credibility of information obtained on the internet can empower citizens to move beyond the informational trash on the internet. Apart from that, accessing the knowledge of trusted community influencers can enhance health message credibility. Not only does this cooperative framework enhance combat against misinformation but also constructs a healthier information environment. Collective action between health communicators, marketers, and community leaders plays a vital role in shaping a more informed society that is immune to the negative effect of misinformation and disinformation (Mahoney et al., 2021; Taraghi and Nima, 2023).

8.5.2. Cultural and Linguistic Barriers

In looking at health communication and social marketing, it is not possible to discount the significant role that cultural and linguistic barriers play in ensuring these efforts are successful. Cultural differences may lead to differences in how health messages are received, typically rendering the flow of information between patients and healthcare providers more challenging. Misunderstandings based on language differences can result in less patient compliance, eventually compromising health outcomes. Thus, the healthcare system must conform to culturally competent modes of communication that address the beliefs and values of the various ethnic groups. Through their embracing of these paradigms, organizations can effectively convey critical health information and provide equal access to care, aiming to close the gap between communities and health-care providers (Lurie et al., 2004). Cultural competence is not merely cross-translation of languages but involves extensive knowledge of the unique experiences faced by ethnic minorities in accessing health services. Barriers in language have a tendency to go in parallel with unfamiliarity with the healthcare system, which itself is found to lead to lower levels of preventive care, such as cancer screening, and an overall lack of health literacy. Such deep divide has a tendency to exaggerate health disparities among populations. Research indicates that the answer to such cultural nuances is essential for more effective health communication. Professionals in the field of palliative care have, in turn, realized that connecting with patients' migration experiences and cultivating trust through individualized approaches of care is essential. These interventions can significantly minimize cultural and linguistic barriers, working towards a more inclusive health system respecting human singularity (Green et al., 2018). Effective social marketing initiatives must recognize and actively bridge cultural and language barriers to optimize health messaging. Practices must incorporate adjusting communications by the demographic characteristics of target groups, simplifying language, and incorporating imagery and narrative that are culturally appropriate.

Engaging community leaders and tapping into local culturally competent actors may help maximize credibility of health messages, acceptance, and trust among communities with diversity. Besides, incorporating family roles in the talk of health will decrease misunderstandings even more because families largely dictate healthcare decisions. By providing a free space where both cultural affiliations and language use are valued, health communication can decrease health disparities and enhance general health outcomes (Lurie et al., 2004).

8.5.3. Resource Limitations in Health Campaigns

Resource limitations severely impede the effectiveness of health campaigns, which are usually implemented under strict fiscal and administrative management. These limitations span across the various aspects of campaign planning and execution, from data collection to community mobilization. For instance, health campaigns that are audience segmented to deliver messages suitably can become prohibitively costly, allocating precious resources that could be committed to other uses. The complexities of segmentation practices require a substantial outlay of financial and professional resources, as the research has also pointed out in elevating expertise to the point of guaranteeing effective interpretation and implementation of these practices (Barnett et al., 2011).

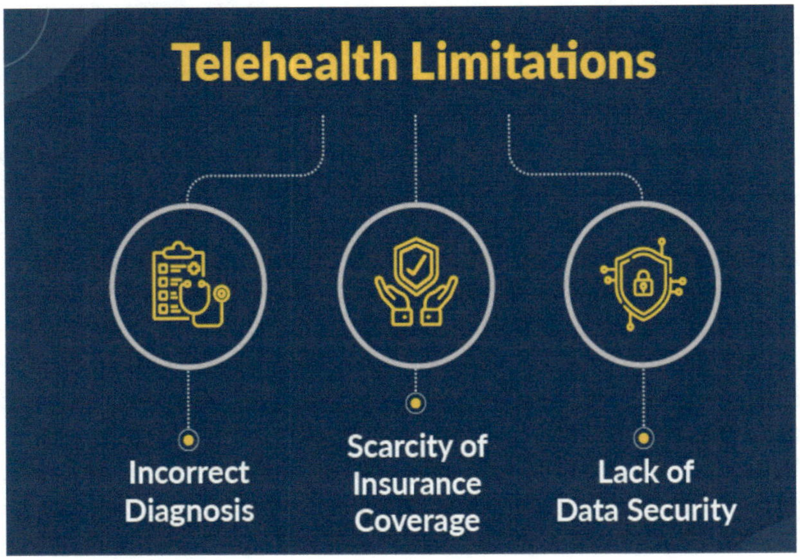

Figure 8.14. Resource limitations in health campaigns.

Source: https://www.selecthub.com/wp-content/uploads/2022/08/Limitations-of-Telehealth.jpg.

This is why the cost component may become a detractor from the overall impact of health communication efforts, with messages being painted in broad brushstrokes that may fail to resonate with target populations. In addition to affecting the budget, the consequences of limited resources extend beyond finance to affect internal organizational processes and relations with stakeholders. When health campaigns overly rely on limited resources, the ability of the staff to innovate and adjust to community needs is compromised, and there are no adaptive mechanisms that can trigger increased participation. Health agencies may find themselves fighting against bad communication among various groups of individuals, the ethical considerations of segmentation methodologies raising doubts about inclusiveness and representation. The potential for reputational damage from such issues may exclude future collaborations or diminish public trust, further confusing the delivery of high-stakes health messaging. Health campaigns must, thus, navigate this thorny intersection of resource limitations in generating authentic relationships with stakeholders to maximize reach potential. Finally, the understanding of the overall socio-political context in which health campaigns operate is key to addressing such resource limitations effectively. Existing orthodoxies and paradigms in the health communication environment have a tendency to constrain novel thought on behavior change as identified in research identifying the constraint imposed on campaign strategy. Such limitations have the effect of inhibiting the delivery of revolutionary practice which could meaningfully engage communities and drive lasting change (Alexander et al., 2014). In response to these obstacles, public health campaigns need to be ready to utilize broader and more inclusive methods, transcending the traditional paradigm to create efficient interventions that communicate to various groups. By thoughtful critique and reevaluation of resource distribution, agencies are better equipped to enhance their overall effectiveness at delivering targeted health messages relevant to the unique needs of various populations (Figure 8.14).

8.6. Future Trends in Health Communication and Social Marketing

The evolving health communication environment is increasingly shaped by technology advancements and changing consumer behavior. Online environments, including social media and mobile applications, will probably change the means through which health information is disseminated and consumed. The trend of individualized communication allows organizations to tailor their messages in accordance with personal choice, leading to higher involvement. For instance, the use of data analytics to determine demographics and health behavior will render outreach more effective. In addition, with more and more individuals searching for health information on the web, public health campaigns will have to use these forums to effectively promote socially. This integration of technology aims not only to enhance communication but also calls for active participation in health-enabling activities, mirroring the possibility of enhanced social influence on health communication interventions. Health and wellness promotion will also be influenced by changing practices in behavior change communication and social marketing. Social norms and peer-influence approaches are gaining popularity, with a community-based approach to public health intervention. Success for such approaches comes in creating trust and building relationships with communities. Moreover, as the trend towards holistic health paradigms takes hold in society, communication approaches must play catch-up by addressing mental, physical, and social health. This cross-cutting approach can enhance the health messages' credibility and encourage diverse groups to engage in health interventions. As Basurto et al. (2018) speculates, other activities and community gatherings, such as pizza night and yoga classes, have the potential to engage individuals and encourage healthier behaviors while also strengthening communal relationships. Future trends in health communication also will be directed towards solving urgent challenges of health equity and access to healthcare. With organizations connecting to diverse populations, it will be necessary to implement inclusive practices that break down barriers to health information and services. This includes recognizing special concerns for marginalized populations and crafting messages in ways that resonate with multiple cultural contexts. Engagement of such communities in the development of health interventions will be imperative to making them effective and appropriate. Moreover, the emphasis on occupational safety and health is a key area of concern, as highlighted in the findings on employee health programs in organizations (Sharma et al., 2018). By being proactive in the area of health communication, organizations are able to create safer communities that not only contribute to employee health but also improve the general community health outcomes (Figure 8.15).

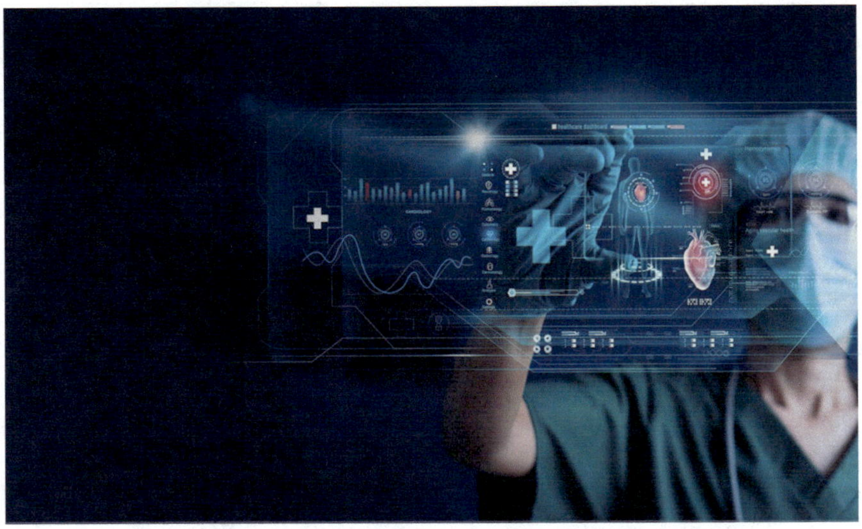

Figure 8.15. Future trends in health communication and social marketing.

Source: https://www.netscribes.com/wp-content/uploads/2023/04/AI-in-healthcare.jpg.

8.6.1. Integration of Artificial Intelligence (AI)

The integration of AI in health communication and social marketing represents a revolutionary shift in the dissemination and consumption of healthcare information. As health care systems continue to integrate sophisticated technological advancements, AI-based instruments, including chatbots, are radically transforming clinician-patient communication. Not only do these instruments enhance the effectiveness of communication tactics but also enhance patient engagement in the form of immediate replies to questions and greater access to health information. Yet the effective integration of such technologies is contingent upon the embracement and approval of healthcare providers who are in closest contact with patient care. To create an integrated strategy that considers technological innovation as well as people-based care, it is critical to learn about clinicians' experiences and attitudes toward such innovations (Dohan et al., 2019). Furthermore, the use of big data analysis complemented by AI technologies provides valuable insights into consumer behavior and epidemiological patterns. This intersection allows healthcare organizations to tailor their communication plans cost-effectively, reaching targeted populations with tailored messaging that addresses specific health needs. Big data, when analyzed with AI algorithms, can detect patterns that are employed by social marketing campaigns and public health programs. Challenges of big data management like data privacy, security, and the need for robust analytical infrastructure still persist. Addressing these issues is at the core of revealing the full promise of big data in health communication. Learning these dynamics and methodologies enables healthcare providers to expand their knowledge-sharing activities and eventually improve health outcomes among the populations they serve (Zhuge et al., 2015). Last but not least, the ethical issues of using AI in health communication need consideration. With autonomous devices becoming more prevalent in AI, there is a requirement for them to function within a system that prioritizes patient autonomy and informed consent. Clinicians should reconcile the utilization of AI for enhanced delivery of service with patient safety and trust. In building this relationship, it is essential to institute training programs that equip healthcare professionals with the skills required to integrate these technologies into their practice while fostering compassion and empathy in practice. By acknowledging the subtle interplay between ethics and AI integration, health organizations may be able to craft a more comprehensive health communication and social marketing plan that not only enhances the effectiveness of services but also sustains the essential virtues of the healthcare profession (Figure 8.16).

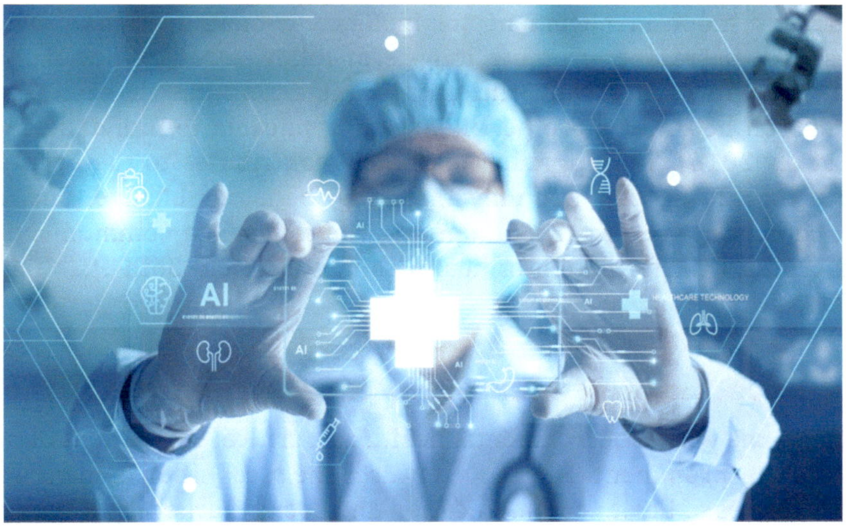

Figure 8.16. Integration of artificial intelligence (AI).

Source: https://www.emaginehealth.com/wp-content/uploads/2023/08/AI-in-healthcare-1024x576.png.

8.6.2. Emphasis on Personalization and Customization

In the fields of social marketing and health communication, personalization and customization are becoming even more important. Customized and personalized health messages tailored to suit individual tastes and needs better make communications more efficient. Personalization encourages a stronger emotional response with the target group so that health campaigns are able to communicate more intensively. By being sensitive to demographic factors, health behavior, and cultural settings, brand marketers can develop campaigns that engage not only a broader base of consumers but also individuals on a personal level. This approach is crucial in the sense of penetrating health literacy concerns as well as varying levels of motivation across groups of individuals. As research indicates, this personalization through communication enhances participation, with the individuals being more inclined to participate in health programs and adopt preventive practices that ultimately lead to improved public health outcomes. Additionally, customization offers a solution to the issues emanating from a heterogeneous population with diverse health needs and wants. In effective health communication, message flexibility based on specific community profiles makes for a targeted approach that maximizes relevance. Personalized communication can be in numerous shapes and forms, from web platforms that leverage algorithms to guide advertising to customized health alerts delivered through health applications. Market researchers can utilize data analysis to identify trends and interests of specific groups, making for more context-specific health messages. The effectiveness of the tailored campaigns is supported by the proof that shows people are more likely to respond positively to messages that appeal to their own experience and values (Dahinden et al., 2008). Tailoring, thus, not only raises user engagement but also enhances the significance of personal agency to decision-making concerning health. Moreover, the potential for customization and tailoring lies in guaranteeing behavior alteration by means of tailored interventions. Health communications that respect individual choices and acknowledge personal circumstances can give people power to be masters of their health. With interventions providing tailored options for eating, exercise, and mood management, for instance, communications provide flexibility for different lifestyles and tastes and promote long-term follow-through. Social marketing studies show that customized approaches can bring significant alterations in health-related behaviors because the information becomes more pertinent and applicable to individuals when tailored to them (McGarvey et al., 2016). The approach ultimately contributes to the eventual aim of social marketing towards educating, and not only inspiring, behavior change, and creating a long-lasting impact on community health. The adoption of personalized communication and tailoring thus represents a crucial transformation of health communication, both enabling individuals and enhancing overall health.

8.6.3. Growing Importance of Mental Health Awareness

With society changing, the perception of mental health as a critical component of overall well-being is becoming progressively prominent. This move towards the recognition of mental health issues has been facilitated by the uses of health communication and social marketing, whose primary function is education and the informing of individuals. By the release of proper information regarding mental health conditions and help that is available, stakeholders can help break the stigma surrounding help-seeking. Educational campaigns that de-stigmatize the symptoms and signs of mental illnesses empower individuals to take their conditions to treatment, making mental health just as important as physical health. The consequences are wide-ranging because increased awareness not only promotes individual wellness but also worker productivity and social cohesion. Moreover, mental health awareness campaigns have become of special significance in fighting special populations that can have special challenges. For instance, marginal communities normally possess barriers that undermine their reach to mental health care, as they widen the existing disparities. Social marketing efforts at these populations can become a powerful support for overcoming these barriers. By employing culturally harmonious messaging along with the leverage of community leaders, these campaigns have the ability to reach target markets penetration. Moreover, the application of platforms such as social media supports the rapid spread of information, which bridges the isolation barriers that usually accompany mental health. This extension emphasizes the interdependence of social marketing and health communication in facilitating equitable mental health care across groups. The recent emphasis on mental health has broad implications for organizational cultures, and the necessity of building mentally healthy workplaces arises. Organizational performance hinges on employees' wellbeing since well employees are more productive, committed, and innovative. The establishment of holistic mental health policies in organizations is therefore imperative. Such policies do not only have to be preventive but should also be a system of intervention when there is mental health. Encouraging openness to discuss mental health can create a culture of belongingness in the workplace where employees feel at ease coming forward about their issues. Furthermore, certain resources, such as training programs and mental health days, can improve overall worker satisfaction and retention, which makes the argument that health should be an organizational priority (Basurto et al., 2018). Such initiatives will ultimately pivot workplaces to recognize mental health as an integral aspect of employee health, aligning with broader public health objectives (Sharma et al., 2018) (Figure 8.17).

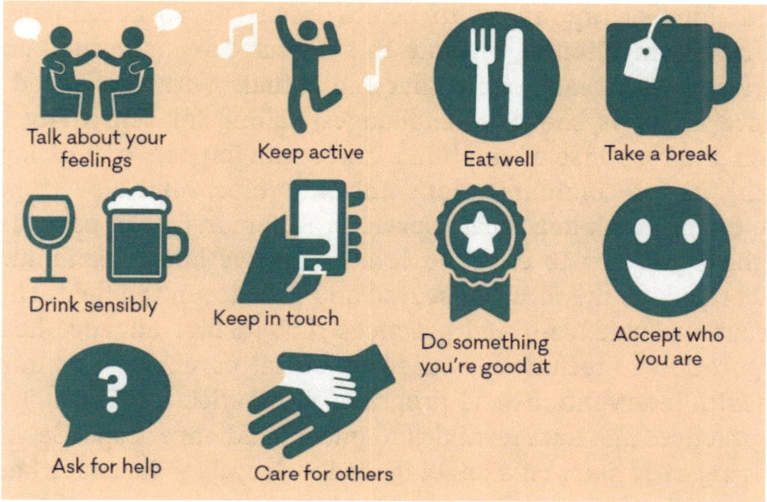

Figure 8.17. Growing importance of mental health awareness.

Source: https://24fingers.co.uk/wp-content/uploads/2017/05/mental-health-awareness-week.jpg.

SUMMARY

In concluding an examination of health communication and social marketing, it is evident that these fields play a crucial role in shaping public perceptions and behaviors related to health. Efficient communication practices can seriously improve awareness and recognition of health issues, thus creating healthier living and well-informed decision-making habits among the population. As noted throughout this work, the synergy between marketing techniques and health communication practices can strengthen their impact when the message is ascertained and targeted to populations. Lastly, an integrated strategy involving these elements leads to increased participation and better health outcomes, especially among underrepresented groups who may have unique barriers to receiving information. Moreover, the psychosocial dimensions of health communication play a key role. As per the research, individuals grappling with health issues do so accompanied by psychosocial distress, and robust communication can negate this aspect. For instance, studies of diseases like Bell's palsy and Parkinson's disease show that individuals with disfigured or distorted facial expressions experience more psychosocial challenges, calling for sensitivity in health messages. Through identification and response of emotional and social impacts of health problems, according to Rasing et al. (2023), health communications not only inform but also empower individuals to access treatment and engage with healthcare services. This marriage of psychosocial consideration with health campaigns is the key to effective comprehensive health communication. Finally, the implications of this work are to the future research and practice in the field. There is always a need for creating and executing evidence-based practices that further advance health communication practices. The incorporation of techniques based on social psychology, as noted by Sadava et al. (1997), can render health interventions and programs more effective. Through the implementation of robust evaluation practices and data feedback to inform audience response, health campaigns are made capable of evolving over time. This ongoing feedback cycle will render health communication responsive to changing societal attitudes and tailored requirements, eventually serving a healthier population with informed choices. Overall, the alliance of social marketing and health communication holds a huge promise to advance public health but requires constant effort and innovation to tap its complete potential.

To create effective strategies in the environment of health communication and social marketing, it is essential to understand the target audiences through segmentation. Segmentation refers to the process of classifying humans into groups based on what they share in common so that it is easier to transmit messages that will appeal to different groups. Successful engagement is greatly based on knowledge of the values, beliefs, and drives of potential recipients of health information. Health institutions focusing on health communication must therefore use segmentation tools fully to grasp the complex layers of public opinion towards health programs. As introduced in the research reports, segmentation is capable of vastly enhancing public engagement activities in health promotion to provide more efficient communication strategies that enhance behavioral change for healthier lifestyles (Barnett et al., 2011). Even the inclusion of a well-proven framework for health communication can also offer the assurance that strategies are not only efficient but also ethical. Health communication must walk the tightrope of persuasion and respect for autonomy. Social marketing organizations must target segmentation with caution, weighing the ethical traps and loss of reputation that can come from targeting specified groups. Allocating significant resources—financial and human—to good segmentation is one demonstration of the commitment required to bring about effective health communication. Also important is the general organizational strategies to the application of these segmentation methods, which are essential to identifying the utility and effectiveness of health campaigns (Barnett et al., 2011). Further supporting the interdependencies of global health communication initiatives, organizations like Northwestern University illustrate the importance of building a vision for the world in their extension activities. By establishing a system that facilitates intensive engagement with diverse populations, health communication approaches can increase institutional visibility within international networks. This two-way emphasis enables institutions to project outward the efforts they are making while also integrating global considerations into their local curricula and practices. Such an approach not only enhances the efficiency of health communication efforts but also promotes a culture of collaboration required to respond to global critical health issues. The integration of these principles promotes the agenda of total comprehension of health communications' contribution towards building positive social change.

KEY TERMS FROM THIS CHAPTER

- Behavior Change
- Message Framing
- Media Advocacy
- Theory of Planned Behavior
- Community Engagement
- Evaluation Metrics
- Interpersonal Communication
- Health Promotion
- Social Norms
- Risk Communication
- Health Belief Model
- Digital Health Campaigns
- Cultural Competency
- Target Audience
- Public Health Campaigns
- Health Literacy
- Audience Segmentation
- Social Media Strategy
- Call to Action (CTA)

CLOSER LOOK

ECONOMIC AND SOCIAL RESEARCH COUNCIL (ESRC)

A closer look at the Economic and Social Research Council (ESRC) reveals its vital role in shaping the landscape of social science research in the United Kingdom and beyond. As one of the UK's leading research councils, the ESRC is responsible for funding and supporting high-quality research that advances understanding of economic and social issues. It plays a crucial role in informing public policy, improving societal outcomes, and driving innovation through evidence-based insights. The ESRC funds a broad range of research across disciplines such as economics, sociology, education, psychology, and political science, ensuring that complex societal challenges are examined through diverse perspectives. It emphasizes the importance of interdisciplinary collaboration and supports both large-scale research projects and early-career researchers, helping to build future research capacity. A key focus of the ESRC is impact—ensuring that research findings translate into real-world benefits by influencing policy, improving public services, and contributing to economic development. Through partnerships with government agencies, businesses, charities, and international organizations, the ESRC helps bridge the gap between academic research and practical application. It also supports data infrastructure, such as longitudinal studies and national data services, which provide researchers with valuable resources to examine trends and inform decision-making. Furthermore, the ESRC is committed to fostering inclusivity and diversity within the research community and addressing global challenges such as inequality, climate change, and technological disruption. By promoting rigorous, ethical, and socially responsible research, the ESRC ensures that social science continues to play a central role in understanding and responding to the needs of society. Overall, the ESRC stands as a cornerstone of research excellence, enabling knowledge creation that not only deepens academic inquiry but also improves lives through informed action and innovation.

REFERENCES

1. Alexander, S., Anable, J., Assadourian, E., Bailey, R., Bamberg, S., Bergman, N., Berker, T., et al. (2014). Prospects for radical emissions reduction through behavior and lifestyle change. https://core.ac.uk/download/29112503.pdf (accessed on 26th June 2025).
2. Almunawar, M. N., & Anshari, M. (2012). Framework of social customer relationship management in e-health services. http://arxiv.org/abs/1207.6179 (accessed on 26th June 2025).
3. Baezconde-Garbanati, L., Byron, M. J., Carroll, D. M., Cruz, T. B., et al. (2019). Pro-tobacco marketing and anti-tobacco campaigns aimed at vulnerable populations: A review of the literature. https://core.ac.uk/download/323062757.pdf (accessed on 26th June 2025).
4. Barnett, C., & Mahony, N. (2011). Segmenting publics. https://core.ac.uk/download/106766.pdf (accessed on 26th June 2025).
5. Barrett, D., & Leddy, S. (2008). Assessing creative media's social impact. https://core.ac.uk/download/71349416.pdf (accessed on 26th June 2025).
6. Basurto, J., & Yaeghoobi, E. (2018). Business activities to use during the low season. https://core.ac.uk/download/187724626.pdf (accessed on 26th June 2025).
7. Bell, J., & Morris, K. (2025). Do future occupational therapists require a different skill set? https://core.ac.uk/download/76980082.pdf (accessed on 26th June 2025).
8. Bolt, C. A. (2017). Environmental education in the public sphere: Comparing practice with psychosocial determinants of behavior and societal change. https://core.ac.uk/download/129153482.pdf (accessed on 26th June 2025).
9. Braybrook, D., Robertson, S., & Robinson, M. (2012). Evaluation of the Choose Life North Lanarkshire Awareness Programmed: Final report. https://core.ac.uk/download/29018946.pdf (accessed on 26th June 2025).
10. Cao, X., Comulada, W. S., Lan, C. W., Li, L., et al. (2016). Report on provider-client interaction from 68 methadone maintenance clinics in China. https://core.ac.uk/download/323311096.pdf (accessed on 26th June 2025).
11. Constantinides, E. (2008). The Web 2.0 as marketing tool: Opportunities for SMEs. https://core.ac.uk/download/pdf/11477173.pdf (accessed on 26th June 2025).
12. Dahinden, U., Gerth, M., Pühringer, K., Rademacher, L., et al. (2008). Challenges to political campaigns in the media: Commercialization, framing, and personalization. http://www.zora.uzh.ch/20005/2/Challenges_to_Political_Campaings_in_the_Media_text.pdf (accessed on 26th June 2025).
13. Dohan, M., Maarup, M., Wu, S., Zhao, X., et al. (2019). Radical technological innovation and perception: A non-physician practitioners' perspective. https://core.ac.uk/download/289123780.pdf (accessed on 26th June 2025).
14. Drabble, L. A., Keatley, J., & Marcelle, G. (2003). Progress and opportunities in lesbian, gay, bisexual and transgender health communications. https://core.ac.uk/download/70410107.pdf (accessed on 26th June 2025).
15. Green, A., Green, M., Jerzmanowska, N., Lobb, E., et al. (2018). "Death is difficult in any language": A qualitative study of palliative care professionals' experiences when providing end-of-life care to patients from culturally and linguistically diverse backgrounds. https://core.ac.uk/download/213607752.pdf (accessed on 26th June 2025).

16. Keys, T. R. (2012). Behaviors that eliminate health disparities for racial and ethnic minorities: A narrative systematic review. https://core.ac.uk/download/56703666.pdf (accessed on 26th June 2025).
17. Lurie, N., & Taylor, S. L. (2004). The role of culturally competent communication in reducing ethnic and racial healthcare disparities. https://core.ac.uk/download/pdf/18491828.pdf (accessed on 26th June 2025).
18. Lyman, D. R., Dougherty, R. H., & Holt, W. (2010). State case studies of infant and early childhood mental health systems: Strategies for change. https://core.ac.uk/download/71355034.pdf (accessed on 26th June 2025).
19. Mahoney, E. (2021). Public health campaigns and the COVID-19 vaccine: An analysis of the role marketing and public relations play in combating vaccine hesitancy and the spread of misinformation on social media. https://core.ac.uk/download/479135550.pdf (accessed on 26th June 2025).
20. Marseille, E., Kahn, J. G., Peterson, K., & Herman, L. (2008). Smarter programming of the female condom: Increasing its impact on HIV prevention in the developing world. https://core.ac.uk/download/71341113.pdf (accessed on 26th June 2025).
21. McGarvey, B., Rath, B., Cushenberry, D., Spangler, D., Griffin, J., Dawson, L. C., Donohue, N. B., et al. (2016). *Seizing the Moment: Realizing the Promise of Student-Centered Learning*. https://core.ac.uk/download/71338651.pdf (accessed on 26th June 2025).
22. Micah, D. J., & Odoemelam, C. C. (2023). Navigating the social media marketing strategies during the COVID-19 era in Nigeria. https://core.ac.uk/download/597809860.pdf (accessed on 26th June 2025).
23. Moreno, A., Navarro, C., Tench, R., Zerfass, A., et al. (2014). Does social media usage matter? An analysis of online practices and digital media perceptions of communication practitioners in Europe. https://core.ac.uk/download/29019023.pdf (accessed on 26th June 2025).
24. Musekiwa, A., Vande Veegaete, A., Avau, B., De Buck, E., Van Remoortel, H., Mosler, H. J., Hannes, K., et al. (2017). Promoting handwashing and sanitation behavior change in low- and middle-income countries: A mixed-method systematic review. https://core.ac.uk/download/141922886.pdf (accessed on 26th June 2025).
25. N/A. (2004). Review of neighborhood revitalization initiatives. https://core.ac.uk/download/71341220.pdf (accessed on 26th June 2025).
26. N/A. (2007). Interactive food and beverage marketing: Targeting children and youth in the digital age. https://core.ac.uk/download/71352321.pdf (accessed on 26th June 2025).
27. N/A. (2011). Handwashing with soap–Two paths to national-scale programs: Lessons from the field: Vietnam and Indonesia. https://core.ac.uk/download/75783149.pdf (accessed on 26th June 2025).
28. N/A. (2016). Report of the Global Strategy Task Force. https://core.ac.uk/download/75760901.pdf (accessed on 26th June 2025).
29. Rasing, N., van de Geest-Buit, W., Chan, O. Y. A., Mul, K., Lanser, A., Erasmus, C., Groothuis, J., et al. (2023). Psychosocial functioning in patients with altered facial expression: A scoping review in five neurological diseases. *Disability and Rehabilitation, 46*, 3772–3791. https://www.semanticscholar.org/paper/df39d3d69ccc1115843457a6070c199396eca110 (accessed on 26th June 2025).

30. Rosidah, R. (2012). Analysis of social marketing for anti-corruption campaign: Case study of film "Kita Versus Korupsi." https://core.ac.uk/download/11521948.pdf (accessed on 26th June 2025).
31. Sadava, S., & McCreary, D. (1997). *Applied Social Psychology*. https://www.semanticscholar.org/paper/c477c73d09c6377492c3d0175b74c664f522e6f3 (accessed on 26th June 2025).
32. Salmon, C. T., Post, L. A., & Christensen, R. E. (2003). Mobilizing public will for social change. https://core.ac.uk/download/71340672.pdf (accessed on 26th June 2025).
33. Sharma, C., & Wood, B. (2018). Health and safety in an organization. https://core.ac.uk/download/187724596.pdf (accessed on 26th June 2025).
34. Taraghi, N. (2023). A conceptual model to protect brand reputation facing "fake news." https://core.ac.uk/download/588606205.pdf (accessed on 26th June 2025).
35. Terris-Prestholt, F., & Windmeijer, F. (2016). How to sell a condom? The impact of demand creation tools on male and female condom sales in resource-limited settings. https://core.ac.uk/download/73982581.pdf (accessed on 26th June 2025).
36. van Dijk, J. A. G. M., Ebbers, W. E., Fennis, B. M., Geest, T., et al. (2005). Alter ego, state of the art on user profiling: An overview of the most relevant organizational and behavioral aspects regarding user profiling. https://core.ac.uk/download/pdf/11463498.pdf (accessed on 26th June 2025).
37. Zhuge, H. (2015). Mapping big data into knowledge space with cognitive cyber-infrastructure. http://arxiv.org/abs/1507.06500 (accessed on 26th June 2025).

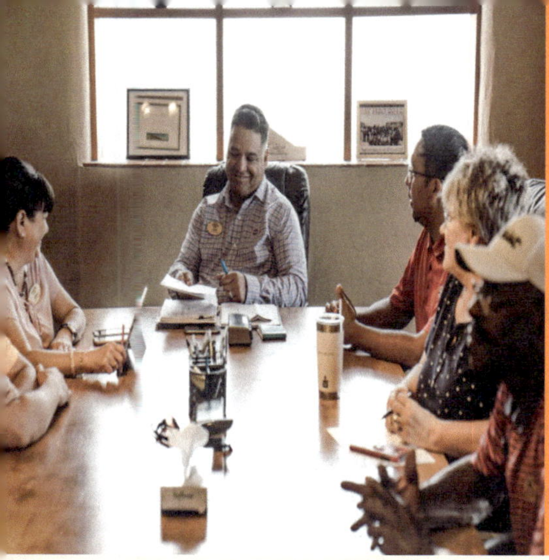

Chapter 9

COMMUNITY-BASED PARTICIPATORY RESEARCH (CBPR)

Contents

Introduction

Community-Based Participatory Research (CBPR) is a new research methodology, emphasizing researcher-community people collaboration. The approach deviates from traditional paradigms, which often neglect the voice of the community people and, instead, promotes their direct involvement in the research. Through the integration of the lived experience and expertise of community members, CBPR not only enhances data collected but also empowers participants by providing a sense of ownership over outcomes. Empowerment is critical, especially in marginalized populations where there has historically been a disconnect between researchers and the population being researched. Consequently, CBPR ensures a more just partnership, making knowledge production a co-created activity and not one that is imposed. Going deeper into the methods used in CBPR, perhaps the most salient feature is its ability to use a variety of participatory methods that are matched according to the needs and situation of particular communities. For instance, multimedia and arts-based approaches have been very successful in involving participants to voice their views and concerns on matters such as risk and safety in a manner that can be understood by broader populations. For instance, through one study, teenagers employed creative forms such as visual arts and blogs to reflect on themselves in the context of community, hence initiating broader discussion of sensitive issues. These methods are significant in establishing a platform for youth voices to allow them to critically reflect on their sociohistorical setting and be capable of articulating their narratives effectively. Through doing so, CBPR is capable of creating not only new information, but also channels of social change, as evidenced by experiences in earlier studies (Cutts et al., 2011). Moreover, the participatory involvement frameworks that are inherent to CBPR hold the potential for systematic impact evaluation and solution-focused collaboration. Through applying whole-systems models with feed-forward from all stakeholders, researchers can potentially specify problem situations more accurately and evaluate probable solutions more rigorously. The SciCafe2.0 Project is shown here to exemplify this process, highlighting how social involvement and participatory research outcome measurement can be facilitated by means of online platforms. These models are not merely conceptual; they actually inform practice and enhance the effectiveness of community engagement processes so that diverse voices are heard and considered. In effect, CBPR represents a research methodological revolution where not only is community voice lifted, but collaboration is fostered that is amenable to enduring social change (Badii et al., 2016) (Figure 9.1).

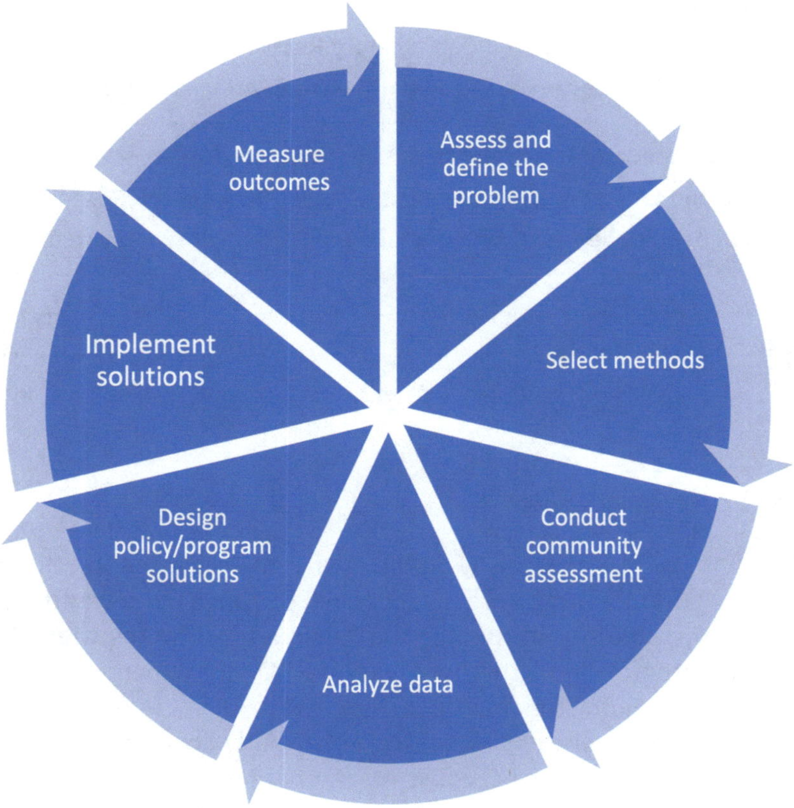

Figure 9.1. Community-based participatory research (CBPR).

Source: https://williamstownma.gov/wp-content/uploads/2021/04/Phases-of-CBPR.png.

Definition of Community-Based Participatory Research (CBPR)

CBPR is fundamentally characterized by its collaborative nature, with the research process involving researchers and community members directly. This is in sharp contrast to typical research methods, typically characterized by a research-driven agenda that unintentionally exclusionary of community input. CBPR emphasizes partnership as a method of health disparity reduction and enhancing research-community trust. Most specifically, the collaboration improves study design and results by infusing contextual and local knowledge into research questions and thereby enhancing relevance and applicability. By recognizing that trust is built on the basis of relational dynamics, it is therefore important to build mutual respect and understanding. There needs to be an operational partnership trust model in order to facilitate effective partnership working, particularly where there has been past distrust on the basis of adverse research experiences among marginalized populations, as highlighted through evidence of how trust develops in CBPR partnerships (Moore de Peralta et al., 2020). The most significant feature of CBPR is its social justice and health equity focus. By working with communities directly at each step of the research—from articulating issues to interpreting results—CBPR empowers members of the community, thus leading to more sustainable and effective health interventions. Furthermore, this model highlights the importance of community knowledge as a legitimate source of information and knowledge, something which becomes very important when culturally responsive solutions are being created. CBPRs focusing on co-learning allows researchers and community individuals to exchange useful information and resources, providing a more complete image of community needs. Not only does such a shared knowledge enhance health practice, but it also serves as a foundation for advocacy and policy-making. Most crucial is the incorporation of community knowledge into policymaking, as can be seen in studies that show the contribution of CBPR collaborations in shaping health policy to eliminate racial and ethnic health disparities (Cacari-Stone et al., 2014). Participation, trust, and shared action form the pillars of CBPR, hence making it a groundbreaking approach in public health research. Community stakeholders will have varying experiences with trust depending on their involvement and the research context, as this captures the complexity of partnership collaborations. It is through direct participation and sustained interaction that researchers can build stronger relationships with the community, which over time mature into increased levels of trust and cooperation. The emphasis on direct contact and continuous interaction is a testament to the fact that trust is built step by step, through commitment and transparency by all stakeholders. Having knowledge of the socio-economic and cultural determinants of partnership trust, scholars are in an ideal position to create spaces for productive co-operation. The knowledge emerged from these collaborations not only contributes to specific health programs but also significantly contributes to overall discourse regarding the effectiveness of participatory research methods in enhancing health equity and social change (Moore de Peralta et al., 2020).

Importance of Community-Based Participatory Research (CBPR) in Addressing Community Issues

CBPR is a critical tool for the identification and resolution of community issues, aiming at partnership between researchers and community stakeholders. By creating a coalition of partnerships through the contribution of input and experience of people impacted by a specific issue, CBPR not only makes the research findings more relevant but also creates a sense of ownership by the participants. This is significant in ensuring that solutions proposed are responsive to the needs and situations of the community. Traditional research methods frequently marginalize communities, leading to unacceptable intervention for the local inhabitants. CBPR, however, focuses on good communication and genuine participation, which allows a deeper understanding of the social processes taking place. By engaging community members as active participants in the research, CBPR encourages trust and confidence building, which is essential in the execution of sustainable development projects. Additionally, CBPR is marked by an allegiance to social justice in giving prominence to marginal voices, which are usually marginalized in mainstream research traditions.

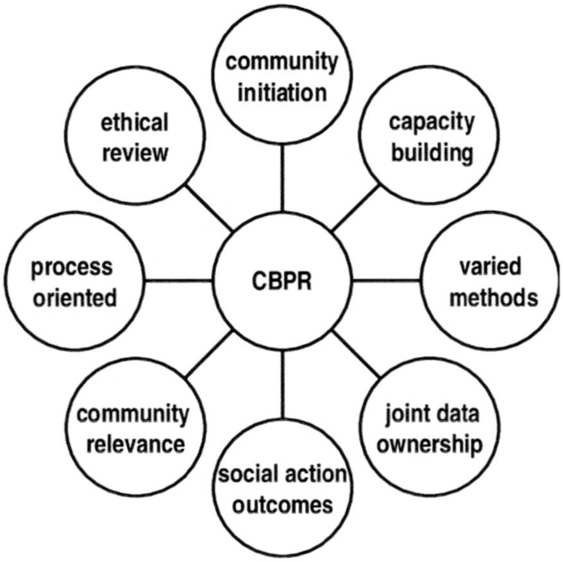

Figure 9.2. Importance of community-based participatory research (CBPR) in addressing community issues.

Source: https://www.researchgate.net/profile/Sarah-Flicker/publication/6392572/figure/fig1/AS:601629254504472@1520451000357/Principles-of-CBPR.png.

It sees that the very individuals most affected by conditions of health inequity, environmental degradation, and social injustice have valuable knowledge that can be used to create better interventions. For instance, researchers and funders increasingly realized that a single discipline alone cannot respond to complex social, health, and environmental problems, as the call for transdisciplinary approaches has highlighted (Cannon et al., 2020). By integrating various perspectives, CBPR does not only augment the research process but also advances greater social purposes, advancing community empowerment. Communities that are themselves participant-observers in research can be placed in a position to challenge structural injustices and prod towards solutions in line with their agendas, winding up with more equitable solutions. Finally, the role played by CBPR in enhancing community resilience cannot be underestimated. In working together in problem-solving and knowledge sharing, CBPR strengthens communities to respond to repeat and emerging challenges. Such a resilience becomes even more important in the case of threats such as climate change, where the impact on regional ecosystems can even increase current health inequities and social inequalities. Participatory research-based interventions not only work towards addressing short-term issues but also promote long-term sustainability by building capacities within communities. Community theatre, as an example, is proposed as a means of engaging residents in dialogue on their marginalization and collectively crafting solutions (Edward et al., 2014). This participatory communication is evidence of how CBPR encourages active engagement and scrutiny of social concerns, ultimately achieving empowered communities that can more effectively navigate their complex worlds (Figure 9.2).

9.1. Historical Context of Community-Based Participatory Research (CBPR)

The evolution of CBPR is firmly rooted in the past of research methods that pursue collaboration and equality between researchers and communities. Historically, there was a past in which research practices isolated power structures and academic institutions collected data from marginalized communities without taking into account their knowledge and experiences. This isolation led to mistrust and cynicism regarding academic research among these communities. As a response, CBPR became a method that actively involves the community members in research activities, hence the sense of ownership and agency. Such collaborative work is essential to decolonize the practice of research so that marginalized individuals can engage and narrate their own stories. This shift towards participatory approaches is also in line with overall social movement campaigns for social justice, representation, and acceptance of local knowledge that are core components of successful CBPR projects (Boeykens et al., 2019). The historical context of CBPR is also better explained through critical examination of cultural and communicative practices in various populations. The traditional Eurocentric paradigm habitually overpowered discussion of knowledge production, excluding the cultural roots and epistemologies that are present within local and indigenous societies. Recent scholarship to our knowledge of communication in varying cultural contexts brings into relief a demand for an epistemological turn that values alternative narratives and knowledge regimes grounded on experience. For instance, in India, communication practices have evolved from a rejection of conventional utilitarian and traditional understandings to a focus on holistic and endogenous solutions respecting local cultures and traditions. Incorporating such knowledge into CBPR ensures that researchers are able to promote culturally contextualized practices that enable communities to set research agendas, and thus, the findings are relevant and empowering (Chaparro et al., 2016). With the growth of CBPR, it has also been influenced by influential waves of scholarship and activism demanding the voice of marginalized individuals be heard in all aspects of research. The historical context of social justice movements, for example, has created a heightened sensitivity to ethical sensibilities necessary in research with vulnerable groups. This has resulted in researchers embracing participatory approaches centered on the everyday realities of community members. Moreover, tools such as participatory action research (PAR) have influenced CBPR strategies by emphasizing co-production of knowledge and collaborative action among community stakeholders. Engaging communities as true partners not only enhances the validity of research results but also facilitates long-term change by linking interventions to realities of most affected populations. Thus, historical evolution in CBPR is a landmark in the ongoing pursuit of just and equitable research approaches (oeykens et al., 2019).

9.1.1. Origins of Participatory Research Methods

The introduction of participatory research methods can be dated back to growing consciousness of constraints associated with traditional research practices. Historically, conventional approaches have privileged researchers' perspectives over the perspectives of the researched populations, and that instilled a disconnect that rendered findings irrelevant. The necessity for methods acknowledging communities' embedded knowledge has compelled the emergence of participatory approaches. This paradigm shift is seen as imperative to achieving research that not only incorporates individuals from various backgrounds but also reflects the interests and values of the various groups, thus making research more meaningful and effective. For CBPR, research methods employed give significant importance to collaboration and co-production of knowledge. The roots of these methodologies lie in other fields, including anthropology, sociology, and public health, where the active participation of community members became core. These methodologies put on the forefront the necessity for cultural interpretation of health and wellbeing, as they acknowledge that each community possesses specific worldviews that condition their experiences. As explained in Hicks et al., (2002), the conceptualization of health within a specific cultural context enhances the dialogue between researchers and members of the community, which ultimately leads to enhanced health interventions. Additionally, the evolution of participatory research has been in tandem with broader social movements that have advocated for democratization and social justice. These have emphasized the intrinsic value of hearing the marginalized and making them part of decision-making. Sanitation and hygiene interventions, for instance, now include participatory methods as part of their core, allowing communities to better engage in behavior change programs (Evans et al., 2010). This is part of a general trend towards empowering local populations by acknowledging respect for their knowledge and enhancing ownership of research results. From this vantage point, the development of participatory research methods reflects a dramatic evolution toward ethical research strategies that focus on community involvement and context knowledge.

9.1.2. Evolution Of Community-Based Participatory Research (CBPR) In Academic And Community Settings

The emergence of CBPR reflects a paradigm shift in the role of researchers within communities and their involvement in the research process. In the past, research has been conducted on societies at their expense, hence the created division between institutions of learning and society. However, with the changes in needs and expectations of society over time, there is increased recognition of the virtues of participatory research methodologies that prioritize contributions and participation by communities. The change not only seeks to increase the relevance of research findings, but it also provides the feeling of ownership to community members. As such, a shift is happening, and technologies such as participatory technologies and digital platforms allow for more participation so that a diverse range of voices have a chance to contribute to knowledge sharing and generation and enhance the community and higher education spaces (Haythornthwaite et al., 2009). University-community partnerships have emerged in recent years as prominent frameworks that help explain the shift in CBPR in academia. Such partnerships bridge the divide between academic learning and practice, particularly in areas such as social work, public health, and environmental science. A good example is the Child Welfare Partnership for Research and Training (CW-PART) and how it represents the effective partnership between a university and the area child welfare agencies. The partnership has the relevance of uniting academic research with community necessity to finally improve social service outcomes. By leveraging federal funding through cooperative efforts, these partnerships illustrate how structured collaboration can yield practical and sustainable benefits for both researchers and the communities they engage with. The CW-PART model epitomizes the potential for CBPR to effect change through shared goals, resources, and expertise (D\u27Andrade et al., 2013). As the landscape of CBPR continues to evolve, it has become ever more crucial to create robust frameworks that encourage ongoing dialogue and reinforce relationships of trust between academic researchers and community stakeholders. The trend has moved in a more participatory direction, in which research is no longer merely an intellectual pursuit but a component of community empowerment. This participatory strategy calls out to community members not just to take part in but also to shape the research agenda, so their specific contexts and experiences are given voice. The use of participatory methodologies, informed by the advent of digital technologies, offers a fluid place for collaboration. Ultimately, these developments bring about a new era in social science and public health research—one of greater accountability, transparency, and equity in its findings, sustaining the principle that involving communities is central to productive scientific research and societal advancement (Haythornthwaite et al., 2009) (Figure 9.3).

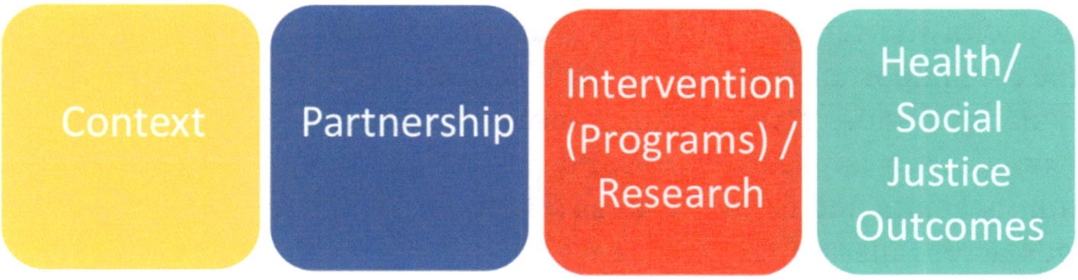

Figure 9.3. Evolution of community-based participatory research (CBPR) in academic and community settings.

Source: https://duckduckgo.com/?q=Evolution+of+CBPR+in+academic+and+community+settings&t=h_&iar=images&iai=https%3A%2F%2Fhsc.unm.edu%2Fpopulation-health%2F_media%2Fphoto-gallery%2Fcpr%2Fcbpr-model2.png.

9.1.3. Key Milestones in the Development of Community-Based Participatory Research (CBPR)

CBPR growth signifies a series of significant steps echoing its essence and practice. The recognition of the prospective benefit of community involvement in public health, particularly in combating epidemics such as HIV, was one of the very first steps. During the second half of the 20th century, coalitions between researchers and affected communities had facilitated unprecedented advances in HIV research, establishing a precedent for collaborative efforts in public health. This early period emphasized the worth of incorporating community voice into research to encourage relevance and usefulness. The guidelines established during this time lay groundwork for scaling up CBPR to various areas of health, and for proving its elasticity and adaptability to conform to the landscape of local communities, a trait still defining successful CBPR work, as outlined in existing literature on its expansion and adoption (Dubé et al., 2020). Another landmark in the development of CBPR occurred through the creation of standardized guidelines and frameworks, emphasizing best practices in community engagement. As researchers began to codify participatory approaches, there was a vast literature emphasizing successes and failures in CBPR methods. The establishment of Good Participatory Practice (GPP) guidelines became focal to describing how researchers approached partnership with communities in mutual respect, equal sharing of power, and listening to the needs of the community. As CBPR took off, it was appreciated that even with available obstacles to participation such as variations in scientific literacy and cultural competency, overcoming these was the key to successful collaboration. The greater focus on surmounting the obstacles enabled a more robust community platform for engagement, facilitating better scrutiny of the co-produced knowledge generated in such partnerships, and subsequently increasing the ongoing development of CBPR approaches (Dubé et al., 2020).

A significant landmark in the application of CBPR is exhibited through the Harvest for Healthy Kids project, demonstrating the co-creation process of the intervention with the community stakeholders. This initiative, intended to increase preschoolers' use of fruits and vegetables through the Head Start program, is a testament to the revolutionary potential of CBPR approaches. Teachers, who were instrumental in assisting in the shaping of the development of the curriculum, ensured that their experience and expertise contributed to the final educational product. Through this participatory process, the curriculum not only incorporated evidence-based practices but also resonated closely with the target community's day-to-day and cultural realities. Such initiatives illustrate how the core importance of community voices is integral to developing health interventions tailored for populations under given circumstances, ultimately leading to more effective research outcomes. By the effective application of CBPR principles, this project illustrates a milestone in fostering community health and demonstrates continuous compliance with the use of participatory research methods across disciplines (Figure 9.4).

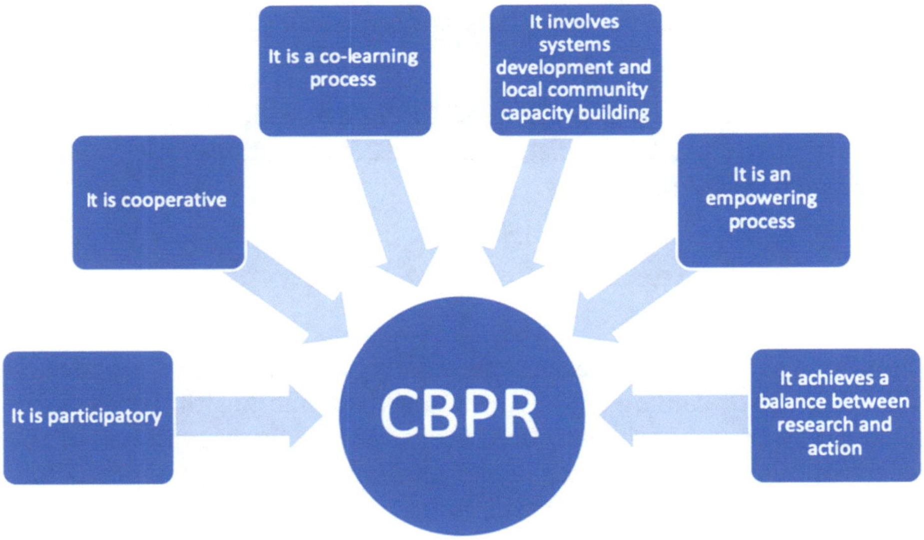

Figure 9.4. Key milestones in the development of community-based participatory research (CBPR).

Source: https://media.springernature.com/lw685/springer-static/image/chp%3A10.1007%2F978-3-030-48277-0_25-2/MediaObjects/496202_0_En_25-2_Fig1_HTML.png.

9.2. Principles of Community-Based Participatory Research (CBPR)

The principles of CBPR are founded on the assumption of having researchers and community people work together, thereby ensuring equity and reciprocal power in the research process. One of the key founding principles of CBPR is the acknowledgment of community knowledge and expertise and necessitates a departure from conventional models of research that have the tendency of disregarding local voices. By valuing the input of the stakeholders in the community, researchers are able to conduct studies that are more responsive and pertinent to the specific issues and needs of the communities. Not only will this enhance the quality and applicability of the research findings, but also the credibility and reciprocity between communities and researchers, and ultimately more sustainable health interventions and outcomes that can be taken up by the community themselves. A key aspect of CBPR is its focus on inclusivity and ethical practices that safeguard vulnerable populations, particularly when there are sensitive topics involved. For example, research into the sexual well-being of young people can be significantly improved by the tenets of CBPR because they open the doors to youth participation and realities in a manner that respects their agency but is also mindful of their vulnerabilities. Mechanisms proposed under the umbrella of CBPR include formalization of youth-friendly mechanisms for consent and working together with local institutions that cater to such youthful populations. In employing these mechanisms, it is ensured that research conducted within the community not only honors the dignity of the community but also meets the ethical standards expected in research as practiced today, thus contributing towards enhanced justice and equality in the conduct of research (Guta et al., 2007). In addition, the ethical implications of CBPR are in lowering the helicopter research model, where communities feel exploited rather than empowered. The model is contrary to the participatory methods adopted by CBPR, where communities are engaged meaningfully throughout the research process. Engaging communities as participants and not objects can contribute significantly towards lowering ethics violations and can instill an ownership attitude over the research outcomes. For instance, in studies conducted with marginalized populations, the researchers are prompted to make participatory methods acceptable that are congruent with community values and address their specific requirements as per CIOMS guidelines and the Denver Principles. Following these guidelines, researchers can optimize an environment in which ethical review procedures are localized, ultimately optimizing the research process and its implications (Brown et al., 2021) (Figure 9.5).

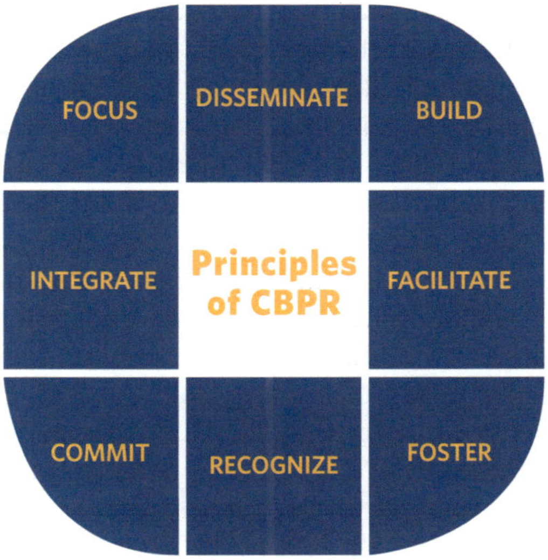

Figure 9.5. Principles of community-based participatory research (CBPR).

Source: https://blogs.ubc.ca/rhsrnbcresearchsupport/files/2022/01/Principles-of-CBPR-1024x1003.png.

9.2.1. Collaborative Partnership Between Researchers and Community Members

The joint researcher-community partnership is a pillar of CBPR, facilitating a model that transcends standard research paradigms. The partnership is characterized by mutual consent to not only address community problems but also to empower the local stakeholders. In such relationships, researchers and stakeholders come together to co-produce knowledge, blending academic rigor with local knowledge to arrive at solutions that are practically viable and culturally relevant. The process involves respect for one another and constant engagement, as both parties navigate the intricacies involved in collaborating. Successful partnerships benefit from having a good model that demarcates roles, duties, and expectations so that the research effectively responds to the needs of the community as well as facilitating scholarly learning. Typically, this partnership strategy builds confidence and sets the stage for continued participation long after a particular research project has concluded. Processes within partnerships often play a primary role in determining the success of community research projects. When members engage with the research process, they bring with them valuable experience and knowledge of living that guide data collection and analysis. Their engagement ensures active participation and ownership in the research findings, which is crucial for the implementation of the decisions derived from them. It has been proven that where partnerships are geared towards member engagement, they build a sense of accountability that enhances the efficacy of the entire project (Lindquist-Grantz et al., 2016). Indicators such as informal judgments of partnership success based on operational partnerships also indicate initial phases of partnership can play a significant role in long-term outcomes. Therefore, fostering a mutual relationship where both the academics and community members contribute inputs can lead to more profound impacts and higher chances of realizing envisaged community-based outcomes. As a prime example of the practical usage of such collaborative frameworks, the experience of the Woman of Faith and Hope (WOFAH) nonprofit organization illustrates the significance of CBPR in addressing community health disparities. In collaboration with La Salle University, WOFAH establishes a sound foundation for educative interventions toward mitigating breast cancer occurrence among Northwest Philadelphias African American community. The partnership is an embodiment of the core values of CBPR, with the programs being sensitively crafted to meet the specific needs of the targeted community. In addition to assisting in the sharing of important health information, the partnership also empowers members of the community with the requisite tools through which they can access healthcare services (Newhall et al., 2013). Therefore, ongoing evaluation of evidence-based programming within academic partnerships ultimately reveals the necessity of keeping programs funded so as to sustain programs with direct impacts on community health, finally justifying the value of collaborative research activities.

9.2.2. Emphasis on Co-learning and Mutual Benefit

Under CBPR, emphasis on co-learning and mutual benefit is a foundation that holds otherwise unequal partnerships between academic researchers and community members together. This democratic approach establishes a context where knowledge is not merely passed on by experts to stakeholders, but instead produced cooperatively by collective experience and diverse perspectives. By engaging community members in the research process, CBPR practitioners legitimize and validate local knowledge so that the research agenda can position itself within the site and circumstances of the community. Such teamwork enhances the validity and utility of research findings, ultimately leading to outcomes that are beneficial to the community as well as the researchers. The scenario of the Community Child Health Network (CCHN) illustrates well the benefits that emerge with a co-learning framework in a CBPR setting. Six salient themes were identified from the qualitative assessment, and from among them, collaboration and perceived benefit were pivotal. When the researchers and community collaborators worked together, they experienced a rich process of learning that shaped their shared knowledge of maternal and child health inequities. Two-way information sharing not only empowered the community members to be research collaborators but also allowed the academic collaborators to develop in-depth contextual understanding that could shape their scientific investigation. The mutual benefit focus therefore undergirds the fundamental goal of CBPR: enhancing health disparities and equipping all the participants with new skills and information translatable to the wider work. For scholars, particularly novices, adopting such behavior to facilitate participation is crucial in times of co-learning. As exemplified in the Community Psychology doctoral students' field experience, embracing traits such as cultural humility, reflexivity, and methodological flexibility fosters a more trusting space for collaboration. These traits enable researchers to approach community engagement with an open mind, opening the door for genuine dialogue and community responsiveness. By putting high emphasis on these traits, researchers maximize their capacity to build sound interpersonal connections with residents of the community and enhance the reciprocities of benefits in CBPR. The learning that arises from such encounters not only enriches each researcher's work but also contributes to continually building soundest practice in community-based study endeavors in upholding the importance of co-learning toward achieving shared goals.

9.2.3. Focus on Social Justice and Equity

The focus on social justice and equity is key in CBPR, as it targets strong involvement of oppressed groups in the research process. Through prioritizing the voices of those typically not heard when making decisions, CBPR seeks to correct the systemic inequalities that exist in society. In this case, the researcher is not a voyeur watching from the outside but is instead a catalytic actor who enables members of the community to define their own problems, define their needs, and work on coming up with solutions. Such an approach to research does not necessarily just make research findings very relevant but also commits the community to ownership and ensures interventions are grounded in the day-to-day realities of the affected community. This equity orientation is important in that it acknowledges social inequalities need to be addressed in order to ensure sustainable change for the benefit of all members of the community. In addition, the guiding principles of CBPR are consistent with the goals of environmental efforts addressing social justice, especially in areas at risk for climate change. The connection between ecological conservation and social justice is best highlighted in studies that are centered on pressing issues such as deforestation, pollution, and access to clean water. As an example, initiatives like community-based waste management and mangrove reforestation illustrate how people's collective action can reap rewards in terms of both environmental restoration and socio-economic dividends. By integrating these elements, as Laudate Deum suggests, scholars are able to enter into on behalf of policies aimed at both environmental sustainability and empowerment of marginalized groups. Both of these priorities reinforce the idea that solutions that work must take account of social setting and involve community members directly in the decision-making process. Using multiple vantage points thus becomes crucial in creating integrated strategies to the complex issues of vulnerable populations (Ingles et al., 2024). In addition to community involvement, CBPR also focuses on the necessities of integrating marginalized voices into broader climate change and social policy governance systems. As the impacts of climate change largely affect marginalized populations, their experience and information need to be made integral to policy-making and planning. This harmonization not only addresses immediate concerns such as food sufficiency and access to safe housing but also promotes long-term safeguarding against climatic disruptions. Engaging marginalized communities in policy-making allows for the integrated understanding of their needs and has a multiplier effect on improving interventions. It resists technocratic approaches generally preferred by academic institutions, which can hinder local knowledge and quotidian reality. By ensuring marginalized perspectives have a role in governance at various levels, thus, CBPR strives to develop more just systems that recognize the interdependence of social justice and sustainability (Perkins et al., 2017) (Figure 9.6).

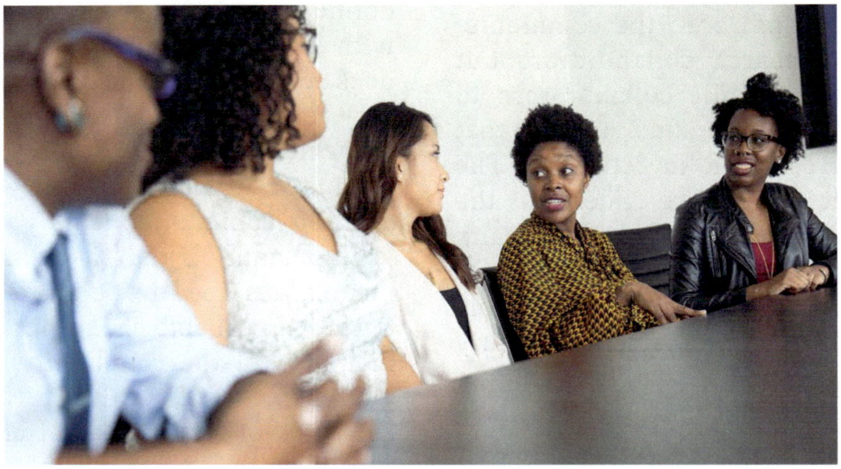

Figure 9.6. Focus on social justice and equity.

Source: https://www.sdfoundation.org/wp-content/uploads/2022/09/sdfnews_raceequityculture1.jpg.

9.3. Methodological Approaches in Community-Based Participatory Research (CBPR)

CBPR employs a wide range of methodological approaches that focus on collaboration between researchers and community members. By incorporating community experiences and voices within the research process, CBPR provides an environment where knowledge is jointly created and not only transferred. The participatory approach guarantees that research findings are not only applicable but also meaningful to real-world situations. It disturbs traditional approaches that have a tendency of excluding the intricate needs of specific communities, instead encouraging approaches that allow stakeholders to engage actively in the research process. By employing CBPR principles, researchers are capable of developing partnership that results in scientific rigor and social utility at the end, thus playing a role in promoting health and providing equal distribution of resources (Becker et al., 2016). The practice-based research networks' contribution demonstrates additional evidence of CBPRs methodological diversity. PBRNs consolidate diverse communities of practice with research academia to solve pressing health questions affecting local populations. The collaborative process leverages the power of both academic expertise and community knowledge in creating action-oriented research findings. Through the application of CBPR principles via PBRN platforms, researchers are able to develop sustainable partnerships that optimize implementation and impacts within tangible settings. As such networks expand, they increase the collaborative spirit required in the health disparities response as well as community resilience building, making the research more inclusive but evidence-base focused (Becker et al., 2016). The integration of social epidemiology elements adds a new layer of complexity to methodology approaches in CBPR. The emphasis on social determinants of health and recognition of systemic inequalities place at the forefront the need for research designs that are participatory and inclusive. By imagining a model with voice at the center, researchers can make ways toward social inclusion that are greater than the academy's disciplinary boundaries. The union of social epidemiology, CBPR, and ICT brings new possibilities to expand people's participation and achieve equitable outcomes. This inter-disciplinary effort is directed at empowering communities through endowing them with tools and resources to actively engage in research activities, hence making research a participatory process that includes in it the aspirations and needs of the populations whose lives it is aimed at impacting (Figure 9.7).

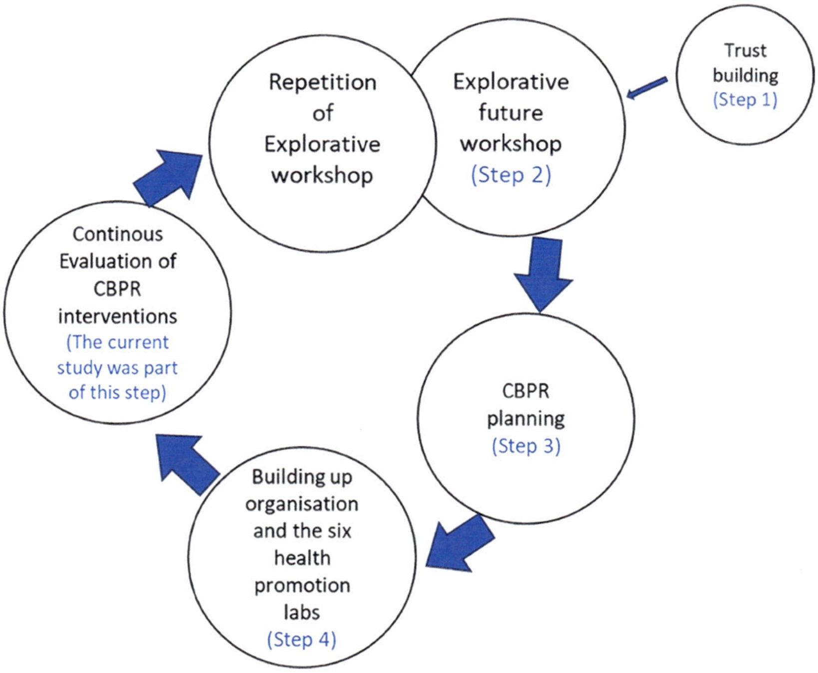

Figure 9.7. Methodological approaches in community-based participatory research (CBPR).

Source: https://www.frontiersin.org/files/Articles/997329/fpubh-10-997329-HTML/image_m/fpubh-10-997329-g001.jpg.

9.3.1. Qualitative and Quantitative Research Methods

The combination of qualitative and quantitative research approaches is crucial in CBPR to facilitate integrated understanding and participation in the community. Qualitative approaches, usually encompassing in-depth interviews, focus groups, and participant observations, provide a closer examination of the stories, experiences, and values of the community. These methods enable scholars to capture the complexity and nuance of communal relationships, revealing cultural understandings and social structures that go unnoticed in quantitative data. As an illustration, participatory workshops have effectively used qualitative approaches to elicit community input, thereby ensuring that research realistically reflects participants' everyday lives. Such methods not only empower the community members but also enrich the research by allowing for different perspectives that contribute to the contextual validity of findings (Hudson-Smith et al., 2016). Quantitative methods, however, provide a much-needed framework upon which the findings from qualitative analysis can be constructed. Through the use of systematic data collection mechanisms, such as statistics and surveys, quantitative approaches allow researchers to measure patterns, test hypotheses, and establish variable relationships within the context of the community.

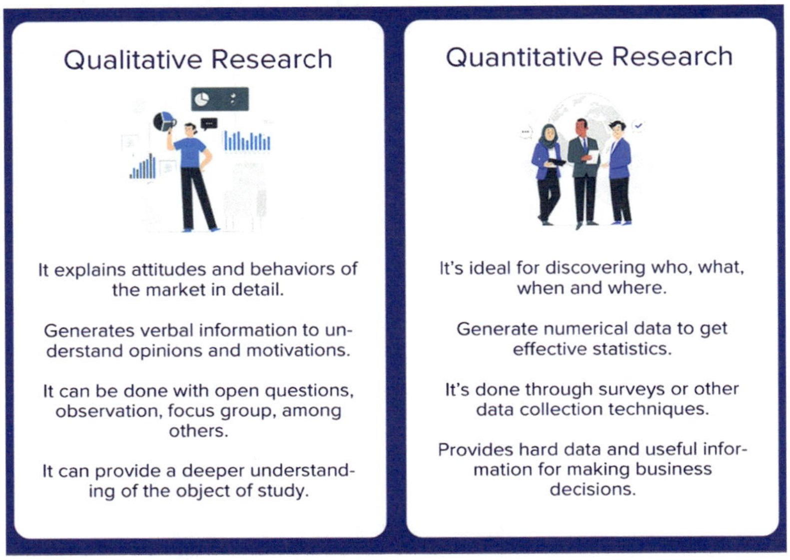

Figure 9.8. Qualitative and quantitative research methods.

Source: https://www.questionpro.com/blog/wp-content/uploads/2018/03/differences-qualitative-vs-quantitative.jpg.

For example, a qualitative and quantitative approach was employed in a study conducted in Khayelitsha, Cape Town, to identify the reasons for hypertension and diabetes among members within the community. This blending of methodologies ensured a more robust comprehension of the health issue, which revealed major insights into economic constraints and cultural determinants of lifestyle. This blending of evidence not only facilitated a more concentrated analytical context but also enhanced reliability and validity of the findings, rendering them actionable for public health interventions (Bradley et al., 2007). Also, combined qualitative and quantitative approaches in CBPR allow for a two-way relationship between community members and researchers. The collaborative approach permits joint evaluation that informs planning as well as the implementation of interventions. For instance, qualitative findings can be used to guide the construction of quantitative tools such that they are culturally valid and appropriate to the daily realities of the community. Consequently, effective CBPR initiatives that effectively incorporate these methods develop local agency since community health workers and members are not merely study participants but active co-collaborators in the process. The collaboration develops trust and establishes the community's interest in research results, demonstrating effective CBPR as so much more than the typical bounds of academic inquiry and rather developing meaningful, actionable change (Hudson-Smith et al., 2016) (Figure 9.8).

9.3.2. Data Collection Techniques Used in Community-Based Participatory Research (CBPR)

Data collection methods employed in CBPR are a key factor in ensuring that the research reflects the needs and perspectives of the community. The most effective among them is qualitative data collection by means of interviews, focus groups, and forums with the community. Such methods facilitate unstructured discussion, and members freely converse in their own words about their experiences and issues. These qualitative approaches not only enable better understanding of issues at the community level but also lay the foundation for two-way knowledge and learning between the community members and the researchers.

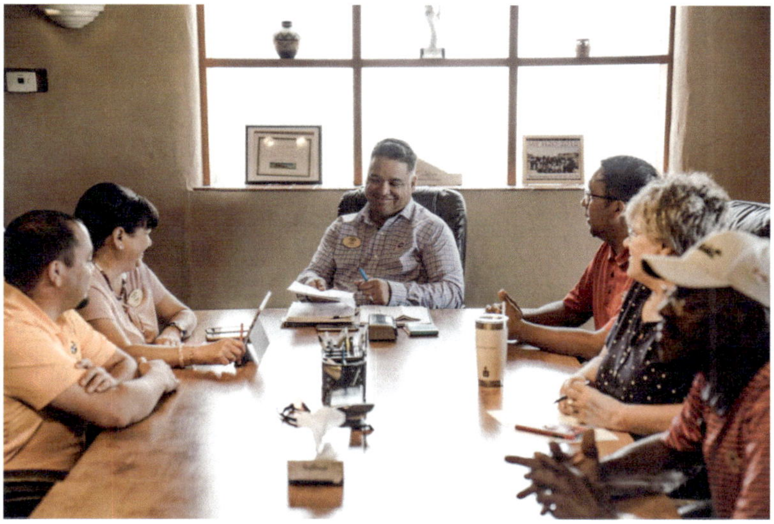

Figure 9.9. Data collection techniques used in community-based participatory research (CBPR).

Source: https://www.communitypsychology.com/wp-content/uploads/2020/04/people-sitting-around-wooden-table-1325766-scaled.jpg.

Through concentrating on local experiences and voices, qualitative approaches in CBPR help in fostering a sense of ownership as well as investment in the research process, leading to more applicable and relevant outcomes in the end. Apart from qualitative methods, quantitative data collection also constitutes a critical element of CBPR in that it provides an added vision that can help enhance the understanding of the dynamics of the community. Surveys and structured questionnaires are common tools in this context, whereby researchers can be able to get quantifiable information on specific variables deemed pertinent to the health, well-being, and socio-economic status of the community. CBPR obviously benefits from a mixed-methods approach, in which qualitative results are utilized to guide the design of quantitative instruments to improve the cultural acceptability of the questions asked. Moreover, the quantification of the qualitative evidence aids in the identification of trends, pre-tests policy recommendations, and illustrates the impact of interventions. This two-stage process of data collection not only improves the research but also improves the evidence base for community health initiatives. New data collection techniques, such as participatory mapping and digital storytelling, are being crafted by the CBPR process, enhancing community residents' participation and inclusiveness. Participatory mapping enables individuals to represent spatially their perceptions of community strengths, barriers, and opportunities, generating mutual understanding among diverse stakeholders. The technique facilitates local engagement while generating informative spatial data to inform community development projects. Similarly, digital storytelling allows community members to narrate their experiences through multimedia media, allowing for emotional engagement and wider community participation. These new methods demonstrate the way in which CBPR can revolutionize and improve through engagement of new technologies and participatory methods, ultimately enriching the data collection process and creating more efficient outcomes for the transformation of communities (Ahmed et al., 2013; Lie et al., 2009) (Figure 9.9).

9.3.3. Ethical Considerations in Community-Based Participatory Research (CBPR) Practices

Ethics are of utmost importance in CBPR in order to ensure that the research has positive effects on both the community and the research participants engaged in information sharing. The interdisciplinary nature of CBPR allows multiple visions to be balanced in overcoming ethical challenges, primarily in bridging the complexities of informed consent and participatory community. Whereas scholars balance research aims with needs in the community, conflicts inevitably occur, primarily when formal review processes prioritize institutional workings over shared decision-making. This calls for ongoing discussions that emphasize the primacy of practical wisdom or phronesis in research activities, whereby ethical issues are a focal point shared by research teams leading to rich solutions (Carmichael et al., 2013). Such dialogue can foster an environment of trust whereby ethical values are not merely adhered to but adapted to respond to the unique culture and social environments of the groups involved. Furthermore, ethics here also involve engaging marginalized populations such as children and young people who are not typically included in dominant research. Engaging young people within disaster-exposed communities, for instance, opens up the promise of empowering youth to the strength of these youth and other spheres of research as well as policy for their plight. Such a participatory method demands of researchers that they be confronted by power relationships that may get in the way of serious youth involvement. Through arts-based methods, researchers can create spaces for inclusive dialogue that respect young people's voice and, ultimately, enhance the validity and meaning of research findings. The ethical imperative is one of permitting young people to build the narrative of their experience and therefore a sense of agency in a place where this is crucial post-disaster (Cox et al., 2016).

These practices ensure that the research process is not only ethical but also transformative to the community participants. Respecting community knowledge and local expertise is one of the other ethical foundations of CBPR practices. Researchers generally come to these collaborations with preconceived notions of what good data is; nonetheless, the proof is in realizing and respecting local wisdom deviating from academic norms. This necessitates a move from conventional top-down methods, clearing the path for a more equal dialogue in which community members become actively engaged in the research process. Ethical transparency regarding the intended results and possible contribution of the research is also necessary to foster trust and allow meaningful participation by the community members. Through establishing environments within which community voices inform research agendas, CBPR legitimates local realities while also enhancing the quality and applicability of research findings. Ultimately, in the long term, addressing these ethical issues has the result of reinforcing the collaboration between researchers and communities, ultimately yielding improved and culturally responsive interventions (Figure 9.10).

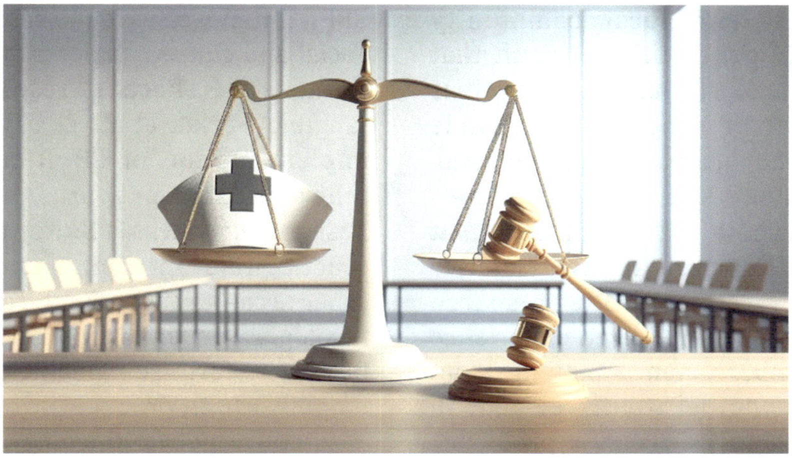

Figure 9.10. Ethical considerations in community-based participatory research (CBPR) practices.

Source: https://cdn.sanity.io/images/tq8eww4k/production/55f5a3feb5da0850ceaf286dc54a1da09b46b2a7-1792x1024.webp?w=1792&q=100&auto=format.

9.4. Benefits of Community-Based Participatory Research (CBPR)

CBPR has a number of benefits, primarily being greater community engagement and empowerment. Through active engagement in the research process by the community, CBPR instills a sense of ownership of the research outcomes and the interventions that come with it. This collaboration ensures that research direction is in response to community needs and priorities. For instance, when local residents are engaged in problem identification such as hunger, they can impact the research questions and methods utilized, and therefore enhance the relevance and usefulness of the results. Community projects developed by such collaboration, as observed by the release of monthly vouchers for better availability of local food, have higher community satisfaction and involvement in healthy dietary practices, portraying how CBPR can best mobilize resources for community development (Constantian et al., 2015). CBPR also adds better coordination among researchers and communities, encouraging a reciprocal exchange of information beyond typical academic fields. This dynamic collaboration not only enhances the research data, but it also enhances the capacity of the two partners to solve complex social problems together. In the social epidemiology system, the use of principles of CBPR reveals the potential of research to be informative and transformative. By emphasizing social inclusion and equity, CBPR establishes a mechanism through which the voices of the people are amplified. This approach can help bridge social epidemiology findings to effective action that is more relevant in community contexts, hence closing systemic gaps (Allen et al., 2019). The integration is indicative of the value of bridging standard scientific methods with local community grassroots activism, generating research that is both action-oriented and empowering. It is the final contribution of using CBPR to include policy making and advocacy. By creating solid, community-grounded data, CBPR provides evidence that is usable to inform policy at various levels. The democratic and collaborative character of CBPR ensures the research findings accurately reflect the lived experience of community members, hence making it an effective tool of public debate. As evident in research responding to food access problems, community partners can use such information to push for policy interventions where they are most needed, thus tackling underlying causes of issues such as food insecurity. Additionally, the participatory process invites communities to take action in engaging policymakers, so that conversation occurs to ensure community health needs are addressed. This synthesis of research with advocacy for policy makes the potential for creating long-term change higher, highlighting CBPR as a vehicle for bridging the gap between academia and successful community action (Constantian et al., 2015).

9.4.1. Enhanced Relevance and Applicability of Research Findings

Research results become useful and relevant to a significant extent when the stakeholders are meaningfully engaged throughout the whole research process, a feature of CBPR. By facilitating partnerships between members of the community and researchers, CBPR ensures that the research focuses on real problems confronted by the communities. Besides enhancing the contextual origin of the data's, this initiative enhances community ownership of findings. This hands-on approach can lead to more effective dissemination measures to ensure that products of research are not left in academic environments but instead utilized to spur change and action at the community level. As reflected in current research, the strength of CBPR is that it can ground research in the specific social and cultural aspects of communities, and so make the effects of research findings more tangible(Becker et al., 2016). Furthermore, the implementation of CBPR concepts can make other research networks, like Practice-Based Research Networks (PBRNs), focused on applying practice-relevant topics to public health and other areas stronger. By the application of CBPR ideologies in such collaborations, researchers can be able to form sustainable collaborations that empower both practice partners and academia. This convergence not only guarantees the co-production of knowledge but also its conversion into actionable practices in communities. The ability of PBRNs to incorporate multiple stakeholder perspectives gives strength to the research process and renders the findings more tangible and supportive of health gains at different levels. Consequently, CBPR is a central model that strengthens the connection between research efforts and the continuously evolving needs of community stakeholders(D'Haeyer et al., 2012). The impacts of increased relevance and utility of research findings extend beyond mere participation; they have practical ramifications towards community resilience and adaptation. Thus, as observed, communities find it easier to adapt to natural resources as well as asserting their rights when they participate as co-researchers. Successful Integrated Natural Resource Management (INRM) is a testament to this complementarity in that local knowledge and traditions are included together with scientific research so that the solutions are both scientifically sound and culturally appropriate.

Through the use of insights from the community, CBPR upgrades the management processes hence contributing towards the greater sustainability of resources. These partnerships create more resilience within communities, allowing them to withstand external pressures and sustain their livelihoods. Consequently, the legitimacy of CBPR activities not only optimizes research influence but also galvanizes constructive change at the community level, ultimately leading to public benefit(Becker et al., 2016).

9.4.2. Empowerment of Community Members and Stakeholders

The empowerment of stakeholders and community members forms a central component of CBPR that enables more democratic and inclusive research. Through active involvement of the community voices in the research process, CBPR encourages ownership and responsibility among the participants, leading to results that are more effective and relevant. Such collaboration of various stakeholders like local government agencies, non-profit organizations, and even the community members is encouraged through this approach. This participation not only enables the ability of communities to voice their needs but also improves capacity and confidence in individuals, ending up enhancing their ability to address local challenges. This empowerment is important since research that reflects community priorities has a greater likelihood of leading to sustainable projects that communicate more strongly with the populations that they aim to benefit, resulting in a healthier and more equitable community overall (Asfahani et al., 2024).

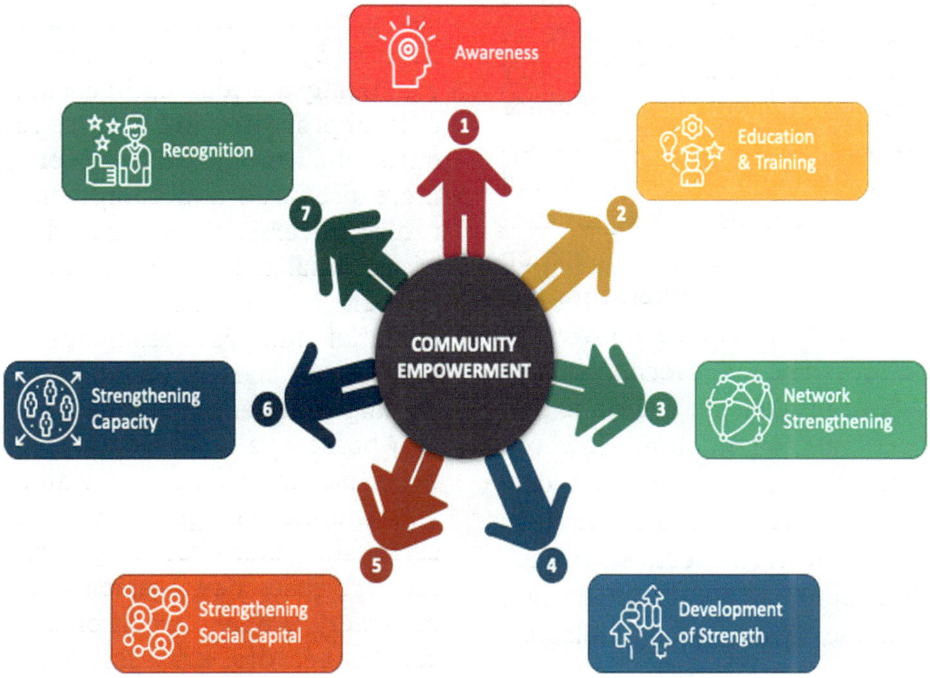

Figure 9.11. Empowerment of community members and stakeholders.

Source: https://cdn.sketchbubble.com/pub/media/catalog/product/optimized1/c/2/c2cab30db6c57cd885aec91b2012ccd7916030ff275d6450ca735a776edcea1c/community-empowerment-mc-slide1.png.

Further, strong empowerment processes are an essential part of identifying and taking advantage of community capacities and assets. As outlined in CBPR models, activating local strengths—social networks, cultural knowledge, or economic capital—enables communities to plan and implement solutions that are meaningful in context. For instance, the utilization of Asset-Based Community Development (ABCD) approaches not only focuses on community capabilities but also builds resilience and autonomy among participants. Empowerment in this context means shifting the emphasis from needs assessments to the recognition of already existing abounding resources within a community. Empowering stakeholders to engage actively in decision-making and research helps make the collective agency increasingly potent and continues to build a more sustainable and autonomous community dynamics (Asfahani et al., 2024). The significance of empowerment in tourism and other industry management further highlights the significance of involvement in governance procedures. ernance in tourism, elaborated udies, indicates the significant participation from the population icy-making and implementation. ocal stakeholders be allowed to discussions on governance, they able of influencing decisions that ffect their communities. However, cates that the majority of local ck the resources and capabilities ecome involved effectively in such processes so that there is little empowerment on political, economic, social, and psychological levels. Through the rectification of such power imbalances and enhanced participatory capability of local institutions, CBPR can assist in empowering a more balanced governance system that recognizes and is willing to incorporate community needs and ideas, thereby facilitating sustainable tourism and development projects that are of benefit to all parties involved (Figure 9.11).

iatives
d Training
ms
ostering Local
eadership
ging Technology

9.4.3. Strengthening of Community Capacity and Resilience

Strengthening of community capacity and resilience forms an essential part of CBPR's framework. CBPR emphasizes mutual learning, cooperation, and active member involvement in the research process. Active involvement lies at the heart not only of fostering ownership but also of enabling communities to find and leverage their internal capacities and resources. These collaborative approaches enhance social networks and community trust, making the community more resistant to adversity. For instance, resource- and training-based programs like those prioritized in the Resilient Baton Rouge project demonstrate that targeted effort can expand local service provision and local health. By aligning research agendas with community agendas, CBPR ensures a full picture of local processes and ensures resilience of the onset of adversity, enabling communities to be more prepared and competent to encounter future adversities. Second, the participation of marginalized group members, particularly women, in decision-making and research is essential to improve resilience in communities. It is not only significant because women possess varying experiences and data but also because they possess valuable local ecological and social expertise. In the case of water management and climate change adaptation, it has been established that effective governance relies on the participatory engagements of all components of society. Women, traditionally a minority in such endeavors, are essential to sustainable resource management and adaptation. By ensuring their engagement, CBPR can enhance collective community capacity to address prominent environmental issues and respond to climate disruption. This representation results in a more representative community dialogue that enhances adaptive capacity in the long term and promotes more sustainable action. Finally, the implementation of people-empowering education programs can also enhance community capacity through enhanced awareness and involvement. As has been the case in some projects, such as the Sister Watersheds project, environmental education provides a foundation for the participation and mobilization of people at the grassroots level. Through offering people information about climate change and resource management, these programs empower individuals with a better-informed view that allows them to stake their claims and effect positive change. This capacity development approach not only addresses present problems but also fosters long-term resilience by constructing solid community relationships and cooperative networks. Granting space for dialogue and cooperative learning enables communities to fit strategies to suit their contexts. Therefore, CBPR not only constructs individual and collective capacity but also fosters a resilient system through which communities can survive, even thrive, amidst adversity (Figure 9.12).

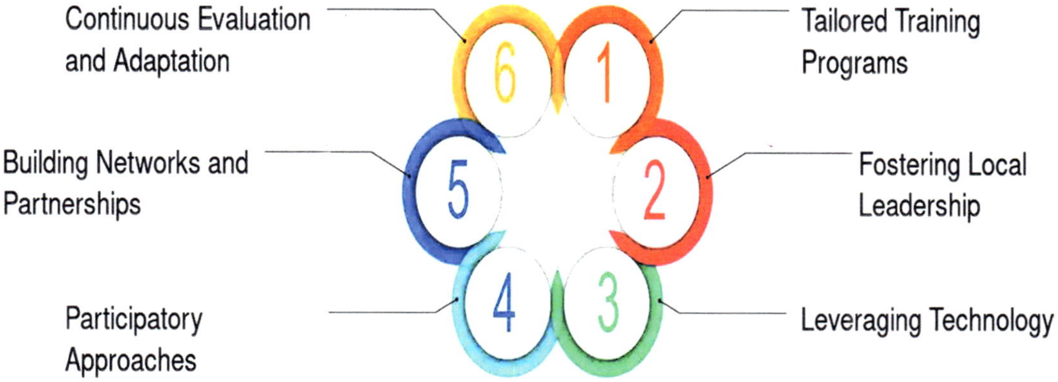

Figure 9.12. Strengthening of community capacity and resilience.

Source: https://fastercapital.co/i/Capacity-building--Building-Resilience--Strengthening-Communities-through-Capacity-Development--Strategies-for-Effective-Capacity-Building-Initiatives.webp.

9.5. Challenges and Limitations of Community-Based Participatory Research (CBPR)

CBPR faces an array of formidable challenges that are likely to impede its efficacy and outcomes. One of the major challenges is in consolidating conflicting stakeholder views. While as much as possible, the involvement of local communities is all about CBPR, the inherent heterogeneity of community perspectives is likely to create tensions that hamper consensus-building. This issue is chronic whenever the research objectives conflict with those of the community, as usual in contributing to power imbalances that exclude some voices. Furthermore, the construction of efficient communication channels between the participants in the community and the researchers is crucial but mostly fraught with miscommunication in terms of words and meaning. As being the focal point of most studies on citizen participation in smart cities initiatives, weighing the scale of participation against relevance continues to be a central issue. Addressing these communication and alignment issues is central to optimizing the potential of CBPR's collaborative model (Barker et al., 2018). Another significant limitation of CBPR is the at times complex logistics of sustaining long-term partnerships among researchers and community organizations. Some of the costs of these include high turnover rates of community leaders or changing organizational priorities that disrupt ongoing research efforts and undermine the foundation of trust that enables successful collaboration. In addition, funding cycles can introduce another level of complication into such partnerships; researchers can have difficulty securing stable sources of funding for community-based programs. This situation is starkly different from the more sequential procedural environments typically confronted with traditional research practice. The shared leadership and co-ownership focus of CBPR models can also lead to fuzzy lines of control, which can make managing the project an issue. Efficient measures should thus address such logistical problems to enhance project continuity and stakeholder involvement (Habron et al., 2009). Outcomes evaluation of CBPR is also a challenge that can limit its potential. Traditional markers of success fail to capture the nuanced changes brought about through community involvement. Quantitative measures may not reflect the tensions and complexities of community empowerment, social cohesion, and relationship dynamics that emanate from participatory processes. Consequently, researchers are often left with limited ability to deliver conclusive evidence of the benefits of CBPR, which is critical in persuading stakeholders and funding agencies to continue investing in it. The intricacy is also amplified by the call for robust ethical considerations, as the participatory nature of the research requires a close adherence to representation and reportage fairness considerations. To take care of these complexities, researchers have to develop innovative evaluation frameworks that bring together qualitative and quantitative approaches, mirroring greater society's influence of CBPRs more accurately (Barker et al., 2018; Habron et al., 2009).

9.5.1. Power Dynamics Between Researchers and Community Members

Power relationships between researchers and community members in the context of CBPR play a tremendous role in shaping the process and outcome of research studies. The spirit behind this collaborative approach is built on the consensus that community partners should exercise considerable influence over all aspects of a research project, ranging from design to application of findings. In spite of this, researchers are sometimes unable to engage with community members, particularly marginalized populations, in fruitful ways. Power imbalances may sabotage these relationships, causing community partners to feel undervalued or disenfranchised, which in turn impacts the richness and value of research produced. According to recent argumentation in the field, bridging these gaps in power is central to creating partnerships that are equitable and serve to augment the research's impact and ensure that concerns and voices of people at the community level are brought to the forefront (Gagnon et al., 2017). Power relations are also made more complex by the intersection of the academic authority with community knowledge, something that can generate discursive tensions antithetical to collaborative CBPR culture. Researchers generally operate from a position of institutional power, a position that frequently produces a disequilibrium that shuts down community voices or overlooks local knowledge that can substantively contribute to research. From a Foucauldian viewpoint, it is apparent that these power asymmetries are not static but rather are dynamic forces that recursively build interactions in research contexts. As with recent writings, it is important that researchers recognize and address these imbalances throughout the process of doing research to counterbalance the threats of oppressive practice in the guise of empowerment (Hanson et al., 2016). Open discussion of these tensions can lay the ground for better balance and more ethical participation in research partnerships. In order to improve the power disparities of CBPR, researchers can employ participatory techniques that are designed to eliminate hierarchies and promote mutual engagement. Techniques such as participatory forums, photo-voice programs, and story circle discussions have proved useful in generating correctives to these power disparities. These strategies not only allow community members to narrate their own accounts and add their own contributions but also provide researchers with better information on local realities and needs. By engaging community participants in the research process actively and respecting their work, researchers have the ability to foster a more inclusive setting that encourages mutual ownership of the project. Eventually, as power relations are consciously reflected on and rearranged, the chance for transformational, impactful research grows, only serving to benefit the academic and community research collaborators (Gagnon et al., 2017; Hanson et al., 2016) (Figure 9.13).

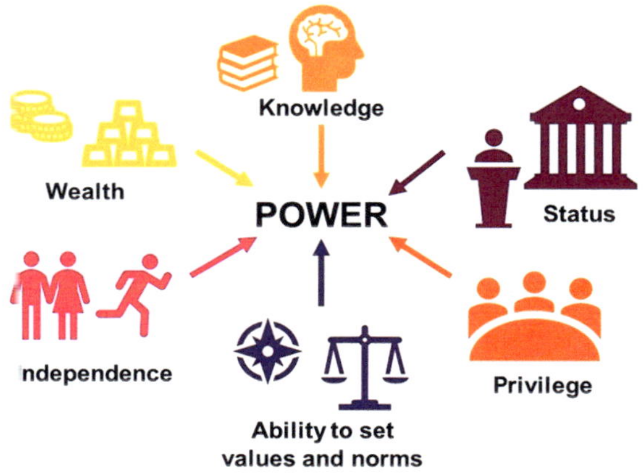

Figure 9.13. Power dynamics between researchers and community members.

Source: https://www.thinknpc.org/wp-content/uploads/2019/04/Power-Ds-e1554805358866.jpg.

9.5.2. Resource Constraints and Funding Issues

Resource shortages and funding issues exert significant impacts on the implementation of CBPR, particularly in limited resource settings. Participatory projects entail not just the observance of community participation but also significant amounts of money to maintain in-depth fieldwork and facilitate ongoing communication. For instance, while research was conducted in two slums of Bangalore, India, there were various challenges that emerged due to underfunding, restricting their presence in the community and earning people's trust over time. The requirement to engage with numerous stakeholders and adapt in light of the changing needs of the different communities demonstrates the disadvantage of the conventional models of funding that center on inflexible timelines and defined results. Without adequate funding, the iterative and exploratory nature of CBPR can be undermined and the benefit of effective participatory involvement lost, further diminishing the impact of the research findings (Meershoek et al., 2018). Furthermore, socio-cultural processes in resource-poor contexts further complicate funding issues in CBPR projects. Language issues and cultural differences create communication challenges and affect participation among community stakeholders throughout the research. These limitations are not mere logistical in nature but relate directly to the viability and sustainability of the project. As highlighted in many studies, appropriate involvement necessitates funds to facilitate translation, interpretation, and culturally sensitive approaches, which are often left out of financial planning. Thus, researchers are then faced with an operating environment where costs constrain the utilization of participatory methods on a sufficient basis. The need for funding strategies that acknowledge and incorporate these socio-cultural subtleties is essential to fostering genuine partnership and achieving enduring change within populations

(N/A, 2012). Lastly, it is critical to reflect on the mechanisms by which institutional frameworks have a tendency to exert constraints on fund disbursements, again hindering the landscape of CBPR. Funding agencies predominantly prefer projects of fixed scope and outcome, inadvertently compromising the adaptive and emergent nature of community engagement research. This inflexibility can create a disconnection between funded research and community priorities, resulting in a mismatch that hinders collaborative work. To address this, mounting pressure is being placed on reconceptualizing funding models to accommodate the fluid, dynamic nature of CBPR. An emphasis on flexibility in study design and funding expectations may facilitate a more responsive approach, allowing researchers to better respond to community needs and facilitate active involvement. By being in a position to tackle these key funding issues, researchers are better placed to develop more impactful CBPR projects that truly reflect and respond to the voices of the communities (Meershoek et al., 2018) (Figure 9.14).

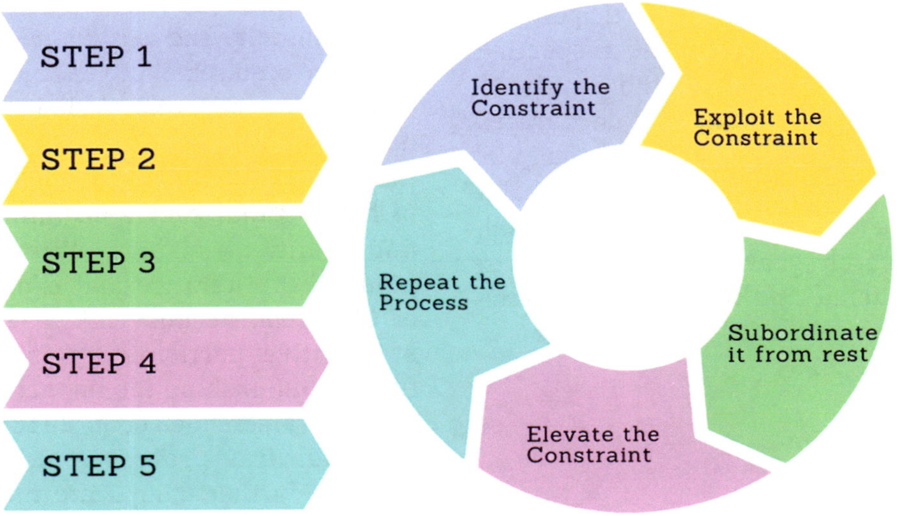

Figure 9.14. Resource constraints and funding issues.

Source: https://lh7-us.googleusercontent.com/dhntuA5-zXRACVKwxbkagGJa2QfdwwPNGt_5PnG0em0qcVB7ou_9003JzOzHZMq-CSumHdlLPIsXxyfE9nBooGd8FT_Upj4Od6bdUys3HpP69qtb_jsd4nAU8hGXXXqNxn6ecNE0E9yx6x83QBj_ncs.

9.5.3. Potential for Conflicting Interests and Priorities

In CBPR, the potential for conflicting interests and priorities among stakeholders is a significant challenge. With different stakeholders partaking in the research activity—ranging from academic researchers to people in the community—their personal interests and goals can become disparate. This disparity can be in terms of different expectations from the research outcome, the methodology used, and resource deployment. Therefore, finding a middle ground becomes essential. The researchers have to navigate these differences dexterously to encourage teamwork and create trust among stakeholders. The need to handle such conflicting interests is highlighted through evidence from transdisciplinary studies, which illustrate that priority conflicts and communication issues can interfere with project implementation, thereby making the research goals more complex and limiting potential benefits to the community (Fang et al., 2020). In addition, successful conflict resolution mechanisms are essential in facilitating effective listening to all voices within CBPR. Unifying diverse perspectives is of highest priority but results in causing conflicts as stakeholders need to reconcile their respective or common interests. Applying participatory planning tools, as indicated through literature, the authors can delineate stakeholder interests systematically, thereby building a systemic approach towards resolving conflicts (Ananda et al., 2010). This facilitates the stakeholder needs to be prioritized and ranked, making it possible to have an environment that can sustain compromises. Through communication as community researchers talk to each other, the potential for building mutual understanding and collaborative decision-making can yield innovative solutions that benefit multiple interests while pushing forward the central research agenda. Lastly, effective CBPR activities hinge on continuous assessment of mechanisms for stakeholder engagement and resolution of ensuing conflict. The strengthening of solid trust-based relationship building is essential; however, this is frequently compromised by incessant competing priorities. Continuous reflective analysis of the collaborative process can help raise recurring difficulties surrounding diverging interests. In cultures where there are several groups with varying goals in terms of the implications of research, models like multiple criteria decision analysis are beneficial to use (Ananda et al., 2010). These models not only describe priority but also empower stakeholders by providing an open forum for the expression of preference. Through such structured engagement, CBPR can facilitate a more just decision-making process that is able to encompass multiple interests as it strives to achieve the collective goals set by the community (Figure 9.15).

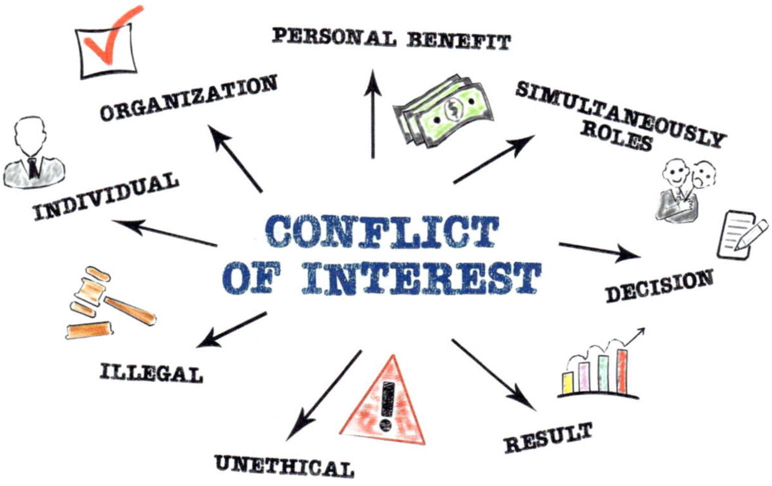

Figure 9.15. Potential for conflicting interests and priorities.

Source: https://research.sdsu.edu/research_affairs/conflict_of_interest/coi_pic.jpg.

9.6. Case Studies of Successful Community-Based Participatory Research (CBPR) Projects

Successful case studies in CBPR emphasize the significance of keeping communities involved as active partners in all phases of the research process. An excellent example is the Fairfield,

Connecticut, Ecological Screen project, which made stakeholder participation central. Through public workshops and surveys, researchers ensured that members' needs and views were considered when designing the projects results. The participatory design process employed was not only transparent but also fostered a sense of high ownership by the participants, thus enhancing the community's active involvement in the success of the projects. The above case illustrates the way holistic participatory methods can lead to effective, community-driven solutions to local environmental concerns that help enhance the significance of CBPR in achieving significant change in the community (Stewart et al., 2017). An equally strong argument can be presented for the Wolcott Park project in West Hartford, Connecticut. It epitomizes the power of using a mixed methods approach in measuring participatory design. In collaboration with social scientist Dr. Miriah Russo Kelly, the researchers employed qualitative and quantitative methods to measure the projects participatory dimensions effectively. The projects incorporated public views through surveys, which provided reliable data on participant satisfaction and participation in decision-making processes. By combining approaches, the assessment not only provided more tangible results but also showed the way that multiple viewpoints could result in better design solutions. This example is a demonstration of how the use of CBPR can strengthen communities while making certain that research is adapted to their special needs and dreams (Stewart et al., 2017). By the observations of non-governmental organizations (NGOs) and capacity building, case studies indicate that it is crucial to connect developmental initiatives with marginalized groups' interests. NGOs labor in these communities frequently, but studies indicate that such efforts are compromised by lacking interactivity with the locals' voices. For instance, by keeping residents out of housing project planning, the benefits promised can be undermined, leading to ineffective effects. Successful NGOs that are practicing CBPR methods take extra effort to build self-sustaining capacity by including community feedback in decision-making. Through such, not only is the appropriateness of the interventions maximized but also a higher degree of linkage is created between communities and NGOs serving them. Finally, these types of cases remind us that participatory processes are vital for obtaining long-term, positive impacts on marginalized populations.

9.6.1. Health Interventions in Underserved Communities

Carrying out health interventions among underserved communities is a key opportunity to address at-level inequities and improve overall health outcomes. At the core is CBPR, which involves community members directly in each aspect of the research process. This approach not only empowers community members but also renders intervention culturally sensitive and contextually relevant. By accessing local knowledge and addressing determined needs, CBPR surmounts barriers typically felt in traditional approaches to research, thus creating avenues for more sustainable health interventions. The evidence for the efficacy of CBPR in facilitating health intervention speaks volumes about its transformative capacity. This community involvement leads to culturally appropriate programs addressing their own unique health concerns, ultimately creating lasting improvements in health and closing the gap between research findings and community health practice (Ayoola et al., 2015). Addressing crucial health disparities, particularly with the case of obesity and related chronic disease, interventions with specific groups can be very effective. African-Americans possess among the United States' highest rates of obesity, which create elevated chronic disease risk factors. Interventions that are specially designed to operate from community settings, including the church, have been effective in the promotion of healthier living. They consider the influential role churches play as community institutions of trust, thereby promoting maximum participation and long-term health promotion participation. Literature emphasizes the importance of respecting sociocultural dynamics and integrating these into health programming. Church leadership in collaboration with health educators during intervention planning increases the possibility of introducing sustainable changes, with a demonstration of a model of improved community health intervention (Mbe and Kougang Anne, 2017). Furthermore, findings of CBPR show that continued involvement requires acknowledging the cultural beliefs held by members within a community about health matters, such as obesity. By working to build genuine partnerships, health educators can create interventions that not only work to shift behavior but also respect and accept the values and beliefs of the community. This integrated strategy does not only guarantee that programs yield short-term benefits but also set the stage for continuous health education and advocacy. As communities actively influence the research agenda and intervention designs, they tend to own the health outcomes, which culminates in greater societal gains. Moreover, such achievements can be replicated as models in future studies, demonstrating the importance of long-term collaboration and the use of cultural and spiritual resources available in diverse communities (Ayoola et al., 2015) (Figure 9.16).

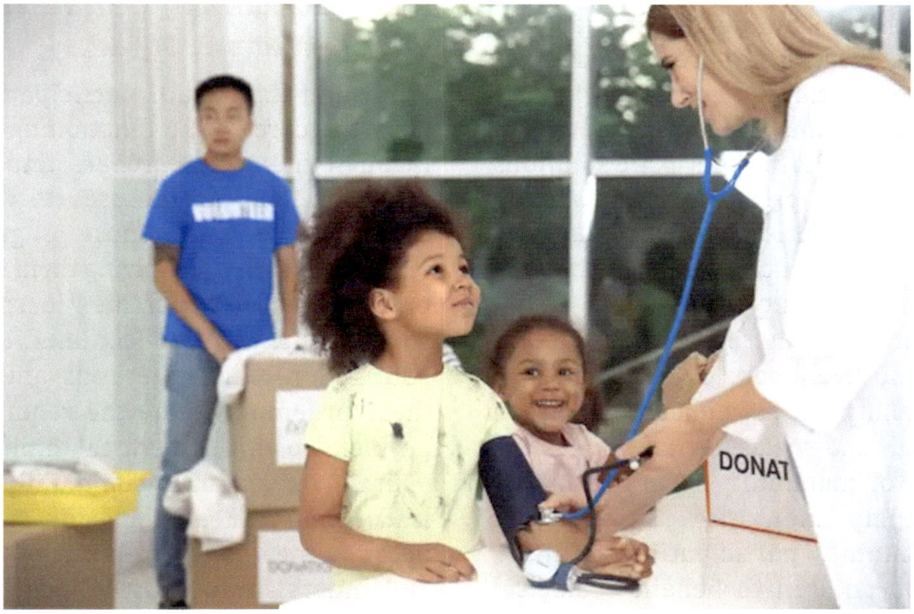

Figure 9.16. Health interventions in underserved communities.

Source: https://flawlessend.com/wp-content/uploads/2023/07/Healthcare-for-Underserved-Communities.webp.

9.5.2. Environmental Justice Initiatives

The integration of environmental justice initiatives into the framework of CBPR is critical to addressing the disproportionate socio-economic impacts of environmental degradation. In the majority of communities, particularly marginalized ones, the burden of environmental emergencies such as pollution, deforestation, and climatic catastrophes is disproportionately shared among the most vulnerable. Utilization of CBPR methodologies allows for a participatory approach, engaging such communities in identifying problems, research questions, and developing solutions. It generates empowerment amongst citizens, allowing them to tap into their day-to-day knowledge and local experience. With collaborative efforts, they are able to define the specific environmental concerns they struggle with, and formulate programs best tailored to their unique socio-economic requirements and cultural settings. Therefore, CBPR presents itself not merely as a research methodology, but as an activist tactic for mobilizing environmental justice action from the grassroots level upwards, and thereby correlating ecological recovery with social equity measures. Moreover, effective environmental justice initiatives are heavily reliant on the principles set forth in documents such as Laudate Deum that give paramount considerations to prompt response, collaborative responsibility, and social justice. Such conceptual axioms have the capacity to bring the focus of CBPR to synergistic solutions that address not just pressing environmental issues but also settle socio-economic injustices. For instance, projects such as reforestation of mangroves and community waste management are beneficial not only environmentally but also in improving the livelihoods and resilience of the local community. Such a connection between ecological health and social justice emphasizes the importance of community agency in project planning and implementation. Through the focus on community participation in CBPR, projects can be tailored to benefit ecological as well as social goals at the same time. This dual approach can assist in making sure that environmental justice initiatives do not simply address symptoms but also the causes of environmental degradation in marginalized groups. With the evolving climate change landscape internationally, the need to engage the marginalized voices in matters pertaining to the environment is increasingly self-evident. Research indicates that the populations most affected by environmental issues have valued knowledge on effective adaptation and resilience strategies. Leaving out these communities from policy-making can render policies ineffective, or even intensify inequalities (Perkins et al., 2017). This concept justifies participation-based governance systems that are sensitive to the wisdom of the marginalized in such fields as urban planning, water management, and health care. By incorporating these perspectives into CBPR systems, environmental justice efforts are strengthened and better situated within context. Finally, empowering local populations to lead climate action fosters not just social equality but also the effectiveness of environmental policy in general, ensuring that it addresses the nuance of the society that it is intended to affect.

9.6.3. Education and Youth Engagement Programs

Education and youth participation programs form the core of the functioning of CBPR, and through them, researchers and members of the community are ensured to work together, especially the youth. These programs not only empower youth by involving them in the research process but also enrich their learning about key social issues in their communities. Involving youth in research methods and approaches, these programs create the required skills like problem-solving and critical thinking. Moreover, youth involvement in community research can lead to more meaningful and relevant results because they carry specificities of perception and understanding. Lastly, putting education in the participatory research context, these kinds of programs bridge the theoretical knowledge-practice gap where youth voices are given due respect and consideration in decision-making. The structure and aim of the youth participation programs tend to capture the essence of CBPR in mirroring equitable collaboration and shared ownership of the research. Through collaborations with schools, community organizations, and local stakeholders, such programs provide a platform for youth to plan their own research projects. For instance, programs focused on community-based engagement revolve around topics like environmental justice, health disparities, or social injustice, allowing students to research issues they face on a day-to-day basis. These experiential learning opportunities foster a sense of ownership in the students, motivating them to become active community members rather than passive consumers of information. These bridges also encourage the merit of representation and inclusivity in the research process, ensuring that solutions can be created that speak to the needs and aspirations of the community, as suggested in the CBPR framework (Munoz et al., 2019). Moreover, integrating education and youth participation into the partnerships of CBPR can lead to revolutionary benefits for members as well as the broader community. For scholars and educators, engaging with youth brings fresh perspectives that can potentially be used to shape research questions and tactics, developing innovative solutions to ongoing social issues. One recent initiative is exemplary of this model, in which interdepartmental faculty members worked with a concentration on community-engaged research, producing publishable case studies that documented successful projects and practices (Center for Clinical and Translational Research and Division of Community Engagement, 2014). Not only are the case studies of value for educational learning, but they also extend the impact of youth engagement by identifying models that will be successful for others to implement. Therefore, education and youth engagement programs, grounded on CBPR principles, enhance a dynamic system that enriches the educational process of the participants and, concurrently, addresses the necessary community needs (Figure 9.17).

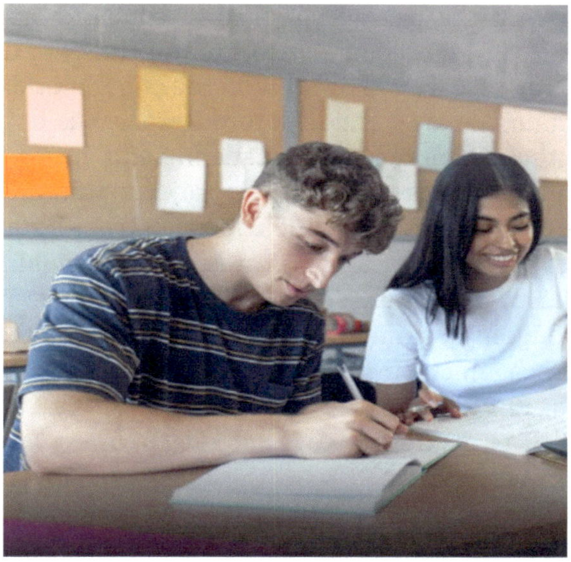

Figure 9.17. Education and youth engagement programs.

Source: https://blackboxresearchandconsultancy.com/wp-content/uploads/2023/04/Education-and-Youth-Engagement-img4.jpg.

SUMMARY

Using the principles of CBPR is highly advantageous in the management of health disparities maximally. Through the formation of partnerships among resident stakeholders and university scholars, CBPR amplifies local knowledge and expertise, making research relevant and actionable. The CCHN research is a demonstration of how such collaborations work. The CCHN examined various child and maternal health influences in multiple communities, highlighting the manner by which community participation in research generated action in the direction of understanding complex health issues. Primary themes arising from qualitative interviews, such as necessary resources and effective communication, highlight the importance of collaborative partnerships in the delivery of effective health outcomes. Ultimately, the existing CBPR approach enhances research validity and empowerment of communities, such as found with the CCHN research (CCHN et al., 2015). Moreover, what are mechanisms discovered through conducting research among some groups, for example, lesbian, gay, and bisexual (LGB) university students, further sheds light on the mandate existing CBPR holds in addressing unique health issues. Through qualitative approaches grounded on CBPR philosophy, researchers can more clearly identify specific barriers placed upon marginalized communities. This tailored approach not only identifies health disparities but also enables researchers and communities to work together to create interventions that are culturally appropriate and functional. The lessons learned from these studies are invaluable; they demonstrate the iterative nature of CBPR, where both the research method and the interaction with the community evolve with the passage of time in order to suit the specific needs of the population being researched. This adaptability speaks to the ability of CBPR to facilitate significant advancements in public health research among vulnerable populations (Stover et al., 2015). In general, the success of Community-Based Participatory Research is dependent on its emphasis on collaboration, trust, and mutual learning among academic and community partners. The success and pitfalls experienced while implementing CBPR projects validate the necessity of building these relationships in addressing health disparities. As seen from both the CCHN and LGB college community studies, the incorporation of community knowledge significantly boosts the research process to produce better health outcomes. The lessons learned from repeated efforts underscore the merit of flexibility and ongoing communication among stakeholders. As growing recognition of the value of community engagement in research catches up with the future projects, they will be grounded on the pillars of CBPR, strengthening its role as a key influencer of enhanced health in various communities (CCHN et al., 2015; Stover et al., 2015).

For CBPR, community partners' involvement is central to the validity of the research process. To make such interaction possible, it is important that community members have a sound grasp of research ethics and human subjects protection. An example of interest describes an innovative educational method whereby a game inspired by the TV show Jeopardy™ was created specifically for young people in a CBPR project. Young people, who were involved in active learning, reviewed infamous cases of ethical breaches—like the Tuskegee Syphilis Study—while playing in teams. This strategy not only fostered immense learning and retention of essential ethics concepts but also illustrated a rich technique for empowering community partners in the research process, again underlining the place of ethics as pivotal to CBPR engagement (Guerrero et al., 2014). Another key aspect in the area of CBPR is the establishment of participatory budgeting (PB) as a model of governance for public engagement. Within a period of a few years, PB has grown very quickly to 46 U.S. and Canadian towns, involving more than 70,000 citizens in making crucial decisions about the allocation of nearly $50 million of public funds. It is an excellent example of a new model for change in how the community is becoming engaged in decision-making about priorities for expenditure, making decisions more civic and transparent. The report Public Spending, By the People provides an overview of such processes and suggests that, although participation is also varied, disparities emerge in representation and the distribution of funds, which reflect the varied degrees of participation of communities among groups (Hagelskamp et al., 2016). Finally, the interweaving of these debates serves to uphold the central principle of CBPR: research must be collaborative and grounded in the local needs and context. Engaging local stakeholders not only strengthens the research evidence but also authenticates community voice in decision-making forums that affect their livelihood. By addressing such challenges as representation and distribution of resources through channels like participatory budgeting and innovative education tools, researchers and citizens can co-produce knowledge that manifests in direct benefits in terms of community health and well-being. Finally, the intersection of ethics, engagement, and inclusion leads us to the ongoing need to adapt and enhance CBPR approaches in ways that serve the communities for which they are attempting to empower.

KEY TERMS FROM THIS CHAPTER

Community Engagement
Empowerment
Shared Decision-Making
Cultural Competence
Participatory Methods
Sustainability
Needs Assessment
Collaboration
Co-learning
Trust-Building
Action-Oriented Research
Local Knowledge
Community Ownership
Translational Research
Equity
Capacity Building
Stakeholder Involvement
Social Justice
Mutual Benefit
Power Sharing

CLOSER LOOK

PARTICIPATORY ACTION RESEARCH (PAR)

A closer look at Participatory Action Research (PAR) reveals it as a collaborative and empowering research methodology that actively involves the people most affected by a problem in every stage of the research process. Unlike traditional research methods where participants are often passive subjects, PAR positions them as co-researchers who contribute to the identification of issues, data collection, analysis, and the implementation of solutions. Rooted in principles of social justice, equity, and community empowerment, PAR seeks not just to understand the world but to change it by addressing real-life concerns in meaningful and sustainable ways. It is particularly valuable in marginalized or underserved communities, where it helps to amplify local voices, validate lived experiences, and challenge power imbalances between researchers and participants. The iterative process of PAR—often described as a cycle of planning, acting, observing, and reflecting—fosters continuous learning and adaptation, making it both flexible and responsive to community needs. One of its strengths lies in its ability to build trust and strengthen relationships within communities while producing knowledge that is contextually grounded and immediately applicable. By engaging participants directly, PAR often leads to more relevant findings and more effective interventions, as those closest to the issue have a deep understanding of the local context. It also contributes to capacity building, as participants gain skills in research, communication, and critical thinking. Despite challenges such as time constraints, power dynamics, and the need for sustained commitment, the benefits of PAR in promoting inclusive and democratic research are substantial. Ultimately, Participatory Action Research is not just a method but a movement toward more ethical, engaged, and impactful research practices. It transforms research from a top-down exercise into a shared journey of discovery and change, creating knowledge that serves the interests of both communities and broader society.

REFERENCES

1. Adebayo, A., & Adebayo, A. (2018). Governance and community participation in the Nigerian tourism sector: A stakeholder analysis. https://core.ac.uk/download/287635122.pdf (accessed on 26th June 2025).
2. Adie, E. U., Okoro, L. A., & Orim, E. G. (2014). Exploring the potentials of community theatre as a tool for social change: The participatory communication method. https://core.ac.uk/download/287611590.pdf (accessed on 26th June 2025).
3. Ahmed, H. U., Allen, C., Arumainayagam, N., Emberton, M., et al. (2013). Multiparametric MR imaging for detection of clinically significant prostate cancer: A validation cohort study with transperineal template prostate mapping as the reference standard.
4. Allen, A., Morello-Frosch, R., Mujahid, M., Petteway, R., et al. (2019). Towards a people's social epidemiology: Envisioning a more inclusive and equitable future for social epi research and practice in the 21st century. https://core.ac.uk/download/323081131.pdf (accessed on 26th June 2025).
5. Ananda, J., Ansell, C., Banville, C., Beierle, T., et al. (2010). Integrating multiple criteria decision analysis in participatory forest planning. https://core.ac.uk/download/11697719.pdf (accessed on 26th June 2025).
6. Asfahani, C., Hanivia, A., Palayukan, H., Rofiah, R., et al. (2024). Optimization community progress through empowerment in the field of sustainable education. https://core.ac.uk/download/642411704.pdf (accessed on 26th June 2025).
7. Ayoola, A., Doornbos, M. M., Topp, R. V., Zandee, G., et al. (2015). Conducting research with community groups. https://core.ac.uk/download/213077570.pdf (accessed on 26th June 2025).
8. Badii, A., Bagnoli, F., Balazs, B., Castellani, T., et al. (2016). Collective awareness platforms and digital social innovation mediating consensus seeking in problem situations. https://core.ac.uk/download/286269669.pdf (accessed on 26th June 2025).
9. Barberis, D., Capello, A., Hallman, J. A., Izumi, B. T., et al. (2013). A community-based participatory research approach to developing the Harvest for Healthy Kids curriculum. https://core.ac.uk/download/84827175.pdf (accessed on 26th June 2025).
10. Barker, M., Brown, R., Forbes, H., Gooch, D., et al. (2018). Amplifying quiet voices: Challenges and opportunities for participatory design at an urban scale. https://core.ac.uk/download/131317312.pdf (accessed on 26th June 2025).
11. Becker, A., Brown, D., de Laine, M., Institute of Medicine, Israel, B. A., Mays, G. P., et al. (2016). Applying community-based participatory research partnership principles to public health practice-based research networks. https://core.ac.uk/download/78919084.pdf (accessed on 26th June 2025).
12. Boeykens, T. (2019). *Exile, Return, Record: Exploring Historical Narratives and Community Resistance Through Participatory Filmmaking in 'Post-Conflict' Guatemala*. https://core.ac.uk/download/225020107.pdf (accessed on 26th June 2025).
13. Bradley, H. A., & Puoane, T. (2007). Prevention of hypertension and diabetes in an urban setting in South Africa: Participatory action research with community health workers. https://core.ac.uk/download/62632892.pdf (accessed on 26th June 2025).

14. Brown, B., Dubé, K., Kuzmanović, D., Long, C., et al. (2021). Ethical reflections on the conduct of HIV research with community members: A case study. https://core.ac.uk/download/519758905.pdf (accessed on 26th June 2025).

15. Cacari-Stone, L., Garcia, A. P., Minkler, M., Wallerstein, N., et al. (2014). The promise of community-based participatory research for health equity: A conceptual model for bridging evidence with policy. https://core.ac.uk/download/323310443.pdf (accessed on 26th June 2025).

16. Cannon, C. E. B. (2020). Towards convergence: How to do transdisciplinary environmental health disparities research. https://core.ac.uk/download/323069074.pdf (accessed on 26th June 2025).

17. Carmichael, P., & Tracy, F. (2013). Research ethics and participatory research in an interdisciplinary technology-enhanced learning project. https://core.ac.uk/download/130975518.pdf (accessed on 26th June 2025).

18. Center for Clinical and Translational Research, Division of Community Engagement. (2014). *Excellence in Community-Engaged Research at Virginia Commonwealth University: A Compendium of Case Studies Developed Through a Faculty Learning Community*. https://core.ac.uk/download/51287407.pdf (accessed on 26th June 2025).

19. Chaparro, M., Das, B., & Landaburu, A. (2016). Epistemología de la comunicación en India: Una aproximación histórica más allá del "desarrollo." https://core.ac.uk/download/288159360.pdf (accessed on 26th June 2025).

20. Child and Community Health Network (CCHN), BeLue, R., Chung, B., Lanzi, R., et al. (2015). Evaluation of the Community Child Health Research Network (CCHN) community-academic partnership. https://digitalscholarship.unlv.edu/cgi/viewcontent.cgi?article=1287&context=jhdrp (accessed on 26th June 2025).

21. Chung, B., Gardner, S., Griffith, K., Grover, K., et al. (2018). Case study of Resilient Baton Rouge: Applying depression collaborative care and community planning to disaster recovery. https://core.ac.uk/download/323077922.pdf (accessed on 26th June 2025).

22. Constantian, E., Dailey, A. B., Davidson, K., Gaskin, D. J., et al. (2015). Healthy Options: A community-based program to address food insecurity. https://cupola.gettysburg.edu/cgi/viewcontent.cgi?article=1000&context=cpsres (accessed on 26th June 2025).

23. Cox, R. S., Fletcher, S., Heykoop, C., Peek, L., et al. (2016). Engaging youth in post-disaster research: Lessons learned from a creative methods approach. https://core.ac.uk/download/213625726.pdf (accessed on 26th June 2025).

24. Cutts, W., Fenge, L. A., & Hodges, C. E. M. (2011). Seen but seldom heard: Creative participatory methods in a study of youth and risk. https://core.ac.uk/download/4899589.pdf (accessed on 26th June 2025).

25. D'Andrade, A., Donoviel, B., Drabble, L., Le, H., et al. (2013). Child welfare partnership for research and training: A Title IV-E university/community collaborative research model. https://core.ac.uk/download/70416065.pdf (accessed on 26th June 2025).

26. D'Haeyer, T., Pirola, E., & Uyttendaele, T. (2012). *Afromaison. Project Objective, Work Progress and Achievements Project Management: Core Part of The Mid-Term Report*. http://agritrop.cirad.fr/567244/1/document_567244.pdf (accessed on 26th June 2025).

27. Dubé, K., Karris, M. Y., & Moore, A. A. (2020). What lessons it might teach us! Community engagement in HIV research. https://core.ac.uk/download/519758850.pdf (accessed on 26th June 2025).

28. Evans, B. E., Peal, A. J., & van der Voorden, C. (2010). *Hygiene and Sanitation Software: An Overview of Approaches.*

29. Fang, M. L., Grigorovich, A., Kontos, P., Sixsmith, J., et al. (2020). An exploration of experiences of transdisciplinary research in aging and technology. https://core.ac.uk/download/286715156.pdf (accessed on 26th June 2025).

30. Figueiredo, P., & Perkins, P. E. (2013). Women and water management in times of climate change: Participatory and inclusive processes. https://core.ac.uk/download/287659514.pdf (accessed on 26th June 2025).

31. Gagnon, V., Gorman, H., & Norman, E. (2017). Power and politics in research design and practice: Opening up space for social equity in interdisciplinary, multi-jurisdictional and community-based research. https://core.ac.uk/download/213625747.pdf (accessed on 26th June 2025).

32. Guerrero, J., Madrigal, D. S., & Minkler, M. (2014). What is ...? A research ethics jeopardy game to help community partners understand human subjects' protections and their importance. https://core.ac.uk/download/323310442.pdf (accessed on 26th June 2025).

33. Guta, A., & Flicker, S. (2007). Ethical approaches to adolescent participation in sexual health research. https://core.ac.uk/download/71340218.pdf (accessed on 26th June 2025).

34. Habron, J., Butterly, F., Gordon, I., Roebuck, R., et al. (2009). Being well, being musical: Music composition as a resource and occupation for older people. https://core.ac.uk/download/pdf/30619262.pdf (accessed on 26th June 2025).

35. Hagelskamp, C., Rinehart, C., Schleifer, D., & Silliman, R. (2016). *Public spending, by the people: Participatory budgeting in the United States and Canada in 2014–15.* https://core.ac.uk/download/75761730.pdf (accessed on 26th June 2025).

36. Hanson, C., & Ogunade, A. (2016). Caught up in power: Exploring discursive frictions in community research. https://core.ac.uk/download/213625713.pdf (accessed on 26th June 2025).

37. Haythornthwaite, C. A. (2009). Participatory transformations. https://core.ac.uk/download/4823230.pdf (accessed on 26th June 2025).

38. Hicks, R. M. (2002). *Health: Sculptured by the Hands of Culture: Exploring the Ecuadorian Worldview of Health: A Thesis Presented in Partial Fulfilment of The Requirements for The Degree of Master of Philosophy of Development Studies at Massey University, New Zealand.* https://core.ac.uk/download/148645846.pdf (accessed on 26th June 2025).

39. Hudson-Smith, A., Hunter, A., O'Brien, J., Psarra, S., et al. (2016). Ensuring VGI credibility in urban-community data generation: A methodological research design. https://core.ac.uk/download/132623739.pdf (accessed on 26th June 2025).

40. Ingirige, M. J. B., Madubuko, L. N., & Sexton, M. G. (2009). The interaction between non-governmental organizations and marginalized communities to build self-sustaining capacity to transfer, absorb and use building technologies in indigenous housing. https://core.ac.uk/download/1666626.pdf (accessed on 26th June 2025).

41. Ingles, A. L. S., Jr. (2024). *Laudate Deum: A Framework for Environmental Stewardship and Social Justice in the Philippines and Southeast Asia*. https://core.ac.uk/download/639390105.pdf (accessed on 26th June 2025).
42. Liboro, R. M., & Travers, R. (2016). Fundamental researcher attributes: Reflections on ways to facilitate participation in community psychology doctoral dissertation research. https://core.ac.uk/download/232208122.pdf (accessed on 26th June 2025).
43. Lie, R., & Mandler, A. (2009). *Video in Development: Filming for Rural Change*. https://core.ac.uk/download/pdf/29251278.pdf (accessed on 26th June 2025).
44. Lindquist-Grantz, R., & Vaughn, L. M. (2016). The journey and destination need to be intentional: Perceptions of success in community-academic research partnerships. https://core.ac.uk/download/213625723.pdf (accessed on 26th June 2025).
45. Mbe, K. A. (2017). Culturally competent health education in African-Americans' faith-based communities for better health outcomes: A literature review. https://core.ac.uk/download/70427442.pdf (accessed on 26th June 2025).
46. Meershoek, A., Krumeich, A., Barnes, D. F., Cleaver, F., Cook, T., Corey, S. M., et al. (2018). Dark clouds in co-creation, and their silver linings: Practical challenges we faced in a participatory project in a resource-constrained community in India, and how we overcame (some of) them. https://core.ac.uk/download/146491135.pdf (accessed on 26th June 2025).
47. Moore de Peralta, A., Smithwick, J., & Torres, M. E. (2020). Perceptions and determinants of partnership trust in the context of community-based participatory research. https://core.ac.uk/download/427167859.pdf (accessed on 26th June 2025).
48. Munoz, J. A. (2019). Community based research/community based participatory research. https://core.ac.uk/download/227028296.pdf (accessed on 26th June 2025).
49. N/A. (2012). *Resilient Livelihoods and Food Security in Coastal Aquatic Agricultural Systems: Investing in Transformational Change*. https://core.ac.uk/download/11024818.pdf (accessed on 26th June 2025).
50. Newhall, T. (2013). Community based participatory research. https://core.ac.uk/download/232012180.pdf (accessed on 26th June 2025).
51. Perkins, P. E. (2017). University-community collaboration for climate justice education and organizing: Partnerships in Canada, Brazil, and Africa. https://core.ac.uk/download/287659513.pdf (accessed on 26th June 2025).
52. Stewart, S. (2017). Evaluating the success of making equitable, predictable, and transparent development decisions by encouraging community and stakeholder collaboration through two participatory design case studies. https://core.ac.uk/download/302392753.pdf (accessed on 26th June 2025).
53. Stover, C. M. (2015). Community based participatory research: The application and lessons learned from a study with LGB college students. https://digitalscholarship.unlv.edu/cgi/viewcontent.cgi?article=1354&context=jhdrp (accessed on 26th June 2025).

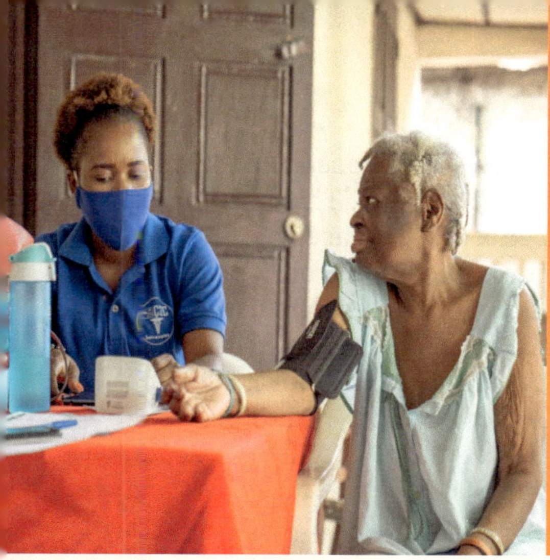

Chapter 10

POLICY AND ADVOCACY IN COMMUNITY HEALTH

Contents

Introduction

Policy and advocacy, within the context of community health, have intrinsic roles in shaping the landscape of healthcare access, equity, and service provision. The mutually influencing relationship between the fields emphasizes the necessity for a concerted approach to mitigating health disparities and enhancing community wellness. As seen in the majority of initiatives, there is also a consensus contribution that includes stakeholders like policymakers, advocates, and community members in comprehending health-related concerns. For instance, the Future of Disability in Alaska Summit highlighted the importance of consensus generation in convening multiplicity to guide future policy directions in important areas such as advocacy, economic well-being, and health (Center for Human Development and University of Alaska Anchorage, 2013). This community engagement not only facilitates the realization of near-term problems but also constructs a vision for sustainable solutions, a precursor to strategic policy development. Community health advocacy cannot be overstressed because it empowers communities and individuals to articulate their needs and influence decisions that determine their health outcomes. It is through advocacy that organizations can create systemic change that connects health policies with agendas at the community level, and closer relationships are established between marginalized people and most required health services. This is mirrored in the results-based approach signified by grantmaking models that encourage measuring advocacy outcomes (Gienapp et al., 2007). By making outcomes tangible, stakeholders are best placed to measure the effectiveness of their work and adjust their approaches accordingly. Lastly, such advocacy activity creates more public awareness and encourages mobilization of resources to ensure that the health of the community remains in the limelight of policy formulation. With healthcare evolving further, knowledge of the interplay of policy, advocacy, and community health grows in importance. Effective advocacy not only informs of health issues but also triggers collective action in order to influence directions in policy at a local, state, and national level. With the depth and richness of these interactions, ongoing dialogue among multiple stakeholders is vital. The common experiences captured in summits like Alaska point to the potential of transformational change where advocacy is informed by an actual understanding of community aspirations and needs (Center for Human Development and University of Alaska Anchorage, 2013). By relating advocacy programs with intentional policy measures, the practice of community health can chart its course toward an understanding that prioritizes equity, access, and broad participation on the part of everyone in the community, establishing a resilient but inclusive system for health (Figure 10.1).

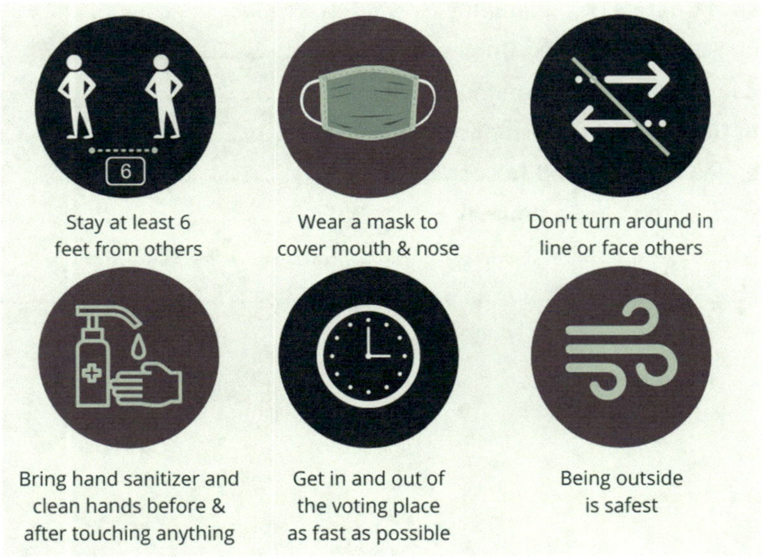

Figure 10.1. Policy and advocacy in community health.

Source: https://www.stlrhc.org/wp-content/uploads/sites/63/2020/12/Generic-votesafe-720x604.png.

Definition of Community Health

Community health can be defined as multidisciplinary practice that focuses on the health consequences of target populations with an emphasis on the social, economic, and environmental determinants of health in the populations. It goes beyond mere medical intervention and includes the promotion of wellness, prevention of illness, and targeting the root causes of health disparities. By involving the people in planning and implementing health programs, community health fosters ownership and participation, which are essential in ensuring effective health interventions. Underlying the process are the principles of universal access, people's participation, and intersectoral action, as stated in various international health platforms, which have a crucial role to play in addressing the various needs of individuals and ensuring that programs are sustainable (Pelaez et al., 2004). In defining community health, attention must be paid to the role of policy and advocacy in shaping the outcomes of health at the community level. Policy developed as a result of advocacy can significantly impact the allocation of funds, resource allocation, and program implementation and thereby shape the health environment of a community. Effective advocacy involves the voice of the community to make their needs and perspectives heard in policy-making. This participatory process not only raises the salience of health policy but also brings about public acceptance of programs meant to improve health outcomes. Understanding community health thus entails examining how grassroots advocacy is tied to policy building, as they converge to create a health equity and wellness-promoting environment (Linzer, 2012). Secondly, community health programs also have a tendency to require intersectoral coordination in a variety of domains, reinforcing the necessity of an integrated strategy for health. This interdependence acknowledges that health is shaped by conditions such as housing, education, and employment, which call for a coordinated strategy of health improvement. Health professionals and community members must work together in interprofessional teams to address these complex determinants of health. For instance, healthy aging initiatives not only take into account medical care but social support networks and physical surroundings as well, all of which have a decisive role to play in allowing for a healthier population. As international discussions on global health have explained, such systematic incorporation of multiple voices and pools of knowledge is essential in advocating for effective community health strategies that can drive change sustainably (Pelaez et al., 2004) (Figure 10.2).

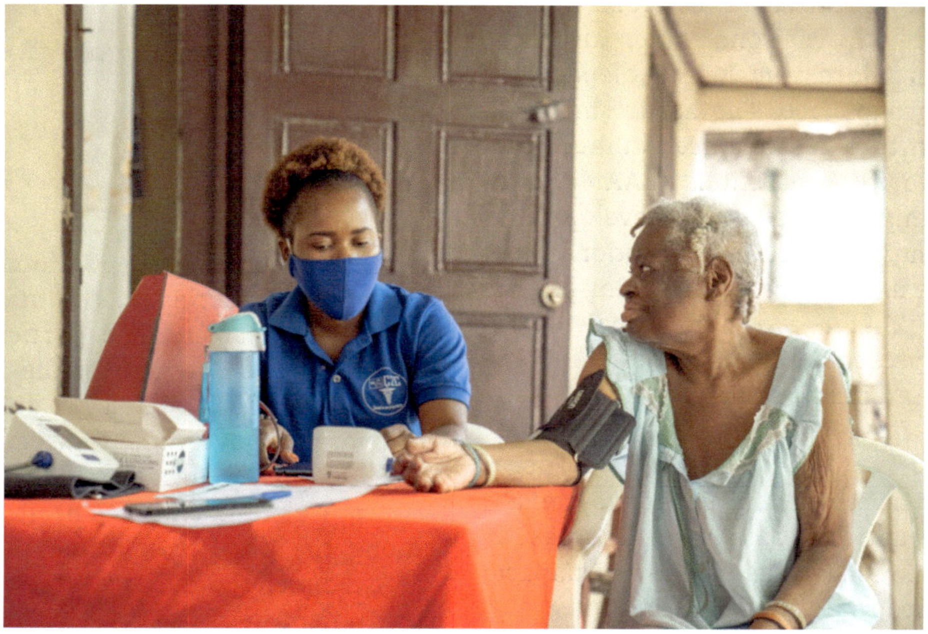

Figure 10.2. Community health.

Source: https://devex.shorthandstories.com/community-health-workers-delivering-frontline-health-innovations/assets/DOWw8Xt4kV/c2c-august-2020-452-4096x2731.jpeg.

Importance of Policy and Advocacy

Policy and advocacy form the crux of driving community health through addressing systemic inequalities that negatively affect marginalized groups. Effective policy interventions can empower communities in a way that they are able to better tackle challenges in access to health and health outcomes. For instance, the Diversifying Leadership for Sustainable Food Policy initiative illustrates how strategic advocacy can reinforce the strength of organizations with people-of-color leadership in facilitating effective policy conversation and policy implementation. By enhancing their ability to identify policy targets and diversify organizational structures, such groups can effectively address structural obstacles that encroach on food access and sustainability. These projects illustrate how combined advocacy efforts translate immediately into improved community health outcomes since policies formulated on the premise of local knowledge are likely to resonate with the interests of populations they aim to serve (Lee et al., 2009). In addition, a healthy environment for advocacy is essential in addressing health disparities that various groups face. The Leadership and Advocacy Institute to Advance Minnesota's Parity for Priority Populations (LAAMPP) is the prime example of leadership development having a strong influence in populations that are likely to be underrepresented during health dialogues. The program, which trains individuals from underrepresented communities—African Americans, American Indians, and LGBTQ members, for instance—benefits not just the advocacy skills of these community leaders but also their networks and support systems. LAAMPP evaluation has shown increased competencies in fellows, as well as the impact of their advocacy, resulting in the passage of vital health policy that benefits their respective communities. This demonstrates the importance of building leadership among marginalized populations in shaping long-term policy reforms in community health (Bosma et al., 2016). In addition, the relationship between policy formulation and advocacy highlights the interweight of community-based health improvement plans and community participation. People are empowered through participatory advocacy-inspired community health programs to influence the policies that shape their health care. This not only enhances community bonding but also facilitates a sense of ownership of health-related decisions. Once communities engage in advocacy, they can combine their experience and expertise and advocate for policies that better address their individual needs, resulting in healthier communities. Policy and advocacy are, therefore, a synergistic formula that can effectively address social determinants of health, improve health equity, and spur transformative change in communities. As such, understanding the power of advocacy and policy is essential to support coordinated health activities that can yield long-term gains in community health outcomes.

10.1. Historical Context of Community Health Policies

Community health policy development is rooted in history, reflecting the values and shared priorities of society at a particular moment in time. In the first half of the 20th century, health care was largely a private matter with little or no government intervention, with much emphasis on infectious diseases that were prevalent in cities. As health emergencies among the population came to be realized, for example, the tuberculosis epidemic, the government began to take a more active role in interventions in health. Social philosophy's power at this time translated into policy developments, emphasizing the necessity of community-based responses and services. Such shifts were a turning point where policies at the community health level began to acknowledge not only physical health but also broader social determinants, thereby laying the groundwork for healthier and more preventative care systems, like in holistic models such as the Saskatchewan Community Living Division jurisdictional study (Blackman et al., 2005). The second half of the 20th century saw radical changes in community health policies, foremost being driven by civil rights movements and a greater focus on human rights. The movement of deinstitutionalization was notably instrumental in calling for the rights of people with disabilities and upholding the philosophy of inclusion rather than isolation. As change was demanded at the system level by advocates, policymakers began to focus on developing services that placed people at the center and respected their individual needs and dignity. This change, with heavy focus on national action and public engagement, emphasized person-centered planning, self-determination, and integration into the community, which was a promise to equity and access in health care by society (Blackman et al., 2005). The cultural context thus changed to support policies promoting community-oriented responses to health care, reducing institutional care. Besides social movements, foundations and non-profits began to have a role in shaping community health policy during the late 20th and early 21st centuries. These entities, including the Kresge Foundation, provided significant funding as well as strategic leadership for enhancing health care equity and, thus, shaped the development of community health programs. The historical backdrop for these attempts at philanthropy was against an increasing sensitization among the public regarding health inequalities and demands for advocacy. This phase was a recognition more generally that community health is not access to the services of a doctor but socio-economic determinants of health. Through the integration of advocacy activities and community health programs, policymakers aimed at remedying structural injustices, thereby offsetting the multi-faceted needs presented by heterogeneous populations (Figure 10.3).

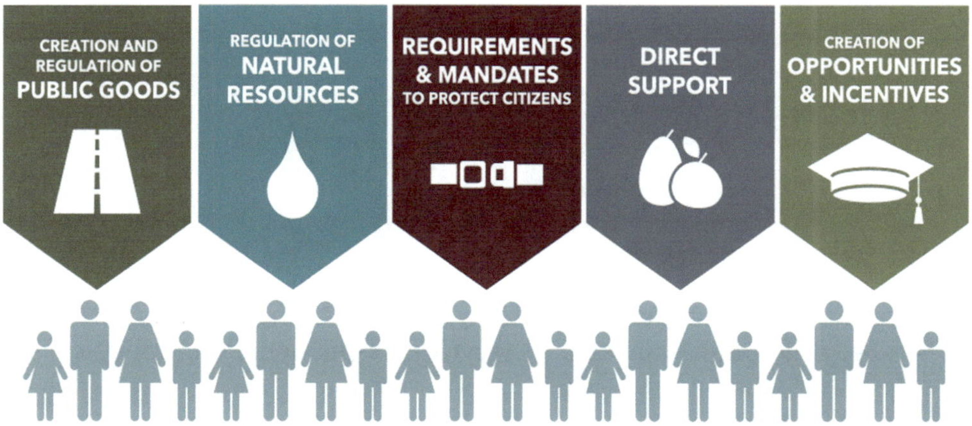

Figure 10.3. Historical context of community health policies.

Source: https://sycamoretn.org/wp-content/uploads/2017/05/5-ways-policy-impacts-health-e1532716467411.png.

10.1.1. Evolution of Public Health Policies

The evolution of public health policies has significantly been influenced by paradigms of shifting health issues and community demands. Initially addressing infectious diseases, the early public health policies attempted to control the spread of these diseases through vaccination and sanitation. Chronic diseases increasingly came under focus, and correspondingly, policies encompassed preventive care, health education, and determinants of socio-economic health. With increasing diversity in communities, public health policies began to exhibit a more inclusive character since they recognize the varying needs of the populations, particularly the marginalized populations. This revolution laid the ground for robust advocacy, enabling stakeholders to address structural inequalities in access and outcomes in health, thereby leveling the playing field for health. Furthermore, data and research have helped in shaping public health policies and advancing effective interventions. Proper collection and analysis of data have facilitated policymakers to identify trends and address specific concerns in health more effectively. For instance, initiatives aimed at the health status of young individuals, and more specifically boys and young men of color (BYMOC), focus on the importance of tailoring public health interventions to address the specific needs of particular populations with characteristic issues. As noted, afterschool professionals are assuming a pivotal role in empowering and organizing BYMOC toward greater equal educational, economic, health, and life opportunities (Gilgoff et al., 2015).

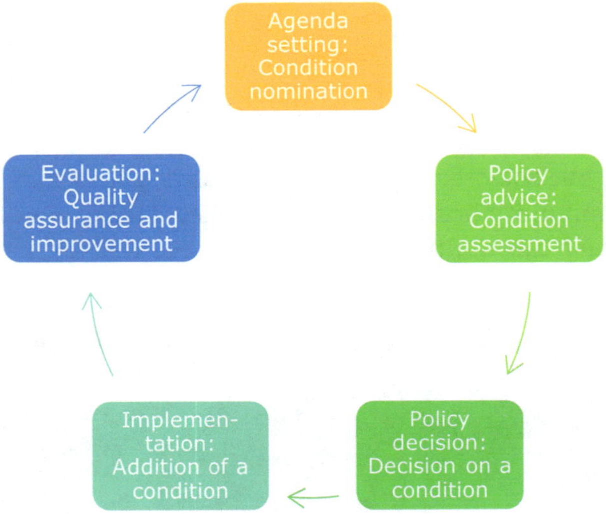

Figure 10.4. Evolution of public health policies.

Source: https://www.researchgate.net/publication/349498815/figure/fig1/AS:11431281187388791@1694197414146/The-public-health-policy-cycle-The-public-health-policy-cycle-consists-of-five-phases.tif.

These targeted initiatives increase community engagement, particularly in environments where more traditional public health frameworks are not well prepared, thus generating a more responsive policy environment. Lastly, bringing advocacy into the framework of creating public health policy emphasizes the requirement of bipartisan endorsement in effecting lasting reform. Strong evidence upon which to demonstrate the efficacy of health interventions underpins successful advocacy and mobilizes political assistance. This complementary relationship between advocacy and policy making is itself demonstrated by initiatives that have moved core data assets into influential tools for promoting health equity. An example is the one-book idea for monitoring child well-being indicators that became a mission-critical resource for the Foundation in securing bipartisan backing for evidence-based practice solutions and policy change (N/A, 2016). The ongoing advancement of public health policies thus underscores the value of informed advocacy that not only benefits existing models but also examines new ways of responding to new health challenges (Figure 10.4).

10.1.2. Key Legislation Impacting Community Health

The advancement of community health is greatly influenced by main legislation intended to tackle most public health challenges. One of the most important pieces of legislation is the Affordable Care Act (ACA), which opened millions of Americans' access to healthcare significantly. By increasing Medicaid coverage and providing subsidies for private insurance, the ACA not only increased the number of people covered but established a system of preventive care and health equity. Further, the law emphasized heavily on community outreach programs needed in health information dissemination and motivating participation among different communities. This act is an indicator of the central role that policy plays in shaping the determinants of health and reducing disparities. The ACA also motivated community-based organizations to integrate their efforts and resources with those for universal access to healthcare, thus strengthening interagency collaborations in public health advocacy. Legislation is also important in addressing specific public health issues, such as domestic violence.

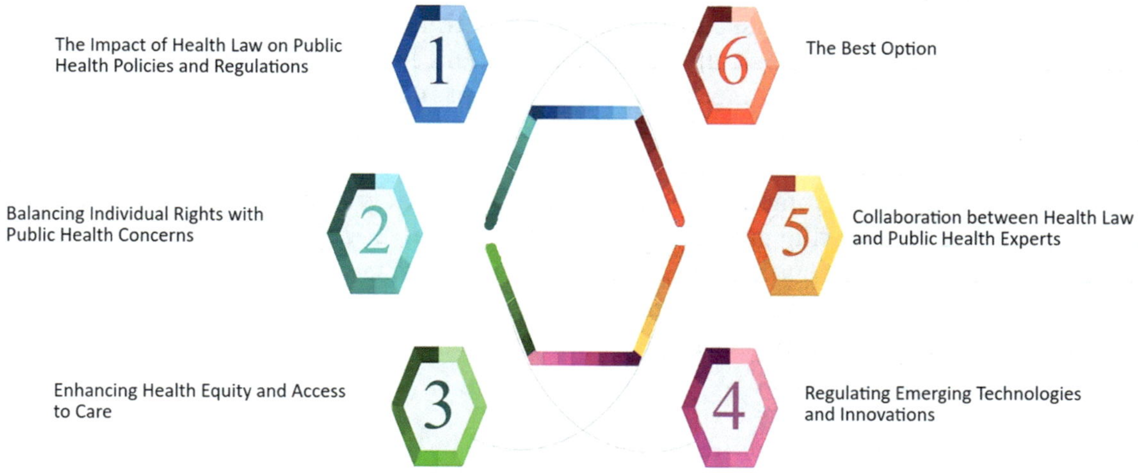

Figure 10.5. Key legislation impacting community health.

Source: https://fastercapital.co/i/Health-law--Healing-the-Legal-System--Understanding-Health-Law-Principles--The-Impact-of-Health-Law-on-Public-Health-Policies-and-Regulations.webp.

Initiatives targeted toward the primary prevention of partner violence emphasize the need for comprehensive strategies that include legislative intervention and community engagement. Policies and laws must embrace approaches for environmental and norms change, particularly in vulnerable groups. The forums in relation to such models of legislation suggest that prevention and intervention must be the focus with an emphasis on culturally suitable practices that resonate with immigrant populations. Through policies that prioritize education and community outreach, legislators are able to create settings that not only empower victims but also engage to prevent instances of violence through intelligent community action. All these efforts are supplemented by cooperative action by foundations providing funding for advocacy efforts, showing the interdisciplinary action involved in community health legislation (N/A, 2010). Moreover, legislations must also tackle the socio-economic determinants of health affecting equity. Policies providing funding for public spaces, nutrition programs, and mental health interventions constitute pillars in providing support for community health. For instance, initiatives to increase access to healthy food and leisure services have long-term implications for physical and mental health outcomes. Action on the broader determinants of this form, the law can allow communities to take back their health as it facilitates long-term change. Immediate recommended action should be the consolidation of funding for community-led health programs and greater legislative support for selective interventions in disadvantaged areas. Lastly, effective advocacy for community health relies on careful examination of how law intersects with social structures that shape health behavior and outcomes so that all members of a community may thrive (Cohen et al., 2007) (Figure 10.5).

10.1.3. Historical Advocacy Movements

Social movements throughout history have played an important role in shaping policy towards community health, opening up channels for marginalized communities through collective work and perseverance. The best example is the women's health movement, which discovered more vitality during the late 20th century. The movement was formed with women challenging the prevailing medical practices that barely addressed their unique health issues. Activists fought not only to be represented more adequately in medical research but also for reproductive health care rights without shame. The intersection of environmental health and reproductive rights has further shown the nuance of health activism. For instance, initiatives such as the Environmental Justice/Reproductive Justice (EJ/RJ) Collaborative indicate the importance of collaborative activism in addressing the multi-faceted issues around women's health, demonstrating how earlier movements can lead to complete approaches considering environmental factors (Khan, 2009). As time went on, the efforts of philanthropy gained more significance as advocacy movements progressed, demonstrating how funding mechanisms could be both facilitators and hindrances of social change. Donors have come to realize that supporting movements requires a nuanced sense of the barriers and possibilities that arise in complex social contexts.

The report, Many Hands, More Impact: Philanthropy's Role in Supporting Movements, provides a framework for understanding these dynamics and guides Grantmakers who wish to maximize their investment in social movements. Philanthropic organizations have the capacity to organize their priorities in a manner that helps them fund community-based programs, hence giving voice to those most affected by healthcare policies. Through the advocacy of coalitions among stakeholders, such movements are in a position to consolidate a larger backing base, hence bolstering advocacy due to past history campaigns (N/A, 2013). These historical advocacy movements have bequeathed a heritage that echoes through contemporary community health policy, all in the pursuit of justice and equality. Examining the trajectories of these movements offers insight into the strategic strategies that have proved successful in mobilizing communities for advocacy. The incorporation of intersectionality in the theories of advocacy has particularly emerged as an important element, as it reminds us to consider the way various identities and social positions determine individuals' health experiences. This recognition makes sure that advocacy is not about specific issues but is inclusive of the diversity of activism needed to tackle systematic disparities. Lastly, the past history of such movements informs current strategies with the aim of creating equitable health policies, emphasizing the important role played by past advocacy towards future and continuous community health initiatives.

10.2. Current Policies Affecting Community Health

Present policies that target the eradication of health disparities among vulnerable groups heavily influence the profile of community health. Policies that promote the development of community-based health programs are important in ensuring inclusive environments that focus on equal access to health. Such examples are programs that focus on building community leadership in communities of color, which are central in empowering the local community to fight for their own health. These interventions are supported by foundation and government sources to create capacity within the community because local leaders are assumed to be aware of their specific needs and better positioned to resolve them.

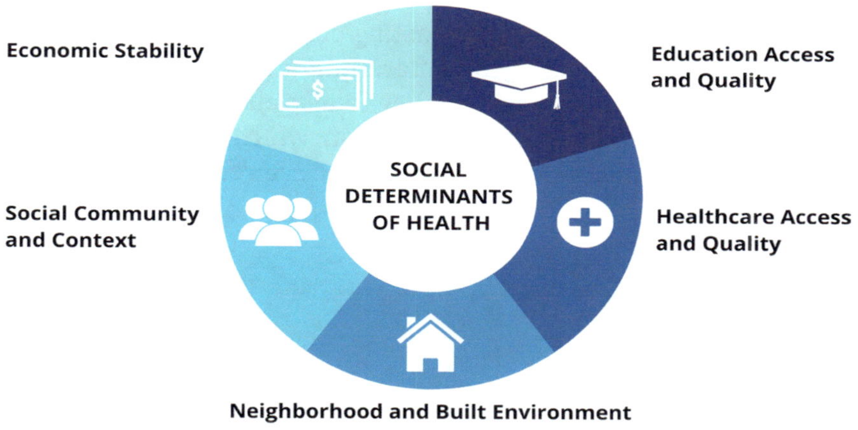

Figure 10.6. Current policies affecting community health.

Source: https://www.voyatek.com/wp-content/uploads/2021/04/SOCIAL-DETERMINANTS-OF-HEALTH-e1663693694195.png.

These policies not only improve health results but also encourage civic engagement and collective action, ending in enduring community health practice (Marsh et al., 2003). Moreover, proper policy implementation which affects the health of communities demands incorporation of sound, evidence-informed approaches. Services for individuals with intellectual disabilities literature underscores the need to combine public consultation with policy development to eliminate barriers in the system. Through scientific analysis of resources available and those needed in a community, policymakers are able to develop tailored approaches that enable inclusivity and improved care for various populations. This includes exploring human rights, advocacy, and individualized funding within community services. By informing policies through sound research and community consultation, stakeholders are able to establish an environment where health services are not only accessible but are planned for within the specific context of community need (Blackman et al., 2005). Finally, utmost importance must be placed on interdisciplinary working when dealing with the multifaceted nature of community health. It is better recognized today that health outcomes are influenced by social determinants like education, employment, and housing stability. Therefore, policy that facilitates coordination between health organizations, schools, and social services can offer more comprehensive solutions to community health problems. Integrated service advocacy can mean increased accessibility and full-spectrum care, addressing the root causes rather than symptoms of health inequities. Therefore, such collaborative policies can create systemic change and empower the communities to build resilience and ultimately advocate for environments conducive to individual and public health goals. By doing so, the framework underlying community health policies can become modified to solve present challenges effectively (Figure 10.6).

10.2.1. Overview of Major Health Policies

United States' health policy is characterized by the enormous volume of legislative actions and regulations aimed at improving public health results. The key policies focus on the convergence of health care access, quality of care, and cost control. Landmark legislation such as the ACA is a cornerstone of moving forward with health equity through expanded insurance coverage and prohibiting discriminatory practices against preexisting conditions. Such policies not only enhance individual well-being but also target structural determinants of health that deal with broader social determinants. Progress in public health policy is also driven by advocacy movements that advocate for participation of people and community action, which subsequently lay the groundwork for the development of effective health interventions that are relevant to the context and culture of various groups.

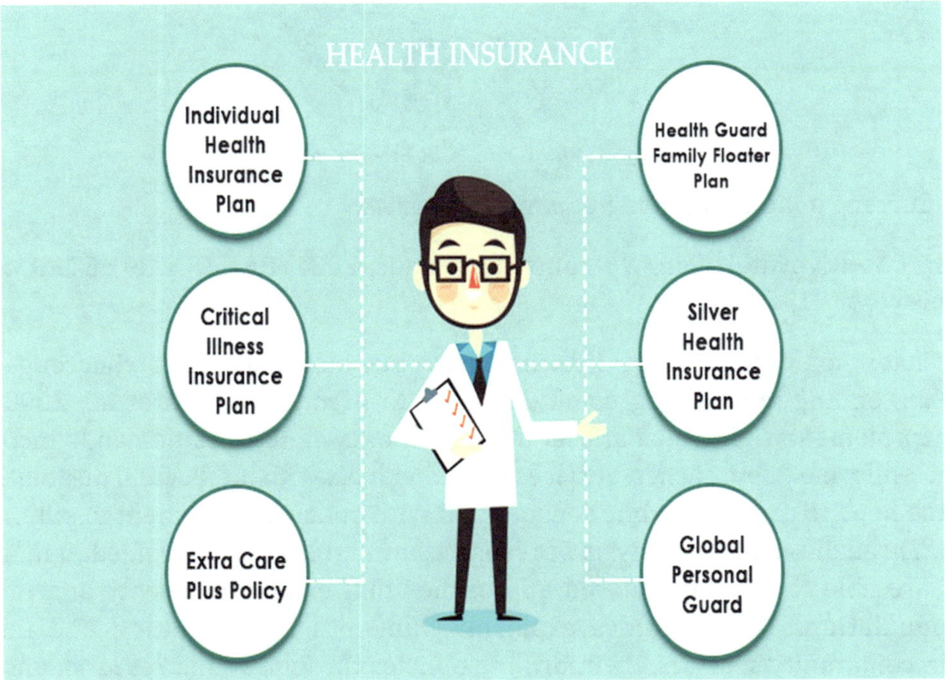

Figure 10.7. Overview of major health policies.

Source: https://www.bajajallianz.com/blog/wp-content/uploads/2020/07/types-of-health-insurance.jpg.

The role of incorporating evidence-based practices is also a major area of concern in health policy since it addresses the need to have adequate evaluation of healthcare programs. Support for such policies is usually based on evidence-based strategies that evaluate the efficacy of interventions. For example, Strong et al. (2011) provides a step-by-step manual of how to assess advocacy projects, focusing on the need to create a logic model and systematic evaluation plans, including the utilization of focus groups and interviews. These methods not only improve program effectiveness but also create accountability for stakeholders engaged in health promotion. As communities try to integrate successful health policies, the incorporation of evaluation into the advocacy process ensures that interventions are effective and sustainable, thus leading to long-term community health improvements. The relevance of health equity has gained significance in policy circles, highlighting the variation in health outcomes among communities. At the center of such activism lies the need to pay attention to social determinants of health, such as income, education, and environment. The State of Health Equity Movement focuses on the collective actions aimed at the erasure of disparity and is a basis for policy of inclusivity. The work of Birnbaum et al. (2011) elucidates that evidence of activities aimed at equitable health practices reflects a collective push for inclusiveness in health systems. To have health policies be in line with equity values is an ever-existing advocacy call by the stakeholders within the communities, thereby affirming policy-making as not merely a top-down process but rather a collaborative effort which should involve those who suffer most from health inequalities (Figure 10.7).

10.2.2. Impact of the Affordable Care Act (ACA)

The ACA has transformed the healthcare landscape in America, impacting health care service access, particularly for vulnerable populations. By expanding Medicaid and establishing health insurance marketplaces, the ACA aimed to reduce systematic disparities that have long plagued the health care system. According to the provisions of the law, millions of previously uninsured individuals were able to access coverage, making it possible for them to receive the necessary medical care and preventive services. This increase in access has led to measurable improvements in health within the population, as seen through higher rates of early detection of disease and better health outcomes within various groups. In spite of this, success in the ACA is also with the ongoing challenges of health equity, where certain groups remain with hindrances to care, highlighting the need for continued advocacy and policy adjustments to remedy such disparities on a comprehensive level. The demographic drift towards an elderly population is one of the principal variables in assessing the impact of the ACA. Since the elderly population is expanding at an exponential rate—particularly those over 85 years who will require extensive health care intervention—the provisions of the ACAs are greatly relevant. The population trend ranks as a gargantuan threat to health policy, necessitating the prioritization of long-term health care and supportive systems that are equitable and sustainable. Specifically, states such as New Hampshire are experiencing a sharp increase in their aging populations, which in turn puts an extra burden on public health programs as well as the healthcare workforce. Good policy advocacy must recognize the unique needs of such elderly populations' diversity by making sure that the infrastructure of ACA is transformed to address the heightened call for geriatric services and care so as to improve the health environment within communities (Davie et al., 2015). In addition, the ACA highlights the intersection of social determinants of health and policy advocacy, with a continued call to action in advancing health equity in community health practices. By the expansion of Medicaid and the provision of funding for preventative care, the ACA has moved towards eliminating health disparities; socio-economic determinants of health such as income, education, and access to health resources, however, remain disproportionate in their impact on health outcomes. Strategies to reduce these inequalities may require intersectoral action across such sectors as healthcare, housing, and education. Integrated strategies that recognize the strengths of community organizations need to be made a priority by policymakers in establishing an environment conducive to a holistic approach to community health and directs efforts to disadvantaged populations. The advocacy function is greatly significant in being at the forefront in advocating for these intersectoral strategies, ultimately enhancing the ACA's effectiveness and ensuring that its benefits extend to all segments of the community (Birnbaum et al., 2011).

10.2.3. Role of Local Health Departments

Local health departments play a critical function in the fabric of community health by acting as the critical link between state and federal health initiatives and local population requirements. Frequently the initial point of contact for health issues, these agencies have the responsibility of putting into place policies and programs that directly respond to the specific health problems facing their communities. Their role is multifaceted and involves carrying out needs assessments, priority setting, and strategic planning to help make health interventions locally relevant. By encouraging partnership with stakeholders in the community, local health departments are improved in that they can create targeted initiatives to facilitate health equity and accessibility.

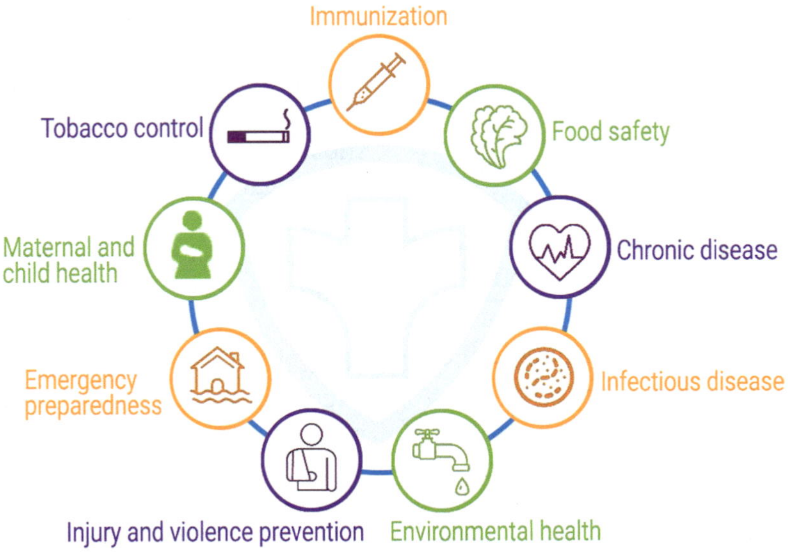

Figure 10.8. Role of local health departments.

Source: https://www.publichealthcareers.org/static/sites/www/files/images/sub/local/in-action.jpg?1723209204.

Their success in shaping health policy and pursuing much-needed systemic reform is made possible by this synchronization of the community's needs and is critical in improving overall public health outcomes (Birnbaum et al., 2011). In addition to operational efficiency, local health departments are important stakeholders in advocacy for health policies that enhance the well-being of marginalized groups. Through community health needs assessment, they identify some health disparities and work towards prioritizing solutions that are evidence-based and community-driven. This prioritization is crucial in strategic planning interventions since it assists in optimal use of resources towards impacting major health issues such as chronic illnesses, infectious diseases, and mental disorders. Secondly, integrating public health programs within the general community agenda helps to increase the impact of health policies as well as foster a culture of cooperation among sectors. As such, local health departments are not just program implementers of health interventions but also forces of health equity driving change that targets the systematic determinants of health disparities (Mueller et al., 2012). They also serve as significant facilitators of the ongoing conversation among policymakers, healthcare workers, and the community at large. Their role as intermediaries heightens the visibility of community health issues in policy discussion, wherein the interest of marginalized populations is represented and expressed. Advocacy allows the local health departments to emphasize the demand for legislative support, appropriations, and resources that underpin community health programs. In this capacity, they often form coalitions and partnerships that spread their influence beyond local geographic boundaries, leveraging pooled resources to drive systemic change. As such, whether or not local health departments are successful at policy advocacy is ultimately dependent upon their capacity to engage and mobilize the community, building a sense of partnership that prioritizes health as a collective societal aspiration (Birnbaum et al., 2011) (Figure 10.8).

10.3. Advocacy Strategies in Community Health

Advocacy strategies in community health have a key role to play in delivering equal health outcomes and bringing about systemic change. Mobilizing constituents is not the only component of advocacy strategies in this regard; it also comprises self-efficacy among constituents. Empowering individuals to exercise their rights and participate in decision-making may support a sense of ownership within communities through advocacy efforts. Programs like New Voices at the Civic Table reflect these principles through the integration of civic engagement with the core function of their model. The six pilot projects in New Voices focused on leadership development, civic education, and hands-on learning and prove that participation is important in creating a sustainable model of health advocacy. Finally, these efforts work to not just amplify community voices but also redefine the way participants understand their place in the broader societal fabric, leading to long-term social change (Nguyen et al., 2009). And further, the intersection of philanthropy and advocacy shows the potential for significant increases in community health outcomes. Foundations are increasingly urged to incorporate advocacy and public policy grantmaking into their portfolio, recognizing that private funding alone can never compensate for structural obstacles to health equity. Effective interventions, while wholesome in a single locale, typically need broader government intervention and investment to achieve their impact at scale. As noted in the debates on strategic frameworks employed by different foundations, public policy grantmaking is a key instrument to utilize resources and streamline them in consonance with advocacy objectives. By integrating such tactics, foundations are able to maximize their leverage to bring about policy changes that enhance access to health resources and services by underrepresented groups (Coffman, 2008). Moreover, advocacy interventions in community health must be responsive to the varying needs of different demographic groups in order to be successful. Advocacy interventions that are reactive to issues related to the community and affinity points guarantee everyone a voice and an opportunity to be heard. The civic activity analysis from the New Voices initiative emphasizes participatory decision-making frameworks that engage several stakeholders within the streams of health advocacy. By facilitating communication and coalition building between various community members, advocacy groups can produce a more comprehensive representation of health problems, overcoming the specific obstacles that face marginalized communities. Ultimately, employing creative and adaptive forms of advocacy can galvanize systemic transformation in community health, not merely providing access to care but also facilitating a more equitable distribution of health resources (Nguyen et al., 2009) (Figure 10.9).

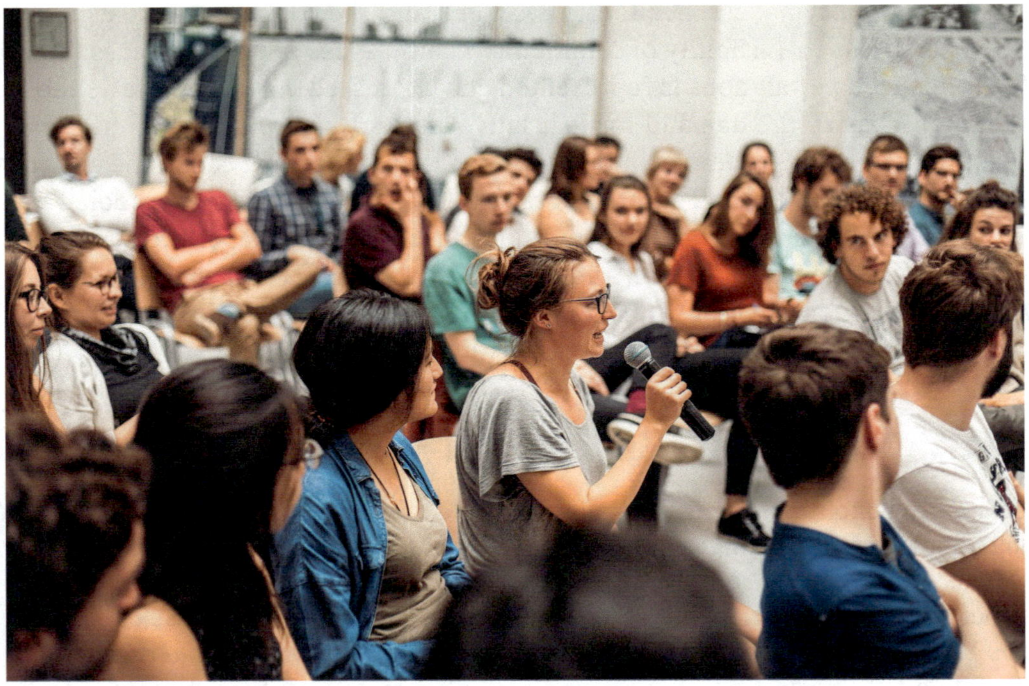

Figure 10.9. Advocacy strategies in community health.

Source: https://www.who.int/activities/awareness-raising-to-protect-human-health-from-climate-change

10.3.1. Grassroots Advocacy Efforts

Grassroots advocacy activities are at the core of shaping community health policies because they are a product of the people and organizations' collective voice at the grass-roots level. Grassroots activities are at the core of eliminating health disparities and organizing communities to fight fundamental health challenges. In tobacco prevention, for example, the National African American Tobacco Prevention Network (NAATPN) has been able to put in sharp relief serious inequities within African American communities when it comes to smoking behavior and quitting behaviors. Grassroots movements can advocate for policies that strongly resonate with marginalized groups' own particular concerns by highlighting community-based interventions, in turn making health programs more relevant and impactful. This community-based approach not only promotes civic participation but also allows citizens to become health advocates so that they may confront systemic problems causing unhealthy consequences, thereby emphasizing the importance of grassroots advocacy for community health (Baker et al., 2017). The effectiveness of grassroots advocacy is also uncovered in how leaders prepare strategic responses to urgent health concerns. Careful evaluation of advocacy initiatives is necessary for ensuring that initiative is fruitful in terms of quantitative health benefits. For instance, stakeholders can employ various evaluation strategies, including the creation of logic models or surveys, to quantify the impact of their efforts on the health outcomes in the community. This systematic approach to evaluation allows advocates to make decisions based on facts, employing evidence from interviews and focus groups to adapt their strategies and better serve their communities. These approaches place value on continuous feedback loops when evaluating grassroots success, rendering advocacy dynamic and responsive to changing health climates. By adopting these approaches, community advocates can demonstrate not just their efficacy but also receive support and funding, overall enhancing their capacity to bring about positive change (Strong et al., 2011). Furthermore, grassroots advocacy work fuels broader social change through incorporating various voices and perspectives that are needed in order to create inclusive health policy. The emphasis on inclusion and diversity in advocacy models, like those offered by NAATPNs, helps in addressing historical inequalities in access and representation to health.

Through the engagement of varied stakeholders, including marginalized groups, grassroots movements have the ability to create more inclusive health programs that reflect the variety of needs of the community. This process leads to ownership by the community members, with the result that they get fully engaged in the policymaking process. Finally, the integration of grassroots advocacy into programs in community health not only heightens the voice of the subject but also erodes system-level oppressions to drive towards more equitable health outcomes that resonate with the lived realities of marginalized groups (Baker et al., 2017).

10.3.2. Coalition Building and Partnerships

Effective coalition building and partnership are cornerstones in defense of policy and advocacy work in community health. Through strategic alliances, different stakeholders, including non-profit organizations, government institutions, and community networks, pool their resources and capacities to address shared health problems. Not only do such collaborations improve the efficiency of advocacy efforts but also foster a sense of shared ownership of health initiatives. By exchanging each other's knowledge and cashing in on each other's abilities, coalition members are in a better position to come up with stronger policy suggestions that capture the actual demand of their communities. Forming such alliances is critical when it comes to interpreting the complexity of health disparities because it pools together different perspectives that can create new solutions. To successfully form coalitions, there is a need to have well-defined objectives and common vision by allies. This alignment comes in the form of mutual goals for all the stakeholders that resonate with one another, thereby promoting uniform advocacy strategies. Mutual communication that is open and ongoing among organizations should be maintained to ensure trust and support, which are core in maintaining long-term alliances. Lessons may be learned from the experiences of successful non-profits in shaping best practices in advocacy. In Alberta, Canada, and other regions, it can be seen through case studies that organized collaboration is involved in the formulation of effective policy change (Krekoski, 2009). These activities will eventually not only contribute to the health of communities but also add to the collective capacity for influencing the health policy at multiple levels. Assessment is equally as important in the success of coalition building and partnerships for community health campaigning. As organizations collaborate to initiate health campaigns, they need to create precise metrics to measure the success of their collective endeavors. Approaches to evaluation such as the development of logic models and the use of focus groups can yield critical information about a coalitions progress and points of improvement. Secondly, collecting evidence and feedback from advocacy efforts enables the organization to better its processes and enhance the relevance of its strategies to meet the needs of the population (Strong et al., 2011). By integrating assessment into the coalition structure, the team can ensure that joint efforts lead to long-term health outcomes and react quickly to the changing landscape of public health challenges. Thus, prioritization of assessment reinforces the foundation for successful partnership relations in the complex space of community health policy and advocacy.

10.3.3. Use of Social Media for Advocacy

Social media has emerged as a revolutionary tool for advocacy in the field of community health, ushering in greater interaction and mobilization of resources. Social media sites like Facebook, Twitter, and Instagram provide a platform for users to disseminate information instantly to many people, galvanizing support for various health campaigns. The immediacy of social media means that research, health alerts, and policy adjustments are disseminated in time. Moreover, it offers channels for engagement between citizens, health professionals, and policymakers, enabling collaboration in addressing public health issues. Its capacity to create specific hashtags and online campaigns allows activists to ramp up their campaigns, creating discussions that may propel real policy reforms. Finally, the robust social media infrastructure serves not only as a vehicle of information transmission but also as an awareness creator and action trigger of community health activism. Apart from enhancing communication, social media platforms are also crucial to bring marginalized voices into the limelight of the community health arena. Mainstream tactics alone efforts in advocacy can overlook the contributions and issues of marginalized communities. Through platforms like Instagram and TikTok, individuals from varied backgrounds can have their voices heard, bringing into the limelight the complexity of health disparities and the imperatives of structural alteration. Such local-level reports appeal to wider audiences and make a convincing argument for policy change. Also, such platforms facilitate outreach in a focused manner, and advocates can deliver messages to targeted populations successfully. Efforts in promoting mental health sensitivity, demystifying mental illness, and promoting preventative health conduct have thrived through the authentic affiliations nurtured within these virtual communities and thus confirming the unique contribution of social media to policy advocacy for community health. A significant detail in harnessing social media for advocacy is the ability it holds to build alliances and collaboration between stakeholders. Connectivity on these sites allows health professionals, community organizations, and advocacy groups to collaborate more efficiently. When viewed cumulatively across case studies of how campaigns mobilized around key health issues—such as vaccination campaigns and mental health campaigns—such efforts have successfully mobilized the public and influenced policy debate. Society for Community Research and Action highlights the importance of developing capacity through social media, as evidence indicates that social media can enhance the effectiveness of advocacy by many folds. Social media not only amplifies campaigns for any one individual but also aids in a sustained movement towards equitable community health policy through networking and best practice sharing (García-Ramírez et al., 2016). Thus, social media is an integral part of the evolving methods employed by champions dedicated to improving community health outcomes (Figure 10.10).

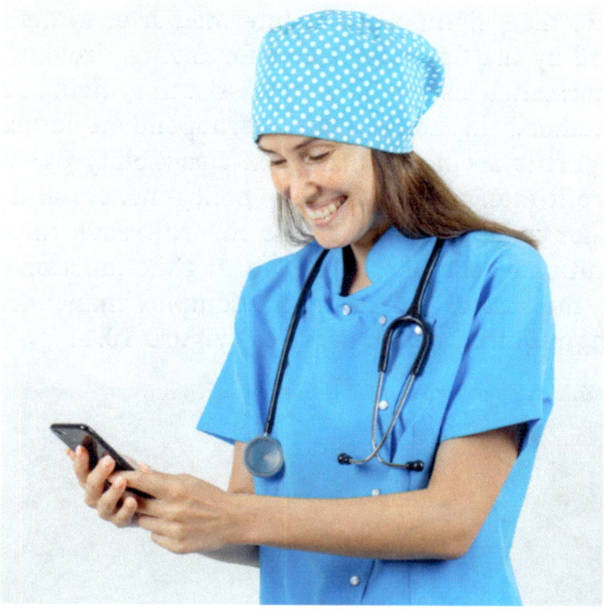

Figure 10.10. Use of social media for advocacy.

Source: https://ihm.edu.au/wp-content/uploads/2022/10/MicrosoftTeams-image-63-scaled.jpg.

10.4. Role of Nonprofit Organizations

Nonprofit organizations are vital in the community health sphere as they act as intermediaries between vulnerable groups and vital health services. These organizations are usually addressing socioeconomic status-based, race-based, and geography-based health disparities, tailoring services to meet the specific needs of the population being served. Through the development of specialized interventions, such as health education programs and preventive care, nonprofits educate and empower individuals to navigate complex healthcare systems. Their placement in communities places them in a position where they can connect with those otherwise disconnected from the mainstream healthcare, thus making significant impacts on population health outcomes. Additionally, their work through advocacy and activism is geared towards advocating for policy changes that try to address system disparities, further showing how much their work is crucial in supporting community health and well-being. The use of technology in the operational frameworks of nonprofit organizations has heightened their potential to initiate change in community health. Technology tools such as neighborhood information systems, electronic campaigning, and digital inclusion programs strive to construct the infrastructure of nonprofits so that they are better at outreach and service provision. For instance, such technologies facilitate organizations to collect and examine data on the needs of community health so that implementation and design of programs can be made more informed. In addition, the combining of internet-based micro-enterprise support can enhance financial stability in communities, with related enhancement of health outcome by mitigating fiscal limitations on care. Through community health projects and equitable access to all populations by organizations like nonprofits, a larger ecosystem with a greater commitment can be ensured (N/A, 2007). Moreover, the role of nonprofit organizations is better understood through research that shows their significance as intermediaries in the healthcare sector. Studies, such as the research funded by the Gateway Center for Giving, provide valuable insights into the functioning of nonprofit intermediaries and how they assist in bringing about improvements in area health. Not only do such studies bring to light the interdependent nature of such entities, but also the part philanthropic support takes in optimizing their capability (N/A, 2011). By understanding the dynamics of the nonprofit intermediary system, policy-makers and funders are able to make more efficient frameworks for collaboration and thus ensure greater impact of nonprofits on policy reform and community health advocacy. Lastly, supporting the function of nonprofit organizations in community health lies at the core of addressing the complex challenges faced by rural and urban populations when accessing required health services (Figure 10.11).

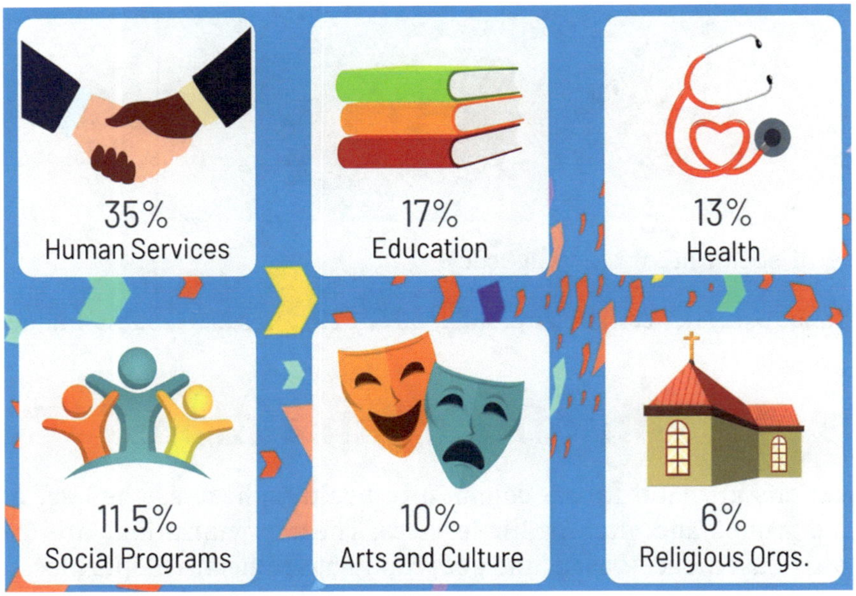

Figure 10.11. Role of nonprofit organizations.

Source: https://learn.g2.com/hs-fs/hubfs/Screen%20Shot%202019-07-09%20at%203.39.01%20PM.png?width=1350&name=Screen%20Shot%202019-07-09%20at%203.39.01%20PM.png.

10.4.1. Contributions of Nonprofits to Community Health

Nonprofit organizations have a crucial role in promoting community health by responding to both acute medical issues and the more overarching social determinants of health. Their impact goes beyond conventional health care services since they mobilize assets to address underlying challenges like poverty, education access, and food insecurity. For instance, the majority of nonprofits offer preventive health interventions, wellness programs, and mental health interventions, which are all aimed at lessening the burden on the public healthcare system. Through stakeholder collaboration, nonprofits not only fill service gaps but also advocate for structural change to improve health equity. The principles of these organizations are local, which enables them to harvest good ideas from the local communities they serve and make sure that their programs prioritize local concerns and needs. This is local customization and engagement, leading to healthier communities and populations. Policy advocacy forms a critical component of the role of the nonprofit sector in community health. Through strategic engagement with policymakers, nonprofits provide credible portrayals of the health needs of their populations, which guide the policymaking decisions that shape resource allocation and health policy. Generally, this practice of advocacy by nonprofits could lead to increased funding for vital health programs, in addition to the passing of policies favorable to health equity. Through the identification of the devastating effects of government budget cuts on nonprofit services, organizations show the need for collaborative arrangements among nonprofits, government agencies, and foundations to address these challenges (N/A, 2010). Not only do these collaborations enhance service provision, but they also ensure that vulnerable populations are offered the support and services they need, illustrating how proactive advocacy can yield tangible benefits for community health. Moreover, strong policy advocacy is not only reliant on grassroots mobilization but also on knowledge sharing and best practices and strategies among organizations. Nonprofits share knowledge with a view to creating strong advocacy, as evidenced in fora such as those mentioned in the guide which examine successful advocacy steps (Krekoski, 2009). By examination of case studies and collaboration on projects, nonprofits are able to organize their efforts to effectively impact policy. These collective steps strengthen the advocacy strength, allowing nonprofits to erect strong demands that address health disparities in their populations. In addition, as nonprofits acquire resources and establish collaborative relationships, they can leverage their combined strength to secure more substantive partnerships with government and private institutions. This robust strategy not only enhances nonprofit activities but also enables richer understanding of the health issues of the population, ultimately contributing to improved health outcomes for various populations (Figure 10.12).

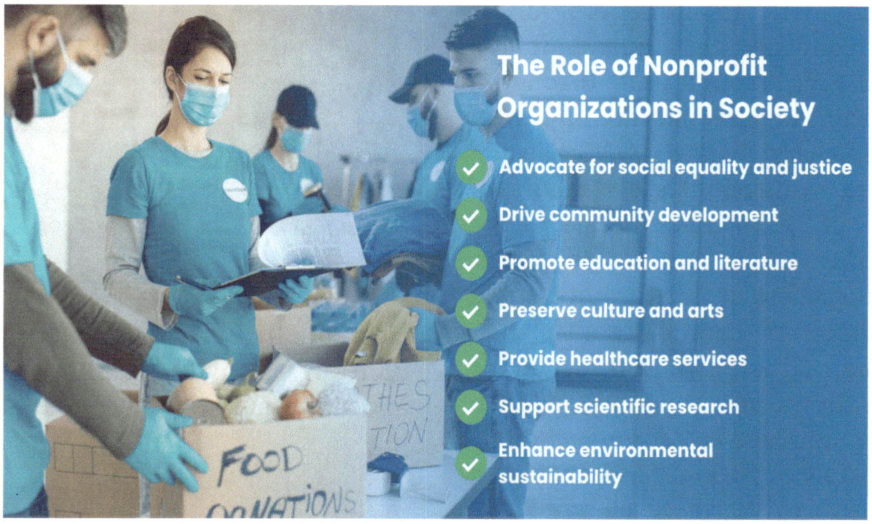

Figure 10.12. Contributions of nonprofits to community health.

Source: https://cdn.azeusconvene.com/wp-content/uploads/Image-02_Convene-GL_WebsiteArticle_What-is-a-Nonprofit-Organization-Overview-Types-and-Best-Practices-A.png.

10.4.2. Funding and Resource Allocation

The efficacy of policy and advocacy interventions in community health cannot be overlooked and has a close relationship with funding and resource allocation. Adequate financing enables health programs to address the multifaceted needs of communities. The EEA Financial Mechanism (2009–2014), for instance, invested a staggering 160.4 million in support of various NGO programs in 16 countries, with an emphasis on civil society development as well as social justice and welfare services. Such investments are significant catalysts for NGOs because they empower them to implement projects that develop democracy, citizen participation, and sustainable development. The grants not only improve the organizational capabilities of these institutions but also help guarantee that vital services are delivered to underserved communities, thereby strengthening the overall system of community health advocacy. In this sense, focused financial resources are essential in order to support organizational functions and advance community health aspirations. Resource allocation within community health also requires systematic assessments in order to guarantee effectiveness and sustainability. EEA Grants NGO Programmes went through a mid-term evaluation to ascertain the impact of their work on beneficiary countries' NGO sector. The two-pronged evaluation had the aim of identifying areas of improvement while, at the same time, guiding future funding priorities. By analyzing the success and failure of funded projects, policymakers can make informed resource allocation decisions and direct funds where they will do the most good. Also, such evaluations can uncover successful models replicable or scalable in various settings. When funding aligns with evidence-based practices, not only is the program more effective but also advocacy for cultivating health equity and community resilience. The same goes for information obtained through Pennsylvania's hunger prevention programs that reveal the critical significance of funding in addressing food insecurity—a fundamental determinant of community health. The Pennsylvania Department of Agriculture regulates significant programs, such as the State Food Purchase Program (SFPP) and The Emergency Food Assistance Program (TEFAP), that build a crucial safety net for underserved communities. These kinds of programs underscore the importance of strategic resource allocation to address food insecurity, thereby directly affecting the health and well-being of residents of Montgomery County and others. Through proper utilization of available funds, such programs not only meet short-term needs but also contribute to long-term improvement in health among affected communities. It is therefore absolutely critical to deal with funding and resource allocation within the policy and advocacy framework to develop effective community health strategies based on multiple aspects of public health and welfare (Figure 10.13).

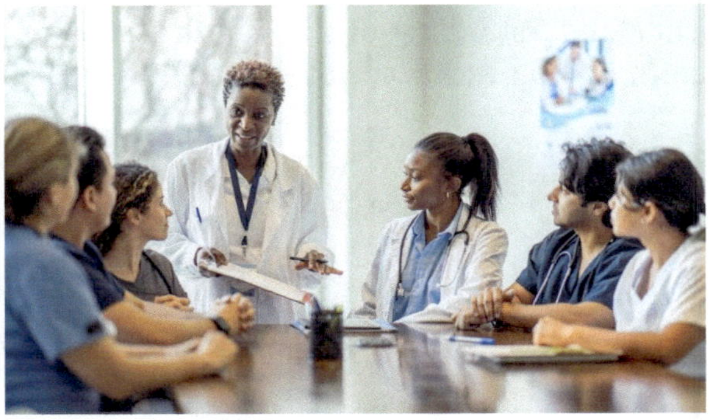

Figure 10.13. Funding and resource allocation.

Source: https://www.careerbeez.com/wp-content/uploads/2023/01/Why-resource-allocation-is-important-in-managing-hospitals.jpg.

10.4.3. Case Studies of Successful Nonprofit Initiatives

Successful nonprofit initiatives are generally exemplary examples of how accurate policy action can yield significant improvements in community health. One such example was the implementation of neighborhood information systems, which used technology to collect and report essential health data. By giving timely data to community organizations, these systems enhanced the effectiveness of these organizations at addressing geographic health inequalities. The effectiveness of this endeavor lies not in the data itself but in organizational capability it creates among nonprofits. According to N/A (2007), technology practices like these have a direct impact on the functional capabilities of community organizations, thereby facilitating more effective decision-making and strategic advocacy responsive to marginalized communities' needs. Another fascinating case study is the Kresge Foundations' complex strategy for funding health-related projects that demonstrates a focus on systemic change through policy advocacy. The foundation's strategy has a broad view of community health, its issues, and solutions that range from access to care and quality of care to social determinants of health. Kresge's thorough reportage—grants summaries and geographic funding distribution—reiterates a methodical approach to maximizing impact on community health. Through aligning resources with what is most needed to address immediate health concerns, the program refunctions what sound funding can do to aid local groups and drive policy changes that benefit society in aggregate, well representing goals outlined in N/A (2012). Last, there was this outstanding project which was focused on digital inclusion programs to bridge the technological gap for underprivileged communities. By providing easy access to digital content, nonprofits were essentially enabling individuals to become active players in their own care. Digital literacy programs not only enhance people's ability to obtain information, but they also provide an element of empowerment needed for effective advocacy. These programs are a part of the overarching narrative of community health in that they position residents on an educated plane as stakeholders, where they are well-positioned to cope with health care systems. Such grassroots empowerment is key in that it lays the groundwork for more effective advocacy that comes from the voice and concerns of the served communities, much like the experience outlined in the observations in N/A (2007).

10.5. Challenges in Policy and Advocacy

The complexity of policy and advocacy in community health is generally heightened by the heterogeneity of public health issues. Among the primary challenges are a mismatch in perspectives between stakeholders, which can lead to uncoordinated efforts in policy. The champions of change usually face indifference or pushback by policymakers who may be ignorant of the given situation in the local community or have conflicting interests. Moreover, the lack of robust empirical data on health disparities may become a hindrance to efficient advocacy. For example, participatory mapping approaches have been promising in engaging communities using the mapping of social and environmental determinants of health disparities, but their implementation is limited. This methodological gap has the potential to lead to insufficient advocacy and lack of proper mitigation of localized health issues, as in the case of South Los Angeles evidence that revealed overlooked variables such as local crime associated with access to public parks (Douglas et al., 2020). Yet another challenge stems from the structural forces in healthcare systems determining policy. Most countries' public health requirements, particularly those transitioning towards universal health coverage, may be overshadowed by the immediacy of economic strain and the prevalence of non-communicable diseases. The Bahrain, Egypt, Lebanon, Qatar, Sudan, and United Arab Emirates cases reflect a common trend in facing insufficient access to primary care and a lack of health professionals (Alnasir et al., 2017). Primary healthcare incorporation strategies into overall health systems continually fail to progress because decision-making is unsupported with comprehensive data. Community-based primary healthcare solutions need to be championed with the overcoming of bureaucratic inertia and inter-agency complexity, in turn calling for a coordinated approach that addresses immediate healthcare and long-term community health planning needs. Lastly, the influence of grassroot organizations on policy advocacy is both promising and greatly challenging. Grassroots movements can influence the voice of marginalized communities and provide representation for community-specific health concerns in policy platforms, but such organizations are often plagued by resource limitation and lack political power to effect change. Including various stakeholders, including academia, health professionals, and local governments, can allow for the establishment of a strong base of support for advocacy. Moreover, heightening public consciousness and knowledge regarding issues in community health through training programs can galvanize support for policy reform. Lastly, integrating participatory approaches, as reflected in community mapping and public health research, can enhance advocacy through the release of valuable information on community needs and wants, facilitating easier policy-making to be more participative in character (Douglas et al., 2020) (Figure 10.14).

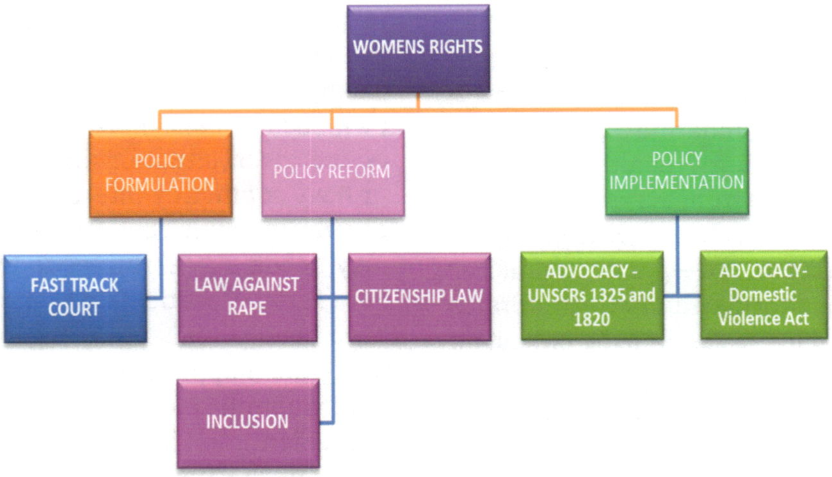

Figure 10.14. Challenges in policy and advocacy.

Source: https://www.researchgate.net/profile/Binit-Gurung/publication/364042022/figure/fig3/AS:11431281087343460@1664547044839/Policy-Advocacy-of-the-NGOs-working-on-womens-rights.ppm.

10.5.1. Political Barriers to Effective Policy

Political barriers to effective policy often impede the formation and success of effective interventions in the area of community health policy. Political party affiliation may greatly influence what issues have priority, with parties prioritizing health issues according to their agendas. Partisanship may inhibit policy innovation and lead to stagnation when offering solutions to urgent health problems among disadvantaged populations. For instance, while politicians are preoccupied with balancing health agendas with political agendas, the pressing concerns of those other segments of a society which are not as represented may still remain insufficiently addressed. Thus, political gamesmanship undermines the ability to speak for all-around health policies, creating a scenario wherein the welfare and health of vulnerable communities become secondary to partisan interests. In addition, the intersection of local and national politics also serves to highlight the challenge of providing effective community health policy. Local institutions may be forced to navigate the balance between federal and state mandates, resulting in piecemeal health programs that do not cater to specific community needs. The fragmentation is especially problematic in communities of color, where the lack of centralized planning may exacerbate existing health disparities. Political barriers also come about where there is under-investment in developing grassroots leadership. There is a need to empower the local leaders to venture into the political landscape, as they possess the wisdom to speak for their people quite well. Budgeting directed towards constructing community-based leadership is important, as indicated in the application of Marsh et al. (2003), to provide options to construct needed advocacy that is sensitive to local conditions. Furthermore, foregrounding health policy with social justice priorities remains an insurmountable political hurdle, always yielding to economic considerations and short-term political gain. In this struggle, policymakers are inclined to subordinate access to important resources such as education, economic empowerment, and sustainable development, especially for underprivileged groups. In so doing, such neglect reinforces existing inequalities, suppressing the health of individuals and families relying on the system. To that end, in this situation, advocacy will need to prioritize framing social justice principles as a way of pushing policy reforms forward. By tackling not just the measures of health but also the social determinants influencing them, advocates can ensure political discourse emphasizes prioritizing health policy that is equitable. The alignment of social justice programs and health advocacy in the community can facilitate more integrated policy responses, required to bridge the political barriers common in health policy formulation, as evidenced by the mechanisms identified in N/A (2009).

10.5.2. Funding Limitations and Resource Scarcity

In the process of community health policy and advocacy, resource shortage and funding constraints represent key challenges that undermine the ability of health programs. As various actors assess the landscape of public health, it is found that philanthropy and state subsidies fall short of financing the urgent health demands of vulnerable populations. This is the situation with the international campaign for lesbian, gay, bisexual, and transgender rights, as witnessed in the coinciding debates among donors and rights activists that reflected actual impediments to achieving fair funding for the provision of essential health services. Ensuring efficient use of financial resources is crucial to tackle health inequities; where funding is lacking, community-based organizations struggle to implement programs that have direct effects on the populations that are underserved, thus continuing the disparities the policy aims to resolve (Simon, 2009). Shortage in resources implies more than the lack of funds; it implies a broader set of constraints that include human capital, infrastructure, and technological capacity. This shortage is particularly critical in developing nations where health outcomes are severely impeded by a scarcity of resources. For instance, water resource management has become the priority of public health policy in urban areas that are facing climatic hardship because poor management of water can be the cause of disease and increasing mortality among vulnerable populations. In countries such as South Africa, Mozambique, and Kenya, water equity challenges are merely symptoms of more fundamental systemic limitations that undermine policy efficacy. The disproportion in the magnitude of public involvement is stark; the most vulnerable individuals subjected to water-related challenges have no means and opportunity to become involved in governance and are thus quite often unable to handle challenges facing their lives (Figueiredo et al., 2013). Initiatives to bridge the gap due to limitation of funds and resources must focus on innovative collaborations between community organizations, NGOs, and local governments. Leverage can be derived from the combined knowledge base and resources of these entities to enhance community participation and advocacy in public health programs. Establishment of participatory workshops and environmental education programs has become an essential method to strengthen local governance capacities, particularly in cities deeply impacted by climate change. Not only do these partnerships facilitate direct empowerment of those communities whose health is impacted by policies, but also inform better decision-making at higher levels, ultimately expanding the reach of resource distribution. With the ever-changing debate on climate change and public health, the issue of how to address the interlinkages of resources, funding, and community involvement is essential in achieving equitable outcomes in health as well as sustaining long-term improvements in community health (Figueiredo et al., 2013) (Figure 10.15).

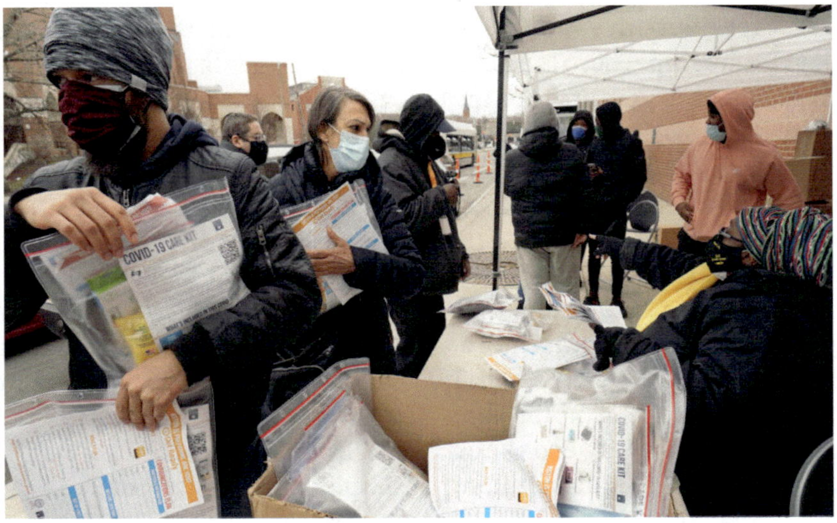

Figure 10.15. Community health funding limitations and resource scarcity.

Source: https://www.statnews.com/wp-content/uploads/2021/06/AP21059722012747-1024x576.jpg.

10.5.3. Public Perception and Misinformation

Public perception plays an important role in shaping health policy and advocacy for interventions in community health. Misinformation, and more specifically misinformation surrounding vaccines and public health measures, can radically alter that perception, with vaccine hesitancy or skepticism regarding key health interventions as a consequence. The Internet and social media, with their rise as a primary source of health information, have also added to that confusing dynamic. While there is much scientifically-based vaccine messaging available, anti-vaccine messaging also comes to dominate through the emotionally engaging and simple-to-communicate nature of the messages. Correcting such falsehoods is not an academic exercise; it is essential to the efficacy of public health campaigns aimed at building community confidence and encouraging vaccination take-up, since active citizenship produces healthier citizens who are more likely to make informed recommendations for good health policy themselves. The role of combating misinformation goes beyond merely presenting correct facts; it involves understanding the emotional landscape behind public attitudes. The vast majority of individuals express a hesitancy to vaccinate not based on a lack of information, but rather through a multifaceted interaction of fears, anxieties, and experiences. This is most commonly exhibited in vaccine-hesitant parents, whom many times seek out their healthcare providers as credible sources of information. To effectively overcome vaccine hesitancy, healthcare providers must utilize communication strategies that appeal on an emotional level and address specific concerns. Evidence suggests that an empathetic style of communication, coupled with the provision of clear and respectful information delivery, has the potential to move undecideds to become champions for vaccination. Placing the conversation in an environment that respects emotions allows health policy champions to work more effectively with populations and establish a culture of evidence-based decision-making through trust. In addition, the intersection of public narrative and disinformation extends beyond the bounds of broad social problems such as climate change to demonstrate parallels between disinformation influence on policy and public consensus. Likewise, how disinformation influences health beliefs, vaccine disinformation can influence health perception. Climate denial is often similarly fueled by narratives being altered by politically motivated campaigns. This polarizes public perception not merely but also complicates advocacy measures for addressing critical health-related ramifications of climate change. Strategies for resisting these trends must involve narrative that evokes empathy and therefore cancels out the emotional resonance of invented stories. Leveraging the potential of narrative to generate more comprehension of the interests involved, so that it presents alternative avenues of communication, is something which campaigners can utilize to displace misinformation efficiently, much as in the case of health campaigns. Lastly, successful public health advocacy depends on a genuine understanding of the manner in which perception serves as the basis for shaping behavior and how error or misinformation affects community health objectives.

10.6. Future Directions in Community Health Policy

Future directions for community health policy debates must ensure a platform that balances advocacy and measurable goals. One of the most important steps into this evolution is having definitive expectations regarding what is effective with successful advocacy. Under a systematic measurement strategy, policymakers and stakeholders can identify precise results that are connected to advocacy movements. This encompasses not only the efficacy of policy reforms but also public awareness and participation in health issues. For instance, leveraging the tools suggested in the new guide to measure policy improvements and public support, advocates can present fact-based narratives that augment activist passion and community support, which is instrumental while moving towards implementing improved health strategies (Gienapp et al., 2007). Ultimately, grounding such frameworks is required to ensure accountability and ongoing improvement in community health policy initiatives. Furthermore, solving in-depth health problems has to entail an intersectional approach of recognition of the intersecting harms to public health. Policies in future community health should strive to address problems of childhood obesity and its spill-over on health in adulthood and healthcare costs. Of particular note in public health advocacy is recognition of the manner in which health outcomes are affected by societal organization, and how they can be better improved through targeted discussion and presentations exposing the impact of restricting food advertising on vulnerable populations (N/A, 2008). By placing health policy within the context of higher-level social determinants of health, stakeholders are best positioned to better advocate for comprehensive change that facilitates healthier environments. This shift not only legitimates community health concerns but also organizes various groups into advocacy action, deepening discourse and bolstering policy capacity. Finally, community health policy must embrace innovative approaches that take advantage of technology and big data analysis to guide and inform future initiatives. By tapping into big data and advanced analytics, policymakers are better able to identify trends and upcoming health issues earlier and more accurately. Such an interactive approach can facilitate the development of specialized interventions and mobilization of resources sensitive to the unique needs of various communities. Interaction with technological interventions can also empower ordinary citizens so they can be engaged in health advocacy more effectively. In creating a responsive policy climate, the integration of analytical tools guarantees optimal optimization of community health initiatives, promoting evidence-based building and collaboration across sectors. As these directions are honed, community health policy will better be able to address contemporary issues, ensuring equitable health outcomes for future generations (Figure 10.16).

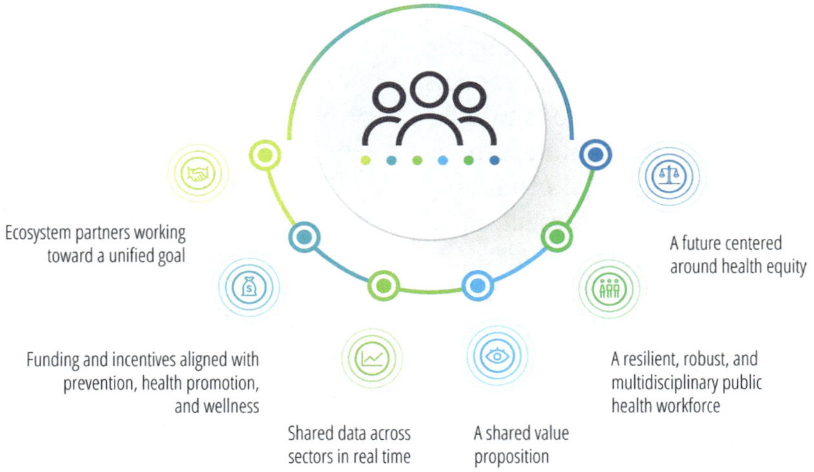

Figure 10.16. Future directions in community health policy.

Source: https://www2.deloitte.com/content/dam/insights/articles/US164606_CHS-the-future-of-public-health/figures/US164606_Figure1.jpg.

10.6.1. Emerging Trends in Health Policy

Evolving trends in health policy are an expression of an increased awareness of the need for equity and for universal inclusion in the health system. With more awareness of the complex challenges of the marginalized groups by the community health practitioners, new trends in health policy seek to integrate strategies dealing with the social determinants of health. This means not only treating illness but addressing the socio-economic determinants that influence health outcomes.

The surge in community-focused initiatives is an exhibition of willingness to empower targeted groups, such as BYMOC, by connecting them with targeted resources and advocacy services. The trend shows the significance of participatory approaches to health policy since it is seeking to remove obstacles and facilitate equal access to health care and education among communities (Gilgoff et al., 2015). Besides, the implementation of the ACA has fueled heated debate about health equity in the United States of America. Trends indicate that health professionals from various disciplines—social workers, community health workers, and public health practitioners—have started collaborating to address systemic disparities impacting health outcomes. The ACAs focus on shifting from fee-for-service to value-based care has hastened such efforts. By redirecting resources and eliminating economic barriers to care, such a policy approach is designed to create a more solid foundation upon which community health initiatives can be strengthened. Health equity is being recognized more and more by advocates as an ethos to inform health reform, promoting policies prioritizing social determinants of health in order to create broad-based enhancements in the provision of health care (Acuff et al., 2017). Finally, acknowledgement of the interdependent relationship between health and policy is a step toward more integrated practices in community health activism. New trends acknowledge evidence-based approaches to monitoring progress and accountability in eliminating health disparities. Developing healthcare dashboards enables providers to monitor their performance in relation to social determinants, thus maintaining institutional promises to health equity. This mechanism of accountability not only fosters transparency but also supports inter-stakeholder collaboration in different sectors. Through their continued influence on health policy, their potential for more inclusive and efficient solutions to health becomes clear, showing the imperative of ongoing advocacy that aims to advance health equity and enhance the life outcomes of all community members (Acuff et al., 2017) (Figure 10.17).

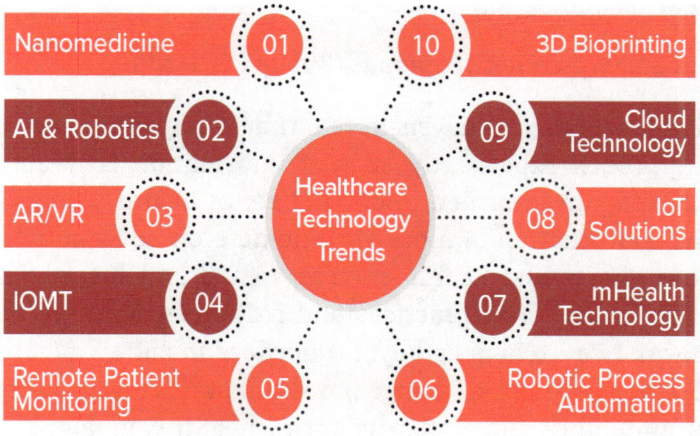

Figure 10.17. Emerging trends in health policy.

Source: https://lh5.googleusercontent.com/yW6x4T2pmJ29ySjrufcIGfqKTmXmm1BNOj4YRYYyVlMtm3mM1ngpYmsCwzKy0Owdhm89qAjbzLYVhyQhpWgkp6_xtCeGqKodozWTdd_eCsJ9bQ1Kdn7KiRT2i0jgGH5jad5DmNSov4ZZMehnjmdk53A.

10.6.2. The Role of Technology in Advocacy

Technology is now a revolutionary power in the context of advocacy, particularly for community health. The availability of digital communication instruments enables advocates to increase their reach for audiences, greatly enhancing their potential in mobilizing support for health activities. Social networking sites, websites, and mobile applications are critical sources for information sharing and raising awareness about pressing health issues. Sanitation and hygiene campaigns, for instance, have employed such technologies to educate communities and prompt action, as noted in the forums organized by the Global Water Futures Project.

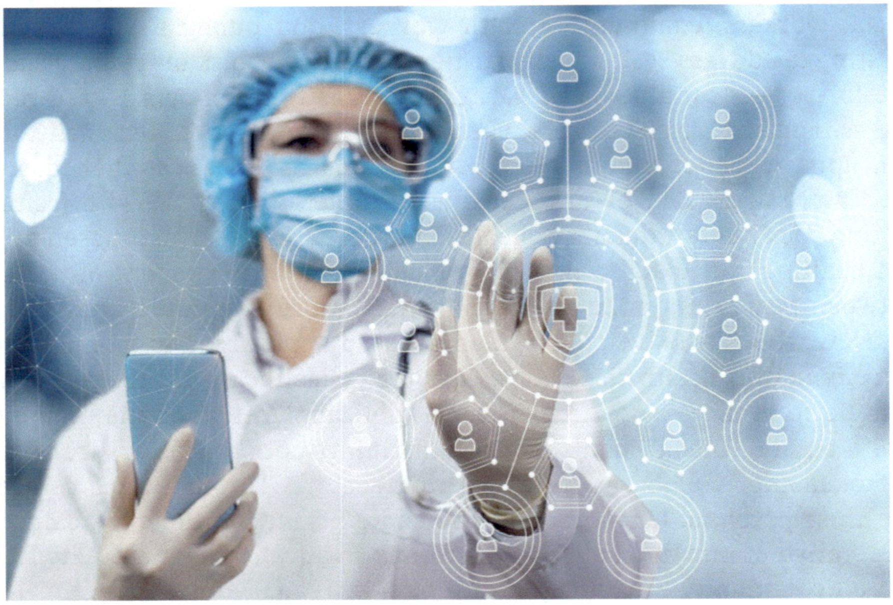

Figure 10.18. The role of technology in advocacy.

Source: https://baggout.com/wp-content/uploads/2021/11/1-1.jpeg.

By integrating data gathering and analysis in real time, campaigning for causes is in a position to better fine-tune its approach expediently, so that information is fresh and persuasive to its constituents, hence promoting an informed public debate of health policy (N/A, 2010). Secondly, technology facilitates the coordination of more stakeholders on advocating for community health. Virtual networking allows for public health officers, NGOs, and local leaders to communicate, creating opportunities for sharing best practices and resources. Some of the tools that facilitate advocates in having informative exchanges beyond borders include virtual webinars and forums online. The capacity to track legislative changes, document advocacy successes, and chart data efficiently enhances accountability and transparency in health campaigns. A case in point is the Paths Forward for the Global Water, Sanitation, and Hygiene (WASH) Sector event, during which technology played a pivotal role to optimize dialogue and decision-making processes regarding global WASH concerns (N/A, 2010). This integration supports a synergistic paradigm of advocacy which is paramount to navigate complex health issues with an urgency to act. The assessment of advocacy impacts has also been revolutionized by technology to ensure that interventions are not only functional but also measurable. The integration of data collection mechanisms into advocacy platforms enables organizations to assess the effectiveness of their actions in a systematic manner. As stipulated in the handbook designed for the Annie E. Casey Foundation, such practical tools as legislative process tracking logs and policy brief stakeholder surveys are significant in assessing changes that arise as a result of advocacy activities. By employing these tools, advocates can enhance their strategy, enhance their approach in the moment, and authenticate their claims to stakeholders as well as funders. Lastly, technology's contribution towards advocacy not only empowers advocates but also reaffirms their commitment towards living up to their word of providing better community health through empowered, data-driven decision-making (Figure 10.18).

10.6.3. Importance of Community Engagement

The role of community engagement takes center stage in driving effective policy and advocacy efforts in community health. By activating engagement from community members, such activity enhances the understanding of community health concerns, thereby designing interventions that address a specific population. Open dialogue permits communities to share their history and insight, which can then be applied to shape public health initiatives and policies. Policy and intervention work prioritizing from community input will have a higher likelihood of making successful health impacts, as they cater to the values and concerns of residents. Secondly, such collaborations raise the social cohesion and empower the individuals, with an emphasis placed on collective action reducing health inequities. The positive synergy between policy advocacy and community engagement serves to bring attention to the importance of involving affected populations in decision making, leading to a better stake in healthier environments and equal access to health care (Byaello et al., 2022).

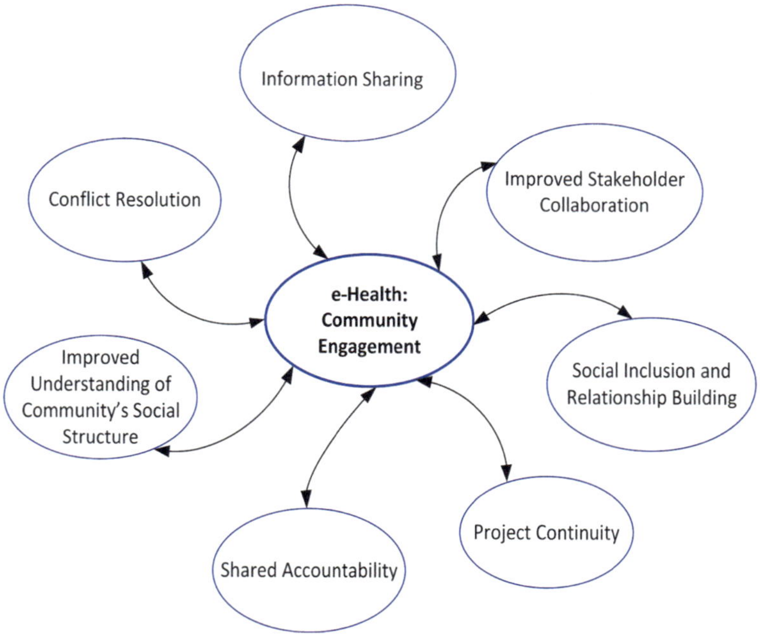

Figure 10.19. Importance of community engagement.

Source: https://www.researchgate.net/profile/Ephias-Ruhode/publication/297709532/figure/fig1/AS:669386285277209@1536605535911/Benefits-of-Community-Engagement-in-e-health.png.

Its strength is that it has the ability to redefine civic responsibility among the participants. Models that incorporate civic engagement systematically empower individuals through the development of leadership, civic education, and experiential decision-making. These models, as identified by the Alliance for Children and Families' New Voices initiative, are distinguished by determining factors that facilitate the exchange of knowledge and active involvement in communities (Nguyen et al., 2009). This process not only encourages self-efficacy and citizen action but also alters how participants conceive their contribution to the larger social sphere. Engaged community citizens become health and social change agents, fostering ownership of the well-being of their community. Empowerment is at the heart of resource mobilization, and what is gleaned from community experience is what informs policy creation that advocates for health equity and social justice. Furthermore, effective community involvement has been proven to produce innovative public health interventions that are sensitive to the ever-evolving health care environment of health concerns. Through the recognition and addressing of the specific needs of diverse populations, community-level initiatives can effectively target health disparities and attain enhanced health outcomes. Where policymakers and public health practitioners collaborate with stakeholders in the community, they can leverage a rich well of knowledge and communal experience that renders their health interventions more potent. The reciprocal relationship of policy activism and community outreach ensures that not only are health programs underpinned with empirical data but also shaped by the lived realities of the communities they seek to serve (Byaello et al., 2022). With communities as engaged players in shaping their health futures, they are advancing the common good of well-being for all and building resilience and sustainability in public health initiatives (Figure 10.19).

SUMMARY

In summarizing an examination of a community health approach to policy and advocacy, it is apparent that these efforts are needed to close the gaps in health and build community well-being. The blending of grassroots mobilization with policy initiatives at the level of the system is instrumental in building a framework that empowers marginalized communities. Through the development of leadership training programs that are specific to communities of color, advocates can effectively ensure that multiple voices are not merely heard but are central to health policy development. This is particularly remarkable given the history of exclusion from decision-making affecting these communities and thus accentuating the need for foundational investment and provision to develop their capacity for leadership (Marsh et al., 2003). Additionally, the charter development and implementation process regarding active living illustrates the complexity of advocacy initiatives. As has been demonstrated in Canadian charter development research, a momentum in the creation of such policies in the first place exists, with ongoing advocacy being necessary for meaningful impacts. Political contexts at the local level and community engagement cannot be overstated, as they largely determine the success and uptake of such charters. This finding emphasizes the need for health professionals and policymakers to not only be proficient in policy-making but also have the capacity to review it frequently and advocate for its enactment, so desired health impacts are attained (Benson et al., 2013). Ultimately, the journey toward equitable community health requires an integrated process that addresses policy review, advocacy strategies, and civic engagement. Effective policy activists must aim at constant evaluation and modify policies based on community sentiments and outcomes observed. Flexible policies will lead to the formulation of effective health policies that are indeed addressing the population's issues it's intended to aim at As we move forward, it is essential that all stakeholders involved are committed to creating an inclusive environment wherein advocacy is not simply one event but a sustained effort towards systems change (Marsh et al., 2003).

In highlighting the relevance of policy and advocacy in community health, some key points illustrate the key role systematic approaches have in encouraging positive health outcomes. At the heart of this discussion is Kairos' recognition of a framework to enable stakeholders to understand and define results pertaining to advocacy work. Such frameworks not only provide a definition of anticipated outcomes but also enable such common language across various audiences, including philanthropic and non-profit organizations. Through standardization of such outcomes, advocates are in a better position to communicate the impact of interventions, driving home the necessity of policy change and community activism as integral components of health promotion. A global approach likewise makes Grantmakers more likely to support programs with the potential to provide measurable improvements in public health policies and community services, which will further promote the field of community health advocacy (Gienapp et al., 2007). In addition, methodological quality in assessing advocacy projects cannot be overemphasized. Strong evaluation processes are paramount to proving the effectiveness of advocacy activities, informing future strategies and fund distribution. Extensive methodologies, including creating logic models and gathering data through various mechanisms—such as focus groups and interviews—are key tools for gauging program performance. The conclusions obtained from such evaluations not only educate stakeholders about their direct impact, but they also sharpen their ability to tailor their strategies for maximum effectiveness. By means of sound evaluation procedures, advocates for community health are able to develop an environment of continuous improvement that not only benefits the specific projects, but also assists in strengthening the overall knowledge concerning advocacy's contribution toward public health (Strong et al., 2011). Finally, advocacy, community engagement, and policy change are complementary to solving system-level differences in health. Raising the public's awareness and prioritization of health issues may involve deliberate efforts to engage members of the public in the process of advocacy. This feeling of belonging not only makes health initiatives relevant but also helps communities identify with their health outcomes. By using measurement tools that assess community attitudes and the salience of health concerns, the advocates can monitor the success of their involvement strategies and make changes as needed. Therefore, the attention to grass roots mobilization and community support can greatly add to the effectiveness of policy activism, setting the stage for long-term health gains at local and national levels (Gienapp et al., 2007).

KEY TERMS FROM THIS CHAPTER

Health Policy	Advocacy Strategies	Public Health Law
Stakeholder Engagement	Community Mobilization	Legislative Advocacy
Policy Development	Health Equity	Social Determinants of Health
Coalition Building	Health Disparities	Policy Implementation
Regulatory Change	Grassroots Advocacy	Health Impact Assessment
Evidence-Based Policy	Civic Engagement	Public Awareness Campaigns
Lobbying	Community Empowerment	Decision-Making Processes
Government Relations	Power Dynamics	Resource Allocation

CLOSER LOOK

VARIOUS INTERNATIONAL HEALTH PLATFORMS

A closer look at various international health platforms reveals a complex and collaborative network of organizations, initiatives, and digital systems working together to improve global health outcomes. These platforms play a crucial role in addressing cross-border health challenges, promoting equitable access to care, and coordinating responses to emergencies such as pandemics, natural disasters, and humanitarian crises. Key players include the World Health Organization (WHO), which provides leadership on global health matters, sets international standards, and coordinates efforts to combat diseases. Other major platforms like GAVI, the Vaccine Alliance, and the Global Fund to Fight AIDS, Tuberculosis and Malaria focus on mobilizing resources and ensuring access to life-saving vaccines and treatments in low- and middle-income countries. Meanwhile, the World Bank and the United Nations Children's Fund (UNICEF) support health infrastructure, maternal and child health, and data-driven interventions. In the digital space, platforms such as Health Data Collaborative, Global Health Observatory (GHO), and DHIS2 facilitate the collection, analysis, and sharing of health data across nations to inform evidence-based policies. These platforms help track disease trends, assess healthcare performance, and identify gaps in service delivery. Additionally, public-private partnerships and regional organizations like the European Centre for Disease Prevention and Control (ECDC) or the Africa Centres for Disease Control and Prevention (Africa CDC) contribute by tailoring strategies to local contexts and strengthening surveillance and preparedness. Despite challenges such as funding limitations, data disparities, and political tensions, international health platforms remain essential for fostering collaboration, innovation, and accountability. They exemplify the importance of coordinated global action in achieving universal health coverage, improving health equity, and advancing the Sustainable Development Goals (SDGs). By uniting countries, organizations, and communities, these platforms create a foundation for a more resilient and responsive global health system that benefits all.

REFERENCES

1. Acuff, C., Antonelli, R., Fox, D., Hirsch, G., et al. (2017). *No Equity, No Triple Aim: Strategic Proposals to Advance Health Equity in A Volatile Policy Environment.* https://core.ac.uk/download/142081335.pdf (accessed on 26th June 2025).
2. Alnasir, F., Howe, A., van Weel, C., Alnasir, F., Goodyear-Smith, F., Saleh, H., Usta, J., et al. (2017). *Primary Healthcare Policy Implementation in The Eastern Mediterranean Region: Experiences of Six Countries.* https://core.ac.uk/download/132609197.pdf (accessed on 26th June 2025).
3. Baker, H. M., Goldstein, A. O., Jefferson, D., Ranney, L., et al. (2017). Identifying outcomes and gaps impacting tobacco control and prevention in African American communities. https://digitalscholarship.unlv.edu/cgi/viewcontent.cgi?article=1434&context=jhdrp (accessed on 26th June 2025).
4. Batalha, K. (2020). Climate, complacency and American culture: The role of narrative in the era of the misinformation amid the Anthropocene. https://core.ac.uk/download/288813359.pdf (accessed on 26th June 2025).
5. Benson, A. J., Evans, M. B., Eys, M., Mitchell, T., et al. (2013). The practitioner's corner: An exploration of municipal active living charter development and advocacy. https://core.ac.uk/download/143690040.pdf (accessed on 26th June 2025).
6. Birnbaum, N., Masterson, E., & Schoomaker, H. (2011). *State of Health Equity Movement, 2011 Update Part B: Catalog of Activities DRA Project Report No. 11–02.* https://core.ac.uk/download/pdf/18491811.pdf (accessed on 26th June 2025).
7. Blackman, D. H. (2005). Current developments in services for people with intellectual disabilities. https://core.ac.uk/download/5124575.pdf (accessed on 26th June 2025).
8. Bosma, L. M., Boyle, R. G., Lew, R., Martinez, A., et al. (2016). Developing capacity, skills, and tobacco control networks to address tobacco-related disparities: Leadership and Advocacy Institute to Advance Minnesota's Parity for Priority Populations (LAAMPP). https://digitalscholarship.unlv.edu/cgi/viewcontent.cgi?article=1394&context=jhdrp (accessed on 26th June 2025).
9. Byaello, K. (2022). Community engagement and public health initiatives in cultivating a healthier future. https://core.ac.uk/download/578907550.pdf (accessed on 26th June 2025).
10. Center for Human Development, University of Alaska Anchorage. (2013). The future of disability in Alaska summit & follow-up survey. https://core.ac.uk/download/162576609.pdf (accessed on 26th June 2025).
11. Coffman, J. (2008). Foundations and public policy grantmaking. https://core.ac.uk/download/71340682.pdf (accessed on 26th June 2025).
12. Cohen, L., Parks, L. F., & Kravitz-Wirtz, N. (2007). Poised for prevention: Advancing promising approaches to primary prevention of intimate partner violence. https://core.ac.uk/download/71346855.pdf (accessed on 26th June 2025).
13. Davie, L. K., Fox, S., & Rataj, A. C. (2015). Collaborating to create elder friendly communities in New Hampshire: A scan of the current landscape. https://core.ac.uk/download/215525830.pdf (accessed on 26th June 2025).

14. Douglas, J. A., Franks, L., Grills, C. T., Johnson, R., et al. (2020). Using participatory mapping to diagnose upstream determinants of health and prescribe downstream policy-based interventions. https://core.ac.uk/download/362660306.pdf (accessed on 26th June 2025).

15. Falconer, A., Ivanova, A., Walek, C., Krushe, D., Genchev, G., Derscanu, I., Tanaka, J., et al. (2014). *Mid-Term Evaluation of Ngo Programmed Under EEA Grants 2009–2014.* https://core.ac.uk/download/80510549.pdf (accessed on 26th June 2025).

16. Figueiredo, P., Lorimer, E., Perkins, P. E., Saad, A., et al. (2013). Strengthening the role of civil society in water sector governance towards climate change adaptation in African cities–Durban, Maputo, Nairobi. https://core.ac.uk/download/287659537.pdf (accessed on 26th June 2025).

17. García-Ramírez, M., Menezes, I., Perkins, D. D., Serrano-García, I., et al. (2016). Community psychology and public policy: Research, advocacy and training in international contexts. https://core.ac.uk/download/580975609.pdf (accessed on 26th June 2025).

18. Gienapp, A., Reisman, J., & Stachowiak, S. (2007). A guide to measuring advocacy and policy. https://core.ac.uk/download/71340679.pdf (accessed on 26th June 2025).

19. Gienapp, A., Reisman, J., & Stachowiak, S. (2012). A handbook of data collection tools: Companion to "A guide to measuring advocacy and policy." https://core.ac.uk/download/84911833.pdf (accessed on 26th June 2025).

20. Gilgoff, J., & Ginwright, S. (2015). Toward more equitable outcomes: A research synthesis on out-of-school time work with boys and young men of color. https://core.ac.uk/download/75786240.pdf (accessed on 26th June 2025).

21. Khan, S. (2009). Climate of opportunity: Gender and movement building at the intersection of reproductive justice and environmental justice. https://core.ac.uk/download/75784987.pdf (accessed on 26th June 2025).

22. Lee, K., Nemes, M., & Zigbi, K. (2009). Setting the table for a sustainable and just food system. https://core.ac.uk/download/10687990.pdf (accessed on 26th June 2025).

23. Linzer, L. (2012). Measuring the work of intermediaries in the St. Louis region. https://core.ac.uk/download/75784677.pdf (accessed on 26th June 2025).

24. Marsh, D. S., Putnam-Walkerly, K., & Daniel, M. H. (2003). Leadership for policy change. https://core.ac.uk/download/71348072.pdf (accessed on 26th June 2025).

25. McGee, L. U., & Suh, J. (2020). Communication strategies to address vaccine hesitancy in healthcare settings and on social media. https://core.ac.uk/download/323216373.pdf (accessed on 26th June 2025).

26. Mueller, C. H., Boddie-Willis, C. L., Folkemer, D. C., Grossman, E. R., & Somerville, M. H. (2012). Hospital community benefits after the ACA: Partnerships for community health improvement. https://core.ac.uk/download/71358452.pdf (accessed on 26th June 2025).

27. N/A. (2007). Bridging the innovation divide: An agenda for disseminating technology innovations within the nonprofit sector. https://core.ac.uk/download/71347273.pdf (accessed on 26th June 2025).

28. N/A. (2008). *New Directions in Obesity Prevention and Treatment: AcademyHealth 25th Annual Research Meeting.* https://core.ac.uk/download/71346805.pdf (accessed on 26th June 2025).

29. N/A. (2009). *A New Generation of Social Change.* https://core.ac.uk/download/71348256.pdf (accessed on 26th June 2025).

30. N/A. (2010). Foundations for civic impact: Advocacy and civic engagement toolkit for community foundations. https://core.ac.uk/download/71351349.pdf (accessed on 26th June 2025).

31. N/A. (2010). Paths forward for the global water, sanitation, and hygiene (WASH) sector. https://core.ac.uk/download/71345815.pdf (accessed on 26th June 2025).

32. N/A. (2010). State budget crises: Ripping the safety net held by nonprofits. https://core.ac.uk/download/71345401.pdf (accessed on 26th June 2025).

33. N/A. (2011). Understand the intermediary infrastructure in St. Louis: Who they are, what they do, and common misconceptions. https://core.ac.uk/download/75784701.pdf (accessed on 26th June 2025).

34. N/A. (2012). Kresge Foundation 2010–2011 annual report. https://core.ac.uk/download/71358585.pdf (accessed on 26th June 2025).

35. N/A. (2013). Many hands, more impact: Philanthropy's role in supporting movements. https://core.ac.uk/download/84911965.pdf (accessed on 26th June 2025).

36. N/A. (2013). *The Hunger and Food Safety Net System: Best Practices and Opportunities for Pennsylvania and Montgomery County.* https://core.ac.uk/download/71361706.pdf (accessed on 26th June 2025).

37. N/A. (2016). From project to platform: The evolution of Kids Count. https://core.ac.uk/download/75784220.pdf (accessed on 26th June 2025).

38. Nguyen, L., & Pinsoneault, L. T. (2009). New voices at the civic table: Facilitating personal and social change. https://core.ac.uk/download/10687991.pdf (accessed on 26th June 2025).

39. Pelaez, M., & Rice, M. (2004). *Primary Health Care and Aging: Edited Proceedings of the Consultative Group Meeting on Geriatric Training in Primary Health Care.* https://core.ac.uk/download/267865253.pdf (accessed on 26th June 2025).

40. Simon, S. (2009). Expanding global philanthropy to support the human rights of lesbian, gay, bisexual and transgender people. https://core.ac.uk/download/71351239.pdf (accessed on 26th June 2025).

41. Strong, D. A., Wooldridge, J., & Honeycutt, T. (2011). Consumer Voices for Coverage: Advocacy evaluation toolkit. https://core.ac.uk/download/71357929.pdf (accessed on 26th June 2025).

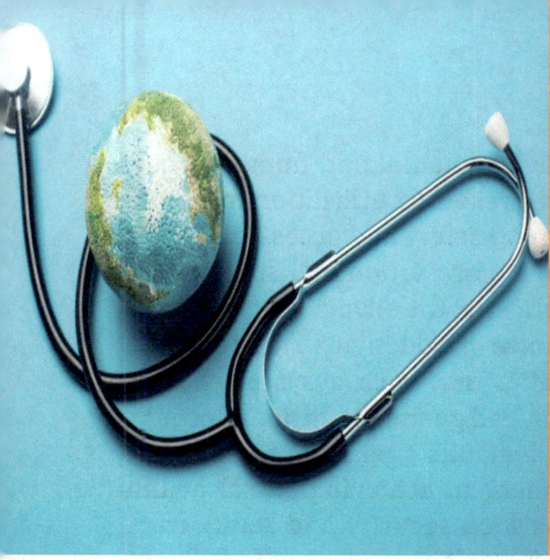

Chapter 11

GLOBAL AND ENVIRONMENTAL HEALTH IN COMMUNITY HEALTH

Contents

Introduction

Global and environmental health is a core discipline that bridges ecological well-being with public health, with emphasis on the relationship between human health and the environment. The global health concerns such as climate change, pollution, and loss of biodiversity must be addressed urgently, particularly in how these concerns affect disproportionately vulnerable populations. These challenges call for adopting a One Health paradigm that brings together human, animal, and environmental health perspectives. This inter-disciplinary approach supports inter-sector collaboration, as well as the development of sustainable solutions toward enhancing community health outcomes. With growing threats to communities from environmental degradation, new practice and strategy must evolve to challenge these interlinks and build resilience against new health challenges. Notably, the agricultural systems that provide food security have significant environmental and human health concerns. Traditional farm methods, which usually involve intensive resource utilization, promote environmental degradation, which further results in compromised food safety and accessibility. For instance, climate change and reduced biodiversity are enhanced by deforestation and soil erosion that accompany conventional farming. One of the promising alternatives is the silvopastoral system, which combines trees and livestock production in order to enhance productivity and conserve ecological health. A Mexican study illustrates the probable benefits that such a system has in maintaining sustainable agriculture, reducing environmental footprint, and guaranteeing food security in the event of global warming and an increase in food resource demands (Villamil et al., 2017). Implementing such advanced farming practices will be a key element to achieving global health goals while supporting resilience among communities. Training on food security and safety from the point of view of One Health is also key to developing appropriate steps that counterbalance both public health and environmental sustainability. Curricula that utilize an interdisciplinary framework and stress the interconnection of food production, safety, and environmental impact are necessary to train the future professionals in this field. Setting up frameworks, like the one offered by the Western Institute for Food Safety and Security, assists instructors in designing comprehensive programs addressing the multidimensional issues of food systems (Angelos et al., 2017). By equipping students with the knowledge and abilities to navigate the complexities of global and environmental health, communities can work towards creating healthier and more sustainable food environments that honor natural resources and achieve health equity (Figure 11.1).

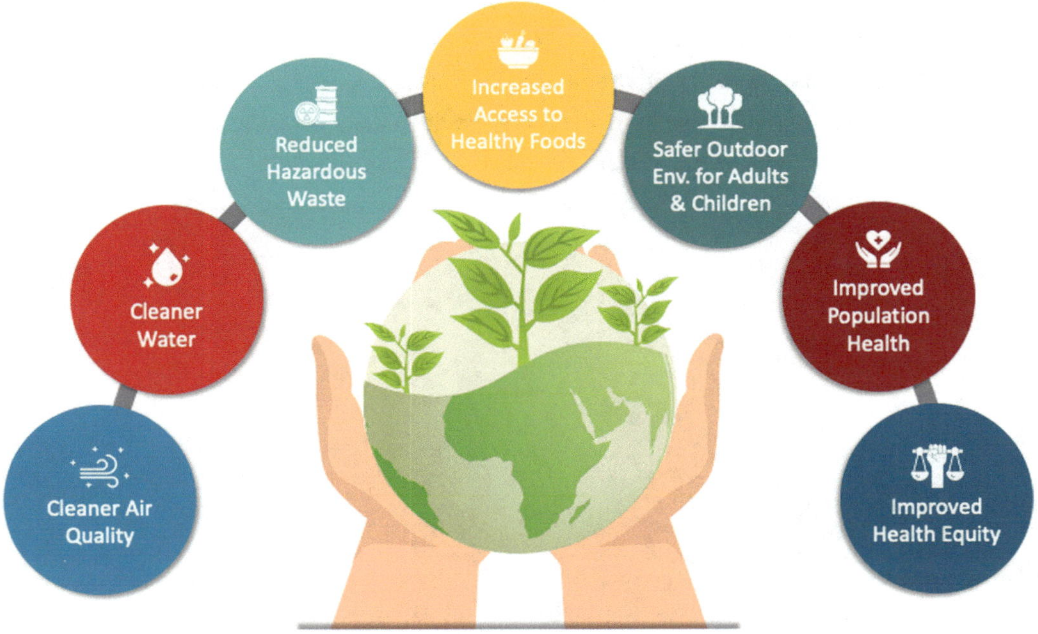

Figure 11.1. Global and environmental health.

Source: https://cdn.sketchbubble.com/pub/media/catalog/product/optimized1/f/4/f43766f062514f09861366753259849382b3ff8eab377714c403541a608bd8e6/environmental-health-mc-slide4.png.

Definition of Global Health

Global health is a term that goes beyond geographical reach, encompassing the health issues that transcend national boundaries and require collective response. It involves studying the determinants of health influenced by globalization, including environmental, social, and economic determinants. In most cases, global health is concerned with the inter-connectedness of health matters, for example, the transmission of infectious diseases, non-communicable disease, and the impact of climate change on health. Pursuing global health all revolves around equity and access to health care, advocating for vulnerable populations all over the world. As the global community becomes increasingly interdependent, it becomes clear that the value of having a broad, comprehensive strategy to health cannot be emphasized too much and recognizes the imperative for action and cooperation among countries for dealing with priority public health issues at the international level.

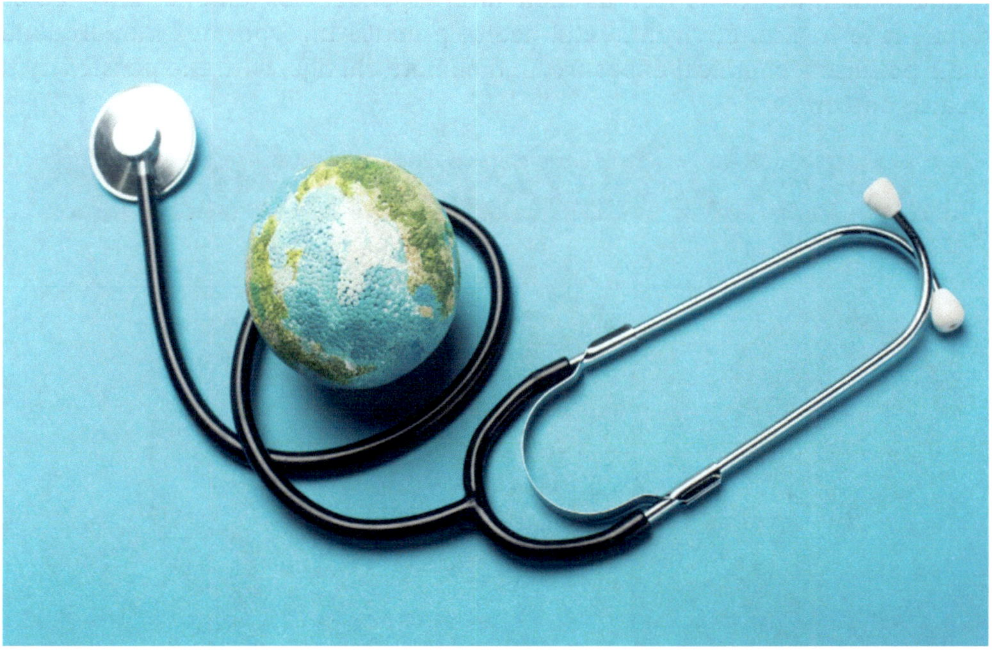

Figure 11.2. Global health.

Source: https://www.cgdev.org/sites/default/files/2023-02/Global_Health.jpeg.

Addressing global health best requires a cross-disciplinary response with inter-sectoral coordination among public health, environmental sciences, healthcare, and policy-making. This collaborative strategy is particularly needed when examining the complex relationship between environmental factors and health outcomes. One instance of this can be observed in the impact food and agricultural policy places on community health, ranging from diet-based illnesses to food security. Furthermore, the application of new practices such as Intensive Comprehensive Aphasia Programs (ICAPs) demonstrates how the adoption of evidence-based practice can be encouraged through international collaboration. As Bright et al. (2019) points out, understanding facilitators and barriers of using such programs across various countries can significantly enhance the efficacy of global health interventions. Equity is the core pillar of global health, given that inequality in the availability of health and quality persists across populations. As community health programs advance, they must recognize and address such disparities to ensure the policies and interventions are inclusive of vulnerable groups. Attempts at improving world health not only require the transfer of effective interventions but also advocacy and promotion of best practice informed by a range of cultural viewpoints. The need for advocacy highlights the promotion of evidence-based practice to bridge these gaps and give all communities fair health resources. By encouraging partnership and collaboration, knowledge that comes from research like Bellon et al. (2025) can illuminate the paths to the achievement of inclusive and sustainable comprehensive health progress and therefore advance the definition and field of global health against environmental wellbeing (Figure 11.2).

Definition of Environmental Health

Environmental health can be defined as the investigation of the interrelation between the environment and human health as well as their interdependencies, emphasizing the contribution of the environment to health. Environmental health practice incorporates numerous factors such as water and air pollution, chemical exposure, and climate change, with the possibility to influence population health outcomes.

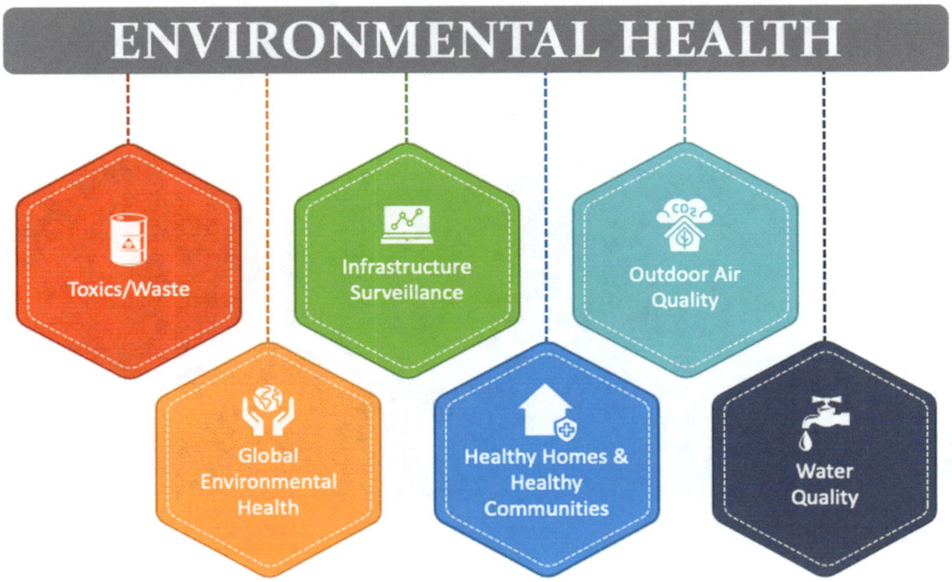

Figure 11.3. Environmental health.

Source: https://www.collidu.com/media/catalog/product/img/b/1/b1d5dd465cb1cd57f802023a2ee05819e4850544169fb23d879b25f081c97fc9/environmental-health-slide1.png.

The World Health Organization highlights that healthy environment is a prerequisite for good health since it has a direct impact on social structures, economic stability, and the extent of disease prevention. With the highly interconnected webs binding environmental determinants to health, it is increasingly evident that enhancing environmental health can achieve better community health outcomes, thus rendering it a key component in public health programs aimed at reducing health disparities and overall quality of life. In the last few years, there has been a significant shift towards recognizing the highly interconnected character of occupational and environmental health within community contexts. Labor-environmental coalitions show the mutual cooperation of activists of diverse backgrounds in seeking health issues as a means of agreement. The blue-green coalitions want to solve problems caused by toxic exposures both within the workplace and the environment, revealing a fundamental link between job-related hazards and environmental health issues. By encouraging stakeholders' dialogue, these coalitions create spaces for innovative solutions that can effectively reduce exposure levels and guarantee safety. This collective effort on environmental health identifies the importance of community engagement and cross-sector collaboration as primary strategies for encouraging progressive social change and speaking a safer, healthier world for all.

Understanding human health and its connection with the environment calls for a multidisciplinary approach, which has emerged as an important methodology in current research. Research recently shows that the pattern change in the relationship between humans and nature affects health significantly. To study such complexity, an interdisciplinary model is suggested by researchers that incorporates data from the fields of environmental science, sociology, and public health. This framework allows for broader examination of underlying processes that affect health at the human-environment interface, ultimately informing the development of more effective health interventions. In addressing these interrelated factors, we are in a better position to appreciate how environmental issues affect physical and mental health, therefore shedding light on mechanisms for enhancing community health programs. Integrating these discoveries into practice is important for the promotion of the definition and use of environmental health in the broader scheme of global health challenges and solutions, as described in Adger et al. (2016) (Figure 11.3).

Importance of Integrating Both Fields in Community Health

The integration of global and environmental health in community health programs is instrumental in addressing complex health challenges that are disproportionately impacting marginalized populations. Because health issues such as malnutrition, disease outbreaks, and environmental degradation are interconnected, a coordinated strategy enables communities to adopt innovative alternatives that are effective and sustainable. For instance, through the integration of health education and environmental measures, individuals within a community can be informed about the contribution of clean environments in avoiding sicknesses. Coordination not only raises awareness but also encourages a culture of responsibility and stewardship for local environments. Lastly, such integration builds resilience in communities so they can neutralize health emergencies in advance through health awareness of the connection between their environments and health outcomes. No less imperative is the integration of local regulatory schemes and community engagement in health programs. As became clear in the latest studies, modern waste management programs do not embrace sustainability principles, worsening public health threats and environmental degradation (Agustin et al., 2024). The rejuvenation of community-centered models, such as the Sharia-embedded Waste Bank of Sunan Ampel State Islamic University, is the best example in this regard. With the integration of local cultural values and sustainability practices, not only are such models avoiding waste but are also safeguarding the health of the community and the environment. This underlines the need for regulatory adherence simultaneously bridging the theory-practice gap in health interventions. Emphasis on local participation guarantees that solutions developed are not only contextually appropriate but also supported by community members, inducing participation and adherence to health programs. Finally, the need for integrated approaches to health, particularly in addressing poverty and disease, cannot be emphasized enough. Efforts aimed at addressing underlying determinants of health such as clean water, sanitation, and diet through an integrated strategy hold great potential to address overall developmental goals (N/A, 2011). Examples from various countries demonstrate that multsectoral efforts combined achieve improved health outcomes because interventions addressing numerous factors of well-being are in a superior position to strike at causes at their base. By prioritizing top the integrated programs, stakeholders can make health systems not only responsive but also preventive, thus promoting a holistic view of community health emphasizing global and environmental health interconnectedness. Integration of this sort serves as a model for how to create healthy, sustainable communities ideally suited to handle challenges of the future.

11.1. The Impact of Climate Change on Health

With climate change accelerating, its public health impacts become more urgent and extensive. Rising temperatures and amplified weather conditions disseminate infectious illnesses and entrench health inequities, particularly for the vulnerable. These groups are likely to be hampered by poor access to healthcare and resources helpful to climate adaptation. The development of the mining sector, particularly in regions like Ontario, provides an applicable example; the sector is of potential worth to green energy technology but has immense health repercussions from environmental decay. Resolution of the competing interests requires more public health advocacy to ensure that policies account for health in addition to economic development. The severity of the weighing of environmental well-being against economic interest further highlights the need for integrated approaches to consider both environmental sustainability and the health of people (Hutchuk et al., 2023). Another critical aspect of climate changes impact on health is that it affects natural disasters, which disproportionately affects coastal and low-income nations.

For instance, South Louisiana towns carry a staggering burden of climate-related events, including hurricanes and flooding, which pose risks not just to physical safety but to social cohesion as well as access to essential services. The organizations play a crucial role in building resilience in such resource-constrained communities. The organizations support individuals in managing public health problems worsened by both climate change and recent pandemics through resource mobilization and networking. However, systemic issues like racism and economic inequality continue to jeopardize such efforts, so it is challenging to construct robust safety nets that promote health equity and healing in communities. The inequalities identified make it necessary to have comprehensive methods that support communities with accumulated health risks (Hancock et al., 2021). Here, the intersection of climate change and health sheds light on what public health institutions and community organizations do to prevent adverse outcomes. With players aware that there are great opportunities hindering climate action, it is clear that interagency collaboration across government agencies, health agencies, and local institutions is crucial. By applying health strategies that are not incorporated into the mining and extractive industries yet, public health workers can introduce thoughtful perspectives that stimulate innovative solutions. Interventions such as greater stakeholder engagement and general policy syntheses have the ability to deconstruct fragmentation and increase community resilience. Lastly, empowering public health to act proactively against climate change not only provides an answer to pressing health concerns but enables sustained sustainability for the affected populations, reasserting the significance of environmental and international health in present community health discourse (Hutchuk et al., 2023) (Figure 11.4).

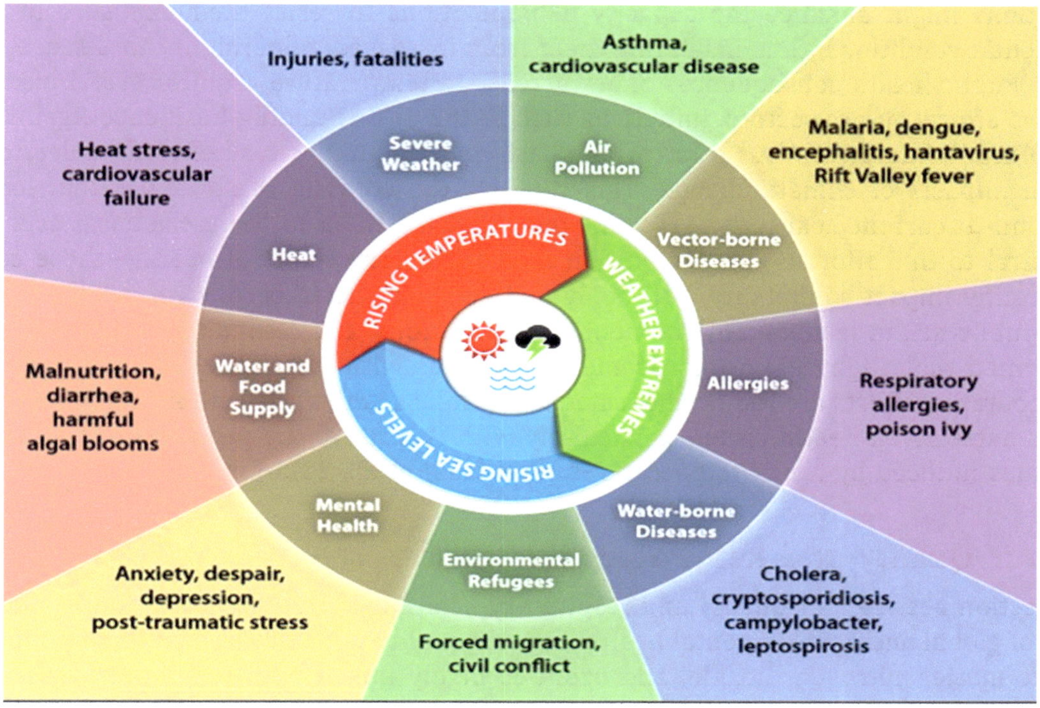

Figure 11.4. The impact of climate change on health.

Source: https://toolkit.climate.gov/sites/default/files/CDC_ClimateHealthGraphic.jpg.

11.1.1. Effects of Rising Temperatures on Disease Prevalence

Rising temperatures across the globe directly relate to a tremendous increase in the occurrence of diseases, as witnessed by the outbreak of various infectious diseases. Climatic factors have a major effect on the life cycle and transmission of vectors such as mosquitoes, causes of diseases such as malaria and dengue fever. Higher temperatures are conducive to breeding, and with that, the range of these vectors can be extended and transmission seasons prolonged. Global health loads of vector-borne diseases are thus expected to rise, impacting not just populations but even communities. It is crucial to understand this correlation between temperature and disease trends if public health planning is going to be effective, particularly in areas where such diseases were not prevalent previously. Besides, increasing spread of these diseases emphasizes the urgent need for strengthened surveillance systems and adaptive health policies in order to protect vulnerable populations from emerging health risks observed as a result of climate change (Petruzelli et al., 2020). The implications of increased temperatures impact vector-borne disease only. Climate change also impacts the spread of waterborne and foodborne diseases, which show dramatic increases during warmer months. Higher temperature can increase water temperatures, supporting the growth of harmful algal blooms that are toxic to human life. In addition, climatological disasters, often caused by global warming, can jeopardize food and water supply chains, facilitating the spread of diseases. Old diseases like cholera that were previously eradicated or controlled are appearing in new habitats, emphasizing the vulnerability of communities that are attacked by such danger. The complexity of such interactions necessitates integrated approaches in public health intervention where actions might enhance the capacity of populations to resist their exposure to changing environmental conditions, thus insulating them from increased vulnerability to disease (Aytur et al., 2014). Public health consequences of an increase in temperature require careful planning and cooperative efforts across sectors. Initiatives such as the CDCs Building Resilience Against Climate Effects (BRACE) framework put a lot of emphasis on community resilience in order to reverse the health impacts of climate change. This calls for the creation of strategies that look ahead and respond to current health threats while also allowing them to be in existence over the long term. Central to this effort is the recognition of social determinants of health—those conditions that inherently impact community well-being and access to healthcare. With coalition formation between public health leaders, environmental organizations, and community leaders, institutions can be formed that align health improvement objectives with climate change adaptation efforts. Such collaborative efforts are required to safeguard public health and maintain communities strong against climate-driven health issues, particularly with regards to the prevalence of disease-borne health issues induced by rising temperatures (Petruzelli et al., 2020).

11.1.2. Air Quality and Respiratory Health Issues

The connection between air quality and respiratory health is a needed priority under the broader umbrella of global and environmental health. Low air quality with elevated levels of pollutants like particulate matter, nitrogen dioxide, and ozone is highly linked with respiratory disease. These contaminants may initiate pre-existing conditions like asthma and chronic obstructive pulmonary disease (COPD) and also increase the rate of respiratory infections. The impact of compromised air quality extends beyond individual health and into the health of communities and economic resilience, most perceptibly in urban areas where pollution will most likely be most dense. An appreciation for these connections is most important to health professionals as they anticipate addressing the anticipated medical consequences of climate change and the attendant environmental concerns (Abouzaid et al., 2009).

Environmental toxins have an influence that extends beyond immediate health effects, causing a cycle of disadvantage in affected populations. Groups most at risk, including children, the elderly, and individuals with pre-existing illness, are particularly susceptible to being negatively affected by worsening air quality. These groups, through being based in low-resource communities, tend to be limited in their ability to meet environmental health issues. Interventions to improve the quality of air are able to minimize health inequalities of the respiratory kind to a large degree. Creating awareness about air quality and its effects and enacting community-based action are able to empower people to take control over cleaner living environments. Along with promoting public health, these interventions help promote social equity, particularly in poor communities where environmental factors compound health inequalities (Aytur et al., 2014). With continued demands on public health systems by climate change, the air quality-respiratory disease nexus becomes increasingly important. Climate-driven phenomena, including increased incidences of heatwaves and wildfires, can amplify air pollution levels, triggering large-scale health crises. Policymakers and healthcare providers must therefore accord more priority to incorporating air quality monitoring in public health planning and community health programs. Employing resources like the BRACE model has the potential to assist communities in formulating steps to develop resilience against climate-related health threats. These steps try to tackle social and environmental determinants of health, thus qualifying as a comprehensive strategy to community well-being in the face of ongoing environmental change. In so doing, improving air quality not only minimizes respiratory health issues but also promotes overall public health objectives in communities (Aytur et al., 2014) (Figure 11.5).

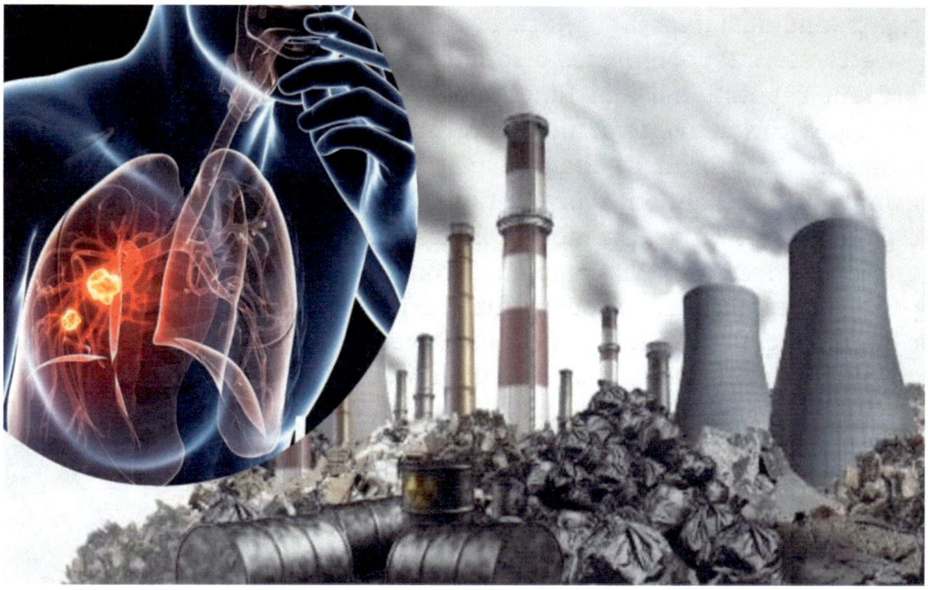

Figure 11.5. Air quality and respiratory health issues.

Source: https://external-content.duckduckgo.com/iu/?u=https%3A%2F%2Fst1.thehealthsite.com%2Fwp-content%2Fuploads%2F2022%2F11%2FLung-Cancer-3.jpg&f=1&nofb=1&ipt=fade702b039356197625d2c2bdb90e3481c6b43f69f3a18d7ce6d88d2bb2e84b.

11.1.3. Water Scarcity and Its Implications for Public Health

Water scarcity is a significant public health issue that has an extremely far-reaching impact on the quality of life in affected communities. Access to clean and safe drinking water is core in the provision of health and well-being, as posited by the United Nations Committee on Economic, Social and Cultural Rights, who has also declared availability of water a fundamental human right essential to the maximal level of well-being. The fear of vanishing water resources not only heightens perceptions of exposure to waterborne illnesses but also expands the divergence in already present health disparities, particularly among marginalized populations. Societies that do not have access to stable water resources are likely to have high incident rates of diseases such as cholera and dysentery that can lead to high mortality. Collective action on the global level is hence necessary in response to water scarcity through policies that ensure equitable access to this precious resource for all regardless of socioeconomic status (Auch et al., 2018). The union of water scarcity and industrial activities, particularly for the production of unconventional energy, is a significant public health concern. Extraction practices common in operations such as fracking require elevated levels of water inputs that significantly strain local water resources and compromise community access to this essential resource. Research indicates that industrial water usage encroachment has brought about a shift in the distribution of resources, bestowing more benefit towards industrial consumption as compared to resident consumption, particularly in regions that have been strongly affected by such behavior. Such an experience not only infringes on the right to water but also goes hand in hand with adverse health impacts on residents since diminished access to clean water affects sanitation and hygiene. As economies expand, the repercussions of public health reach further afield and call for an urgent discussion of water management, rights, and sustainability (Auch et al., 2018). Government is not solely responsible for confronting water scarcity; companies also have a critical role in ensuring they manage their water use to prevent reputational and functional harm. The implementation of efficient water management strategies can alleviate some of the pressures off regional water resources, where companies are incentivized to adapt themselves to sustainable practices appropriate for their respective environments. Multinational corporations, in case studies, demonstrate diverse reactions to bridging the global water crisis, promoting intersectoral cooperation to create solutions. This sense of cooperation is necessary as companies compete to minimize their ecological footprint while fulfilling their water needs. Through this, businesses are able to contribute to positively affecting public health in communities through improved access to water, thereby having an overall improvement on public health outcomes (Figure 11.6).

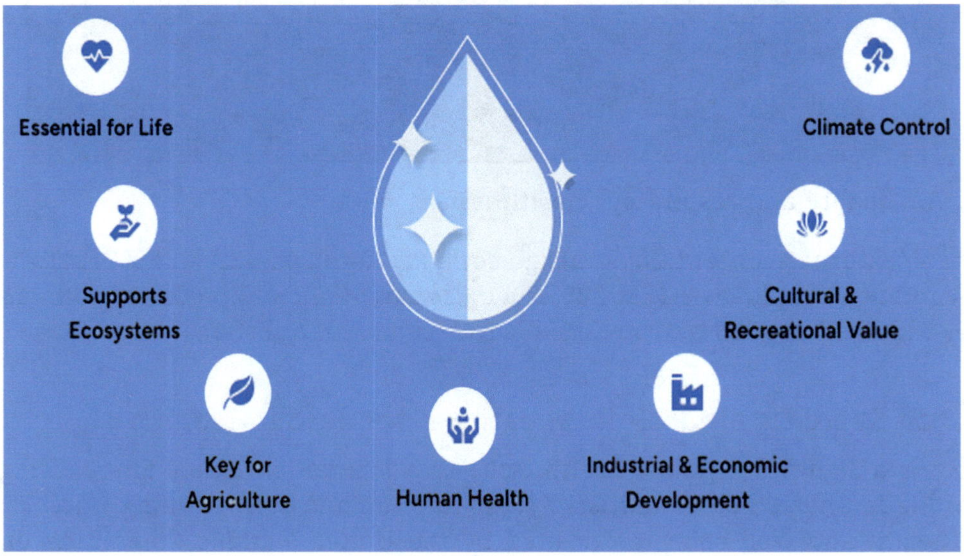

Figure 11.6. Water scarcity and its implications for public health.

Source: https://teamtweaks1-blog.s3.us-east-2.amazonaws.com/blog/wp-content/uploads/2024/05/28174545/01-3.jpg.

11.2. Global Health Initiatives and Their Role

Global health initiatives lead in the reaction to immediate health issues on an international scale, particularly in regard to the environmental determinants of health. Global health initiatives, which are financed by national and international organizations, have the objective to reduce health inequalities while providing fair access to health services. One significant aspect of these initiatives is their ability to integrate various fields of study, including public health, environmental science, and even the arts. By advocating for comprehensive approaches to health challenges, global health initiatives foster collaborative networks that transcend geographical and cultural boundaries. These partnerships are critical to design and implement effective interventions addressing both the immediate health issues and the structural determinants of health disparities, constructing a more holistic understanding of community health. Furthermore, the intersection between climate change and public health highlights the importance of an integrated response across global health systems. As established in new studies, climate change is not only an environmental issue; it has significant implications for human health, which affects the distribution of diseases and overall population health. The call to incorporate oral health programmes in climate adaptation policies shows that attention needs to be given to addressing health in the context of environmental change. As populations face increasing environmental challenges, promoting climate-resilient health practices is imperative.

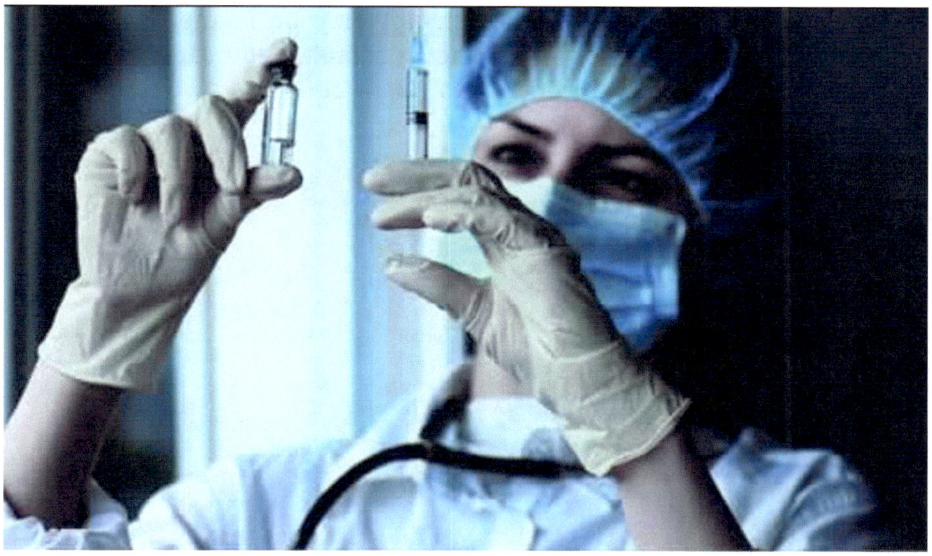

Figure 11.7. Global health initiatives and their role.

Source: https://s3.amazonaws.com/global-db-public/global-db-public/publication/translation/image/1674/GlobalHealthInitiativeBrochure.jpg.

This can include the establishment of mobile clinics and increased tele-dentistry care that removes barriers to access, ensuring targeted groups receive needed care while adapting to the new environmental factors affecting their performance in healthcare (Shrivastava et al., 2025). Additionally, the incorporation of the arts in global health programs is a novel approach to reducing health disparities and encouraging community engagement. By employing the use of artistic representations, health campaigns are made more effective to engage in relation with various groups of people, enhancing public awareness and promotion of health programs. The arts have the capacity to promote mental and physical well-being, particularly among marginalized communities where traditional health communication is minimal. Notwithstanding this, arts-based interventions are usually restricted by funding and cultural prejudices. Effective case studies in the sector demonstrate the potential gains to health realized when innovative approaches and conventional ones are applied at the same time. Empowering interdisciplinary collaboration and leveraging digital platforms will be the way forward to enhancing the role played by the arts in global health initiatives to effect a more holistic approach toward improvement in overall health outcome within communities (Ugwu, 2025) (Figure 11.7).

11.2.1. Overview of Major Global Health Organizations

Global health is driven by major organizations whose mandate concurs with public health needs across the world. These include the World Health Organization (WHO), a major international coordinator of response to health matters. Established in 1948, WHOs primary function is to direct and coordinate global health actions, faced with a wide spectrum of health issues, ranging from infectious diseases to emerging threats from the environment. Its robust structure helps member nations develop effective health policies and even advises on practice in health toward improving community well-being. By initiatives like the Global Action Plan on Antimicrobial Resistance, WHO demonstrates how global health organizations can not only be in the forefront of dealing with health crises but also take the leadership in advancing sustainable health behaviors that consider the impact of the environment on health outcomes (N/A, 2007).

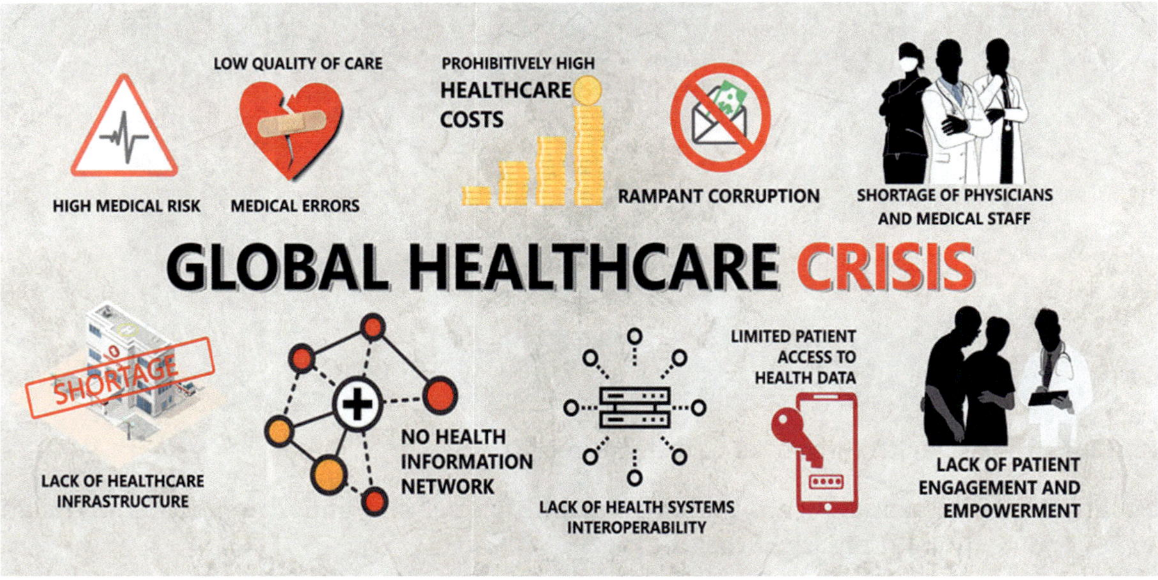

Figure 11.8. Overview of major global health organizations.

Source: https://transformglobalhealth.org/wp-content/themes/boss-child/front-page-assets/images/problem-illus-v1.jpg.

In addition to the WHO, agencies like the Centers for Disease Control and Prevention (CDC) also offer significant feedback on how local community health efforts are connected with global health. CDC's emphasis on evidence-based public health interventions equips community health organizations with the capability to combat disparities in health. Such a linkage between the CDC and local institutions illustrates the necessity to integrate international models of health into community health care, particularly due to globalization. Through a prevention and public awareness approach, the CDC enables communities to view the overall implications of global health policy on local health, bridging otherwise existing gaps between policy creation and community application. These initiatives indicate the role played by health organizations collaborating with each other, as shared knowledge has the potential of enhancing the effectiveness of health interventions in different populations (Hricko et al., 2011). Other organizations, such as Médecins Sans Frontières (Doctors Without Borders), also indicate the multi-dimensional roles played by international health organizations to address health concerns. While best known for their medical response in crisis situations, Médecins Sans Frontières is also engaged in advocacy to promote social and environmental determinants of health. Through their activities, they highlight the influence of socioeconomic inequality and environmental degradation as determinants of global health outcomes. By putting the health-environment interdependence at the forefront of their endeavors, these organizations establish, induce action on, and champion urgent global concerns such as climate change and health inequalities, all that support the important role played by community health programs in providing better health globally. This interdependent approach lends power to the argument that effective global health interventions must address the environment, therefore addressing the immediate and root causes of health issues (N/A, 2007) (Figure 11.8).

11.2.2. Key Initiatives Aimed at Improving Community Health

As the impact of urbanization and environmental pollution grows, key initiatives aimed at improving community health have become a necessary reaction. One of the key priorities is combating air quality and its impact on public health, particularly in urban communities where the rates of pollution are absurdly high. To counter these challenges, societies are embracing comprehensive measures that include stricter air quality regulations and the creation of green areas. Initiatives such as the development of public transportation and the encouragement of electric vehicles significantly reduce air pollution. These integrated steps not only tackle environmental health determinants but also foster community action, turning residents into motivated stakeholders in the quest for cleaner air. Through the integration of advanced technologies with policy platforms, such efforts aim to minimize air pollutions adverse health effects, thereby enhancing collective community well-being (Kapoor et al., 2024). Apart from air quality, the intersection of maternal health and climate change has spurred unprecedented action towards enhancing community health. Climate change is full of pitfalls for expectant mothers, whose lives and those of their offspring can be permanently damaged by high temperatures, natural disasters, and stressors that ensue. These challenges need programs that aim at healthcare access, mental health care, and building resilience in climate change-impacted families. Those programs incorporating scientific information with community-based initiatives, especially those with local religious organizations, will be able to enhance mitigation efforts effectively. By developing an environment where mothers feel empowered and can access appropriate health care, these programs aim to safeguard maternal health outcomes and ensure healthier future generations, in line with global sustainable development goals (Mashara et al., 2024). Lastly, community-based health programs increasingly emphasize the importance of mental health, as well as physical health, recognizing that both play a role in overall well-being. Curricula for educating the community regarding mental health problems, particularly those exacerbated by the environment, are central to a comprehensive approach to well-being.

Improved provision of mental health facilities and support infrastructures, including counseling and stress management training, enables individuals to manage the psychosocial burden imposed by climate-related challenges. Further, community participation programs encourage a supportive environment under which people can share experience and build resilience as a collective. Programs that combine education, outreach, and resource access not only improve mental health but also enhance the capacity of the community to deal with the interconnected problems of global and environmental health (Kapoor et al., 2024).

11.2.3. Success Stories from Global Health Interventions

The intersection of various health interventions has been crucial in addressing global health concerns, particularly in the Third World. A classic case is evident in the collaborative approaches towards advancing primary healthcare, the availability of clean water, and proper nutrition. Such interventions not only meet targeted vulnerabilities in a population but also push for an overall approach that supports sustainable development. By incorporating these dimensions, numerous countries have achieved significant reductions in disease incidence and poverty levels. The report based on these essential areas gives 17 countries that have successful examples, which give the scenario of how well-coordinated activities can result in tangible health improvements (N/A, 2011). The combined model is a shift in strategy whereby resource deployment and program operation are conjoined, thereby guaranteeing their overall cumulative impact on health outcomes and overall community well-being. Second, hygiene promotion as a public health intervention is unparalleled. Focused hygiene programs in nations such as South and Southeast Asia and targeted African nations have been hugely successful.

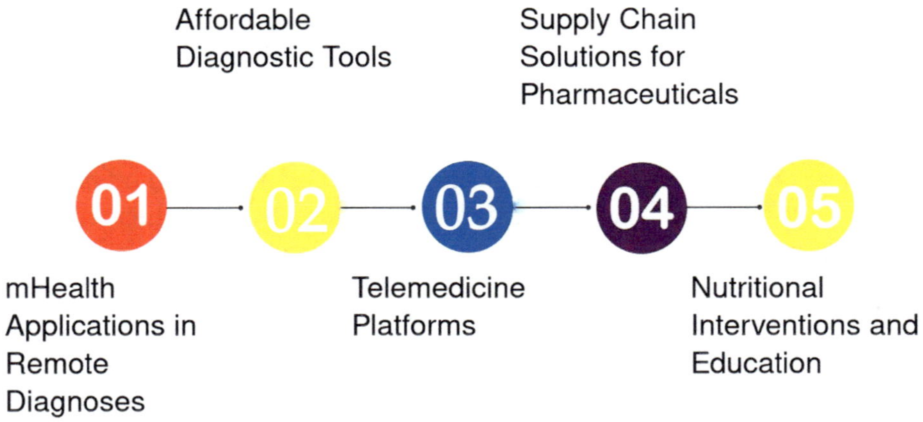

Figure 11.9. Success stories from global health interventions.

Source: https://fastercapital.co/i/Global-health--Business-Opportunities-in-the-Global-Health-Sector--Success-Stories-in-Global-Health-Ventures.webp.

These projects address the specific needs of different populations, allowing intervention with reach to targeted groups. By ensuring local people's participation and offering chances for behavior change, such projects promote individuals to adopt improved hygiene behaviors. Experience gained from these projects shows that gaining an understanding of the cultural setting and issues being faced by communities significantly enhances prospects for long-term behavior change (N/A, 2011). These success stories support the theory that health programs have to be contextually relevant to provide sustained impact on public health. The reported accomplishments from global health interventions indicate the need for the public and private sector collaboration to further strengthen community health outcomes. Investing in integrated health systems incorporating education, resource focusing, and community mobilization enables stakeholders to create a more sustainable health infrastructure. For instance, initiatives that bring together sanitation, nutrition, and healthcare in an integrated approach have been more effective than efforts taken individually. Just like in the lessons across various countries, collaborative effort by the governments and organizations is a keystone foundation upon which sustainable health achievements can be established. Together, these stories illustrate that the response to global health problems through a collaborative approach does not only alleviate current health emergencies but also paves the way for the attainment of long-term health equality and improved quality of life among vulnerable populations (Figure 11.9).

11.3. Environmental Determinants of Health (EDH)

The relationship between EDH and community health is complex and important. Environmental determinants encompass a range of factors, such as the quality of air, water, housing, and climatic factors, which collectively influence the overall health environment of populations. According to recent evidence, approximately one-quarter of the entire global burden of disease could be attributable to such environmental risk factors. These determinants are particularly crucial within the framework of the 2030 Agenda for Sustainable Development, in light of the fact that economic growth, environmental sustainability, and social equity are interconnected. The fact that these determinants interact can allow evidence-based interventions aimed at minimizing health risks, particularly in high-risk zones like sub-Saharan Africa, where the disease burden remains disproportionately high (Dietler et al., 2020). Policies to treat EDH can produce better health impacts by emphasizing comprehensive environmental evaluation and community-based approaches. Mining activities are an example of the double-pronged potential for certain industrial processes to be drivers of both economic growth and health hazards, making their role in community health more complex. For instance, while mining activities will enhance infrastructure and employment rates, they will also add to more air and water pollution that has a direct effect on public health. Thus, research has highlighted how, while industrial mining might enhance access to basic services, its benefits to health hardly trickle down to all levels of the community equally. Studies in sub-Saharan Africa reveal that more impoverished households gain less from infrastructural improvement associated with mining (Dietler et al., 2020). It is essential that health effect assessments consider these diversified outcomes holistically so that the interests of those most affected are adequately represented in discussions surrounding mining and health. This integrative approach can enable the discovery of indirect pathways through which mining influences health, therefore allowing more effective policy interventions. Furthermore, transnational corporations (TNCs) that operate in extractive industries also have a profound influence on the environmental determinants of health. Through their impact on forms of production, regulatory policies, and social conditions, TNCs have the capacity to empower or disempower community health. Case studies, such as Rio Tinto, show that business operations can offer good employment opportunities alongside negative health impacts through insecure types of work and environmental pollution. Despite potential benefits, such as good jobs, the biggest challenge lies in addressing corporate responsibilities in a way that is interested in health equity as well as environmental preservation. To be effective health champions, an improvement in regulations governing the operations of TNCs and community involvement in assessing health impacts is crucial. Through a collective debate among corporations, communities, and policymakers, stakeholders can work together towards balancing corporate interests and public health goals, ultimately leading to improved community health.

11.3.1. Role of Housing and Urban Development

The role of housing in city development lies at the heart of actualizing the broader implications for global and environmental health. Urban areas are economic and cultural centers but also deal with issues related to living conditions, which significantly affect the wellbeing of the population residing there. Housing of poor quality could be to blame for most of the diseases like respiratory disease and mental illness, a problem enlarged by socioeconomic disparities. For instance, poor housing estates have few links with clean water, sanitation, and good nutrition, which contribute to the poverty and decline in health. The housing deficits form a critical part of the urban development strategy since enhanced living conditions not only enhance an individual's well-being but also a healthier community. Granting equal access to housing is a crucial measure towards ensuring sustainable cities that support both social justice and health equity. Plans for urban development should also consider the environmental impacts of infrastructure and housing. Accelerated urbanization witnessed globally presents both possibilities and pitfalls. Cities, becoming densely populated and highly heterogeneous, have an immense influence on the health of urban as well as non-urban populations. Sustainable urban planning can minimize detrimental impacts on the environment while maintaining public health through green spaces, efficient public transportation, and reduced pollution. Research indicates that properly planned cities with systems of development planned in a prudent manner can decrease adverse effects of overpopulation and environmental degradation. An interdisciplinary approach with incorporation of public health perspectives into housing policy has the potential to improve living conditions and address far-reaching urban problems. By embracing such frameworks, cities can facilitate better health outcomes and resilience among their population and eventually support a more sustainable future.

Besides that, community engagement offers an essential element in addressing urban health issues around development and housing. Effective urban health interventions rely on the engagement of stakeholders, be it residents, policymakers, or leaders of organizations. Community-driven approaches foster ownership of health initiatives, which enhances sustainability and success. For example, in interventions on childhood obesity among multicultural populations in inner cities like London, cross-sections of community contributions to such programs gain insights crucial for effective solutions. Such collaborations can enhance nutrition outcomes among various demographic populations by valuing the specific socio-cultural contexts they inhabit, according to previous studies (Al-Khudairy et al., 2018). Further, urban health systems, which are informed by residents' diverse experiences, can embrace integrated solutions, which address underlying determinants of health while assuring that urban development promotes equity and improves the well-being of the whole population (Freudenberg et al., 2005).

11.3.2. Influence of Access to Clean Water and Sanitation

Clean water and adequate sanitation are the pillars of world and environmental health, and they have a profound impact on well-being and community development. Where such needs are lacking in communities, health profiles actually deteriorate and lead to an incidence of water-borne diseases such as cholera and dysentery. Aside from the physical damage caused by such illnesses, such issues also strain local health systems and economies. Poor sanitary facilities also aggravate the condition of vulnerable groups such as women and children, who normally end up drawing water from inappropriate places. Restricted availability of clean water and sanitation has direct relationships with increased rates of morbidity and compromised quality of life, such that interventions and policy changes that prioritize these services are an urgent need for the development of public health in disadvantaged groups.

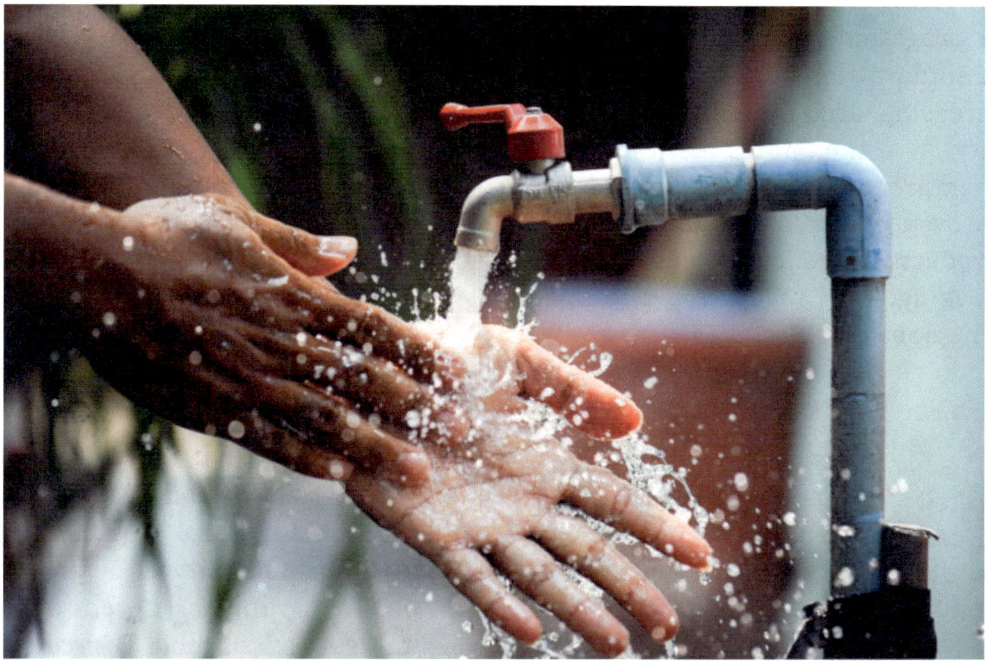

Figure 11.10. Influence of access to clean water and sanitation.

Source: https://www.brookings.edu/wp-content/uploads/2022/03/shutterstock_1688502520_small.jpg.

The influence of unsanitary conditions on womens health further increases the imperative for enhanced access. They suffer disproportionately from sanitation problems, with increased risk of urinary tract infections and maternal complications due to their lack of access to clean and sanitary sanitation. In addition, poor sanitation may prevent girls from advancing their studies as most of them are forced out of school during menses due to a lack of proper facilities. This continues to nurture a cycle of poverty and gender inequality, preventing socio-economic progress. As maintained in recent studies, addressing such sanitation issues is not just a health issue but a human rights issue that requires concerted action from governments, businesses, and civil society to establish an enabling environment where everyone can access basic commodities to maintain their health and dignity (N/A, 2013). Strategic investments in clean water and sanitation infrastructure are critical to achieving worldwide health goals, such as those defined within the Sustainable Development Goals (SDGs). World access to these essential services is within our grasp, and therefore concerted action on innovative partnerships and financing is required to assist with funding these projects. Groups like WaterAid note that political commitment is required to sustain momentum towards attaining this (N/A, 2013). Connecting community engagement with health programs will additionally allow local stakeholders to advocate for their agenda, increasing accountability and long-term viability. As communities feel the actual benefits of improved water and sanitation, such as improved public health and increased economic productivity, concerted effort toward universal coverage will result in a healthier, more resilient global population (Figure 11.10).

11.3.3. Impact of Food Security on Community Health

The multifaceted issue of food security has deep meaning on community health since it is one of the major determinants of good health and wellbeing. Inadequate access to nutritious food leads to a series of conditions like malnutrition, obesity, and diseases resulting from lifestyle. For instance, the hunger-obesity paradox identifies that individuals in food-insecure environments would consume larger portions of calorie-rich, low-nutrient foods due to availability limitation, exacerbating the health issues. Food-insecure environments are predisposed to higher rates of diet-related illnesses, eventually placing a strain on healthcare systems and undermining local public health programs. This intricate interconnectedness underscores the imperative of community interventions that address food security to create healthier communities, particularly in economically disadvantaged communities where both hunger and obesity are deplorably prevalent (Gutschall et al., 2021). Community intervention on food security is a vital step towards local health enhancement. Collaborative initiatives, such as community-academic partnerships, can bridge resource and knowledge divides and supply durable solutions that promote general health within communities. For instance, partnerships between local groups and universities have the potential to provide nutrition education, healthy food systems, and healthcare-based food security screening. Not only do these programs enable consumers to make more healthy food choices, but these programs also aim to change community policy influencing access to food. The success of these interventions relies on active community member engagement, where they can engage in efforts to obtain changes and become resilient to future food insecurities (Gutschall et al., 2021). Through strengthened relations within and between systems and increased information about food-related health issues, communities can begin to respond to the adverse effects on health associated with food insecurity.

Moreover, environmental determinants embedded within food security also strongly affect community health outcomes. Local food systems sustainability is of primary concern in ensuring uninterrupted availability of healthy sources of food. Overcapacity as well as governance issues in food production worsen challenges for vulnerable groups. With effective management methods, including those illustrated by innovative fisheries practices, communities can enhance food security while maintaining environmental integrity. Sustainable methods not only ensure the availability of food resources but also contribute to long-term community well-being. Integrating environmental health factors into food security initiatives can create a synergistic advantage, both enhancing ecological balance and improved public health outcomes. Thus, food security and environmental health have a critical synergy to achieve in terms of building healthy, thriving communities (Figure 11.11).

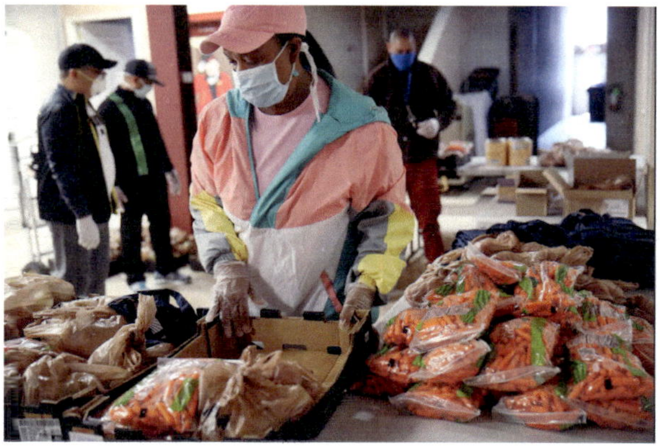

Figure 11.11. Impact of food security on community health.

Source: https://www.association-chrysalide.org/wp-content/uploads/2024/10/USHunger.webp.

11.4. Health Disparities and Vulnerable Populations

Health disparities are most forcefully realized among vulnerable populations, who in turn tend to stay there due to systematic disparities. Such groups include low-income groups, racial and ethnic minorities, and other vulnerable populations who often have difficulty accessing health care, adequate nutrition, and safe living conditions. These disparities are exacerbated by the socioeconomic determinants of health outcomes, including education, employment, and environment. Furthermore, the emergence of climate change brings about other threats that affect these vulnerable groups disproportionately. For instance, inhabitants of the less resource-rich regions are found in environmentally hazard-prone locations, thus further perpetuating health disparities. All of these must be addressed with an organized strategy that includes health policies that seek to prioritize accessibility, equity, and actively involve affected populations in decision-making. Current studies recognize disproportionate climate change impacts on disadvantaged groups, with a demand for intervention that targets their unique needs. The Climate Gap describes unequal climate-related health risks for low-income and communities of color in such areas as heat waves and decreasing air quality. They lack the abilities to reverse these sufficiently, thereby making them more vulnerable and causing related health issues. It is essential to document these disparities within a framework that not only reveals the urgent challenges but also explores potential solutions. Collaborative efforts must focus on integrating climate action with social equity, ensuring that policies aim to alleviate both environmental and health disparities simultaneously. With the understanding and resolution of the intersectionality of climate and health, effective plans can be crafted to ensure the overall wellness of the most vulnerable populations (Sadd et al., 2009). The roadmap to carbon neutrality brings an imperative opportunity to reduce health disparities and foster equity. The Boston Green Ribbon Commissions Carbon Free Boston project illustrates how green solutions can be designed to factor in social considerations so that no vulnerable group is left behind as the world moves towards a greener future. By emphasizing energy efficiency and equitable access to resources, the project seeks to reverse existing imbalances exacerbated by climate change. A just carbon neutrality strategy requires a policy design with intentionality, prioritizing the interests of long-marginalized communities. Therefore, urban planning and environmental health policies must incorporate equity frameworks centered on how enhanced infrastructure can create a healthier environment. Ultimately, the elimination of the health disparities that affect vulnerable populations by comprehensive environmental strategies not only builds a healthier community but also a more just and equitable society (Boston University Institute for Sustainable Energy et al., 2019).

11.4.1. Socioeconomic Factors Affecting Health Outcomes

Socioeconomic determinants take on an essential role in deciding health results in various populations, showing the need for targeted interventions toward disparity reduction. Individuals in lower socioeconomic status are more likely to have higher risks for adverse health conditions due to their lack of access to resources such as quality healthcare, healthy diets, and sanitary living conditions. These disparities clearly manifest when comparing maternal health outcomes, with education, income, and marriage playing active parts in determining pregnancy results. For instance, research confirms that mothers with certain demographic features suffer different levels of exposure to harmful environmental contaminants, the etiology of preterm and low birth weight, respectively. Public health interventions aimed at minimizing such adverse effects depend on an understanding of such determinants for the case of marginalized groups of individuals living in urban areas where there is excessive environmental contamination, underlining interdependence between socioeconomic status and health inequity (Carman et al., 2009).

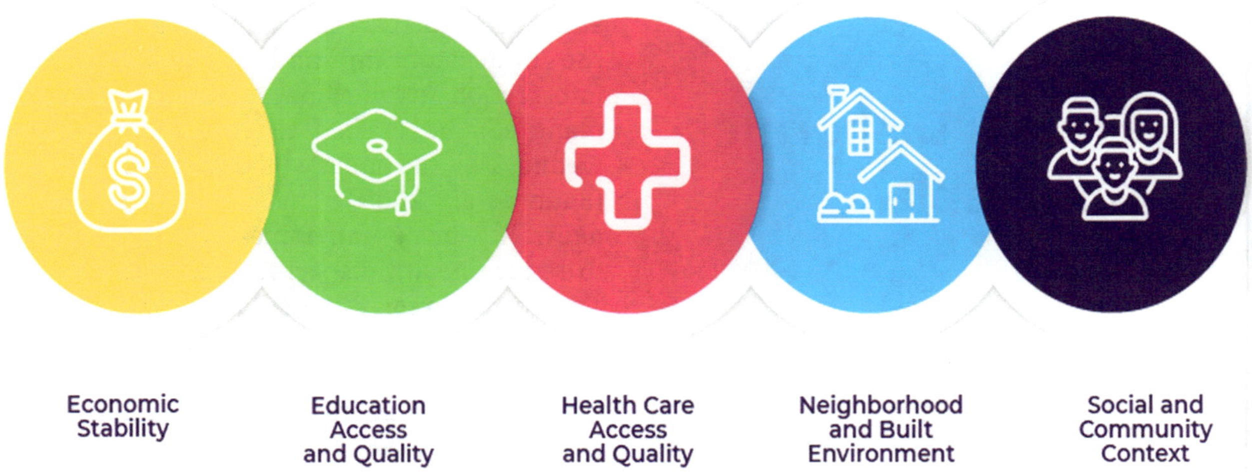

Figure 11.12. Socioeconomic factors affecting health outcomes.

Source: https://info.totalwellnesshealth.com/hubfs/SDOH-01.png.

Also, the effect of living conditions on health should not be overlooked since they incorporate physical and social elements impacting lifestyle patterns. Recent studies have expanded the focus on childhood obesity to broader socioeconomic and environmental determinants rather than solely personal behaviors. Influences such as access to healthy food in the neighborhoods and play spaces are particularly important in mediating the role of socioeconomic status on obesity among children, particularly among Hispanic minorities that carry the disproportionate burden. Housing segregation also complicates this issue since it can limit quality access to resources and physical exercise spaces. Such environmental contexts contribute to significant health disparities, highlighting the urgent need for community interventions that consider both existing structural inequities and individual behaviors to foster healthier outcomes for residents (Ahmed et al., 2017). Lastly, addressing these socioeconomic determinants involves a multifaceted approach that requires collaboration across sectors, including health, education, and urban planning. Policies intended to expand healthcare access, food security, and secure safe physical environments are necessary to counteract the effect of socioeconomic determinants on health outcomes. Community health initiatives must empower the residents as well through education and awareness building about the significance of healthy lifestyle choices, as well as providing residents with tools to overcome the barriers of socio-economic status. By connecting research findings and practice, policymakers can create integral frameworks that not only focus on resolving health inequalities but also support sustainable community health. Ultimately, it is necessary to address the complex interaction of socioeconomic factors in order to develop fair health outcomes in diverse communities, paving the way to healthier communities around the world (Ahmed et al., 2017) (Figure 11.12).

11.4.2. Disparities in Access to Healthcare Services

Healthcare service inequities are a key topic of discussion in global and environmental health research within paradigms of community health. There are multiple factors that contribute to these inequities, including socioeconomic status, location of residence, and racial or ethnic status. Individuals residing within impoverished communities often have extreme access barriers to quality health care, such as limited transportation, inferior health insurance coverage, and limited health literacy. Such difficulties are further exacerbated by geographical disparities, considering that rural dwellings lack adequate health facilities and qualified practitioners, leading to poorer health outcomes. The resultant effect is therefore that marginalized populations with poor care access exhibit a high prevalence of preventable conditions and poorer health status overall, and thus the necessity for targeted intervention targeting such health disparities in access to healthcare facilities is even more critical. The effect of these variations is not just limited to personal health, but it also filters down to the rest of society and maintains prevalent public health problems. When parts of the population have no exposure to healthcare services through systematic limitations, the whole community suffers with increased rates of disease and cost liabilities on healthcare. One portion of poor health can even translate into increased morbidity and mortality rates, which ultimately contribute to the burden of public health systems. Moreover, redress of these disparities is not only one of equity, but one of economic viability; healthy communities equal healthier economies. Policymakers and institutions must take priority in making equitable access to healthcare services in line with a series of recommendations from health equity organizations (Birnbaum et al., 2011) as well as effective practices of closing gaps in service provision (Birnbaum et al., 2011). Structuring inequalities of access to healthcare requires a multi-dimensional intervention addressing the heterogenous needs and contexts of affected populations. Multi-sector collaboration among healthcare providers, community organizations, and policymakers should be employed in planning and implementing effective interventions. Through partnership building involving grassroots communities, stakeholders are facilitated to identify constraints to access and resolve them appropriately. Interventions such as enhancing public transportation coverage, increasing the supply of community health workers, and expanding telehealth coverage are useful in reducing access barriers. Moreover, health education and outreach programs aimed at improving health literacy can empower people and communities to receive the care necessary, culminating in improved health outcomes. Here, bridging the access gap to healthcare not only benefits the health of the individual but also the social fabric as a whole, leading to an overall healthier society.

11.4.3. The Role of Marginalized Communities in Health Advocacy

Marginalized groups are now at the forefront of health advocacy, particularly in the case of global health and environmental health. These communities, constantly exposed to systemic disadvantage that reinforces health inequity, hold a rich reservoir of experiential knowledge that contributes to effective intervention strategies. Engaging with these communities not only produces a perception of belonging but also leads to healthier, more culturally sensitive health programs that speak within their own needs and dreams. These groups' advocacy strategies are critical in resisting dominant health discourses and thus gaining more voice in public policy arenas. As noted in the literature, the task of fostering critical consciousness of the populace is amongst the important mandates for enhancing health advocacy for marginalized groups, emphasizing how pivotal they are as visionaries of a society which is more equitable and where health equity prevails, as noted in Liboro et al. (2015). Additionally, the nexus between health advocacy and environmental justice is unveiled when there is consideration of the particular vulnerabilities that face marginalized communities. Environmental degradation, often linked to socio-economic inequalities, has direct impacts on public health outcomes. Studies indicate that the vulnerable groups bear disproportionately the adverse effects of pollution, climate change, and habitat loss, leading to a range of health complications. This sets the context for inclusive responses to address both the health and environmental problems. Such interventions like the waste management at a community level have been discovered to be promising towards establishing ecological sustainability as well as enabling public health, in terms of how empowering marginalized communities can establish twin benefits. Through a participatory approach that connects health promotion with environmental protection, communities might improve their overall resilience, as a reflection of the principles established in the study on the Philippines and Laudate Deum framework highlighted in Ingles et al. (2024). Lastly, the participation of marginalized groups in health advocacy offers a means of creating a united front against structural injustices that frustrate health outcomes. Through the creation of political will and shared vision by group members, the groups can mobilize resources and alliances to effect meaningful changes. This is a process necessary to subverting barriers and access to health resources on an equal basis. The advocacy function is not just a function of heightening consciousness but also for arguing for achievable strategies which resonate with the people's immediate socio-economic needs. Through empowerment programs that strengthen community networks, such marginalized groups are the impelling forces behind paradigm-breaking health policies with international appeal. Lastly, the integration of these perspectives in health advocacy is required to create a better and more sustainable future because it upholds the significance of shared responsibility as viewed in Ingles et al. (2024).

11.5. Policy and Regulation in Environmental Health

Policy and regulation of environmental health have a crucial link for the sake of public health protection and sustainable development promotion. Effective policies are blueprints that guide action and decision-making that affect the environment and therefore human health in both direct and indirect ways. In community health, they aim to minimize the threats caused by environmental hazards such as pollution, exposure to chemicals, and climate change. Effective regulations hinge on collaboration between government agencies, private sector, and communities. Participatory framework enhances compliance and imbues stakeholders with the feeling of ownership of their contribution towards enhancing environmental health. Participatory forces are essential to unveil innovation in public health solutions as well as to address effectively emerging environmental issues jeopardizing public wellbeing. Frameworks must adapt based on the constantly evolving context of environmental health challenges, indicative of the imperative for integrated assessments and monitoring mechanisms. Rigid or reactive policies often fail to address long-term health outcomes effectively. Responsive regulations that blend scientific evidence and community input can thus facilitate proactive measures, addressing potential health problems even before they escalate into public health crises.

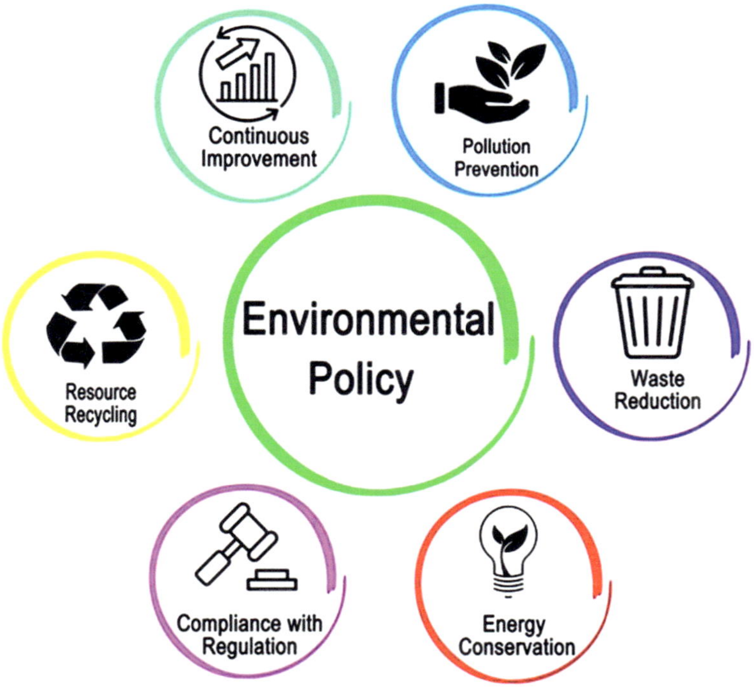

Figure 11.13. Policy and regulation in environmental health.

Source: https://storack.in/images/Picture5.jpg.

For instance, including environmental health considerations in urban planning can minimize the effects of urban heat islands and improve the overall living environment. This model not only enhances residents' wellbeing but also aligns with broader public health goals. The constant cycle of assessment, adjustment, and implementation is thus instrumental to effective environmental health policy that reverberates through community health activities. Implications of regulatory practice extend beyond the local environment, as global environmental health concerns emphasize global interconnectivity of communities. Problems such as climate change, biodiversity loss, and pollution have a tendency to be international in scope, requiring coordination for effective regulation. International conventions and policy arrangements are important to promote collective action towards environmental wellness issues. For example, the development of organic agriculture, as highlighted on debates of sustainable agriculture, demonstrates how policy can privilege environmentally friendly practices while taking into account the effects of markets (Dabbert et al., 2003). Whereas organic farming has prospered in congenial regulatory settings, there is also tension between market success and obeisance to underlying ecological and public health principles (Banks et al., 2003). It is the signature of the dilemma involved in developing policies that promote economic growth at the same time as retaining environmental stewardship and community welfare principles (Figure 11.13).

11.5.1. Overview of Environmental Health Policies

Environmental health policy has become obligatory frameworks offering guarantees for the protection and promotion of public health in expanding urban settings. With the growth of urbanization, the interdependent relationship between environmental determinants and health results assumes growing importance, necessitating efficient policy interventions that span what conventionally had been imagined as health domains. These policies strive to prevent the adverse health consequences of environmental risks, ranging from air and water pollution to climate change. Multisectoral responses have been described as successful responses in this regard, since these enable various sectors—e.g., agriculture, urban planning, and health—to collaborate in order to reduce the determinants of health which are beyond the reach of health care itself.

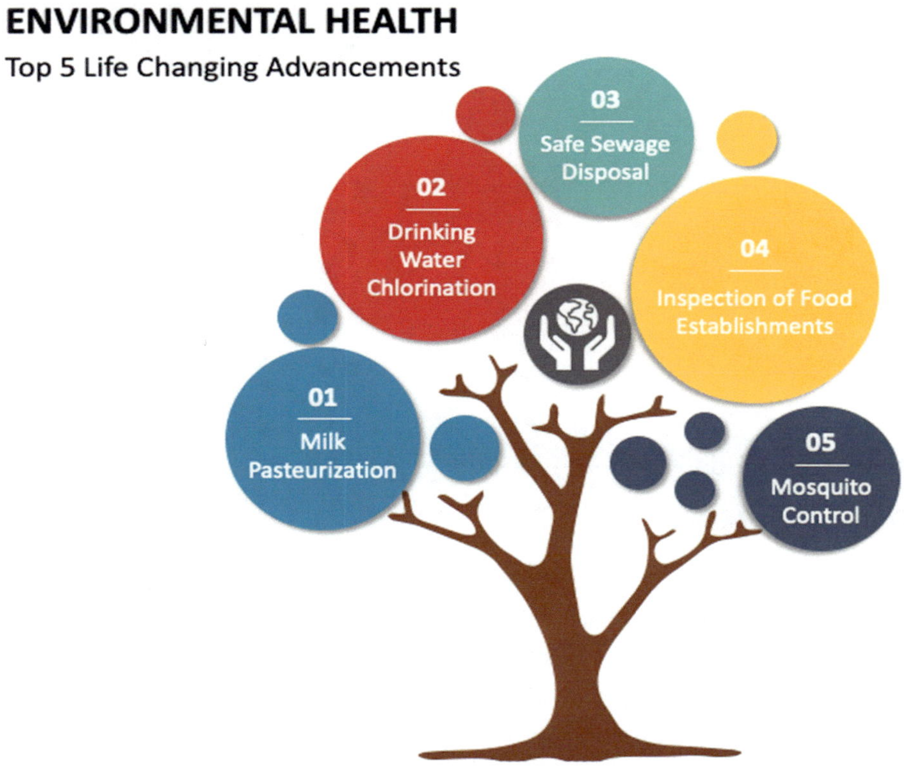

Figure 11.14. Overview of environmental health policies.

Source: https://cdn.sketchbubble.com/pub/media/catalog/product/optimized1/b/2/b285be83c720883c86f1b02279b869dd42cea128a9227d13a001534d157a4fca/environmental-health-mc-slide1.png.

Such a holistic perspective is encouraged particularly in regions of high urbanization, where health equity has not yet disappeared from the agenda, because there are so many policies which continue to be ineffective for the most vulnerable communities (Bhagtani et al., 2024). Moreover, the incorporation of environmental health policies on governmental agendas demonstrates a growing recognition of the intricate relationship between human health and the environment. For instance, the New Zealand disability and health system plays an active role in responding to environmental determinants of health, advocating for policies that not only deliver health services but also address the socio-environmental determinants of health inequities. Programs directed toward enhancing community health are increasingly focused on preventive strategies that promote health, like expanded access to green space, clean water, and reduced pollution. The establishment of environmental determinants in health policy reflects a pivotal shift toward sustainability and preventive care in response to current and future health priorities in a setting of resource constraint. With shifting policies, the emphasis on availing community participation will be even greater in implementing effective environmental health interventions that are appealing to communities (N/A, 2025). In conclusion, environmental health policies work best if they encourage collaboration among several sectors while maintaining ongoing emphasis on health equity as well as community participation. Previous research highlights significant gaps in existing interventions, particularly in developing nations, whereby resource limitations and infrastructural defects still persist. Prioritizing health equity in policy results and processes enables stakeholders to decide and implement interventions that better reflect the requirements of the community, finally enhancing public health outcomes. With the growing demand for multisectoral interventions, ongoing research and dialogue will become crucial in constructing a sustainable framework that provides health and protects the environment. This proactive approach not only will boost global health outcomes but will also empower communities to take an active role in shaping the policies influencing their health and wellbeing (Bhagtani et al., 2024) (Figure 11.14).

11.5.2. The Role of Government in Regulating Pollutants

The role of the government in regulating pollutants is crucial in the conservation of both environmental and public health. Through environmental policy setting and implementation, governments aim to discourage the adverse effects of pollution on ecosystems as well as human populations. In the United States, there have been significant frameworks that involve the Clean Air Act and the Clean Water Act, which provide regulatory authorities like the Environmental Protection Agency (EPA) with power to set and enforce air and water quality standards. Through these acts, governments can put in place stringent National Ambient Air Quality Standards (NAAQS), which are imperative in addressing pollutants that have a considerable impact on public health and climate change. The accomplishments of the Clinton Administration are notable in that they were focused on establishing tougher environmental objectives, which had a positive impact on the general air quality and environmental safeguard, further validating the necessity of an effective regulatory system in the assurance of public welfare (Hahn et al., 2025). Economic analysis principles also play a crucial role in influencing environmental legislation. Benefit-cost analysis has been a contentious point for policymakers, particularly in the 1990s, when effective resource allocation to environmental ends became increasingly top-heavy on the agenda. Although such analyses are meant to reason the highest-priority public health risks and increase the effectiveness of regulation, they must consider vulnerable populations as well. Marginalized groups are disproportionately subjected to toxic exposures, which suggests an acute conflict of interest in environmental policy. The balancing of economic efficiency over health equity might inadvertently ignore such groups, with the effect of less than adequate protection from the bads of pollution. Policy-makers must deal with these challenges carefully to ensure that the benefits from pollution reduction are shared equitably across all groups of populations (Swanston et al., 1994). In the face of these facts, government's role extends beyond enforcing the laws to include dealing with the special susceptibilities located in various communities. Regulatory bodies must introduce innovative approaches that target vulnerable groups, such as low-income and minority populations, which ultimately bear the largest burdens of environmental exposures. It is important to recognize the increased vulnerability of these groups to pollution-related health risks in order to create appropriate public health responses.

With evolving policies, it is important that policymakers engage with the affected communities and stakeholders so that environmental policies not only be comprehensive in nature but also equitable in implementation. With participatory consultation and community voice, governments can create improved regulatory frameworks that enhance public health while reversing the systemic injustices brought about through environmental degradation (Swanston et al., 1994).

11.5.3. Community Involvement in Policy-Making Processes

Participation of people in policy-making is a vital mechanism to make sure that the interest of different stakeholders is represented, particularly matters related to international and environmental health. When the citizens are actively involved to shape policies which affect their livelihoods, they offer valuable local knowledge and precious perspectives that can make policies more practical. Such engagement creates a sense of responsibility and ownership among the people in the communities, thus generating a spirit of teamwork that can result in creative solutions to complicated health problems. In addition, incorporating the experiences of minority groups, policy-makers can customize interventions according to the particular needs of the communities, enhancing health outcomes overall.

Thus, enhancing community participation is not only beneficial to policy implementation but also adds substance to the democratic process, allowing citizens to shape decisions that affect their health and lives. Another significant aspect of community participation in policy making is that it can empower silenced majorities, who are invariably disproportionately affected by international health problems. Engaging such voices makes sure that the policies created address their biggest issues, such as access to water, sanitation, and health care. For instance, reported, womens experiences are crucial in understanding the effects of water and sanitation policies on public health. Through such experiences, policy-making is more comprehensive and informed, thus improving the delivery of health services and resource allocation within communities. This empowerment is more than token consultation; it actually reverses the power and decision-making dynamics to serve those who historically have been marginalized in their health and environment decisions, resulting in policies that actually reflect the community's desires and needs (N/A, 2015).

Climate change also poses a significant threat to global health, so citizen engagement in policy-making is more critical now than ever before. The climate vulnerabilities most disproportionately affect marginalized populations whose own experience can provide rich lessons for adaptive fruitfulness. These populations most suffer the consequences of environmental change, most urgently in relation to increasing food and water insecurity due to extreme weather events.

Their experience can guide the crafting of policies that are not only responsive but also sustainable given the dynamics of variable climates. Engaging these groups in the health-aspect policy governance will enhance local-level resilience, and ultimately, regional environmental health objectives. By incorporating local knowledge into regional and international plans, policymakers will be in a position to formulate context-relevant but functional interventions, and bridge the gap between international health problems and regional and local concerns with precision and compassion (Perkins et al., 2017).

11.6. Education and Awareness in Community Health

Education and awareness are key to promoting health at the community level since they allow individuals to make healthy choices regarding health. Central to such an education campaign is the dissemination of information that is readily available and relevant to the specific challenges of health among various communities. The health challenges vary significantly in various communities, necessitating the use of specific health education programs. Societies that promote health literacy have lower incidences of avoidable disease and higher rates of compliance with healthy practices. Involving the local population in education programs can help instill a sense of responsibility for health, which will eventually translate to overall improved health of the population. Hence, a strategic investment in education becomes imperative to enable communities to respond both to global and environmental health challenges, ensuring resilience against health challenges like climate change and health inequities.

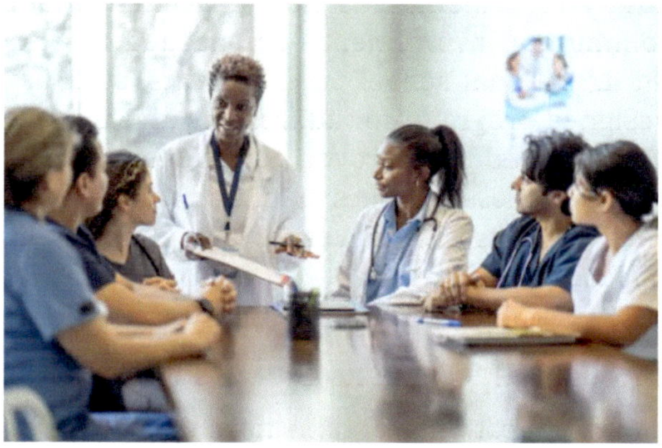

Figure 11.15. Education and awareness in community health.

Source: https://innewsweekly.com/wp-content/uploads/2023/02/Education-in-Public-Health.webp.

In programs with the objective of advocating for education and sensitization, youth involvement is a key driver of ensuring health interventions that will be effective. Youths, constituting a substantial portion of the population, have diverse insights and capacities contributing towards innovative solutions to health issues. As noted, value for youths as equal participants in development processes aligns with the natural inclination of the youths to help positively contribute to change. When empowered through education, the youths become advocates for the communities that they lead in terms of bringing about change through sensitization campaigns and helping to make decisions on public health interventions. Young people programs do not only validate their voice but also direct their energy and ingenuity towards tackling critical health concerns. Acknowledgment and affirmation of youth engagement thus become an obligatory aspect in enhancing the health education that concurs with broader community efforts towards sustainable health goals. Finally, the crossroads of community health and education is crucial in tackling health equity since education aids in dismantling barriers that are experienced by marginalized populations. These at-risk populations, which tend to have health inequities, are very assisted through intensive education efforts focused on health awareness and access to services. Looking at various community health programs, such as the ones provided in the State of Health Equity Movement, it is clear that multifaceted strategies—pairing educational components with community involvement—are needed to bring about change. Learning can be obtained outside the traditional school environments, such as outreach and community workshops in specifically designed programs for addressing diverse populations' needs. Such a focus creates collective action that can lead to improved health results and social well-being. In general, emphasis on education and awareness becomes essential in the fight against global and environmental health in community environments as it moves towards securing higher equity in the access and achievement of health (Figure 11.15).

11.6.1. Importance of Health Education Programs

Health education programs form the core of building community health as they provide individuals with the information and ability to make educated health decisions. Through a strategic education program, societies are able to deal with various health issues, including those nurtured by environmental factors such as climate change. For instance, being aware of the relationship between rises in temperature and the transmission of diseases like malaria can allow populations to be proactive about prevention. Based on a literature review, complex technology and global teaching systems for health workers and populations are essential to combat the impact of climate-related health issues, particularly in regions significantly affected by diseases like malaria. By giving health education a priority, communities can establish a culture of awareness and an active practice of controlling and managing health, ultimately translating to declining morbidity rates and improved public health outcomes among geographically isolated areas, particularly among marginal communities (Nara et al., 2013). Aside from this, interdisciplinary health education courses have an important role in addressing global health inequities brought about by globalization and migration. These initiatives, where institutions and communities partner, offer the opportunity for health professionals to work with different populations and become aware of their unique health concerns. For example, at the University of Wisconsin-Madison, its global health center, an interdisciplinary center, offers students adequate courses and field experiences that broaden their education on global health concerns. Through country partnerships, students are able to explore the intricate relationship between culture, community health development, and health, thereby enhancing their ability to improve health equity. These models of education highlight the power of health education in promoting bridging and resilience in communities experiencing health disparities (Baumann et al., 2008). In the end, investment in health education programs lies at the heart of establishing sustainable community health infrastructures. These initiatives not only enhance individual understanding but also enhance community-level resilience to emerging health challenges, particularly those related to environmental changes. Climate literacy initiatives could lead to higher public awareness of personal behavior's influences on environmental health, thus enhancing active community action. By empowering people with the means to know and act on public health issues, communities can make substantial advances toward health improvement. However, the plea for more comprehensive studies and funding for such initiatives is still pressing, as learned in recent public health assessments. Continuous monitoring and adaptation of health education programs can ensure that they are responsive to the dynamic global health situation and thus make communities resilient to the varied challenges with which they have to struggle (Nara et al., 2013) (Figure 11.16).

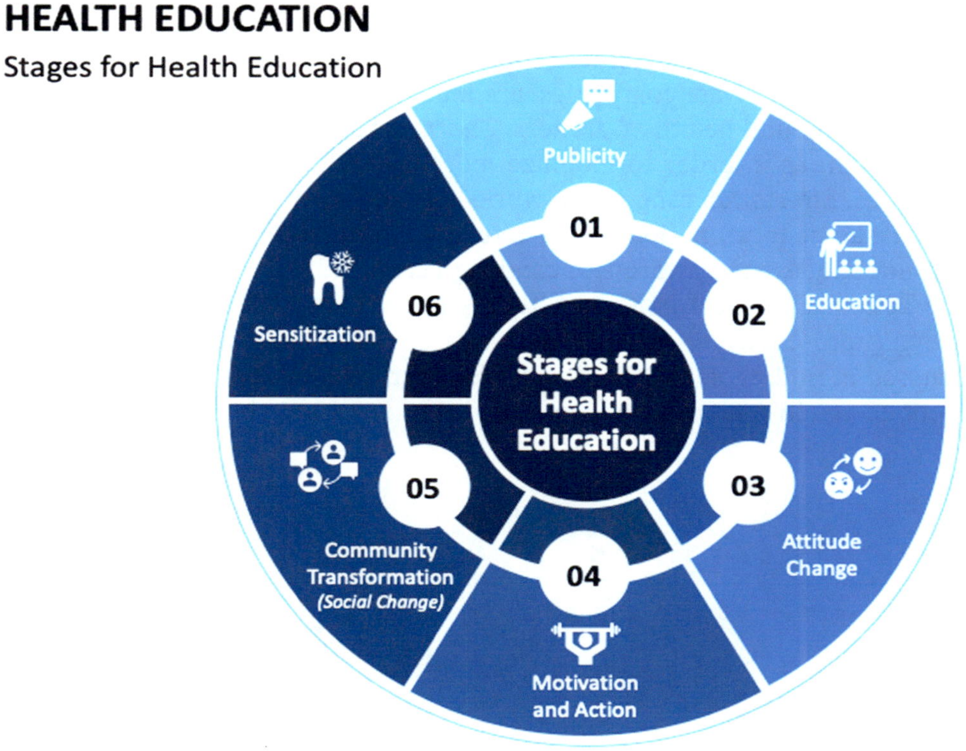

Figure 11.16. Importance of health education programs.

Source: https://cdn.sketchbubble.com/pub/media/catalog/product/optimized1/7/5/7543af18d6c8b6d54681753854feb1a1636ba62988f5453cbf221f016acbe8ff/health-education-slide1.png.

11.6.2. Strategies for Raising Awareness About Environmental Health

Effective strategies for raising awareness about environmental health rely upon a multi-dimensional intervention involving various sections of society. Community-oriented intervention is an important starting point because it utilizes local knowledge and tailors messaging to address local issues. Involving residents in problem identification increases ownership and maximizes the impact of intervention. Local schools can be leveraged to support integration of environment health themes into the curriculum, building awareness early on. By promoting public activities such as workshops and clean-up drives, organizations can mobilize citizens while also providing hands-on training that supports in-depth knowledge. Grassroots action not only increases awareness but also builds a more informed citizenry that is better equipped to support healthier environmental approaches in their community. Environmental health awareness can be significantly enhanced by leveraging digital platforms and social media. Increasingly, the internet is a good channel for conveying information quickly and extensively. Social media campaigns reach younger groups, breaking down complex environmental health issues through images, charts, and interactive conversation. Virtual platforms facilitate real-time communication, allowing quick response to emerging environmental crises and public action. However, the effectiveness of online outreach relies on the correct information shared; therefore, the use of evidence-based data and collaboration with health professionals. The emphasis on accurate information helps build confidence and encourages individuals to adopt good health practices of their environment. This strategically harnessed online media plays a vital role in shaping the attitude and mindset of people towards environmental health matters. Finally, associations with other stakeholders, including government institutions, non-governmental organizations (NGOs), and private companies, are indispensable in bringing forward a coordinated effort towards environmental health awareness. The associations have the ability to bring together resources and capabilities in order to mobilize more powerful educational campaigns that reach various communities. Efforts can range from workshops to policy action, that environmental health is an actionable issue at local, national, and international levels. These alliances, in their cross-sectoral nature, not only expand awareness campaign scope but also ensure a shared responsibility for sustainable action. Empirical behavior studies show that such shared strategies are indeed effective in driving pro-environmental behavior based on established relationships and shared values, as discussed in Bolt et al. (2017). Therefore, leveraging on these alliances is a key approach in advancing public action and knowledge on environmental health issues (Figure 11.17).

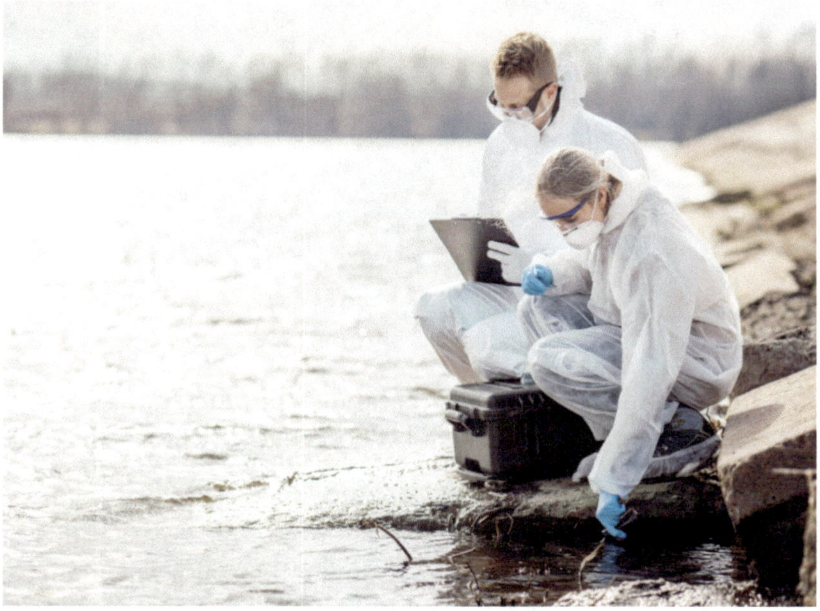

Figure 11.17. Strategies for raising awareness about environmental health.

Source: https://www.masterspublichealth.net/wp-content/uploads/2020/06/5-Characteristics-of-a-Great-Environmental-Health-Officer-2048x1365.jpg.

11.6.3. Role of Community Leaders in Promoting Health Initiatives

Community leaders have an important role to play in promoting health progress, as they are key intermediaries between government health policies and the specific needs of their local communities. Their role informs them of the cultural, economic, and social determinants of health behaviors and outcomes in their communities. Using their influence and credibility, these leaders are able to effectively mobilize citizens to engage in health-promoting activities such as vaccination campaigns, health checkups, and education workshops. Community leader participation in these activities not only generates awareness but also instils a sense of ownership among the residents towards their own health and well-being, which is imperative for long-term success. Besides mass mobilization, there is also the role of community leaders as health equity champions, raising awareness about disparities to be addressed among at-risk populations. In this case, through driving awareness about such inequalities, they can push for resources and policy intervention necessary to promote health access to every member of their communities. It can take countless forms, from public forums to direct opposition to policymakers. Research highlights the importance of such programs, echoing the effect that community leaders can have in the spheres of initiating significant changes in public health policy and resource priority (Birnbaum et al., 2011). As trusted leaders, they play the role of intermediary between healthcare services and marginalized groups, allowing for the dividends of health programs to reach the most disadvantaged. Secondly, collaboration as health organizations and community leaders is also essential in finding solutions to international and national health problems. Collaboration with such organizations can enhance the effectiveness of health programs such that there is enhanced data collection, program evaluation, and resource allocation. The inclusion of the leaders in planning and executing programs boosts their recommendations to more culturally sensitive interventions that carry significant value to the people within the community, thereby boosting the level of participation. Community participation projects have the tendency to offer better health outcomes, as in the case of the majority of health campaigns (N/A, 2007). Community leaders can involve health workers with whom they can make the project responsive to the particular needs of their community and hence create a more sustainable model for health promotion in terms of environmental and global health.

SUMMARY

In conclusion, the intricate relationship between global and environmental health has far-reaching implications for international community health programs. While public health professionals navigate climate change issues, recognizing the economic and environmental benefits of the latest healthcare technologies like telemedicine is not a choice, but an imperative. Evidence shows that telehealth not only facilitates increased access to healthcare services, particularly for marginalized groups, but also to significant greenhouse gas emission reductions. For context, a study revealed that telemedicine for maternity care saved over 204 miles and 96.6 metric tons of emissions during a specified timeframe, demonstrating the double dividend of improved health outcomes combined with maintaining the environment (Valverde et al., 2024). This convergence makes visible the imperative of policy systems embracing technology-facilitated care to propel healthier communities in the face of increasingly dire environmental crisis. Moreover, the mental impacts of climate change add complexity to the health dynamics of communities. While communities grapple with the fact that they are facing extreme weather and the accompanying distress, care should be taken to recognize the mental health implications related to environmental decline. A research conducted in Indonesia revealed a straight correlation between the problems of climate change and increasing levels of anxiety and depression, and it was suggested that the crisis of mental health has an inherent relationship with environmental factors (Shareeff et al., 2024). This indicates the importance of establishing mental health welfare systems alongside traditional health intervention, in order to enable a more integrated approach to health at a community level. Mental health provision is not a frill to add to physical health initiatives; it is an indispensable factor to incorporate to facilitate the resilience and stability of communities faced with the double threats of climate change and public health concerns. In addressing appropriately these intertwined issues, a multi-faceted strategy is needed in creating resilience among communities. This necessitates collaborative efforts from governments, health organizations, and community members in setting up enduring infrastructures that accommodate the provision of healthcare and environmental management. By leveraging new technologies and integrating healthcare strategy with environmental goals, a great deal can be done towards the enhancement of community health outcomes. Thus, programs that incorporate mental health education and reduce carbon footprints must be accorded top priority to foster a comprehensive concept of health outside the confines. Emphasizing such integrative approaches will not just reduce the immediate health crises but also promote long-term community resilience in the face of recurring global environmental hazards.

Global and environmental health convergence directly affects community health, and it gives us a multi-dimensional framework through which we can look at and address health inequities. A significant aspect of this discourse is around socioeconomic determinants that affect risk perception. Evidence indicates that poorer populations will concentrate on proximal threats, i.e., food unavailability, over more distant global challenges like climate change. This characteristic identifies a central dissonance between global health policies and community priorities, where risks are measured against temporal and spatial distance. It becomes crucial to comprehend these dynamics in order to create successful health interventions to tackle the most urgent needs of various socioeconomic groups, because risk perceptions can vary widely among the groups and determine health outcomes in tangible ways (Jewitt et al., 2011). Further exploring the role of water, sanitation, and hygiene (WASH) in community health reveals a key area for intervention.

The UNICEF strategy emphasizes 10 of the most significant areas for WASH impact, ranging from newborn and maternal health to nutrition and menstrual hygiene management. Not only do these impact individual health outcomes, but they also overlap with broader environmental health concerns. For instance, improved WASH behaviors can prevent disease that disproportionately targets the vulnerable, and this in turn enhances resilience at a community level. This underlines the importance of mainstreaming WASH programs into overall health policy in a manner that addresses intervention in both immediate public health issues and the underlying environmental causes of health inequities (Mills et al., 2016). Furthermore, the link between community health and environmental sustainability calls for an integrated understanding of determinants of health. The inequalities in health observed among different communities underscore the significance of policies promoting equality in resource and opportunity access. Positioning a systems-oriented strategy at the forefront, health intervention can better converge concerns regarding sustainable use of the environment with pressing concerns regarding vulnerable populations. As the nature of global health concerns evolves, with additional considerations in light of climate change, action concerning these inequalities becomes increasingly critical. Therefore, the encouragement of the collaboration between different levels of stakeholders can lead to more effective strategies that not only build community health but also assist in solving broad-ranging environmental issues (Jewitt et al., 2011; Mills et al., 2016).

KEY TERMS FROM THIS CHAPTER

- Environmental Justice
- Water Sanitation
- Food Security
- Occupational Health
- One Health Approach
- Disaster Preparedness
- Deforestation
- Environmental Policy
- Climate Change
- Vector-Borne Diseases
- Sustainable Development
- Urban Health
- Global Burden of Disease
- Ecosystem Health
- Climate Resilience
- Community Resilience
- Air Pollution
- Global Health Equity
- Waste Management
- Environmental Exposure
- Environmental Risk Factors
- Renewable Resources
- Infectious Disease Control

CLOSER LOOK

BUILDING RESILIENCE AGAINST CLIMATE EFFECTS (BRACE)

A closer look at Building Resilience Against Climate Effects (BRACE) reveals it as a strategic public health initiative designed to help communities adapt to the growing health impacts of climate change. Developed by the U.S. Centers for Disease Control and Prevention (CDC), BRACE provides a five-step framework that enables health departments and local governments to anticipate climate-related health risks and implement evidence-based interventions. The core idea behind BRACE is to move from reactive responses to proactive planning by integrating climate science with public health practices. This involves identifying climate-sensitive health outcomes—such as heat-related illnesses, respiratory conditions, and vector-borne diseases—and using localized data and projections to assess vulnerabilities. The process also includes evaluating public health capacity, developing and implementing adaptation plans, and assessing the effectiveness of those strategies over time. A key strength of BRACE is its emphasis on cross-sector collaboration, bringing together experts in climate science, health, urban planning, emergency management, and community organizations to build more cohesive and context-specific solutions. Equity is also a central concern, as BRACE aims to protect populations that are most vulnerable to climate impacts, including the elderly, children, low-income communities, and people with preexisting health conditions. By focusing on adaptation rather than just mitigation, BRACE acknowledges that many climate effects are already unavoidable and that communities need tools to cope with current and future challenges. The framework is flexible, allowing jurisdictions to tailor strategies to their specific climate threats and population needs. In doing so, BRACE strengthens community resilience, enhances public health infrastructure, and fosters long-term sustainability. Overall, BRACE serves as a practical model for climate resilience planning, demonstrating how public health systems can be a frontline defense in protecting communities from the increasing health risks posed by a changing climate.

REFERENCES

1. Abouzaid, S., & Sarfaty, M. (2009). The physician's response to climate change. https://core.ac.uk/download/46966943.pdf (accessed on 26th June 2025).
2. Adger, N., Ashford, L., Badyaev, A., Bahn, M., Baird, J., Barton, D., Baum, J., et al. (2016). The human–nature relationship and its impact on health: A critical review. https://core.ac.uk/download/163076696.pdf (accessed on 26th June 2025).
3. Agustin, R., Arista, S. R., Fitrianto, A. R., Gibbons, A., et al. (2024). Revitalizing the on-campus waste bank: Promoting community environmental awareness and improving waste management efficiency. https://core.ac.uk/download/639388624.pdf (accessed on 26th June 2025).
4. Ahmed, N. U., Chang Martinez, C., & Natale, R., et al. (2017). Residential segregation, neighborhood social and physical context in obesity disparities in Hispanic preschoolers: A conceptual model. https://digitalscholarship.unlv.edu/cgi/viewcontent.cgi?article=1493&context=jhdrp (accessed on 26th June 2025).
5. Al-Khudairy, D., Dregan, A., Assari, S., Bronfenbrenner, U., Atherton, C., Elia, C., Elia, C., et al. (2018). Global cities and cultural diversity: Challenges and opportunities for young people's nutrition. https://core.ac.uk/download/159081490.pdf (accessed on 26th June 2025).
6. Anaf, J., Baum, F., Fisher, M., London, L., et al. (2019). The health impacts of extractive industry transnational corporations: A study of Rio Tinto in Australia and Southern Africa. https://core.ac.uk/download/188741941.pdf (accessed on 26th June 2025).
7. Angelos, J. A., Arens, A. L., Cadriel, J. L., Johnson, R., et al. (2017). One Health in food safety and security education: Subject matter outline for a curricular framework. https://core.ac.uk/download/323068605.pdf (accessed on 26th June 2025).
8. Ashton, M., Bartlett, R., Davila-Ortega, L., Farmanesh, A., et al. (2025). Youth and the Millennium Development Goals (MDGs): Challenges and opportunities for implementation. https://core.ac.uk/download/pdf/7296591.pdf (accessed on 26th June 2025).
9. Auch, W. E. T., Palmer, R., & Short, D. (2018). The human right to water and unconventional energy. https://core.ac.uk/download/161233181.pdf (accessed on 26th June 2025).
10. Aytur, S., Bucci, J., & Wake, C. P. (2014). An assessment of the impact of climate change on human health in New Hampshire. https://core.ac.uk/download/84123597.pdf (accessed on 26th June 2025).
11. Banks, R., Haylor, G., Macfadyen, G., Mazaudier, M., et al. (2003). Background paper on the international seafood trade and poverty. https://core.ac.uk/download/11017269.pdf (accessed on 26th June 2025).
12. Baumann, L., Bousquet, G., Brown, L. D., Conway, M., et al. (2008). Creating a center for global health at the University of Wisconsin-Madison. https://core.ac.uk/download/287623788.pdf (accessed on 26th June 2025).
13. Bellon, S., Deverre, C., Geniaux, G., Powell, B., et al. (2025). Sustainable development indicator frameworks and initiatives. https://core.ac.uk/download/pdf/6517845.pdf (accessed on 26th June 2025).

14. Bhagtani, D., Boscott, R., Dalzell, S., Dambisya, Y., et al. (2024). Multisectoral interventions for urban health in Africa: A mixed-methods systematic review. https://core.ac.uk/download/603239260.pdf (accessed on 26th June 2025).
15. Birnbaum, N., Masterson, E., & Schoomaker, H. (2011). State of Health Equity Movement, 2011 Update Part C: Compendium of Recommendations DRA Project Report No. 11–03. https://core.ac.uk/download/pdf/18491812.pdf (accessed on 26th June 2025).
16. Bolt, C. A. (2017). Environmental education in the public sphere: Comparing practice with psychosocial determinants of behavior and societal change. https://core.ac.uk/download/129153482.pdf (accessed on 26th June 2025).
17. Boston University Institute for Sustainable Energy, Castigliego, J., Cleveland, C., Fortune, D., D'Janapha, A., et al. (2019). *Carbon Free Boston: Social equity report 2019.* https://open.bu.edu/bitstream/2144/39229/1/CFB_Social_Equity_Report_053119.pdf (accessed on 26th June 2025).
18. Bright, F., Cruice, M., Jagoe, C., Le Dorze, G., et al. (2019). Increasing the intensity and comprehensiveness of aphasia services: Identification of key factors influencing implementation across six countries. https://core.ac.uk/download/196222625.pdf (accessed on 26th June 2025).
19. Carman, A. E. (2009). Ambient air toxic releases and adverse pregnancy outcomes in Allegheny County, Pennsylvania. https://core.ac.uk/download/12206720.pdf (accessed on 26th June 2025).
20. Dabbert, S., & Lampkin, N. (2003). Organic farming–can policy and markets mix? https://core.ac.uk/download/10925762.pdf (accessed on 26th June 2025).
21. Dietler, D. (2020). Impact of mining projects on environmental determinants of health and associated health outcomes in sub-Saharan Africa: Insights for guiding impact assessment practice. https://core.ac.uk/download/511532385.pdf (accessed on 26th June 2025).
22. Erales Villamil, J. A. (2017). Silvopastoral system for sustainable cattle production in the tropics of Mexico. https://core.ac.uk/download/354387298.pdf (accessed on 26th June 2025).
23. Freudenberg, N., Galea, S., & Vlahov, D. (2005). Cities and population health. https://core.ac.uk/download/323072008.pdf (accessed on 26th June 2025).
24. Froggatt, A., Happer, C., & Wellesley, L. (2015). *Chatham House Report: Changing Climate, Changing Diets: Pathways to Lower Meat Consumption.* https://core.ac.uk/download/42367153.pdf (accessed on 26th June 2025).
25. Gutschall, M., NC DOCKS at Appalachian State University. (2021). Hunger, poverty and health: Community-academic partnerships that improve food and nutrition security in rural Appalachia. https://core.ac.uk/download/475606942.pdf (accessed on 26th June 2025).
26. Hahn, R. W., Olmstead, S. M., & Stavins, R. N. (2025). National environmental policy during the Clinton years. https://core.ac.uk/download/pdf/6665197.pdf (accessed on 26th June 2025).
27. Hancock, J., Haywood, C., Johnson, A., Meyers, D., et al. (2021). Impact of the COVID-19 pandemic on resilience to climate change in underserved communities. https://core.ac.uk/download/617035086.pdf (accessed on 26th June 2025).
28. Harris, C., Agnew, D., Leotte, F., Arthur, R., Walmsley, S., Davies, T., & Peatman, T. (2013). Fisheries and aquaculture and their potential roles in development: An assessment of the

current evidence. https://core.ac.uk/download/75777502.pdf (accessed on 26th June 2025).

29. Hricko, A., De Lara, J., Matsuoka, M., & Gottlieb, R. (2011). Global trade impacts: Addressing the health, social and environmental consequences of moving international freight through our communities. https://core.ac.uk/download/71358287.pdf (accessed on 26th June 2025).
30. Hutchuk, N. (2023). Exploring the role of public health in climate change initiatives and the mining industry in Ontario, Canada. https://core.ac.uk/download/581135735.pdf (accessed on 26th June 2025).
31. Ingles, A. L. S. (2024). *Laudate Deum: A Framework for Environmental Stewardship and Social Justice in The Philippines and Southeast Asia.* https://core.ac.uk/download/639390105.pdf (accessed on 26th June 2025).
32. Jewitt, S., & Baker, K. (2011). Risk, wealth and agrarian change in India: Household-level hazards vs. late-modern global risks at different points along the risk transition. https://core.ac.uk/download/pdf/14329685.pdf (accessed on 26th June 2025).
33. Kapoor, A. R., Patel, A., & Nair, V. P. (2024). Exploring the neurobiological mechanisms mediating the impact of air pollution on cognitive and emotional health in urban residents of New Delhi. *Studies in Psychological Science.* https://www.semanticscholar.org/paper/204fbb16f1c567f6bf59cbd544d990ef75ec67c2 (accessed on 26th June 2025).
34. Liboro, R. M. (2015). Forging political will from a shared vision: A critical social justice agenda against neoliberalism and other systems of domination. https://digitalscholarship.unlv.edu/cgi/viewcontent.cgi?article=1380&context=psychology_fac_articles (accessed on 26th June 2025).
35. Mashara, J. N., Thuranira, M., & Kathambi, F. (2024). Health risks of climate change and variability to maternal health. *International Journal of Research and Innovation in Social Science.* https://www.semanticscholar.org/paper/a862cbc69d9912ce1cf608e43bc224028c9debe5 (accessed on 26th June 2025).
36. Mayer, B. (2009). Blue-green coalitions: Fighting for safe workplaces and healthy communities. https://core.ac.uk/download/5125790.pdf (accessed on 26th June 2025).
37. Mills, J. E., & Cumming, O. (2016). The impact of water, sanitation, and hygiene on key health and social outcomes: Review of evidence. https://core.ac.uk/download/75761114.pdf (accessed on 26th June 2025).
38. N/A. (2007). Nathan Cummings Foundation–2004 annual report. https://core.ac.uk/download/71353343.pdf (accessed on 26th June 2025).
39. N/A. (2009). Why water? https://core.ac.uk/download/71345832.pdf (accessed on 26th June 2025).
40. N/A. (2011). Join up, scale up: How integration can defeat disease and poverty. https://core.ac.uk/download/71359748.pdf (accessed on 26th June 2025).
41. N/A. (2011). Promoting good hygiene practices: Key elements and practical lessons. https://core.ac.uk/download/71358782.pdf (accessed on 26th June 2025).
42. N/A. (2013). Everyone everywhere: A vision for water, sanitation and hygiene post-2015. https://core.ac.uk/download/71361302.pdf (accessed on 26th June 2025).
43. N/A. (2013). We can't wait: A report on sanitation and hygiene for women and girls. https://core.ac.uk/download/75783160.pdf (accessed on 26th June 2025).

44. N/A. (2015). Women, WASH, and the Water for Life Decade. https://core.ac.uk/download/75783060.pdf (accessed on 26th June 2025).

45. N/A. (2025). Briefing to the incoming Minister of Health 2014. https://core.ac.uk/download/pdf/30673327.pdf (accessed on 26th June 2025).

46. Nara, S. (2013). Current and future impacts of climate change on malaria in central and western Africa. https://core.ac.uk/download/33559639.doc (accessed on 26th June 2025).

47. Perkins, P. E. (Ellie). (2017). University-community collaboration for climate justice education and organizing: Partnerships in Canada, Brazil, and Africa. https://core.ac.uk/download/287659513.pdf (accessed on 26th June 2025).

48. Petruzelli, N. (2020). The influence of climate change on disease and public health. https://core.ac.uk/download/322826252.pdf (accessed on 26th June 2025).

49. Sadd, J., Pastor, M., Morello-Frosch, R., & Shonkoff, S. B. (2009). The climate gap: Inequalities in how climate change hurts Americans & how to close the gap. https://core.ac.uk/download/71342763.pdf (accessed on 26th June 2025).

50. Shareeff, N., Pramono, R. K., & Saliha, A. (2024). Climate change and mental health: Exploring the psychological impacts of environmental distress in Indonesia. *Scientia Psychiatrica.* https://www.semanticscholar.org/paper/54a1ead54a6b2d813ffa9071395f910b3830e483 (accessed on 26th June 2025).

51. Shrivastava, S., Bobhate, P., & Kukde, M. M. (2025). Oral health and climate change: Working toward adaptive strategies to the changing environment. *Journal of International Society of Preventive & Community Dentistry, 15*, 192–195. https://www.semanticscholar.org/paper/7c617d71fd80dfbc36686c7c09a4d55b21cff6cd (accessed on 26th June 2025).

52. Swanston, S. F. (1994). Race, gender, age, and disproportionate impact: What can we do about the failure to protect the most vulnerable? https://core.ac.uk/download/144228527.pdf (accessed on 26th June 2025).

53. Ugwu, J. N. (2025). The role of arts in global health initiatives: Opportunities and challenges. *Newport International Journal of Research in Medical Sciences.* https://www.semanticscholar.org/paper/cb514fc0b6a2e53f72145fa213b812c2843598d9 (accessed on 26th June 2025).

54. Valverde, V. M. L., Althaus, E., Horton, L., La Rosa, M., & Haeri, S. (2024). Economic and environmental pollutant impact of maternal–fetal telemedicine. *American Journal of Perinatology.* https://www.semanticscholar.org/paper/92407947ef4c607a7b3bef56a4f68c4ca07e8349 (accessed on 26th June 2025).

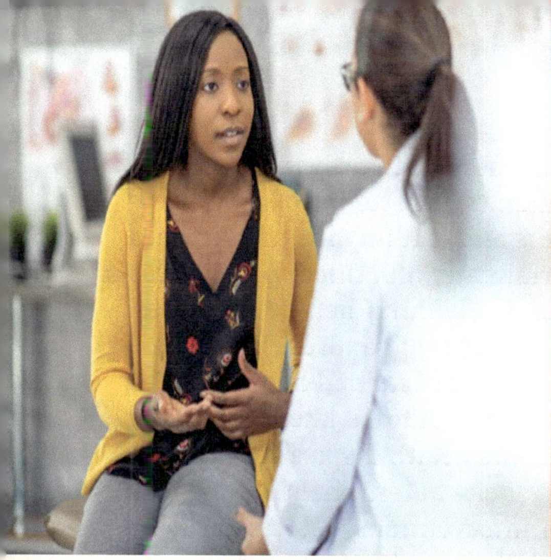

Chapter 12

HEALTH DISPARITIES AND SOCIAL DETERMINANTS

Contents

Introduction

Understanding health disparities is indispensable with an extensive analysis of social determinants, which encompass the various conditions and structures in biological, physical, built, and social surroundings. These determinants significantly contribute to health outcomes, social functioning, and quality of life in different populations. For instance, the use of standardized measurement procedures for social determinants of health can enhance health disparities and minority health research. The PhenX Toolkit is one such initiative that provides standardized measures involving individual and structural factors in varied environments. This baseline approach is crucial in advancing the science of health disparities, as good data collection has the potential to lead to better public health policy and interventions. By thoroughly documenting the social determinants and resulting health outcomes, researchers can develop targeted strategies that maximize health equity in disadvantaged groups, evidencing commitment to strong and equitable public health initiatives (Breen et al., 2023). The Appalachian region is a particularly apt example through which the discussion of health disparities and social determinants can be made more complex. Residents of Appalachia have had to live with overwhelming morbidity and mortality rates that surpass national rates, primarily the result of unequal exposure to a variety of social and environmental determinants. A recent scoping review did acknowledge necessary relationships between such determinants and leading health outcomes like cancer, diseases of despair, and diabetes. Leading health determinants identified were access to care, rurality, and education, all of which had substantial roles in defining health outcomes. Through these specific determinants, stakeholders can create interventions that address the unique issues in Appalachian communities. Additionally, the findings indicate that sustained and impactful public health interventions need to be created by multidimensional interventions like educational interventions and technological advancements to mitigate these chronic health disparities (Cattell-Gordon et al., 2023). Ultimately, addressing health disparities using social determinants is the way forward in the creation of sustainable and effective public health interventions. Efforts must be directed toward infusing culturally sensitive approaches that are relevant to affected communities, particularly in regions like Appalachia, where standard health interventions are not sufficient. With collaborations between researchers, healthcare providers, and grassroots champions, efforts can be designed which not only address immediate health concerns but also allow communities to take charge of their own health trajectory. Continual monitoring and quality improvement of these programs, based on evidence-based research, will ensure that the most pressing health concerns are treated with an evidence-based intervention. This comprehensive vision of health disparities—based on the various social determinants—presents the door to a more equal healthcare environment for every population (Figure 12.1).

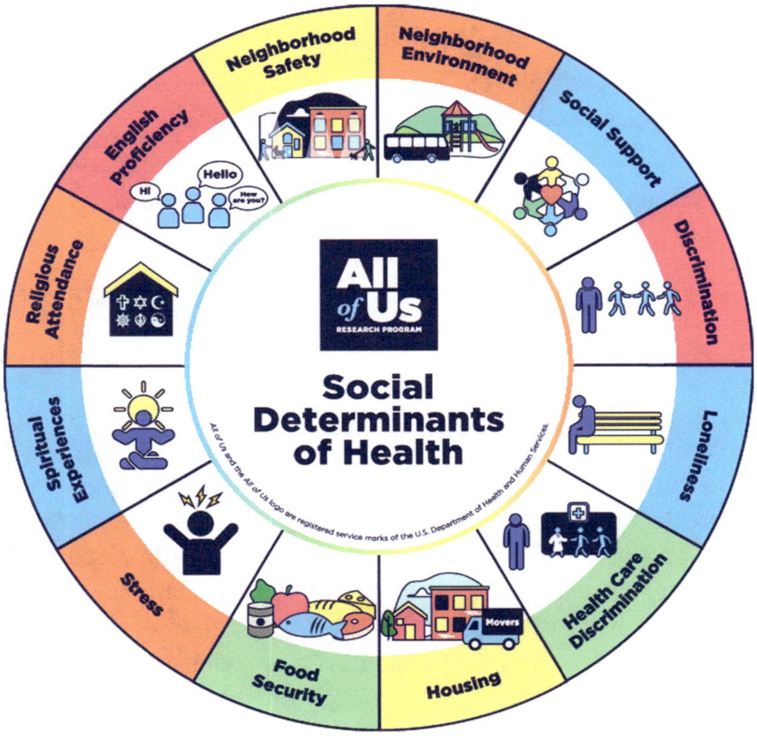

Figure 12.1. Health disparities and social determinants.

Source: https://aahd.us/wp-content/uploads/2022/05/SDOH_Icon_Wheel_%E2%80%93_Web-668x668-1.png.

Definition of Health Disparities

Health disparities are the undesirable and discriminatory health status variations and differences in access to healthcare services that occur among different populations. Such disparities typically have a direct relationship with social determinants of health such as socioeconomic position, education, race, and residence. For instance, there are usually disproportionate numbers of chronic illness and mortality among marginalized groups due to structural inequities in health care, including reduced access to proper care and preventive treatment. Identification of health disparities is necessary, as it forces policymakers and public health specialists to address the determinants that continue to keep health outcomes unequal, thereby instilling higher levels of awareness of the intersectionality of social issues and their applicability to health. In addition, the articulation of health disparities is often supported by poor communication and culturally insensitive care practices. Effective delivery of healthcare does not only mean that services are available but also that health workers can work with diverse populations in a manner that appreciates and respects their everyday experience and cultural identity.

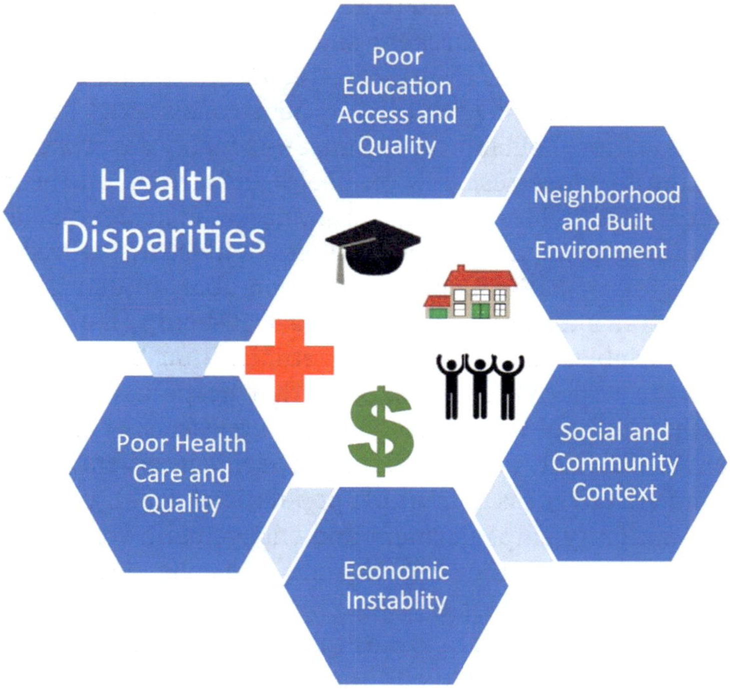

Figure 12.2. Health disparities.

Source: https://www.jaci-global.org/cms/10.1016/j.jacig.2024.100350/asset/e2067f96-f704-4aac-8864-ae9d8c7da6b3/main.assets/gr1_lrg.jpg.

For instance, developing clinical communication models adapted to the unique requirements of oppressed groups, e.g., the Aboriginals, can enhance communication during healthcare interactions. By focusing on critical self-reflection and awareness of relational processes, health workers can maximize their interaction and, ultimately, health outcomes for such populations, in trying to eliminate health access and quality disparities (Hudson et al., 2018). Citizenship through involvement in democratic activities like voting is an important factor in health equity that should not be overlooked. The civic engagement barriers, such as voter suppression, also differentially impact marginalized communities and therefore the racial health disparities. Civically disenfranchised individuals who are restricted by barriers such as the law of restrictive voting do not only suffer from disenfranchisement but also negative health outcomes since these barriers result in less representation and bargaining for necessary health resources. In understanding and deconstructing health inequities, health impact of civic engagement needs to be addressed. In developing a framework connecting civic engagement to health status, researchers are able to differentiate more sharply between mechanisms by which social engagement impacts well-being and shed light on where intervention can be sought (HIng et al., 2020) (Figure 12.2).

Importance of Studying Health Disparities

Concepts of health inequalities are significant in the development of effective public health policy and interventions to decrease inequity in access to healthcare and outcomes. Disparities are often produced by a composite of factors, including socioeconomic status, race, and geographic location, that define systematic disparities that may lead to negative health states among varying populations. Investigating these differences helps researchers and policymakers identify who is at risk and in need of targeted intervention, such that health care resources can be effectively utilized. Studies focusing on the social determinants of health (SDOH) have consistently identified that intervening in these determinants—education, housing, for instance—is highly associated with health outcomes and is a sound justification to place research on health disparities on the priority list of public health agendas (Carlos et al., 2025). Moreover, the examination of health disparities enables broader understanding of contextual determinants of inequalities. To illustrate, research focusing on specific areas, e.g., the Andean region of Latin America, has been able to identify significant ethnic and regional variations in children's nutritional status and well-being (Carlos et al., 2025). Through a study of the effects of variables like location and ethnicity on health outcomes, scientists can gain further insight into the underlying mechanisms that perpetuate health inequities. Through a holistic framework that not only acknowledges the intricacies of health disparities but also enables the development of culturally and contextually specific interventions, academics are able to optimize their efficacy and effectiveness in multiple populations. Finally, education regarding health disparities encourages community empowerment and engagement. When individuals are aware of what is behind their health outcomes, they can organize and collectively address these disparities. Community participation is responsible for creating effective public health policy because it ensures that policies are not based on a single set of issues that will not be representative of the particular problems of different segments of society. In addition, an understanding of health disparities leads to public debate regarding social justice and health equity, which prompts legislature to act on system issues. Lastly, this knowledge equips communities with the skills necessary to handle their health concerns, highlighting the importance of considering disparities in health as inherent social justice issues demanding collective action and informed advocacy (Ajani et al., 2023).

Overview of Social Determinants of Health

Social determinants of health are a broad range of determinants that influence the health and outcomes of individuals at the population level. These determinants include socioeconomic status, education, physical environment, and social support systems, in addition to access to health care services. The World Health Organization emphasizes that such conditions bear a profound impact on health disparities and inequities across populations. It is critical to realize how such factors influence one another because they operate at multiple levels—individual, community, and society—to impact health in numerous ways. For instance, individuals with lower socioeconomic status are likely to face challenges in reaching quality food, housing, and health care, thus being at greater risk of developing chronic diseases. These social determinants need to be addressed while formulating effective public health policies that contribute to reducing health disparity and enhancing health equity across different demographic segments. Measurement and analysis of the social determinants of health accurately are essential for the development of health equity programs. Estimating disparities in terms of social positions requires high-quality data and analytical approaches with sufficient flexibility to pick up on the various aspects of health inequities. This requires a multidimensional approach that includes social as well as structural determinants in addition to health outcomes, as conceptualized in recent health equity research.

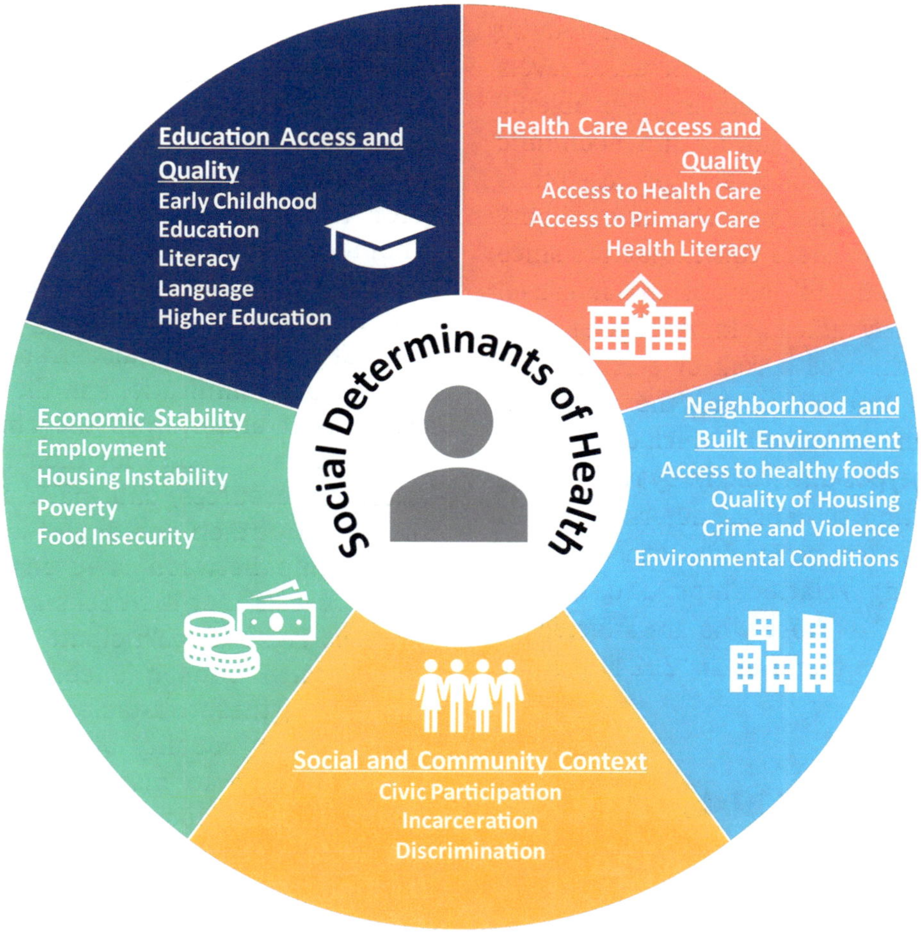

Figure 12.3. Overview of social determinants of health.

Source: https://res.cloudinary.com/dpmykpsih/image/upload/c_fill,f_auto,q_auto/marcus-daly-site-390/media/316c56290400413bb47e08ce88563fab/social-determinants-of-health-wheel.png.

Researchers recommend clear justification for methodological choices and with an accompanying classification of groups across a plurality of social statuses to allow for comparability. The incorporation of such vast data facilitates stakeholders to develop more efficient health interventions, hence offering the foundation for policy reforms to address causative determinants of disparities rather than treating symptoms of undesirable health circumstances. With such approaches, actual progress toward health equity is possible, as viewed in recent research (N/A, 2025). Also, considering the case of specific experiences of marginalized communities, such as Black men, clearly illustrates the powerful impact of social determinants on mental health outcomes. Their lives are often shaped by structural avenues that result in increased levels of psychological distress because of problems such as racial discrimination and economic marginalization. Mental health professionals must perform rigorous social risk assessments that take account of these context factors since automatic assessments overlook major causal factors. If they lack sufficient knowledge of these determinants, there is a risk of perpetuating inequalities by not addressing the causes of mental health manifestations, which can solidify negative stereotypes unwittingly. By recognizing and incorporating the social determinants of health into practice, counselors can establish stronger helping relationships and deliver stronger services to those who are affected by systemic injustices (Sami et al., 2024) (Figure 12.3).

12.1. Historical Context of Health Disparities

The historical context of health disparities is a complex interdependence of systemic forces that has created chronic inequities in different populations. From the impact of colonialism and institutional racism to socioeconomic disparities, historical events have had a significant impact on vulnerable populations' health outcomes. For instance, Indigenous people have suffered poor health outcomes ever since colonization commenced, frustrating their customary way of life, and engraving unequal treatment into health systems. It is especially so in the context of medical education, because it has routinely ignored the unique health needs of these people and thereby continues to perpetuate the cycle of inequality. Recognition of colonization, racism, and privilege as central to determining Indigenous health emphasizes the required educational reform that incorporates holistic Indigenous health programs with a focus on dismantling the barriers creating inequality in outcomes (Calam et al., 2018). Beyond education, civic participation stands as an influential but often overlooked health inequality determinant among people of color. Historical voter suppression tactics—inhomogeneous voter ID requirements and reduction of polling sites—have systematically disenfranchised marginalized groups from the political process. Such disenfranchisement has very serious ramifications in the public health arena, as it undermines the ability of these groups to have a voice for their rights, receive access to resources, and make decisions that directly affect their health and well-being. The relationship between civic engagement and health reveals that if citizens are denied their inherent right to participate in governance, their health consequences are impacted. Eliminating these obstacles is vital not only for improving equality but also for the sake of giving voice to historically marginalized groups in discussions regarding health policy and social determinants (HIng et al., 2020). Examining the origins of health inequalities in the past is a reminder of the indispensable importance of intersectionality in understanding the complex experiences of various populations. The cumulative effect of past injustices such as segregation and discrimination has developed chronic injury in communities of color that results in long-term illnesses that are belittled as simple statistical anomalies. In an effort tc deal with these inequalities, it is imperative to acknowledge past legacies that have created the existing health inequity terrain. With the integration of existing knowledge on history into existing health policy and research, stakeholders are able to develop better interventions that are sensitive to the needs of impacted populations. Such an orientation serves to promote greater understanding of how historical injustices influence the present situation and reinforces the necessity of a multi-dimensional strategy in addressing health disparities based on historical factors (Calam et al., 2018; HIng et al., 2020).

12.1.1. Evolution of Health Disparities in the United States (U.S.)

The emergence of health disparities in the United States is a complex issue shaped by historical, social, and economic factors that have shaped the various groups differently. Years have witnessed structural disparities that have continued to exclude marginalized communities from accessing the fundamental health care services. Health disparities often reflect broader socioeconomic determinants such as income, education, and employment that have disproportionately affected racial and ethnic minorities. As chronic diseases have become one of the top reasons for morbidity and mortality in such populations, understanding the underlying barriers becomes important in establishing effective public health programs. Recent research shows that most state chronic disease programs have recognized such disparities but are not finding it simple to integrate health equity into their systems due to inadequate funding and training resources, thereby indicating the necessity for system reforms (Adunola et al., 2017). The recognition of health disparities has motivated movements in attempts to respond to systemic inequities in access and quality of health care. Initiatives to promote health equity have been increasing in the field of public health, operating to empower vulnerable populations via specific strategies and community participation. An example is the establishment of strategic frameworks by organizations like the National Association of Chronic Disease Directors, which underscores the necessity for health departments to prioritize health equity as a goal of chronic disease programming. All of the above notwithstanding, implementation remains uneven. Fewer than half of state chronic disease directors see their efforts as doing enough to address health inequities, and this indicates that significant obstacles, such as underfunding and a lack of prioritization on equity, remain in health departments. These obstacles signal the necessity for continuous advocacy as well as policy change to advance large-scale health equity measures (Birnbaum et al., 2011). Besides, the relationship between health disparities and social determinants of health requires a multidisciplinary approach, involving knowledge from various disciplines, including sociology, economics, and public health. Through scrutiny of the intricacies of such disparities, researchers and policymakers are better placed to establish effective interventions to support vulnerable populations. Intervention in social determinants such as housing quality, education, and healthcare access is required in dismantling systemic impediments that perpetuate health inequities. Whereas public health agencies expand their focus from mere curing of diseases to addressing the causes of health disparities, there exists the possibility to construct a healthier more equitable environment. The commitment to equity must also be followed by concrete actions and policy reforms that avail every group the means to optimize health outcomes towards a better and more just society (Adunola et al., 2017).

12.1.2. Impact of Systemic Racism on Health Outcomes

Systemic racism in healthcare provision has a significant impact on worsening health disparities in minority populations. Racial and ethnic minorities are also impacted by limitations in accessing quality care, leading to lower health outcomes. Black and Latino children with asthma, for instance, are more likely to be hospitalized in emergency departments and hospital care than their White counterparts. This disparity is a reflection of structural challenges brought about by systemic racism, which affects socio-economic status, access to healthcare facilities, and the quality of care provided. Conceptual frameworks of today emphasize that these differences are sustained by unequal exposures to social determinants of health and not just economic but also environmental factors. Therefore, the impact of systemic racism is achieved as it produces biologic changes throughout the life course and sustains morbidity and mortality cycles in such vulnerable populations (Apter et al., 2024). In looking at health outcomes by racial groups, it is clear that systemic barriers go beyond one's individual socioeconomic status to include more societal factors. The disparities in cancer care, for example, point out how systemic racism is evidenced in treatment access and effectiveness. Lower socioeconomic patients often face financial toxicity and access issues to necessary screenings that impact their cancer outcomes. In addition, geographic disparities exacerbate the problem of these populations, particularly in medically underserved or rural environments, where a lack of advanced cancer care contributes to delayed diagnosis. These system-level considerations highlight the urgent need for interventions that finally begin to stem the complexity of race- and ethnicity-related health disparities. Healthcare policy structural reform is essential to ensure equal access to effective interventions and to combat the negative impacts of systemic racism in cancer treatment centers (Owusu et al., 2025).

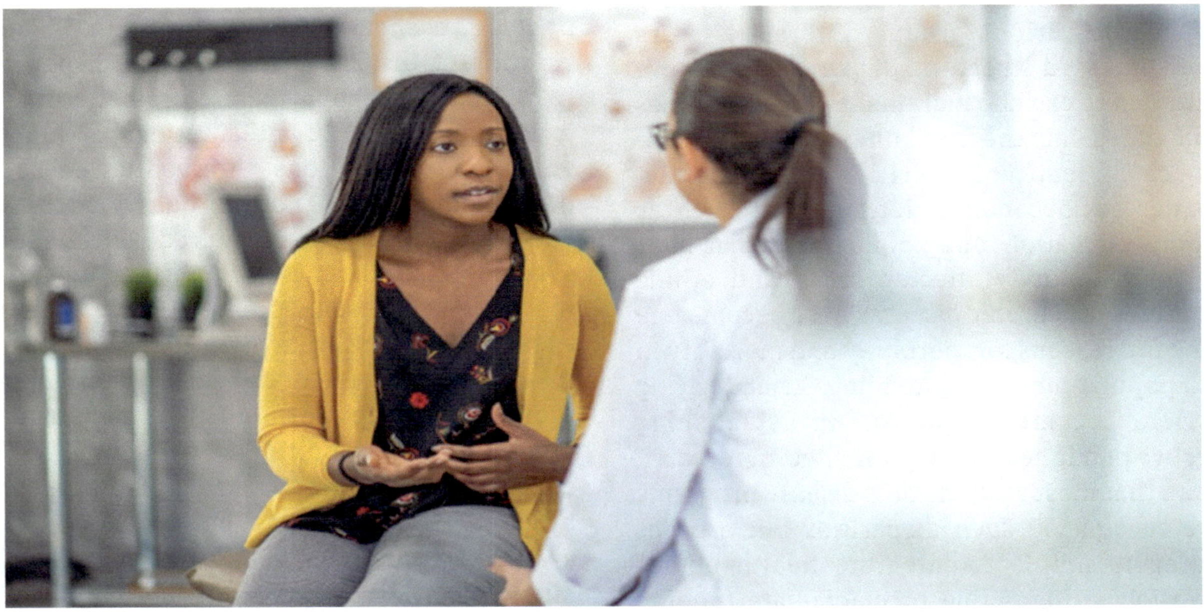

Figure 12.4. Impact of systemic racism on health outcomes.

Source: https://images.journals.lww.com/tnpj/SocialThumb.00006205-202302000-00006.FU1-6.jpeg.

Elimination of systemic racism in the healthcare system requires multi-dimensional intervention, with policy-based interventions and community engagement. Medicaid expansion and patient navigation programs are policies that have the potential to promote increased access to healthcare among marginalized groups. In addition, community-level and culturally targeted health education and interventions can make citizens their own health advocates and enhance awareness of available health resources. Health education's role in including social determinants of health in models of healthcare is important for understanding barriers faced by racial and ethnic minorities. Future research will have to strive towards designing particular interventions that address the consequences of systemic racism such that all populations are assured health equity. Through the acknowledgment and addressing of these systemic inequities, healthcare systems can improve overall health outcomes and create a more egalitarian society for all (Owusu et al., 2025) (Figure 12.4).

12.1.3. Historical Policies Affecting Marginalized Communities

Historical policies adopted throughout American history have significantly influenced the health status of marginalized groups, often exacerbating social and economic disparities. Such laws as redlining have systematically denied racial and ethnic minorities access to quality housing, healthcare, and education. These systems have institutionalized cycles of poverty that are associated with poor health outcomes. The effects of housing instability are particularly severe, as evidenced by the lack of access to stable and secure living conditions, which are an underlying health determinant. This discrimination is then compounded when one takes into consideration the manner in which complex policies regarding civic participation, including voter ID requirements and early voting restrictions, have disenfranchised people of color overwhelmingly. The outcome is that the civic engagement barriers aggravate the health inequities, where targeted populations are excluded from involvement in policies that influence their health, as a way of augmenting disenfranchisement and equity (HIng et al., 2020). Aside from policy on housing, public health interventions have never effectively addressed the specialized needs of oppressed groups. For instance, the San Francisco HIV epidemic had a clear emphasis on laying out critical gaps in support and care for individuals from marginalized socio-economic groups. Whereas the city's Getting to Zero campaign is aimed at stopping new HIV infections and their accompanying stigma, it fails to capture the critical role of housing instability in determining health outcomes.

The convergence of race, class, and health is most explicitly brought to the fore within the oppressed groups, where the lack of stable housing restricts access to routine medical treatment, support networks, and community services. The understanding of the complex relations of race and socio-economic status within public health campaigns is therefore vital for correcting such historical inequalities. Lastly, these cases point to the need to revisit public health policy to integrate a more holistic approach that puts housing and socio-economic stability at the center as critical determinants of health (Zaragoza et al., 2019). To resolve existing policies on marginalized individuals calls for a general rethinking of the relationship between socio-economic status and public health problems. Structural inequities created by policies, whether through discrimination in housing or voting, actually more fundamentally indicate an inability to perceive the significance of historical context in addressing present health disparateness. Promoting civic engagement and empowerment of disenfranchised groups can offer a critical element towards the reduction of these disparities. Being involved in policy reform that ensures not only access to healthcare but also to the socio-economic conditions enabling health is critical.

This demands a multi-dimensional approach that involves an appreciation of past injustice and an eagerness to remove barriers that hinder health equity. When these elements are harmonized, future policy will be successful in reducing disparities, thereby enhancing overall community well-being and health.

12.2. Socioeconomic Status (SES) as a Determinant

SES plays a pivotal role in determining health outcomes and is a top determinant in the health disparity context. Lower SES persons typically have handicaps in their capacity for accessing quality health care, and this contributes to inferior status of health. This impact is multifaceted; it takes place through a number of channels, some of which include limited resources, poor education, and lack of access to quality food. Research continuously proves that individuals with higher SES are healthier because they have better access to health care services and improved living conditions. In contrast, those of lower SES are more likely to live in environments with stressors such as crime, substandard housing, and unavailability of health centers.

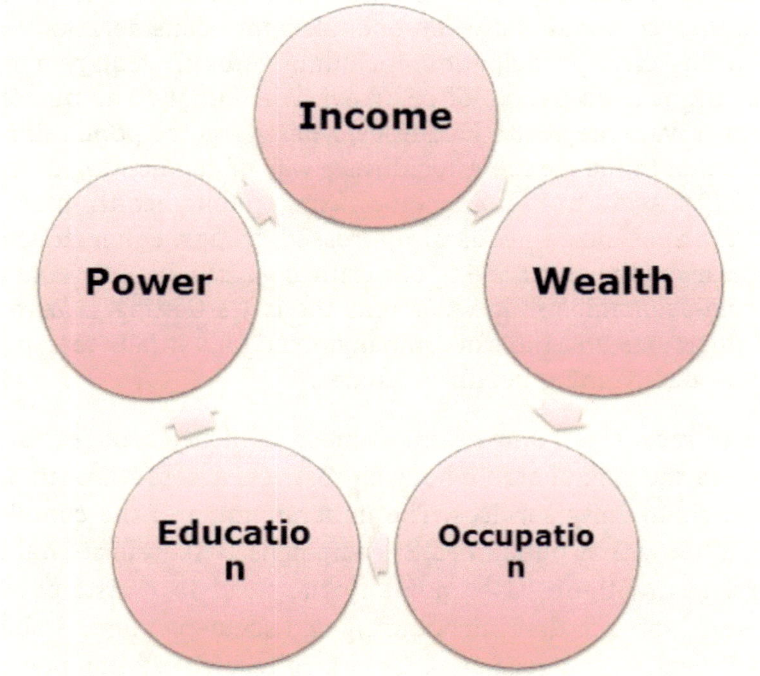

Figure 12.5. Socioeconomic status (SES) as a determinant.

Source: https://slideplayer.com/slide/4509483/15/images/6/Five+Determinants+of+Socioeconomic+Status.jpg.

These disparities highlight the need for policies addressing such socio-economic challenges to reduce health inequities and maximize overall public health response in poor populations. In the case of particular disease conditions, socioeconomic concerns are particularly noted in the management of chronic diseases, such as asthma. Asthma management disparities (AMD) point to the urgent overlap of low SES and health statuses. Evidence suggests that African Americans disproportionately experience barriers to optimal asthma care, a condition exacerbated by socioeconomic determinants of poverty and bad healthcare services access. According to research models assessing AMD, individual and community-level determinants play an important role in such disparities. Exposure to violence, stress, and indoor air quality are issues that affect low-income populations, reflecting how socio-environmental determinants may have a detrimental effect on health management plans. To deal with these determinants through multilevel interventions may assist in neutralizing AMD, improving the health and well-being for such affected groups since they are often the most vulnerable segments of society (Evans-Agnew et al., 2012). In addition, the power that social networks have on health for poor sectors indicates another aspect of intricacy with respect to socioeconomic status. Support systems are able to stimulate mental health quite effectively, facilitating escape from poverty and into the workforce. For instance, women on welfare tend to experience depressive symptoms that discourage their employability. However, strong social networks have been shown to provide important emotional as well as instrumental support, which reduces these adverse effects. It is shown through research that those who possess larger networks or closer affiliations with their society have reduced depression rates and, perhaps most notably, healthier outcomes. But the intricate process between SES, social networks, and depression symptoms renders policies for social support systems all the more important in achieving healthier communities and promoting economic security among low-income populations (Davidson et al., 2012) (Figure 12.5).

12.2.1. Relationship Between Income and Health Outcomes

Income levels and health outcomes interact to be a significant driver of health inequities in society. Individuals with lower incomes are likely to face many difficulties that work negatively against their health. Repeated research has shown that limited financial means restrict access to suitable health care, nutritious food, and health education, leading to decreased long-term outcomes for health. For instance, lower income can result in greater levels of stress, which has been associated with a wide array of negative health outcomes. In addition, the ability to pay for preventive care and medical check-ups lowers, and there is greater reliance on emergency care with resultant higher morbidity rates. Thus, income sets the health trajectory of individuals and governs an important social determinant influencing total community health and well-being. A careful examination of the nuances of the relationship reveals that education is a conduit that mediates the impact of income on health outcomes. Higher levels of education associated with higher income levels tend to produce better knowledge of health and good healthcare practices. Educated individuals place greater value on their health, are effective at navigating healthcare bureaucracies, and engage in prevention, which lowers health risks. Furthermore, parents education has been shown to create a ripple effect in children's educational and health prospects, cementing health inequality cycles across generations. This exchange emphasizes that improving education accessibility and quality is, in essence, a strategy to combat health inequalities linked with income inequalities. The relationship between income, education, and health status promises a knotty system of social determinants to which focused intervention methods must be directed in order to enhance population health. Additionally, the psychological stress associated with economic insecurity has a considerable influence on health outcomes. Low-income individuals are typically subject to ongoing stressors, such as economic insecurity and limited access to goods and services, that can lead to both psychosocial and physical health issues. Stress has been clearly linked to numerous health issues, including preterm delivery and other pregnancy-related complications, as supported by research showing the relationship between cortisol levels and risk of preterm birth among low-income communities. Research outlines how individuals with lesser privileged backgrounds, particularly Black women, are more susceptible with compounded stress owing to socio-economic disadvantage. Remediation of these psychosocial determinants of health inequities related to income calls for a multi-faceted approach integrating mental health treatment with economic assistance to foster more equitable health in various populations (Jallo et al., 2015).

12.2.2. Education Level and Its Impact on Health Literacy

Level of education is a key determinant of health literacy, whose importance has direct consequences on one's capacity to understand and react to health information. Increased education usually accompanies enhanced health literacy, as educational institutions provide critical thinking, better reading comprehension, and higher ability to comprehend complex systems of healthcare. The population with low education often has barriers to accessing and interpreting health-related information, thereby inequalities in health outcomes. This convergence focuses on the need for targeted interventions to improve education services, particularly among disadvantaged groups, to thereby empower individuals with competencies for effective self-management of their health. Encouraging educational programs can therefore serve as a key strategy in responding to broader health disparities and improving overall community health.

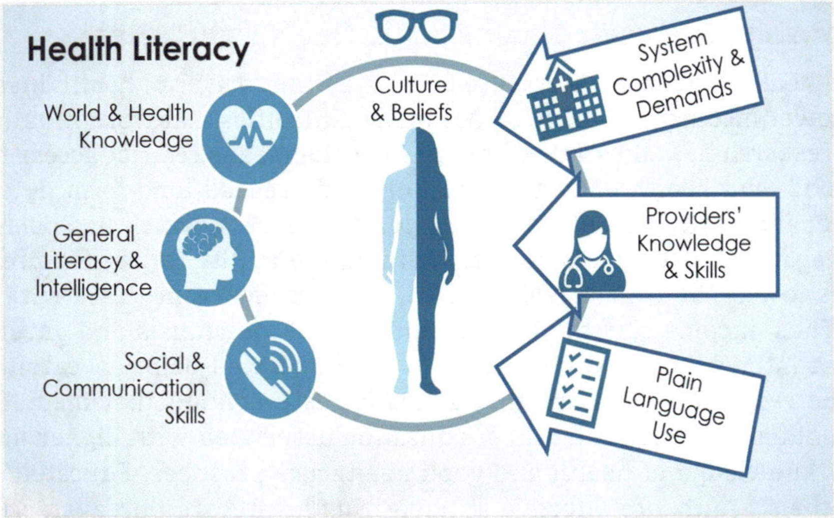

Figure 12.6. Education level and its impact on health literacy.

Source: https://media.licdn.com/dms/image/v2/D4D12AQHA7Chmm2yKHA/article-cover_image-shrink_720_1280/article-cover_image-shrink_720_1280/0/1714008490775?e=2147483647&v=beta&t=p28ByY2y9xTCnikw_W6_Zj1G9VoKbQncPQTqIKlXcrw.

In addition, education's contribution to health literacy is not limited to individual capacity to influence community health assets and outcomes. More educated populations are better able to make demands for primary care and public health policy. Such activism tends to enhance health care access and quality because highly educated people are better able to communicate with health care providers, make knowledgeable decisions about treatment, and practice prevention. Therefore, the bettering of overall educational attainment within a population can manifest as an elevated overall level of health literacy, producing a healthier population with reduced health disparities. Education and public health efforts should therefore work to increase educational attainment, particularly where socioeconomic hardship is the standard, in order to provide settings in which health literacy is maximized and health inequities are decreased. Starting programs to bridge the gap in education is essential towards encouraging health literacy, particularly among susceptible populations. Adaptive educational programs, such as health literacy classes or community health education, can train individuals to better access healthcare. Such programs can focus on developing competencies to understand medical information, complete healthcare forms, and negotiate one's own health needs. Furthermore, integrating health education into schooling can enable children to gain the knowledge to make healthy choices throughout childhood. As evident from studies on disparities in asthma management, where socioeconomic status and education intersect in significant interaction, enhancing educational interventions can address systemic determinants of such disparities. By establishing a context of educated individuals, communities are then equipped to successfully counter and break down barriers to realizing equal health outcomes, leading to healthier societies overall (Birnbaum et al., 2011; Evans-Agnew et al., 2012) (Figure 12.6).

12.2.3. Employment Status and Access To Healthcare

The relationship between employment status and access to care is a vital aspect of health disparities that is likely to occur along socioeconomic lines. Individuals with secure employment typically have greater access to a range of health benefits, including vast health insurance coverage. This is strongly typical in formal labor markets where employers provide medical benefits as part of compensation. The unemployed, underemployment, and informal sectors workers are typically not offered such health benefits, and thus might end up relying on emergency services rather than preventive care. Thus, such limited access not only exacerbates already present health issues but can even create a cycle of ill health and poverty as the health uninsured can avoid treatment they require, further entangling their overall health condition and well-being. Moreover, discrimination in healthcare also reduces the availability of care for marginalized populations, further making it more difficult to link work with health outcomes. For example, a study targeting African-American veterans revealed that individuals who perceived racial discrimination in healthcare settings reported lower patient satisfaction and poorer health outcomes. Discrimination was especially found to have an adverse impact on ratings of perceived quality of care and satisfaction, providing insights into the negative consequences of bias among healthcare access (Amaro et al., 2012). This development signals that employment status is but one factor, but that also included in the determination of health inequities are the equity and quality of health experiences. The intersection of employment-related benefits with institutionalized discrimination reminds us that policy change must work to overcome the complicated barriers that obstruct access to quality health care within minority groups. There is a need for a multifaceted approach through policy change and societal change to address issues of work status and health access. Recommendation from health equity movements calls for improving healthcare access regardless of work status, for example, approaches offering universal healthcare coverage or subsidies to the poor (Birnbaum et al., 2011). Deconstructing obstacles such as employer-sponsored health insurance, which disproportionately excludes the most vulnerable, can allow society to progress toward a fairer healthcare system. In the long run, improving employment opportunities and ensuring full access to healthcare can improve the health of different population segments, thereby correcting the social determinants behind health disparities. Effective interventions must grasp and address these complex linkages to improve health equity comprehensively (Figure 12.7).

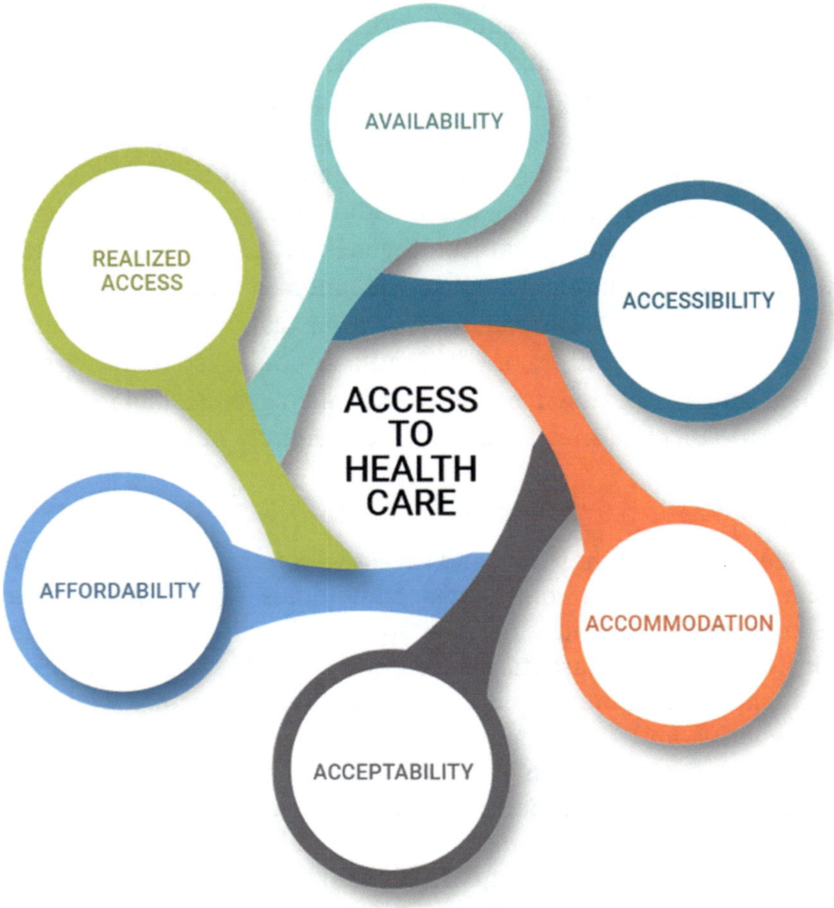

Figure 12.7. Employment status and access to healthcare.

Source: https://www.accesstocarela.org/wp-content/uploads/2020/10/access-to-health-care-la.png.

12.3. Geographic Location and Health Access

Geographic location and health access have significant application to health disparities among various communities. Areas having high rates of preventable hospitalizations reflect inadequacies in local primary health care services that adversely affect vulnerable populations disproportionately. For instance, African American populations often have greater rates of preventable hospitalization than their white counterparts. The Maryland study indicates that these disparities are not scattered at random but rather reflect intense geographic clusters where access to healthcare is specifically constrained. Identification of these spatial clusters enables a more focused deployment of health resources and interventions, addressing strategies to the unique needs of different populations within the multiple geographic regions. Therefore, understanding spatial health access dynamics is crucial towards recognizing systemic inequalities inherent in American healthcare systems because they call for certain interventions and policies aimed at those most affected by geographic healthcare deficiencies (Bell et al., 2018).

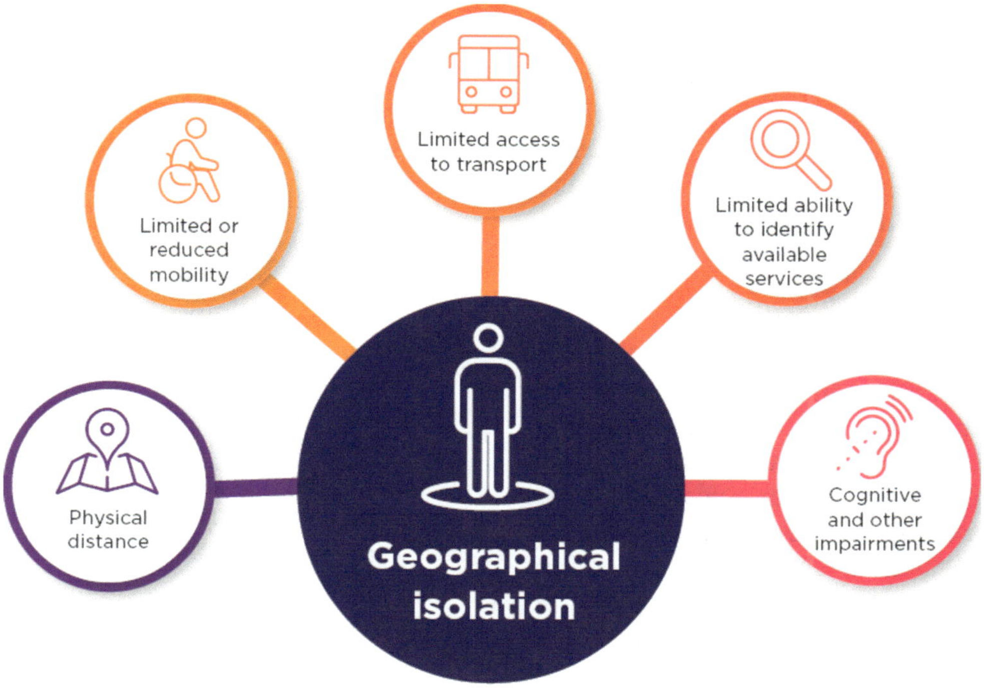

Figure 12.8. Geographic location and health access.

Source: https://aifs.gov.au/sites/default/files/2023-12/SS3_graphics1.png.

Geographical variations in health access also inform us about the interconnected nature of social determinants and racial/ethnic healthcare disparities. The implication is that just expanding healthcare coverage, unless it is combined with removing the underpinning determinants associated with geographic disparities, will not suffice to bridge the gap. Certain suggestions point towards the necessity for dedicated committees to assess the needs of communities, obtain relevant information, and establish quality indices for improving healthcare accessibility in such disadvantaged areas. By doing so, healthcare systems can create a structured framework for minimizing racial and ethnic health disparities in healthcare delivery, which are often exacerbated by geographical isolation. Thus, approaching health access on a geographical plane requires a nuanced understanding of the socio-economic and socio-cultural forces molding these areas to ensure interventions work as well as are equitable in implementation (Green et al., 2009). When addressing geographic dimensions of access to health, there is a need to engage local populations in the development process of healthcare interventions. Local involvement can lead to culturally relevant approaches that address the specific aspects of targeted groups. Disparities in health, especially those related to geography, need inputs from many different stakeholders, such as healthcare providers, community organizations, and policymakers. By establishing relationships within these communities, health programs are better able to target the daily lives of residents, enhancing participation and outcomes. Furthermore, lasting alterations in access to health require ongoing evaluation and revision according to changing needs for accessibility by diverse geographic populations. By providing priority to a community-based solution to overcoming these inequalities, healthcare systems become capable of approaching an inclusive strategy that addresses and acknowledges the complexities of geographic access to health (Bell et al., 2018; Green et al., 2009) (Figure 12.8).

12.3.1. Urban vs. Rural Health Disparities

Urban-rural disparities in health are deep-seated and well-established and mirror a complex array of social determinants of health. Urban residents typically have greater access to health care services, and thus more directly influence health outcomes. Rural residents will experience a scarcity of health care professionals and required services and hence increased mortality rates. The social determinants in these kinds of settings include socioeconomic determinants such as education and levels of earnings, which have also been shown to have a profound impact on health outcomes. For instance, in rural areas, socioeconomic disadvantages play an even stronger role in health, particularly because of more amenable causes of death, such as cancer, thus the need to address these inequalities (Topping et al., 2020). Colorectal cancer (CRC) is one illustration of the extreme health disparities between the two geographic areas. Research indicates vast inequalities in incidence and mortality rates of CRC, with higher rates among rural compared to urban communities. Socioeconomic factors such as poverty, educational attainment, and behavioral traits such as smoking and alcohol consumption contribute to these disparities. The confluence of these social determinants makes preventive health practices and early detection services unattainable for rural people who are unable to access these services needed to improve the health outcomes. Statistical analyses have indicated that the impact of health behaviors on CRC mortality and incidence is disproportionately more pronounced in rural communities, demonstrating systemic vulnerabilities that must be addressed by targeted health policies to this population (McDaniel et al., 2022). Fixing health disparities requires a multifaceted solution that considers the unique problems of rural communities. Effective health policies must not only augment access to medical care but also touch on the underlying socioeconomic factors that contribute to poor health outcomes. The measures may include more investment in rural health centers, and programs to improve education and economic prospects. Efforts at public health should equally be focused on augmenting preventive behaviors and health education specifically tailored for rural dwellers. Health promotion programs relating to the risks of cigarette smoking and drinking, and enhanced screenings for diseases like CRC, can play a significant role in encouraging health equity. Last but not least, bridging the gap in health care accessibility between urban and rural areas is essential to reduce inequalities and improve public health as a whole (McDaniel et al., 2022; Topping et al., 2020).

12.3.2. Availability of Healthcare Facilities in Different Regions

Availability of facility has a significant role to play in the determination of health outcomes of various regions and plays a great part in differing access and quality of health. Urban areas are usually associated with the availability of more advanced healthcare facilities, while rural areas lack even basic services. This disproportionate distribution of resources is one of the main determinants of serious inequities in health outcomes, as population members in underserved communities tend to experience obstacles in terms of longer travel distances, reduced availability of healthcare professionals, and little access to specialty services. These inequities are also compounded by socioeconomic factors, which further fuel the issues of accessing appropriate medical care. Addressing these differences requires strategic action that not only increases the number of healthcare establishments in rural areas but also prepares them to meet the diverse needs of the respective communities (Birnbaum et al., 2011). Additionally, health equity has a direct relationship with policies responsible for regulating healthcare distribution across different areas. Assessments of state policy models illustrate the disparities in quality and coverage that arise from alternative proposals for healthcare reform. Successful measures to increase comprehensive access to quality healthcare must consider geographical and socio-economic factors, keeping in mind the special barriers faced by underserved populations. These policies must address transportation issues, physician shortages, and the type of services available in healthcare institutions. Through policy development and implementation that increase full health insurance coverage and address the social determinants of health, an equitable system can be realized that ensures the marginalized communities gain equal access to healthcare resources (Fish-Parcham et al., 2008). Besides, innovative methods are required to end the gap in access to healthcare, particularly among previously disenfranchised communities. Telemedicine, mobile health centers, and community health programs have been found to be potent tools in overcoming geographical barriers that most face. Through such remedies, there is increased communication between the providers of healthcare and the people residing in under-served communities, allowing for a more proactive approach towards health. By augmenting the availability of such healthcare services through technology and mobile health facilities, health disparities are significantly reduced, with a better comprehension of health equity. But systemic change is of highest priority, requiring investment in infrastructure and care for healthcare workers in these regions. Such efforts, combined with supportive policy, can ultimately lead to a worthy shift in the general healthcare picture (Birnbaum et al., 2011) (Figure 12.9).

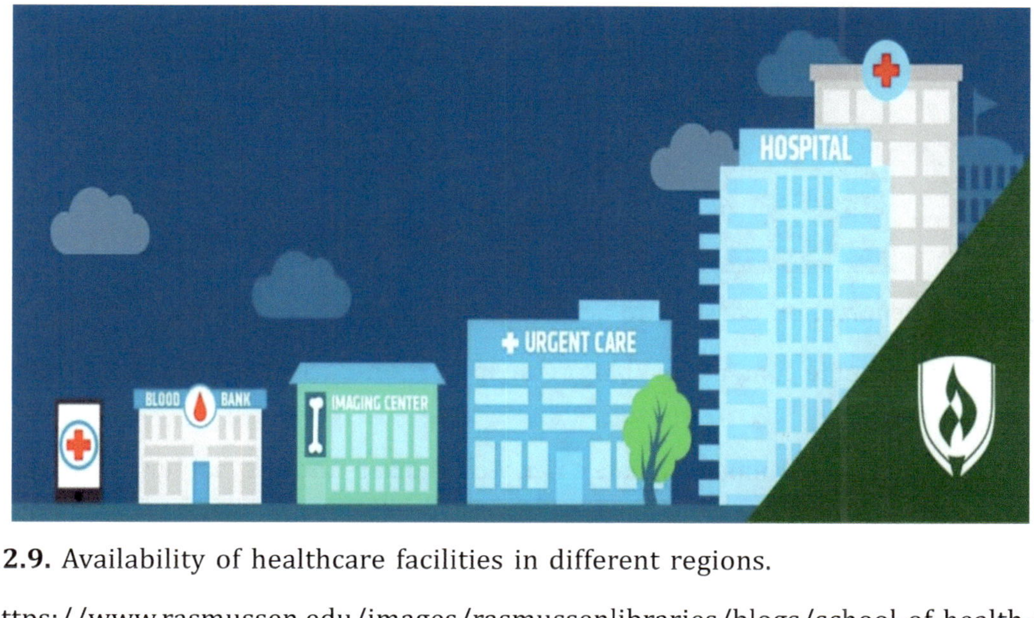

Figure 12.9. Availability of healthcare facilities in different regions.

Source: https://www.rasmussen.edu/images/rasmussenlibraries/blogs/school-of-health-sciences/types-of-healthcare-facilities.jpg?sfvrsn=81a73034_1.

12.3.3. Transportation Barriers to Accessing Healthcare

Transportation barriers significantly prevent access to healthcare, perpetuating health disparities between various communities. Citizens of rural or poor urban communities often experience the challenge of ineffective public transportation systems, rendering access to healthcare facilities difficult. Such a challenge is further worsened by the integration of geographic and socioeconomic determinants in that low-income communities lack adequate transportation. Consequently, patients end up delaying or missing important medical appointments, which can exacerbate their conditions and boost emergency healthcare needs. The implications are particularly severe for pregnant women, who might struggle to access necessary prenatal care, thus compromising infant and maternal health outcomes (Bryan et al., 2016). Breaking down these transportation barriers is crucial to achieving health equity and to the provision of timely and necessary healthcare services to vulnerable populations. More than mere logistical issues, the impact of transportation barriers also typically results in the exposure of underlying systemic inequities that impact health outcomes. Inequities in access to transport are rooted in more extensive social determinants like economic insecurity, education, and discrimination. Poor populations, for instance, can not only be without a personal vehicle but also face additional barriers like scarce healthcare provider availability and cultural or language barriers to the healthcare system (Carlson et al., 2016).

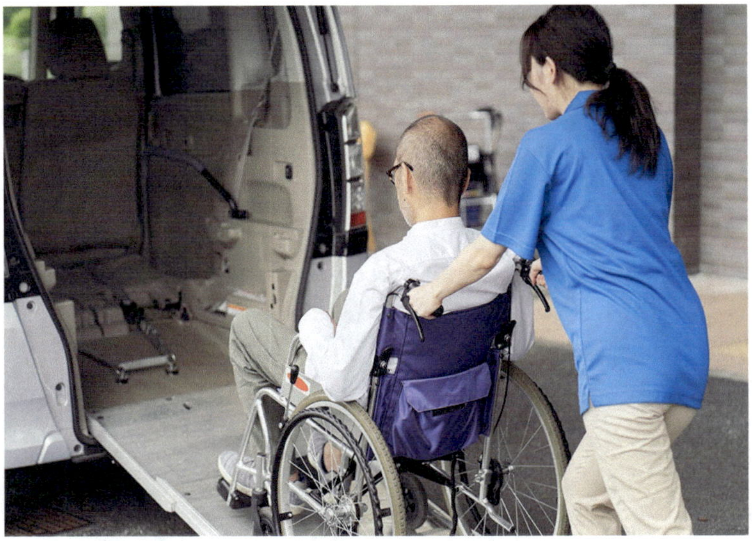

Figure 12.10. Transportation barriers to accessing healthcare.

Source: https://routegenie.com/media/blog/Transportation-Barriers-To-Healthcare-Access-And-Their-Cost_EalUiw1.jpg.

These intersectional determinants create a rich web of disadvantages that further marginalize and exclude marginalized groups from access to healthcare. It becomes critical for health organizations and policymakers to value the multifaceted nature of such challenges and implement targeted interventions addressing transportation as a social health determinant. By supporting initiatives that improve transportation systems in underprivileged communities, we can make concrete steps toward reducing health disparities. Further, new solutions exist to alleviate transportation barriers and enhance healthcare access for the most affected. Community-based interventions, such as patient navigation services and mobile health clinics, have also been effective in bridging the gap between patients and medical care providers. Such interventions can help guarantee that people successfully make it to appointments and access appropriate health services, resulting in improved overall health outcomes. Transportation options, from ride-sharing agreements to community volunteer transportation programs, can do much to break down the barriers to care among targeted populations (Bryan et al., 2016). Through incentivizing and investing in these community-based interventions, health systems can not only activate patients better but also make a more equitable health context where equal access to care is not an afterthought (Figure 12.10).

12.4. Race and Ethnicity in Health Disparities

In regard to health disparities, the dynamic between race and ethnicity is a central factor in determining general health outcomes. Urban communities of color are subjected to systemic problems that make them more susceptible to risk factors for health. Poverty, lack of good access to healthcare, and environmental pollutants disproportionately impact these communities, thus contributing to higher rates of chronic illnesses. The system-based aspect of such disparities lies within the social determinants of health, which are deeply entwined with race and ethnicity. Awareness of this intersection is imperative to design specific interventions to reduce health disparities in racial and ethnic groups. These differences are answered by recognizing the unique challenges of these populations so that more tailored public health efforts can be put in place to more appropriately appeal to different groups (Quinn et al., 2008).

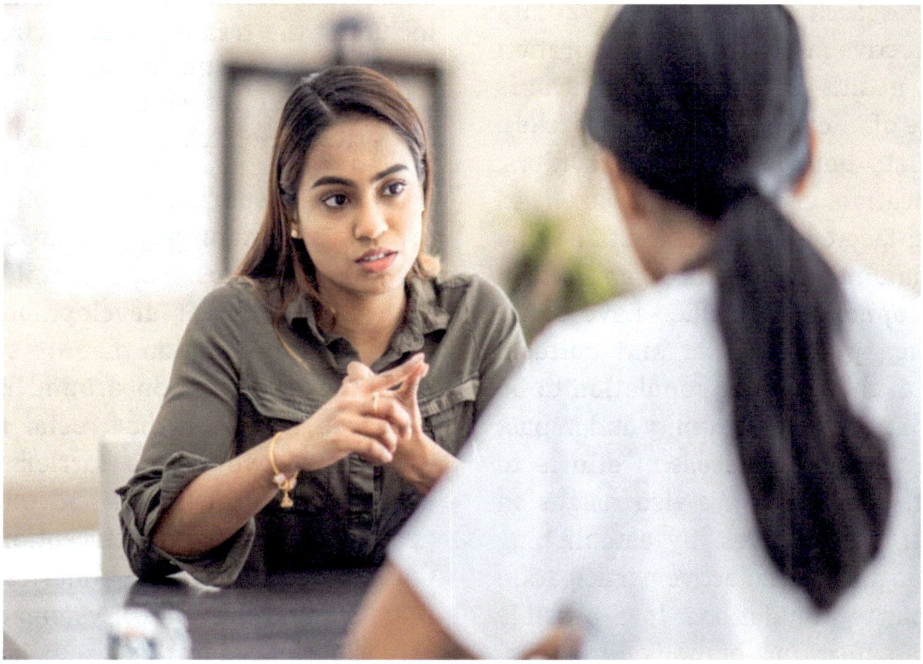

Figure 12.11. Race and ethnicity in health disparities.

Source: https://images.squarespace-cdn.com/content/v1/5ab90fe81137a689f2342048/1639692837231-305VZGBCALVWSG97D4HK/iStock-1150732836.jpg.

In addition, research endeavors towards eradicating health disparities stress the critical necessity for comprehensive knowledge about social determinants that influence minority populations. Giant health organizations, like the U.S. Department of Health and Human Services and the World Health Organization emphasize that variations in socioeconomic factors such as income, education, and health insurance coverage have key roles to play in shaping health outcomes across various racial and ethnic populations. Through integrating education models that place emphasis on the importance of social determinants into professional healthcare education, a future generation of research scholars and practitioners who are better equipped to close such gaps is possible. Such endeavors not only empower learners in the healthcare industry but also lead them to think critically about social determinants as fundamental building blocks of health practice and research (Bartlett et al., 2018). In addition, effective multi-sector collaboration in addressing health disparities underscores the significance of interdisciplinary approaches. Collective efforts between health providers, schools of education, and community agencies can yield multi-faceted strategies that entwine education, community action, and organizational capacity development. Strategies have to be tailored to the specific social and cultural environments of the targeted population to be attained and thus enhance the utility and impact of health interventions. Successful efforts to diminish health disparities are also reliant on interdisciplinary approaches. By establishing community engagement and active participation by health disparity populations, it is possible to develop resilience and empower minority populations to be their own voice for their health needs. In essence, eradicating health disparities depends on solid partnerships and commitment to understanding the intricacy of race and ethnicity in the entire spectrum of social determinants of health (Quinn et al., 2008) (Figure 12.11).

12.4.1. Disparities in Health Outcomes Among Racial Groups

The persistent racial group inequalities in health status are inextricably bound up with social determinants that affect access to care and overall health. The inequalities are manifested through various aspects, such as disease rates, quality of care received, and availability of basic health care. Racial and ethnic minorities usually experience barriers such as socioeconomic disadvantage, poor quality education, and unsuitable health care infrastructure, which increase their susceptibility to adverse health outcomes. Such disparities, in line with contemporary research, persist regardless of numerous public health interventions aimed at correcting them. It is increasingly evident that addressing health through a holistic approach, including the treatment of environmental and social determinants of health, is required to develop effective solutions to achieve such disparities (Bolnick et al., 2015).

Certain specific vulnerabilities are also present in certain groups that further deepen health disparities. For example, individuals with intellectual or developmental disability (IDD) are a population that are often excluded from the conversation around health equity. Research indicates that racial minorities in this group have unique barriers with respect to access to oral health and quality of care, necessitating targeted interventions. Comparing Caucasians and African Americans with IDD, there is identification of systematic barriers to care experienced by this group, including social stigma, economic hardship, and inaccessibility of culturally competent healthcare providers. These barriers contribute significantly to the poor health outcomes seen in such a population.

and it highlights the importance of health policy reforms aimed at addressing the special needs of vulnerable populations (Williams et al., 2024). Last but not least, eliminating health disparities by race necessitates a critical examination of healthcare practice and education. Embedding anthropological and genetic understanding within medical school programs can equip the next generation of health caregivers with an advanced understanding of the complexities of race and health inequality. Educational reform along these lines will better position medical physicians to recognize and react to the genesis of the disparities they encounter clinically. Further, building a culture of cultural competence can enhance communication and trust among racially diverse patients and clinicians, which can enhance health outcomes in the long run. In order to combat the perpetuation of these disparities, it is crucial that the healthcare system evolve by embracing new approaches that take into consideration the multifactorial nature of health as well as the social determinants that influence outcomes among racial groups (Bolnick et al., 2015).

12.4.2. Cultural Factors Influencing Health Behaviors

Understanding cultural determinants of health behavior is instrumental in the response to health disparities and social determinants. Cultural practices, norms, and beliefs build people's perceptions of healthcare availability, disease, and health. These cultural determinants largely manifest together with socioeconomic aspects, giving rise to differential health effects in various populations. For instance, in marginalized groups, cultural stigma of some diseases deters individuals from getting proper medical care, and therefore exacerbates their conditions. This is a stark reflection of the necessity for mainstreaming cultural competence into the healthcare system so that the medical professionals can communicate and connect with patients who belong to different cultures. Writing curricula aimed at cultural competency, as outlined in studies utilizing models like the Tool for Assessing Cultural Competence Training (TACCT), can enhance medical graduates' ability to navigate and bridge these cultural barriers in patient care significantly (Jernigan et al., 2016). In addition, cultural determinants tend to align with social determinants of health, shaping lifestyle choices and strategies of managing health. For instance, among South Asians, the prevalence of type 2 diabetes is common due in part to culturally ingrained dietary practices, social support systems, and economic concerns. Providers have documented that barriers associated with settlement as well as socioeconomic concerns frequently command more attention than the management of chronic conditions like diabetes (Banerjee et al., 2022). This suggests that health interventions must not only be focused on individual behavior change but also consider the wider socio-economic and cultural setting that dictates these behaviors. Addressing these determinants suggests a multi-faceted approach that involves cultural sensitivity, specially tailored education, and community-based interventions that resonate with the values and practices of the groups affected. Finally, cultural influences on health behavior must be more than simply acknowledged; they must be addressed through health care policy changes.

Cultural incompetence among health care providers can result in health care providers misunderstanding patients' needs and perpetuating bias and inequality. By providing culturally appropriate health care services, health care organizations can begin breaking down barriers that create disparities in health outcomes. For instance, the application of culturally aimed diet and exercise interventions can promote change in patients from diverse backgrounds. Moreover, system-level reforms such as an advocacy for equitable employment policies can eliminate some of the external stressors that exert a significant influence on health outcomes. Identifying the central intersection of culture, social determinants, and health behaviors is critical in developing proper public health strategies that maximize equity and overall health among diverse populations along the continuum (Banerjee et al., 2022) (Figure 12.12).

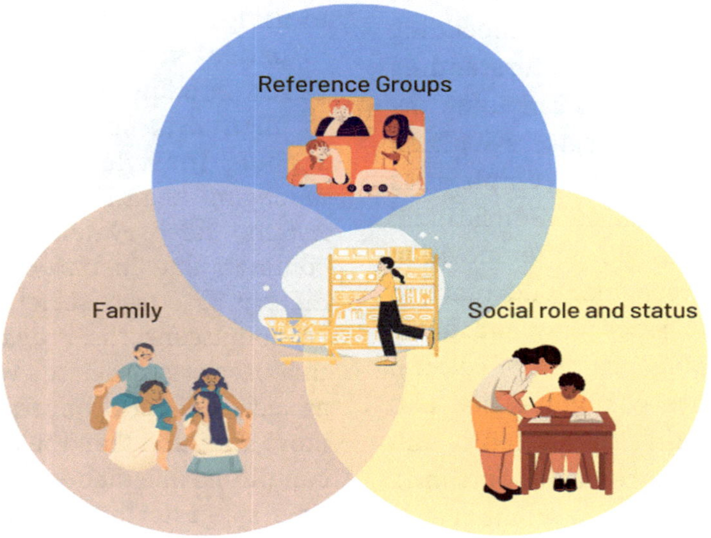

Figure 12.12. Cultural factors influencing health behaviors.

Source: https://www.superheuristics.com/wp-content/uploads/2023/02/Sage-Green-Abstract-Floral-Social-Networking-Venn-Diagram-Graph-1-768x576.png.

12.4.3. Discrimination in Healthcare Settings

Discrimination in healthcare is a key driver of health disparities, and it mostly affects disadvantaged populations. In other studies, systemic prejudices have been seen to lead to discriminatory treatment as well as unequal health outcomes based on race, ethnicity, and socioeconomic status. The disparities are usually caused by unconscious biases held by healthcare providers, which can compromise the quality of care received by patients from varied backgrounds. For instance, if patients are dealt with disrespect or their worries belittled, the ensuing distrust can dissuade them from placing further requests for important healthcare services. Therefore, efforts to stop discrimination in healthcare facilities are necessary since it not only impacts individual health patterns but also maintains more general social disparities that are well rooted in society (Dizon et al., 2017). Adding another layer of complexity is the convergence of several social determinants affecting individuals' ability to access care. People who reside in lower socioeconomic environments often find not only fiscal barriers but also structural barriers that limit their ability to access proper care. A current study illustrates how minority racial and ethnic groups endure higher infant mortality rates, indicating considerable disparities in prenatal care that are not necessarily clinical interventions but are also care perceptions and experiences (Bryan et al., 2016). The majority of patients report being ignored or dismissed by healthcare providers during encounters, which ultimately result in undiagnosed conditions and untreated diseases. This lack of patient-oriented care is capable of perpetuating systematic disparities, an issue particularly requiring policy reform in prioritizing equitable treatment for all patients, regardless of background (Bryan et al., 2016). The presence of stigma over some health conditions, such as HIV, extends the discrimination experienced in healthcare settings. Individuals living with HIV are likely to endure societal stigma that translates into poor health outcomes due to discrimination in healthcare settings. Evidence indicates that in spite of increased resource allocation towards HIV care and prevention, societal attitudes can ultimately reverse the impact of these resources by negatively affecting the overall quality of life of victims (Dizon et al., 2017). Stigma not only perpetuates patient discrimination but also discourages patients from seeking care and adhering to treatment as advised. Recognizing and working with the stigma of health issues is key in reducing discrimination and improving healthcare encounters for all, particularly marginalized groups. This demands an inclusive strategy where healthcare practice and policy intervene at both the individual and structural levels of discrimination to build a more equitable health system (Dizon et al., 2017) (Figure 12.13).

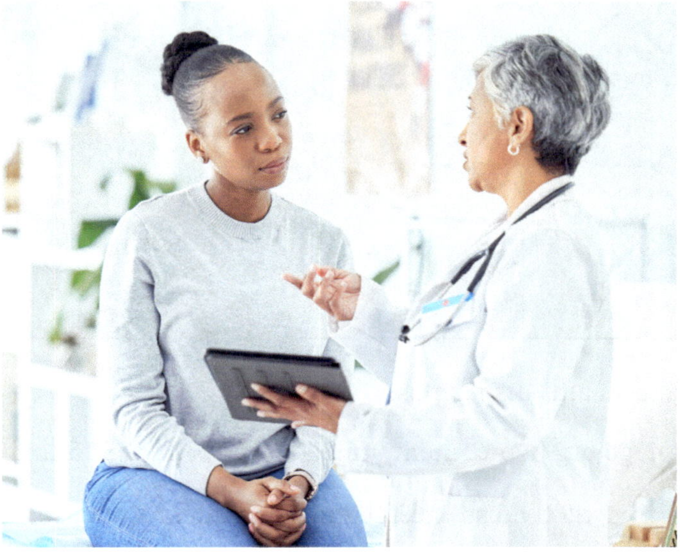

Figure 12.13. Discrimination in healthcare settings.

Source: https://publichealthpost.org/wp-content/uploads/2025/01/R_V.Wang_Discrimination-in-Medical-Settings-1536x1229.png.

12.5. Gender and Health Disparities

Gender is the pivot around which health disparities revolve since biological and sociocultural determinants overlap to generate differential health status among men and women. Disparities assume various forms, including access to health care services, modes of treatment, and health-related outcomes. Women, for instance, are disproportionately underrepresented in clinical trials, an occurrence that leaves gaps in knowledge regarding the special health needs of women patients. In addition, gender norms can impact health behaviors, as men eschew medical care because societal forces frame vulnerability as a weakness. The effects of these trends are most poignant among marginalized populations, where dominant gender roles exacerbate health disparities. Reducing these inequalities requires a greater consideration of how gender impacts health and commitment to policies that seek health equity, being mindful of these specific factors. The interaction of gender with other social determinants, such as socioeconomic position and race, contributes to the complexities of health disparities. Women of color are usually subjected to the worst disparities since they face the double-edged stigma of sexism and racism.

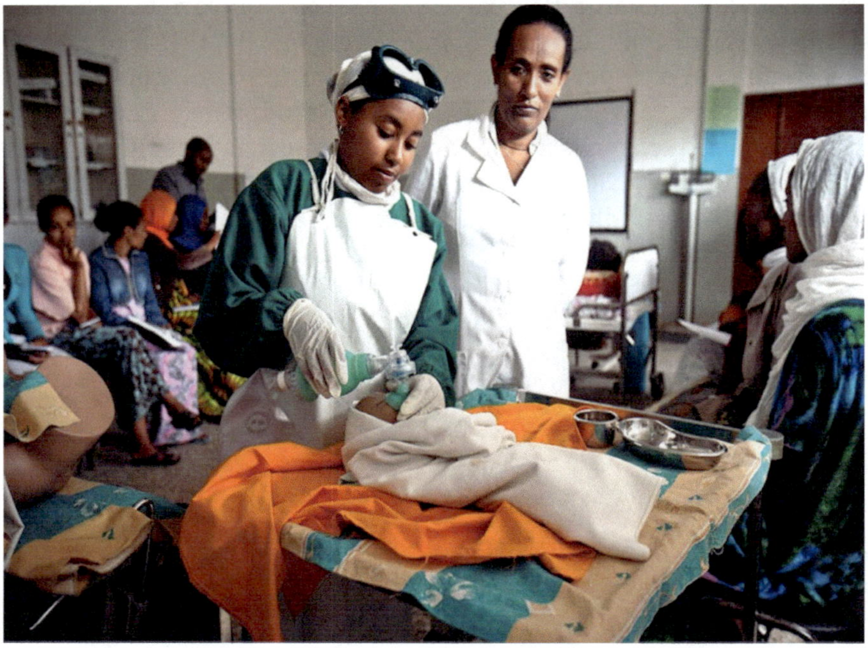

Figure 12.14. Gender and health disparities.

Source: https://www.jhpiego.org/wp-content/uploads/2016/01/2526-image-001-1.jpg.

The evidence indicates that these intersections result in increased occurrences of chronic illnesses such as diabetes and hypertension among women of color. Moreover, social determinants such as educational level and economic status play a significant role in determining womens health outcomes. For instance, lower socioeconomic status has been found to have reduced access to quality healthcare services, healthy dietary options, and health education, which in turn sustains cycles of poor health. Comprehension of the interaction among these determinants lies at the heart of designing targeted interventions to reduce health disparities along the gender continuum, to ensure that each individual receives care and support equally. In addressing health and gender inequities, systemic interventions need inclusive policies and practices that support health equity. The U.S. Department of Health and Human Services Healthy People 2020 program emphasizes the necessity of addressing disparities through social determinants that impact health outcomes (Balser et al., 2020). By creating equal and inclusive settings, public health interventions are in a better place to reach vulnerable groups, tearing down the barriers they face in accessing healthcare. These interventions not only enhance the well-being of individuals and societies but also the resilience of society at large. Advocating for models of gender-responsive healthcare that acknowledge the differentiated experiences of the two sexes is necessary in addressing these disparities. Lastly, health equity is promoted through collaborative effort that allows communities to deal with their own unique issues while developing an interconnected perception of health as a social construct influenced by multiform determinants (Balser et al., 2020) (Figure 12.14).

12.5.1. Differences in Health Outcomes Between Genders

The gender differences in health outcomes are shaped by a complex combination of biological, environmental, and social determinants. Men and women have varying health profiles, shaped mainly by social expectations and norms about health behavior and access to care. Females in studies will report more chronic illnesses, such as autoimmune disorders and depression, whereas males will report a greater prevalence of hypertension and coronary heart disease. These differences are not merely reflections of biological variation but are often accentuated by social factors like gender roles, economic status, and access to medical care. The convergence of these determinants serves to underscore the need for gender-specific public health interventions that treat gender-specific health requirements in addition to the structural inequalities that have a disproportionately large impact on one gender compared to another. In addition, socioeconomic status plays a vital role in affecting health outcomes in both genders. Research has proven that individuals living under the poverty line are much more likely to be exposed to adverse health conditions, including chronic kidney disease and cardiovascular disease. The impact of socioeconomic status on health disparities can be defined using the case of cardiorenal syndrome, where increased cholesterol levels have strong correlations with adverse health outcomes. Specifically, hyperlipidemia was noted to have higher risks for cardiorenal syndrome, particularly in the lower socioeconomic segment. This further emphasizes how important it is to include socioeconomic determinants in health assessments and interventions that can detect populations at risk and enhance equal access to healthcare services for both genders, meeting their respective health needs (Banerjee et al., 2020). In addition, gender differences in health outcomes are influenced by the varying impacts of lifestyle characteristics and health-seeking behaviors. For instance, men are less likely to seek medical attention until illness is acute, which could lead to late diagnosis and poorer health outcomes. Women, in turn, use more healthcare but with their own barriers, i.e., underdiagnosis of particular states of illness. The health behavior differences indicate the necessity of education of men and women in anticipatory management of health as well as the provision of access to those resources that facilitate early medical treatment. Thus, in addressing the multi-dimensional nature of gendered health outcomes, the response has to be at the systems level and emphasize the social determinants, accessibility of medical care, and education to facilitate a healthier population overall (Birnbaum et al., 2011).

12.5.2. Gender-Specific Health Issues and Access to Care

The intersection between health issues related to gender and healthcare access is crucial in describing health variation among various groups. Not only does gender influence what type of health issues one may experience, but one's capacity to receive the necessary care as well. Women, for example, most often experience issues like reproductive health complications and conditions like osteoporosis, which are exacerbated by lack of proper healthcare access. Moreover, women from oppressed groups might have other barriers to overcome, like socio-economic barriers and cultural prohibitions. For LGBTQ+ communities, particularly transgender individuals, the health environment is usually plagued by more impediments— absence of clinician training in gender-affirming care and non-availability of accepting health care are significant determinants of lower health outcomes for them than heterosexual ones (Winter, 2012). Thus, an understanding of these gender-specific needs is essential in the pursuit of improving health equity. Access to care is also made more complex by structural biases embedded in healthcare systems that can disenfranchise marginalized gender identities. Transgender and gender non-conforming people, particularly Native Americans or Native Hawaiians, often face intense prejudice within medical environments that can dissuade them from obtaining care at all. Research among American Indian and Native Hawaiian transgender individuals highlighted access to healthcare as a notable issue, as negative interactions with providers and the lack of gender-specific services increase systemic health disparities (Jackson et al., 2013). These barriers not only affect short-term health results but also prevent long-term well-being, underlining the importance of culturally competent healthcare providers who have been educated to address the unique issues of different gender identities. Furthermore, social determinants that affect gender-specific health results cannot be overstated. Education, economic status, and community assets are significant determinants of affecting access to healthcare. For instance, individuals in poor families are likely not to afford health insurance or reside in areas with limited access to health centers, which supports their health disadvantage. For gender minorities, the intersection of the social determinants of health might doubly disadvantage them; they might experience discrimination that affects their physical well-being in addition to their emotional and mental well-being. Addressing these interconnected determinants is necessary to encourage an inclusive healthcare system that recognizes and responds to the diverse needs of all genders. This combined approach is imperative to shattering barriers and facilitating health equity among populations (Figure 12.15).

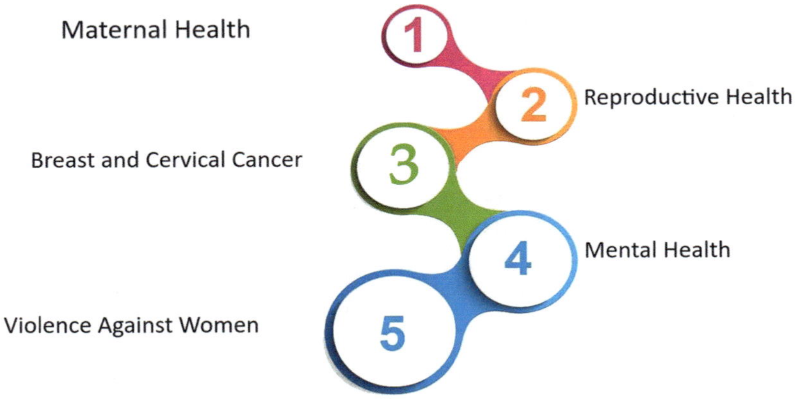

Figure 12.15. Gender-specific health issues and access to care.

Source: https://fastercapital.co/i/Arab-League-Women-Empowerment--Championing-Gender-Equality--Addressing-Gender-Specific-Health-Challenges.webp.

12.5.3. Societal Roles and Their Impact on Health

The social roles occupied by individuals are crucial in determining health outcomes, particularly among vulnerable communities. For instance, CHWs can bridge the healthcare delivery system gaps through provision of core services such as education, advocacy, and navigation assistance to disadvantaged populations. Their extensive knowledge of community dynamics enables them to adequately address the social determinants of health, thus enhancing prevention and treatment services. Initiatives such as Accion Para La Salud show how effective it can be to train CHWs to work on chronic disease prevention through community work and advocacy, showing how societal roles can lead to better health outcomes by aligning efforts at health promotion with community needs and priorities (Carvajal et al., 2014). In understanding the interconnectedness of individual, community, and environmental determinants of health, these functions are integral to the broader public health system. Education is also at the center in the role of closing health disparities, especially as it pertains to the medical workforces competence and cultural sensitivity in the care of a diverse patient population. The evidence implies that health outcome disparities between Indigenous and non-Indigenous groups can be minimized through the application of medical education as an equity-enhancing force. Health institutions must engage in addressing deeper problems such as colonization, racism, and privilege that pervade schooling institutions. Developing a comprehensive Indigenous health curriculum and strengthening it consistently will significantly contribute to advancing health equity. This commitment not only improves the medical practitioner's capacity to effectively provide services for Indigenous communities, but it also propels more holistic advocacy for structural shifts in health and society that counteract inequities (Calam et al., 2018). Thus, education social roles can redefine health outcomes and challenge system barriers that sustain disparity. The social roles encompassed in community and institutional leadership also exert a strong influence on health disparities via policy reform and advocacy. Health organizations and health equity-focused community leaders create a conducive environment for improved health outcomes, which demonstrates the impact of leadership on social health dynamics. For instance, initiatives that strengthen grassroots leaders to push for systemic change in health policy can dismantle barriers to access, particularly for marginalized populations. Together, in collective advocacy, these leaders can put the necessity of addressing social determinants of health and ensuring investment in sustainable outcomes at the forefront. As illustrated by efforts that empower CHWs and revolutionize medical education, the nexus between health advocacy and social roles is paramount to effectively resolving and preventing health disparities. Through a concerted effort at different levels, society can make significant strides towards achieving health equity for all individuals.

12.6. Policy Interventions to Address Disparities

Policy interventions against health disparities must be directed at the social determinants which play so great a role in health outcomes among varying populations. A review of interventions indicates that successful policies address intermediary determinants such as housing stability and access to care, which are bridges that span structural determinants and link them to individual health. Recent studies indicate a strong correlation between these social determinants and the progression of disease, most prominent in such diseases as asthma, where disparities continue to manifest along racial and ethnic lines. Importantly, while interventions addressing proximal factors will immediately be rewarded, the systemic determinants of health disparities require focus on the upstream structural determinants as outlined in the WHO Conceptual Framework for Action on the Social Determinants of Health. Promoting mass-scale policy solutions to address such deep-seated structural issues may eventually become important in bridging the gap in health equity, as evidenced by present findings in the literature (Sullivan et al., 2020). Equitable tobacco control policies are an illustration of successful intervention measures that can narrow health disparities with their roots in social determinants. Extensive tobacco prevention efforts—i.e., smoke-free laws, tax increases, and availability of cessation—are in large part misplaced unless they penetrate the most susceptible populations. Susceptible populations, particularly those that are less educated and of lower incomes, disproportionately shoulder the burden of tobacco use due to systematic health inequities in policy impact. Interventions therefore need to be tailored accordingly to address overall public health objectives. Efforts to integrate social determinants into tobacco control programs illustrate that equitable policy implementation has the dual benefit of declining tobacco consumption and reducing related health inequities, highlighting the necessity of a justice-oriented approach to health policy (N/A).

Further, the effectiveness of policy interventions in alleviating health inequities relies on efficient cross-sector partnership among actors. By drawing from multiple sectors, such as housing, education, and health, policymakers can structure comprehensive strategies that tackle the root causes of health disparities in a holistic approach. For instance, housing policies to improve conditions and access to quality healthcare can synergistically enhance the health status of vulnerable populations. The interrelation of multiple social determinants makes it more manageable to obtain focused insights into health disparities and enable innovative solutions that yield long-term effects. As research keeps unfolding the intricate aspects of health inequities, they point towards the importance of comprehensive policy interventions with a focus on equity and community engagement that eventually shape public health objectives and improved outcomes for all (Sullivan et al., 2020).

12.6.1. Overview of Current Health Policies

The existing health policies within the United States are increasingly shifting toward addressing health disparities through comprehensive frameworks that consider various social determinants of health. These policies aim to reveal and rectify systemic inequities that have a profound effect on health outcomes based on race, ethnicity, economic standing, and geography. The integration of social determinants into policy for public health is an acknowledgment of the complex interrelation between personal choice and environmental factors. By putting health equity first, existing policies aim to provide everybody, irrespective of background, with the resources and opportunities needed to achieve optimal health. This shift in paradigm is particularly important because it tackles disparities not just through healthcare access but through a broader vision of health as shaped by places people live, learn, work, and play. As determinants of health have gained more recognition, federal programs, such as those created by the Federal Interagency Health Equity Team (FIHET), are promoting cross-sector partnerships.

These partnerships utilize resources and capacity from various government and community agencies to approach complex health-related challenges. The importance of mission alignment and capacity building was underscored in a recent FIHET Roundtable, along with a need for innovative funding strategies to maximize community health infrastructure. Conferees mentioned barriers to successful partnership and emphasized the need to develop common aims and vocabulary among stakeholders. Breaking down these barriers is important in building an enduring model for health equity, ultimately leading to improved health outcomes for different populations, as systemic barriers still limit access to resources and care for marginalized groups. Moreover, the work of institutions like the Robert Wood Johnson Foundation (RWJF) is important in disseminating information regarding the impact of social conditions on health disparities. Through initiatives such as the Commission to Build a Healthier America, RWJF takes complicated information and turns it into compelling messages that engage a wide audience, tracking the routes through which social and environmental determinants lead to disparities in health. By bringing these conversations forward, current policies can be informed by evidence-based research that highlights the link between place and health outcomes. These initiatives aim not only to educate policymakers but also to mobilize the public's involvement in the conversation about health equity, making them more alert and outspoken. Together, these initiatives reaffirm a comprehensive model of health policy that extends beyond traditional models of medical care and acknowledges the broader set of determinants driving health disparities (Figure 12.16).

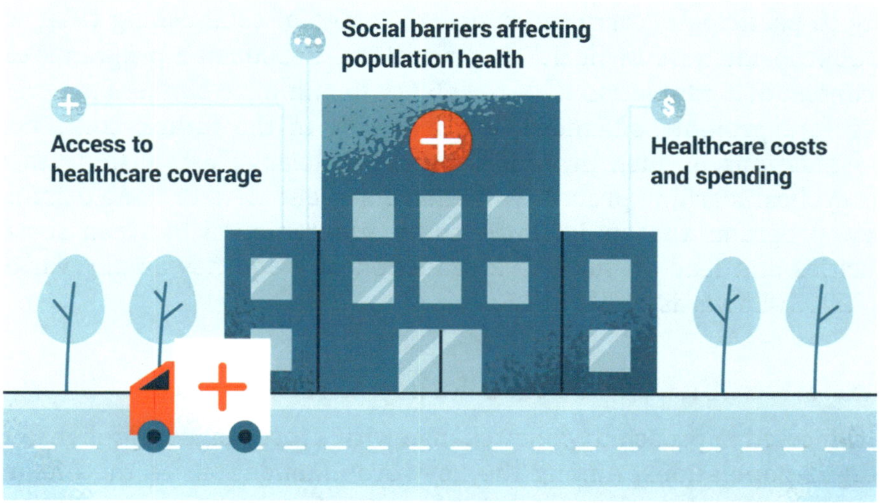

Figure 12.16. Overview of current health policies.

Source: https://www.usa.edu/wp-content/uploads/2021/10/three-major-issues.gif.

12.6.2. Successful Case Studies of Intervention Programs

Effective intervention programs have been crucial in enhancing health disparities linked with social determinants. A good case in point is the implementation of structural interventions to reduce the rate of HIV infections among women, particularly among vulnerable groups. It is evidence that the rate differences are staggering, with the data revealing that, in 2010, black women were 20 times more likely to have new HIV infection than their white counterparts, and Hispanic women four times as likely. Interventions have centered on economic empowerment, decreasing gender-based violence, and integrating health services into providing a holistic approach of care that is responsive to womens experience and needs. The merging of these contextualized approaches has been found to prevent HIV vulnerability through the intervention not just of health behaviors but also of the risk-perpetuating social conditions, thus offering a replicable model for the solution of other health disparities (Edwards et al., 2015). Another success story in the prevention of health disparities is also the interventions for individuals with IDD. Such groups have in the past faced disproportionate difficulty in accessing quality care because of socio-economic determinants, systemic failure, and social neglect. Recent focus has been on preparing health care providers to recognize and address the unique health needs of individuals with IDD. Training programs have facilitated active lifestyles and encouraged the inclusion of individuals with IDD into public health and wellness programs, ultimately reducing the health disparities that they face. Despite this progress, continued study is essential to identify and reproduce effective interventions, monitor chronic conditions prevalent in this group, and develop effective strategies for healthcare provision (White and Beiter, 2013). Holistic such initiatives must be implemented to deliver equitable health outcomes to people with IDD, addressing both their specific needs and the broader socio-cultural determinants (Anderson et al., 2013). Secondly, the integration of best practices from successful case studies provides useful lessons for future interventions addressing health disparities. Interventions that integrate evidence-based practice with community participation have achieved significant improvements in health outcomes. Participatory-based programs, for instance, which involve engaging members of the community to participate, carry the extra advantage of establishing trust while promoting greater cultural appropriateness of health interventions. Responsive programs to the particular socio-economic context of a population have the ability to minimize barriers to access to healthcare services and therefore promote enhanced health equity. In the future, continued emphasis on evidence-based evaluations of such programs will be crucial in establishing their impacts and replicability. This cyclical learning process will enable stakeholders to hone existing interventions and fine-tune new programs that address the complex interaction between social determinants and health disparities and lead, in turn, to a reduction of inequities among various populations (Anderson et al., 2013; Edwards et al., 2015).

12.6.3. Recommendations for Future Policy Changes

It requires a multi-faceted approach to policy change with a focus on comprehensive measures that target disadvantaged populations. Among the key recommendations is the integration of health equity principles into all aspects of public health policy. This entails an examination of existing programs and initiatives from the vantage point of their impact on various demographic groups, with particular attention to those that are marginalized on socioeconomic, racial, and geographic grounds. Through implementation of policies that have particular regard for health disparities, stakeholders can create tailored interventions that target reducing barriers to receiving care and improving health outcomes among vulnerable groups. A resource allocation emphasis is necessary in this business to spend funds in high-need areas to the extent outlined in Birnbaum et al. (2011). In addition, enhanced accessibility of good quality employment and education opportunities plays a vital role in creating a foundation that can be long-standing in sustaining health equity. Educational gaps should be addressed as a priority through programs that aim at it since education is key in determining health outcomes. Policyholders need to invest in education programs that target communities and equip individuals with the knowledge and skills to navigate healthcare systems efficaciously. Moreover, job opportunities can be enhanced through targeted economic development strategies that reach historically disadvantaged communities. These kinds of policies establish an environment where people are capable of making better choices and will come for preventive care, ending up addressing underlying causes of health inequalities as noted by Birnbaum et al. (2011). Finally, a good framework of community engagement is essential in formulating sustainable change in health policy. It is important that policymakers involve members of the community in decision-making in a manner that makes it possible for the voices of the affected to be heard. Partnerships between the government, health institutions, and community organizations facilitate trust building as well as a comprehensive understanding of the needs of the population within the area. Such an inclusive process ensures not only that policies are contextually relevant and culturally sensitive but also allows communities to claim their health outcomes.

SUMMARY

In addressing the more underlying causes of health disparities, one must recognize the fundamental role that social determinants play in shaping the state of health among varying populations. Health communication, so directly tied to socioeconomic status, becomes a powerful determinant of individual and community health. Evidence indicates that inequalities in health communication are brought about by factors such as family income and education, which directly impact one's capacity for accessing and understanding health information. In the absence of specific communication strategies designed to close the gaps, marginalized groups end up facing the worst health outcomes, thus maintaining the cycle of disadvantage. As the case in Japan illustrates, addressing such disparities in terms of greater access to good health information can go a long way towards mitigating health disparities as well as enhancing public health efforts among marginalized groups (Hayashi et al., 2012). In addition, examination of oral health disparities among individuals with IDD emphasizes the unique needs of racial and ethnic minorities in this subpopulation. The intersection of social determinants such as access to care, education, and personal status complicates the health environment further for these patients. As measures are taken towards reducing disparities, most of the barriers continue to exist, and the underprivileged communities continue to be vulnerable to inadequate dental care. The disparities not only indicate systemic disparity but also necessitate immediate interventions that cater to the specific needs of minority groups in the IDD population. These include mobile dental clinics and health education outreach, which can specifically address the barriers these populations face (Williams et al., 2024). In general, eliminating health disparities demands a multifaceted approach that takes into account the interplay of social determinants as well as the diverse needs of different populations. By putting health communication first, expanding access to care, and individually adapting interventions, stakeholders are working towards a more equitable system of health care. These disparities are not only an ethical imperative but a necessity in working towards comprehensive health equity. Involving evidence-based methods that speak to socioeconomic and contextual factors will be necessary in leading to marked improvement in health outcomes. As we progress in our understanding of health disparities, it is important that continuous research keeps a focus on innovative solutions that engage marginalized communities and close the gap of health inequities (Hayashi et al., 2012; Williams et al., 2024).

Understanding of health disparities involves taking into consideration the social determinants of health that affect the health outcomes within populations. These determinants include factors like socioeconomic status, education level, and housing, all which have a combined effect on individuals' capacities to reach optimal health. From evidence, it is clear that inequities in health are not the result of choices made by individuals but deeply rooted within inequalities in systems that perpetuate unfair distribution. Addressing these social determinants enables stakeholders to implement policies to alleviate health disparities, hence realizing an equal state of health. As highlighted in health equity program debates, comprehensive understanding of such interrelated determinants is significant for developing effective interventions and policy measures to ensure the maximum joint well-being of deprived groups. Cross-sectoral partnerships are accorded top priority as a foremost strategy for responding to the complex social determinants for unequal health situations. This approach involves coordinating various sectors like government, enterprise, and community organizations to align effort and resources towards particular health equity aims. Latest venues like the Roundtable brought together by the FIHET have placed the approach under the spotlight as it seeks to overcome barriers to collaboration and innovation. Critical recommendations emerging from such discussions include convergence of mission, infrastructure investment, and goal convergence among stakeholders. Through the establishment of collaborative platforms, such programs seek to break through institutional barriers and effectively deploy resources in a bid to reduce health inequities among diverse populations, thereby providing improved health outcomes. Furthermore, translating knowledge about social determinants into usable insights is essential in a bid to enlighten diverse publics about health disparities. Robert Wood Johnson Foundations Commission to Build a Healthier America is a model practice in the translation of empirical studies into informing public opinion and policy. Recognizing the prevalent force of settings in which individuals reside, learn, work, and play, the Commission presented a persuasive argument for modifying these determinants in healthcare intervention. These initiatives create a basis for public discourse and enable system reform that can promote health equity. By reaffirming the importance of addressing social determinants, stakeholders can initiate meaningful advances in public health for everyone while eroding present gaps along racial and ethnic lines.

KEY TERMS FROM THIS CHAPTER

Health Inequities	Income Inequality	Access to Healthcare
Racial Disparities	Education Level	Housing Instability
Food Insecurity	Employment Status	Chronic Disease Disparities
Cultural Barriers	Health Equity	Discrimination
Transportation Access	Neighborhood Safety	Environmental Racism
Healthcare Utilization	Language Barriers	Mental Health Inequities
Policy Interventions	Social Exclusion	Insurance Coverage
Vulnerable Populations	Structural Racism	Life Expectancy Gap

CLOSER LOOK

SOCIAL DETERMINANTS OF HEALTH (SDOH)

A closer look at the social determinants of health (SDOH) reveals how deeply social, economic, and environmental factors influence individual and population health outcomes. These determinants—such as income, education, employment, housing, food security, access to healthcare, and social support—play a far greater role in shaping health than medical care alone. Where people are born, grow, live, work, and age significantly affects their opportunities to live healthy lives. For instance, individuals living in poverty or unstable housing often face barriers to nutritious food, safe environments, and quality healthcare, leading to higher risks of chronic illness and mental health challenges. Similarly, low levels of education are often linked to limited health literacy and reduced access to well-paying jobs, further compounding health disparities. Racial and ethnic minorities frequently encounter systemic discrimination and structural racism, which also impact their health through chronic stress and unequal access to services. Addressing the SDOH requires a shift from treating disease to promoting health equity through cross-sector collaboration, policy reform, and community engagement. Interventions must go beyond clinical settings to address the root causes of health disparities—such as improving access to affordable housing, investing in early childhood education, increasing minimum wage, and ensuring safe neighborhoods. Public health agencies, healthcare providers, schools, governments, and non-profits all have a role to play in creating environments that support well-being. Data collection and community-based research are also essential to understanding local needs and guiding targeted action. Ultimately, recognizing and addressing the social determinants of health is key to achieving more just and sustainable health outcomes. By focusing on upstream factors and promoting equity, societies can reduce health disparities, improve quality of life, and build healthier, more resilient communities for all.

REFERENCES

1. Adunola, DDS, MPH, F., Brandt, EdD, MPH, E., et al. (2017). An assessment of funding and other capacity needs for health equity programming within state-level chronic disease programs. https://digitalscholarship.unlv.edu/cgi/viewcontent.cgi?article=1668&context=jhdrp (accessed on 26th June 2025).
2. Ajani, S. N., Bahulekar, A., Dabade, T. D., Kakade, R., et al. (2023). Examining the social determinants of health in urban communities: A comparative analysis. https://core.ac.uk/download/599214699.pdf (accessed on 26th June 2025).
3. Amaro, H., Dominguez, S., & Rickles, N. (2012). Perceptions of healthcare, health status, and discrimination among African-American veterans. https://digitalscholarship.unlv.edu/cgi/viewcontent.cgi?article=1024&context=jhdrp (accessed on 26th June 2025).
4. Anderson, L. L., Humphries, K., Larson, S., Marks, B., et al. (2013). The state of the science of health and wellness for adults with intellectual and developmental disabilities. https://core.ac.uk/download/267563158.pdf (accessed on 26th June 2025).
5. Apter, A., Beck, A., Bentley-Edwards, K., Berkowitz, R., et al. (2024). Research priorities in pediatric asthma morbidity: Addressing the impacts of systemic racism on children with asthma in the United States. An official American Thoracic Society workshop report. https://core.ac.uk/download/622190771.pdf (accessed on 26th June 2025).
6. Balser, A., O'Brien, S. P., & Wittman, P. (2020). Doing it right: OT meeting population needs with COVID-19. https://core.ac.uk/download/344949446.pdf (accessed on 26th June 2025).
7. Banerjee, A., Chaze, F., Dhillon, P., D'Silva, S., et al. (2022). Service provider perspectives on exploring social determinants of health impacting type 2 diabetes management for South Asian adults in Peel Region, Canada. https://core.ac.uk/download/534394364.pdf (accessed on 26th June 2025).
8. Banerjee, K., Banerjee, S. K., MD, PhD, Diegel, B., et al. (2020). Effect of poverty level on the relationship between hyperlipidemia and cardiorenal syndrome. https://digitalscholarship.unlv.edu/cgi/viewcontent.cgi?article=1912&context=jhdrp (accessed on 26th June 2025).
9. Bartlett, R., Coakley, T. M., Kelley, A., Randolph, S., et al. (2018). Integrating students into interdisciplinary health and health disparities research teams. https://digitalscholarship.unlv.edu/cgi/viewcontent.cgi?article=1677&context=jhdrp (accessed on 26th June 2025).
10. Bell, C. N., Bowie, J. V., & Thorpe, R. J., Jr. (2018). Race and "hotspots" of preventable hospitalizations. https://digitalscholarship.unlv.edu/cgi/viewcontent.cgi?article=1506&context=jhdrp (accessed on 26th June 2025).
11. Birnbaum, N., Masterson, E., & Schoomaker, H. (2011). *State of Health Equity Movement, 2011 Update Part B: Catalog of Activities DRA Project Report No. 11-02.* https://core.ac.uk/download/pdf/18491811.pdf (accessed on 26th June 2025).
12. Blue Bird Jernigan, V. (2016). An examination of cultural competence training in US medical education guided by the tool for assessing cultural competence training. https://digitalscholarship.unlv.edu/cgi/viewcontent.cgi?article=1426&context=jhdrp (accessed on 26th June 2025).

13. Bolnick, D. A. (2015). Combating racial health disparities through medical education: The need for anthropological and genetic perspectives in medical training. https://core.ac.uk/download/56688593.pdf (accessed on 26th June 2025).

14. Breen, N., Cullen, T., Darity, W., Entwisle, B., et al. (2023). The PhenX Toolkit: Measurement protocols for assessment of social determinants of health. https://core.ac.uk/download/617033193.pdf (accessed on 26th June 2025).

15. Bryan, J. K., D'Angelo, K. A., & Kurz, B. (2016). Women's experiences with prenatal care: A mixed-methods study exploring the influence of the social determinants of health. https://digitalscholarship.unlv.edu/cgi/viewcontent.cgi?article=1425&context=jhdrp (accessed on 26th June 2025).

16. Calam, B., Crowshoe, L., Curtis, E., Ewen, S., et al. (2018). Educating for Indigenous health equity: An international consensus statement. https://core.ac.uk/download/213607778.pdf (accessed on 26th June 2025).

17. Carlson, C., Sholk, J., Nanni, J., Peterson, K., Smith, L. A., & Bhavaraju, N. (2016). Breaking the barriers to specialty care: Practical ideas to improve health equity and reduce cost–Helping patients engage in specialty care. https://core.ac.uk/download/75785773.pdf (accessed on 26th June 2025).

18. Carvajal, S., PhD, MPH, & Guernsey De Zapien, J., BA, et al. (2014). Developing an action learning community advocacy/leadership training program for community health workers and their agencies to reduce health disparities in Arizona border communities. https://digitalscholarship.unlv.edu/cgi/viewcontent.cgi?article=1164&context=jhdrp (accessed on 26th June 2025).

19. Cattell-Gordon, D. C., Driscoll, D. L., O'Donnell, H., Patel, M., et al. (2023). Assessing and addressing the determinants of Appalachian population health: A scoping review. https://core.ac.uk/download/596874112.pdf (accessed on 26th June 2025).

20. Davidson, T. C., & Singelmann, J. (2012). Determinants of depressive symptoms among women on public assistance in Louisiana. https://digitalscholarship.unlv.edu/cgi/viewcontent.cgi?article=1022&context=jhdrp (accessed on 26th June 2025).

21. Dizon, S. P. (2017). Reducing stigma-driven health disparities in people living with HIV (PLWH): A literature review. https://core.ac.uk/download/129533005.pdf (accessed on 26th June 2025).

22. Edwards, A. (2015). Recognizing the influence of social determinants on HIV risk behaviors and the need for structural interventions to prevent HIV in women. https://digitalscholarship.unlv.edu/cgi/viewcontent.cgi?article=1276&context=jhdrp (accessed on 26th June 2025).

23. Evans-Agnew, R. A. (2012). Asthma management: An Eco social framework for disparity research. https://digitalscholarship.unlv.edu/cgi/viewcontent.cgi?article=1011&context=jhdrp (accessed on 26th June 2025).

24. Fish-Parcham, C., Panares, R., & Adland, S. (2008). Identifying and evaluating equity provisions in state health care reform. https://core.ac.uk/download/71352106.pdf (accessed on 26th June 2025).

25. Green, A. R., Betancourt, J. R., & King, R. R. (2009). Improving quality and achieving equity: A guide for hospital leaders. https://core.ac.uk/download/71352207.pdf (accessed on 26th June 2025).

26. Hayashi, H., Ishikawa, Y., Nishiuchi, H., Viswanath, K., et al. (2012). Socioeconomic status and health communication inequalities in Japan: A nationwide cross-sectional survey. https://core.ac.uk/download/28940828.pdf (accessed on 26th June 2025).

27. Hing, A. K. (2020). The right to vote, the right to health: Voter suppression as a determinant of racial health disparities. https://digitalscholarship.unlv.edu/cgi/viewcontent.cgi?article=1894&context=jhdrp (accessed on 26th June 2025).

28. Hudson, N., McKivett, A., & Paul, D. (2018). Healing conversations: Developing a practical framework for clinical communication between Aboriginal communities and healthcare practitioners. https://core.ac.uk/download/213607715.pdf (accessed on 26th June 2025).

29. Jackson, T., & Vernon, I. S. (2013). Closing the gap: A research agenda for the study of health needs among American Indian/Native Hawaiian transgender individuals. https://core.ac.uk/download/84404197.pdf (accessed on 26th June 2025).

30. Jallo, N., Kinser, P. A., Masho, S. W., Price, S. K., et al. (2015). Racial disparities in the association between stress and preterm birth. https://digitalscholarship.unlv.edu/cgi/viewcontent.cgi?article=1358&context=jhdrp (accessed on 26th June 2025).

31. Larrea, C., Montalvo, P., & Ricaurte, A. (2025). Child malnutrition, social development and health services in the Andean region. https://core.ac.uk/download/pdf/9315033.pdf (accessed on 26th June 2025).

32. McDaniel, J. T., Nuhu, K. M., & Ruiz, J. I. (2022). Colorectal cancer, socioeconomic distribution and behavior: A comparative analysis of urban and rural counties in the USA. https://core.ac.uk/download/522897570.pdf (accessed on 26th June 2025).

33. N/A (2009). Breaking through on the social determinants of health and health disparities: An approach to message translation. https://core.ac.uk/download/71346249.pdf (accessed on 26th June 2025).

34. N/A (2009). Education matters for health. https://core.ac.uk/download/71346552.pdf (accessed on 26th June 2025).

35. N/A (2025). *Nicotine Tob Res.* https://core.ac.uk/download/144202194.pdf (accessed on 26th June 2025).

36. Nweke, O. (2017). A roundtable on cross-sector collaboration and resource alignment for health equity: Meeting summary. https://digitalscholarship.unlv.edu/cgi/viewcontent.cgi?article=1681&context=jhdrp (accessed on 26th June 2025).

37. Owusu, M. A., Oyeleke, M., & Yusuf, R. (2025). Cancer and social determinants of health: Examining the impact of economic, geographic, and racial disparities in treatment outcomes: A review. https://core.ac.uk/download/654538576.pdf (accessed on 26th June 2025).

38. Quinn, S. C., & Thomas, S. B. (2008). Poverty and elimination of urban health disparities: Challenge and opportunity. https://core.ac.uk/download/pdf/11541635.pdf (accessed on 26th June 2025).

39. Sami, W. Y. (2024). The unequal distribution of social risk for Black men across the lifespan. A novel framework. https://core.ac.uk/download/619723173.pdf (accessed on 26th June 2025).

40. Sullivan, K., & Thakur, N. (2020). Structural and social determinants of health in asthma in developed economies: A scoping review of literature published between 2014 and 2019.

https://core.ac.uk/download/323073611.pdf (accessed on 26th June 2025).

41. Topping, M. S. (2020). Rural-urban cancer disparities in mortality: The role of physician supply. https://core.ac.uk/download/480755290.pdf (accessed on 26th June 2025).
42. Williams, D. (2024). A comparative analysis of oral health disparities among Caucasians and African Americans with intellectual disabilities. https://core.ac.uk/download/599632121.pdf (accessed on 26th June 2025).
43. Winter, C. (2012). *Health Equity Series: Responding to LGBT Health Disparities August 2012.* https://core.ac.uk/download/71362140.pdf (accessed on 26th June 2025).
44. Zaragoza, G. (2019). Getting to zero HIV cases San Francisco: Reconceptualizing housing as HIV prevention and HIV treatment. https://core.ac.uk/download/287624137.pdf (accessed on 26th June 2025).

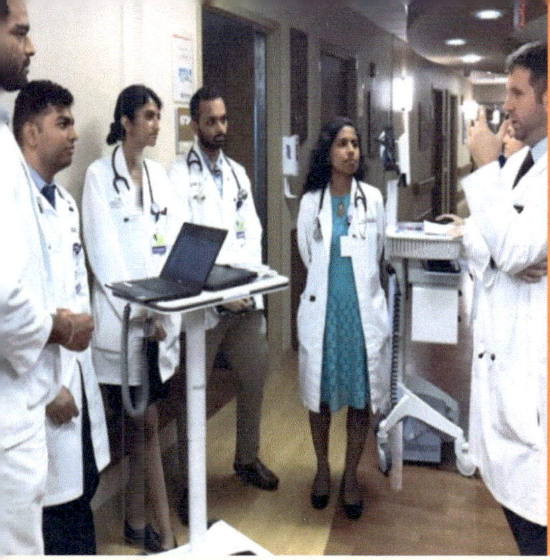

Chapter 13

EMERGENCY PREPAREDNESS AND COMMUNITY RESILIENCE

Contents

Introduction

The increasing frequency of natural disasters, coupled with the worsening impacts of climate change, have resulted in an urgent necessity for effective emergency preparedness and community resilience systems. Poor and rich communities alike from around the world are susceptible to destructive events. For instance, inundating one of the most prevalent natural disasters affects developing and developed nations similarly in causing extensive economic as well as social dislocation. While addressing such problems, there is a need to explore effective actions that enhance the resilience of communities. This question not only ensures improved preparedness for some disasters but also fosters a culture of resilience that can weather a variety of shocks. They are necessary in enabling societies to bounce back quickly and resiliently, thereby safeguarding their future in an increasingly uncertain climate (Amaratunga et al., 2013). Parallel to realizing the importance of resilience is realizing the methodologies upon which effective emergency preparedness planning is conducted.

Contingency planning is an overdue addition to the disaster control toolkit, but practice failures reflect a theoretical deficit in the models that support such interventions. For instance, as the theory has come on, in practice the process of contingency planning in nations like those in southern Africa reveals a gap between intended and actual achievements on the ground. Studies show that response activities largely do not correspond with expected events, and it is suggested that contingency planning funds are regularly inadequate. Such a mismatch undermines efforts to build disaster-resilient communities, and the role of empirical knowledge in bridging the theory-practice gap is emphasized (Mabaso et al., 2013). A comparison of two substantially divergent case studies—one from the developed world of Cockermouth in Cumbria, UK, and another from the developing world of Patuakhali in Bangladesh—offers a comparative context against which we might observe effective strategies in emergency preparedness. Both case studies have their own specific challenges and solutions depending on the underlying socio-economic conditions and stakeholder relationships. By comparing these case studies' results with well-established frameworks such as the UNISDR's ten-point checklist under the "Making Cities Resilient Campaign," lessons learned can be applied to inform city development plans and enhance stakeholder engagement. The ultimate goal is to create a resilient infrastructure that not only prepares communities for future disasters but also promotes an ethos of preparedness and adaptability across communities in the face of the uncertainties of modern life (Amaratunga et al., 2013) (Figure 13.1).

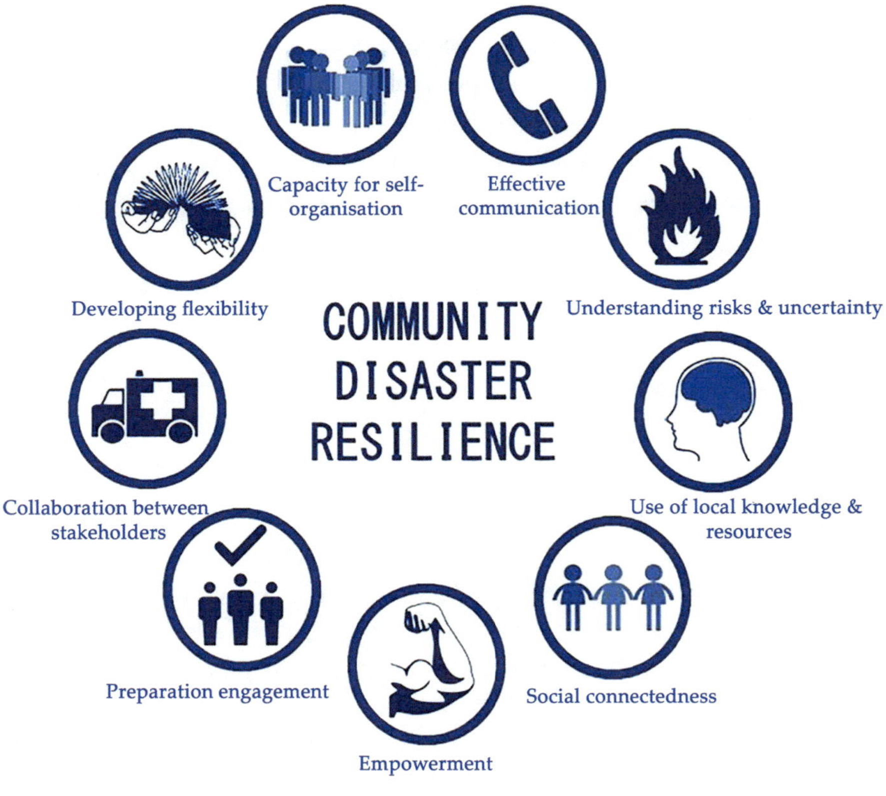

Figure 13.1. Emergency preparedness and community resilience.

Source: https://www.researchgate.net/publication/328655434/figure/fig1/AS:11431281240310085@1714717089728/Factors-important-for-community-disaster-resilience-as-identified-by-the-authors-review.tif.

Definition of Emergency Preparedness

Emergency preparedness is a defining framework designed to prepare individuals and communities to respond effectively to sudden disasters and emergencies. It entails all sorts of forward-looking activities, from risk assessment to public education, resource mobilization, and training. By identifying hazards—either natural disasters like floods or human-made emergencies—communities are able to craft customized emergency plans that better equip them to be resilient. Emergency preparedness also involves coordination across sectors, from government ministries to non-governmental organizations and local enterprises. These collaborations enhance data exchange and resource sharing, hence enabling a cooperative means of handling crises. This pillar of emergency preparedness is the foundation for the general goal of community resilience in that it not only provides one with preparedness for prompt response, but also creates a platform for long-term recovery and adaptation when facing future adversity. Central to the concept of emergency preparedness is the role of communication, particularly in multilingual and multicultural societies. As different groups of people are likely to encounter various forms of challenges during emergencies, effective crisis communication strategies should incorporate language translation as a core element of preparedness. Unfortunately, the need to translate key information is underestimated, and this creates enormous loopholes in emergency response efficiency. Federici et al. (2019) emphasizes the need for focus on language translation right away since this not only maximizes the response in the short run but also ensures trust among communities. When everyone from the community can access information related to their safety and obtain emergency preparedness, these efforts become more holistic and effective, and ultimately, more valuable during disasters. Moreover, learning from past emergencies as well as individuals' personal experiences can be extremely effective in strengthening emergency preparation arrangements. Research like the one conducted on behalf of the Civil Contingencies Secretariat demonstrates how learning from real events, such as the 2007 Hull flood, can inform future policy and intervention. Deeming et al. 2011) emphasizes the importance of adopting a bottom-up approach which attempts to put people's own experiences of surviving disasters first. Contrasting these experiences, emergency planners are able to identify vulnerabilities in current protocols and develop targeted interventions that enhance recovery capacity at the community level. This iterative process of learning from past scenarios ensures that preparatory efforts remain relevant and useful, ultimately creating a more resilient society able to withstand and recover from various types of emergencies.

Importance of Community Resilience

Community resilience is a foundation element in the overall emergency preparedness system with an emphasis placed on the capacity of individuals and communities to innovate and recover from adversity such as natural disasters and public health crises. This resilience is not only driven by infrastructure but also by social connectivity and local engagement. For instance, initiatives like the Los Angeles County Community Disaster Resilience (LACCDR) project demonstrate that participatory practices can successfully enhance resilience among varying community groups. Through the practice of cross-sector collaboration and mutual learning, residents grasp the essence of partnership in enhancing readiness for prospective disasters. By putting community involvement first, resilience becomes a collective objective, allowing residential areas to harness their special assets and capacities to counteract disruptions and recover well in their wake, strengthening social connections and overall well-being overall (Bromley et al., 2017). Additionally, the growing role of technology in community resilience models cannot be ignored. Information and communications technologies (ICT) have transformed emergency preparedness efforts through the utilization of optimum communication measures and the ability to quickly send information. The ability to leverage real-time data in the event of a crisis, especially through mobile networks and social media, allows community members to respond to well-informed decisions quickly. These technologies not only aid in the effective building of early warning systems but also facilitate higher levels of local constituents' participation in response efforts. With these information and communication technologies, communities can be more anticipatory in responding to emergencies, which can soften the blow of disasters and widen the scale of recovery. Hence, the inclusion of ICT in community resilience planning is a watershed development in enhancing communal readiness and responsiveness to unexpected challenges (Amaratunga et al., 2015). Community resilience is not only a matter of rapid response to emergencies; it creates a long-term vision of sustainability and recovery. Resilient communities are entrepreneurially and more adaptable and can respond to socio-economic disparities that have the tendency of aggravating disaster impact. By creating a culture of continuous learning and coordination, community resilience initiatives can enable the engagement of local stakeholders and agencies in driving inclusive strategies that recognize and empower vulnerable populations. These initiatives enhance the level of investment in communities, promoting trust and cooperation that are critical during crises. Lastly, building community resilience not only facilitates rapid recovery but also fosters a more equitable society with each individual having the means and network to weather crisis. This multi-tiered approach underlines the premise that community resilience is central to the greater objective of emergency preparedness programs (Bromley et al., 2017) (Figure 13.2).

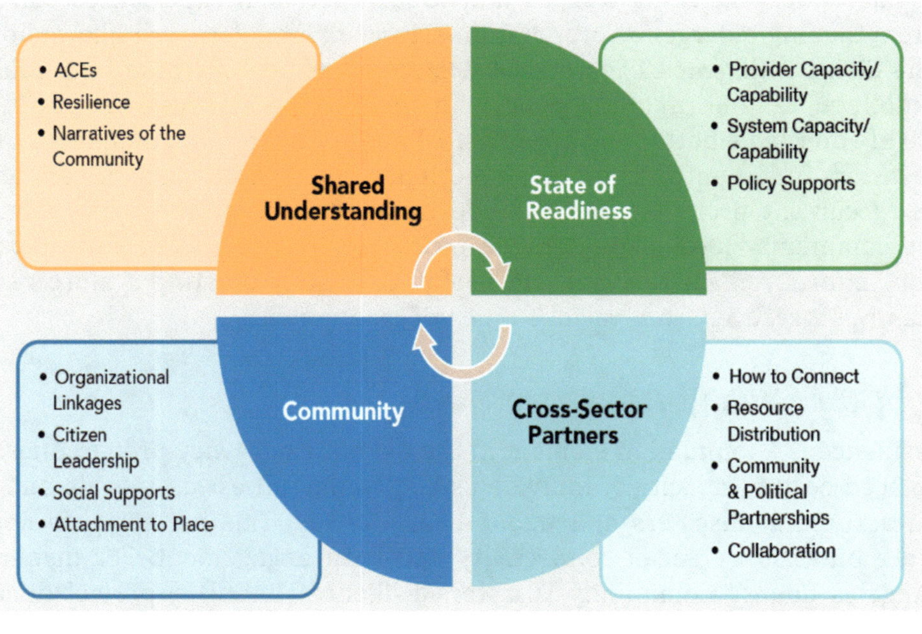

Figure 13.2. Importance of community resilience.

Source: https://ccr.publichealth.gwu.edu/sites/g/files/zaxdzs4361/files/2022-05/case-study-graphics-1.png.

13.1. Historical Context of Emergency Preparedness

The historical context of emergency preparedness is a complex process that has been determined by societal need, technological progress, and shifting political influences. Casual systems were employed to manage local catastrophes in ancient societies that had great variabilities in feelings of the community and their shared traditions. With growing urbanization came the greater demand for more systematic emergency systems, as evident in the aftermath of devastating disasters such as the 1906 San Francisco earthquake. The severe loss of lives and property in such tragedies urged the establishment of official agencies and procedures aimed at minimizing follow-up calamities. These historical foundations laid the basis of the contemporary emergency preparedness frameworks emphasizing community resilience and active disaster management by way of organized planning and resource deployment, emphasizing how to improve response to more complex emergency situations. With the dawn of the 20th century, the connectedness between emergency preparedness and community resilience was accelerating, particularly as a result of World Wars and natural disasters.

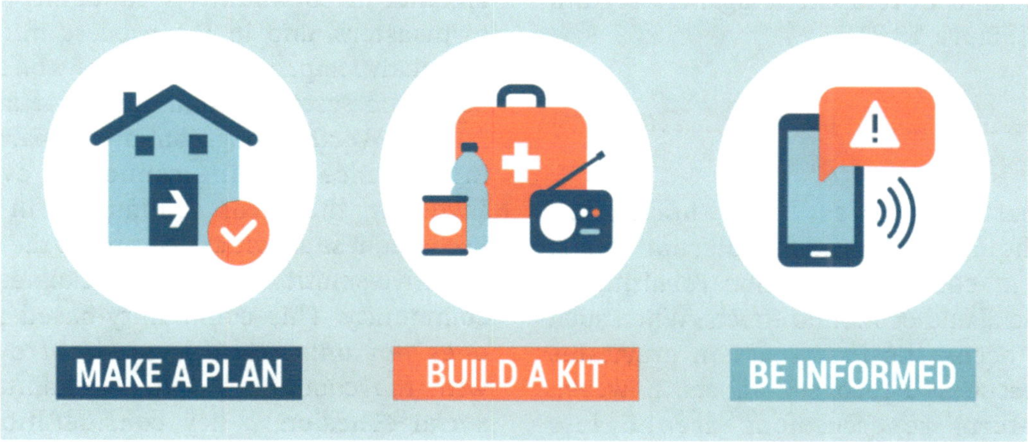

Figure 13.3. Historical context of emergency preparedness.

Source: https://www.eldoradocounty.ca.gov/files/assets/county/v/1/images/public-safety-amp-justice/istock-1146766974.jpg.

The strict enforcement of actions such as the establishment of the Federal Emergency Management Agency (FEMA) in 1979 was a shift towards greater centralization of disaster management in America. This was an age not only of timely response but also one that encouraged community resilience through preparedness education, resource mobilization, and interagency coordination. Studies like those of Kontar et al. (2017) indicate how proactive flood management, say, becomes indispensable in marginalized or infrastructure-poor contexts. Embracing an in-depth study of natural as well as anthropogenic causation of vulnerabilities has become the backbone of effective emergency preparedness in today's society. In the past decade, disaster risk reduction and readiness efforts have increasingly incorporated the preservation of cultural heritage as a critical element in building community resilience. According to the Hyogo Framework for Action, the integration of cultural heritage into disaster management is an indication of the significance of community identity and continuity. The recognition of the fact that heritage can be an asset to build resilience is core in informing strategies which not only respond to physical protection but also psychological and social rehabilitation. Albrito et al. (2013) emphasizes the dual nature of cultural heritage within disaster risk management as something which is vulnerable to be conserved and also an asset capable of building coherence in a community during recovery phases. Subsequently, contemporary preparedness measures now involve a broader perspective that inspires the conservation of cultural heritage, thus increasing overall community resilience and establishing pillars for sustainable development against certain disasters (Figure 13.3).

13.1.1. Major Disasters and Their Impact on Communities

Major disasters such as floods, hurricanes, and earthquakes drastically disrupt social cohesion in communities, thus resulting in serious social and economic effects. When such accidents occur, the first reaction gravitates toward rescue and recovery efforts; however, the long-term repercussions are no less significant and may extend for many years. The most devastating repercussions normally befall vulnerable populations, including poor working individuals and marginalized groups, and normally appear in the forms of loss of housing, means of living, and access to essential services. Research has shown that the effects of such calamities are not uniformly distributed; instead, they exacerbate existing imbalances in societies to continue to disproportionately burden those least able to respond and recover. In our analysis of the dynamics of disaster impact, it is essential to recognize the necessity of interventions able to reverse such disparities and ensure a more equitable recovery process within afflicted communities. Here, the need for effective emergency preparedness measures and community resilience interventions comes clearly into focus. Effective preparedness is not just the development of response systems but also infrastructures strong enough to survive future disasters. Findings have shown that communities with effective disaster preparedness plans, in the form of early warning systems and community-based education programs, recover more quickly and sustainably. By building on public-private partnerships, as in various case studies of flood response interventions, stakeholders can implement measures responding to immediate needs but also seeking to create long-term resilience. For instance, the foregoing studies reveal how some strategies, when adopted collectively, can enhance a community's capability to adapt to disasters, and in the process mitigate the cumulative impact of such disasters on social and economic systems (Amaratunga et al., 2013a, 2013b). Worth noting, community participation in resilience building cannot be overstated. Involving the local community in disaster preparedness activities guarantees the culturally sensitive solutions and the special needs of the community. This community-based approach does not only foster a sense of ownership with the community but also capitalizes on social cohesion, a key consideration in the recovery. If individuals are kept involved and committed to their communities' preparedness plans, they would be encouraged to actively play their roles in readiness efforts and look after one another during times of need. The lessons learned from successful case studies indicate that the inclusion of community-based information in emergency planning is essential for the development of robust systems that are capable of withstanding catastrophic impacts effectively. Lastly, community resilience needs to be developed in a complex array of interventions that take account of the interlinked roles of public engagement, preparedness planning, and social vulnerability in responding to large-scale disasters.

13.1.2. Evolution of Emergency Management Practices

The evolution of emergency management practice has been highly influenced by increasing rates and intensities of natural disasters, which have pushed society to adapt in many ways. Historically, emergency management has been predominantly reactive, with attention to crisis response after the incident. But the recognition that disasters can never be completely prevented has shaped the paradigm towards resilience and emphasized the importance of developing societal capacities to resist and recover from such events. This is a sign of the broader understanding of risk management, where good governance and concerted response efforts are the key towards the development of sustainable community resilience. With heightened flood dangers due to climate change, strategies like Flood Emergency Management Systems (FEMS) have been implemented across Europe, detailing the complex cultural, political, and geographical environments that control emergency management policy among different nations (Alexander et al., 2016). In recent years, integrating advanced technology into emergency management has revolutionized operations with emerging solutions being delivered to increase preparedness and resilience in communities. The use of information and communications technologies (ICT) is a foundation in modern emergency management systems.

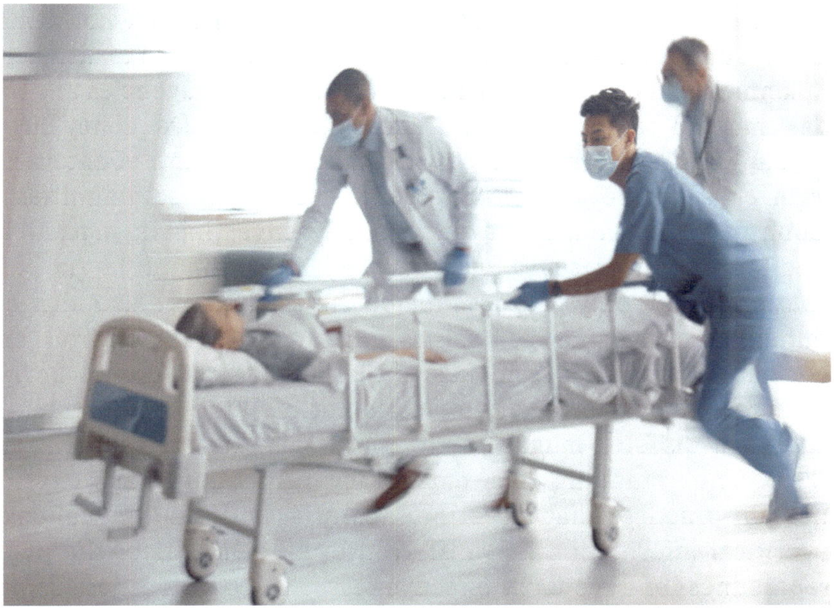

Figure 13.4. Evolution of emergency management practices.

Source: https://agipatna.in/wp-content/uploads/2024/05/15.png.

Internet platforms, online social media, and warning systems enable real-time communication and dissemination of vital information to the public, thereby enhancing situational awareness and enabling proactive decision-making. These technologies also offer empowering tools and facilitation for individuals and organizations across different hierarchies to meaningfully participate in the emergency response process. As societies increasingly use ICT, the contributions of ICT to improving disaster management practices and resilience need to be examined. Moreover, the positive impact from strategically deploying data-oriented practices and networks enables an interconnected disaster preparedness strategy, further reshaping the emergency management scene (Amaratunga et al., 2015). Lastly, the advancement of disaster management practices is marked by growing focus on community engagement and capacity building. As it is well known that local communities play a central role in emergency response, community-level training and preparedness programs are becoming popular. This trend comes on the heels of the development of stakeholder-based models of governance that are focused on collaboration, facilitating the incorporation of community knowledge and resources in emergency management. While institutionalized formal mechanisms may be the cornerstone of emergency response, community-led action can be instrumental in creating resilience by fostering social solidarity and support systems. As it is observable in a number of examples, such as the successful utilization of community preparedness schemes in flood-prone areas, collective action among local stakeholders can lead to a widespread safety net for vulnerable individuals. Thus, the evolution of emergency management practice shows a comprehensive understanding of the aspect that resilience does not just pertain to technology and governance but also includes the agency and engagement of the communities themselves (Alexander et al., 2016) (Figure 13.4).

13.1.3. Lessons Learned from Past Emergencies

Knowledge of what was learned through past emergencies is crucial when consulting on future emergency preparedness and community resilience. Historical responses to disasters have shown the necessity of better planning and coordination between government agencies and local communities. For example, lessons that can be derived from increasing disaster frequency suggest that existing structures need to adapt in an effort to effectively manage risks and counteract new challenges. As laid out in Bergin et al. (2014), developing resilience among communities does not always equate to just responding to systems but, additionally, investing in proactive initiatives that empower people and localities to recover and adapt. By integrating different strategies, societies can have a strong basis that not only prepares for possible crises but also mitigates their adverse impacts. Cross-communication in times of crisis is also a valuable lesson from experience. One of the critical aspects that tends to be overlooked is the language difference between populations, and this can hinder access to very critical information at the time of a disaster. The contribution of language translation in disaster management is now an extremely urgent issue, as noted in Federici et al. (2019). Understanding this, emergency responders have a priority to embrace inclusive communication practices that target multicultural and multilingual communities. These efforts ensure that critical information is transferred to all elements of the population and thus enhance overall preparedness and response effectiveness. This consciousness compels communities to approach linguistic diversity as a vital aspect of their emergency planning. Lastly, long-term development of facilities within vulnerable areas provides another key lesson from past emergencies. The persistent destruction caused by natural disasters highlight the need for strong structures and systems that can withstand extreme forces. The economic aspect is also high, with estimations indicating higher costs from such occurrences, as set out in Bergin et al. (2014). Investment in resilient infrastructure saves not only short-term damage but also fosters long-term stability and growth of populations. Through reflection on lessons learned from past events, decision-makers can make resilience-bolstering efforts that ultimately support communities against subsequent crises. This comprehensive approach, founded on historical lessons, is vital to success in creating a culture of resilience and preparedness against more uncertain challenges.

13.2. Key Components of Emergency Preparedness

Effective emergency preparedness depends on the establishment of efficient early warning systems, which are an essential risk assessment and dissemination tool. They enable timely dissemination of information, thereby enabling individuals and groups to prepare proactive responses ahead of emergencies. Through harnessing the potential of information and communication technology innovations, such as mobile and internet-based platforms, communities can transform their preparedness frameworks. Their use facilitates the concurrent interrogation of data across the various hierarchies of society, effectively undermining long-entrenched power structures within emergency management frameworks.

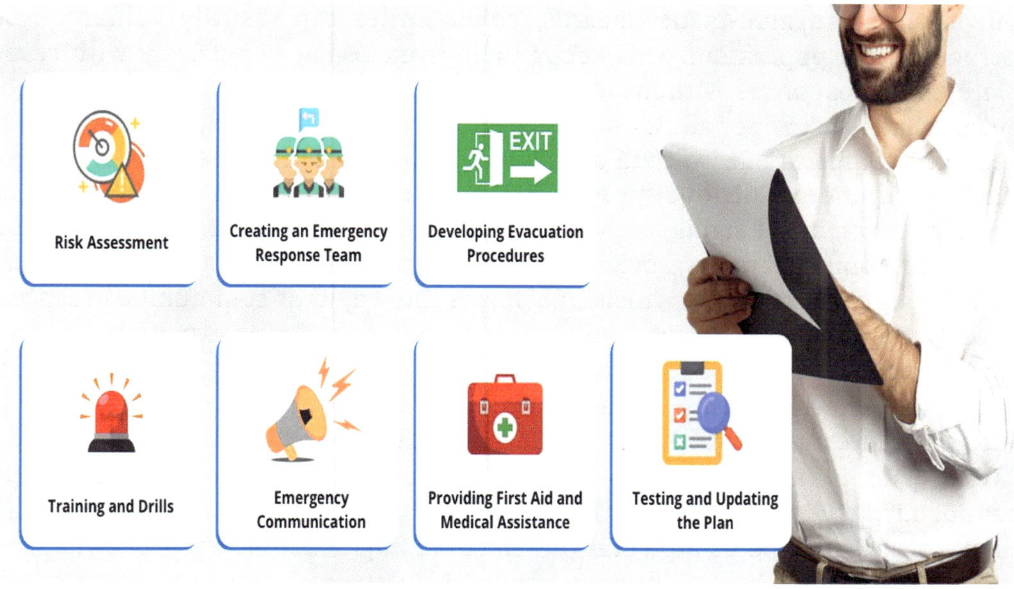

Figure 13.5. Key components of emergency preparedness.

Source: https://vizito.eu/images/blog/infographic-emergency-readiness.webp.

As highlighted in Amaratunga et al. (2015), the networks result in an informed public, ultimately enhancing resilience through facilitating individuals to react swiftly to imminent threats. Another crucial aspect of emergency preparedness is contingency planning, in which there is the development of formal plans with the aim of handling potential disaster scenarios. Successful contingency planning in the majority of locations, especially where there are frequent recurrent disasters, is capable of minimizing risks and building resilience in the community. Empirical research indicates a disparity between model theory and actual plan implementation. A study carried out in southern Africa indicates that response operations rarely conform to expected circumstances, and the provision of resources negates the success of strategies as in Mabaso et al. (2013). Such paradoxes must be resolved; otherwise, communities are left vulnerable and poorly prepared for the next impending crisis. Further, ongoing training and simulation is what ensures that community preparedness is enhanced. By regular exercises and drills, residents are aware of their emergency protocols and response strategies, bolstering their overall capacity to react in an emergency. Such readiness programs, potentially as collaborative initiative among city or township governments, non-profits, and neighborhood associations, contribute to a stronger society. Engaging the community in preparedness efforts promotes a culture of preparedness and awareness, enabling people to understand what kinds of threats they are vulnerable to and how to respond. Ultimately, the integration of early warning systems, contingency planning, and proactive community training is an overall strategy for emergency preparedness, which fortifies the platform for long-term resilience in the face of adversity (Figure 13.5).

13.2.1. Risk Assessment and Hazard Identification

Effective hazard identification and risk assessment are at the heart of enhancing emergency preparedness as well as community resilience. Through the systematic evaluation of potential threats from natural and man-made hazards, communities can identify vulnerabilities within their infrastructure and population. This keeps them from acting impulsively with resources and asking for mitigation responses without identifying specific risks. For example, detailed mapping of flood or earthquake-risk zones allows for more effective urban planning and resource allocation. Communities with complete hazard data are also able to communicate effectively about risk and are more likely to promote individual preparation activities as supplements to larger community schemes. The application of ICT significantly enhances risk-assessment and hazard-detection systems. Through the use of mobile networks, social media, and data analysis, release of key information and real-time monitoring are facilitated, which transforms the way that communities respond to risks. Specifically, early warning systems are a good illustration of this transformation using an array of hazard warnings, risk estimates, and communication channels allowing for residents to respond in a timely manner. These systems are not only vital for delivering key information in a crisis situation but also create an informed citizen that makes decisions conducive to general community resilience. With communities increasingly making use of digital platforms, the deployment and establishment of such technology is integral to risk management impact. Furthermore, the evolving nature of digital technology holds a pivotal role in reshaping traditional power dynamics involved in emergency preparedness. By facilitating interoperable data exchange via semantic technologies, decision-making stakeholders at every level can be simultaneously made available with pertinent data, thus decentralizing the decision-making process. This access promotes an open environment in which communities are able to engage in collective response and planning, representing a shift towards more participatory models of governance. Interdisciplinary coordination is highlighted in conference deliberations on climate change and disaster impact reduction, for instance, the UK – South Asia Young Scientists and Practitioners Seminar on Climate Change and Disaster Impact Reduction conference in 2008, which highlighted the need to integrate technological advancement in risk analysis frameworks (Aryal et al., 2008). Lastly, enhanced risk estimation and hazard identification with the help of advanced technology must be achieved to build resilient communities that are more equipped to handle future issues.

13.2.2. Emergency Response Planning

Effective emergency planning is needed for communities facing the emerging danger of natural hazards. Urban areas are also experiencing rising threats, particularly floods, with far-reaching implications for urban governance in the face of climate change. For example, comparative studies of research in Toronto and Calgary have highlighted differences in responses during floods and emphasized the need for comprehensive strategies involving structural and non-structural methods. Such planning involves the development of policies, public participation, and decision-making structures that facilitate collaborative efforts by government institutions, non-governmental institutions, and the broader population. Through the mitigation of weaknesses and uncertainties, cities can enhance resilience to the impacts of floods through interventions like preparedness packages, live flood maps, and permeable surfaces, eventually culminating into an efficient emergency response system (Asrat et al., 2015). Coordination of multiple stakeholders' opinions in emergency response planning highly increases community resilience. Involvement of the public in emergency preparedness fosters a culture of mutual responsibility, which is crucial for the effective mitigation of risks. Research has established that the shift to a more participative method from isolationist emergency management can empower society to deal with disasters more efficiently. For instance, the UK emergency management system encourages an outward orientation with all stakeholders participating in the process of social learning, thereby making society more resilient. Involving citizens in drills, training, and policy-making not only makes them aware of potential dangers but also allows them to contribute actively to their community's safety and recovery strategies (O'Brien et al., 2008).

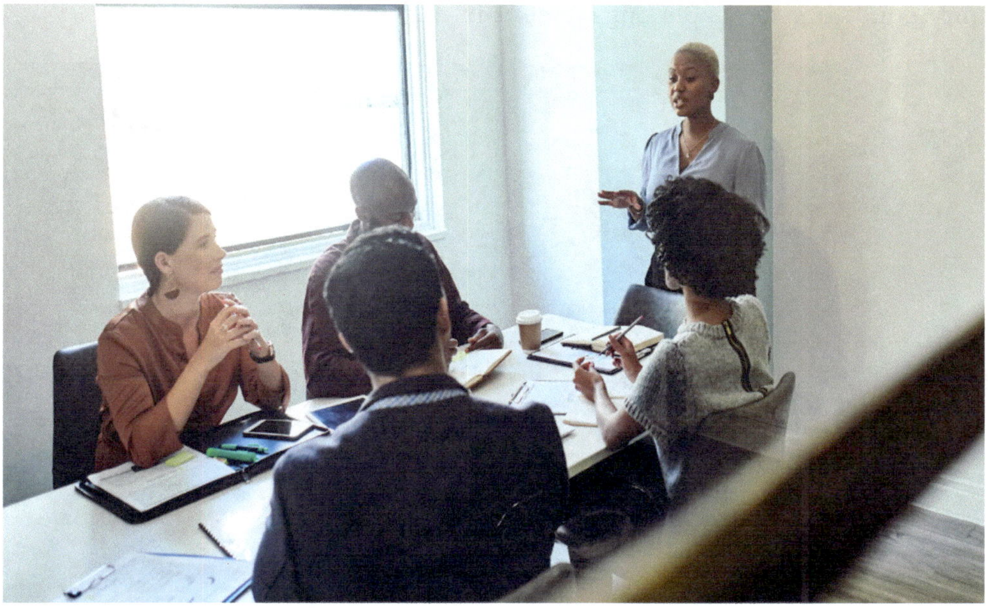

Figure 13.6. Emergency response planning.

Source: https://www.alertmedia.com/wp-content/uploads/2023/10/Blog-Emergency-Response-Plan.webp.

Continuous education and awareness schemes are also critical components of effective emergency response planning. Implementing measures that prepare the public about the realities of climate threats allows communities to pre-adapt to potential catastrophes. For instance, the residents can know how to identify warning signs, know the evacuations routes, and make proper use of available resources in times of emergencies. Research indicates that effective communication measures along with pre-emergency preparedness can greatly enhance community capacity to respond quickly and effectively to disasters. In general, cultivating a culture of preparedness equips communities with the knowledge and gear necessary to mitigate threats and raise overall resilience to escalating environmental threats, most significantly by flooding (Asrat et al., 2015; O'Brien et al., 2008) (Figure 13.6).

13.2.3. Training and Education for Community Members

Training and education for community members form the pillars upon which emergency preparedness and resilience programs are constructed. A community's resilience and capability to recover from disasters is very high if its citizens are endowed with the appropriate knowledge and skills. The programs are aimed at educating individuals in first aid, emergency response planning, and mitigation measures that directly influence their environments. Programs tailored for community needs enhance a sense of responsibility within a community and enable residents to respond proactively during a disaster. For instance, training individuals to prepare communities for resilience doesn't merely prepare the individual but also improves social networks and creates a more cohesive and proactive community that can better withstand crises (Bromley et al., 2017). The Los Angeles County Community Disaster Resilience (LACCDR) program is one such illustration of best practices for training methodology. This initiative engaged the expertise of public health nurses and community educators to enable engagement in multiple coalitions.

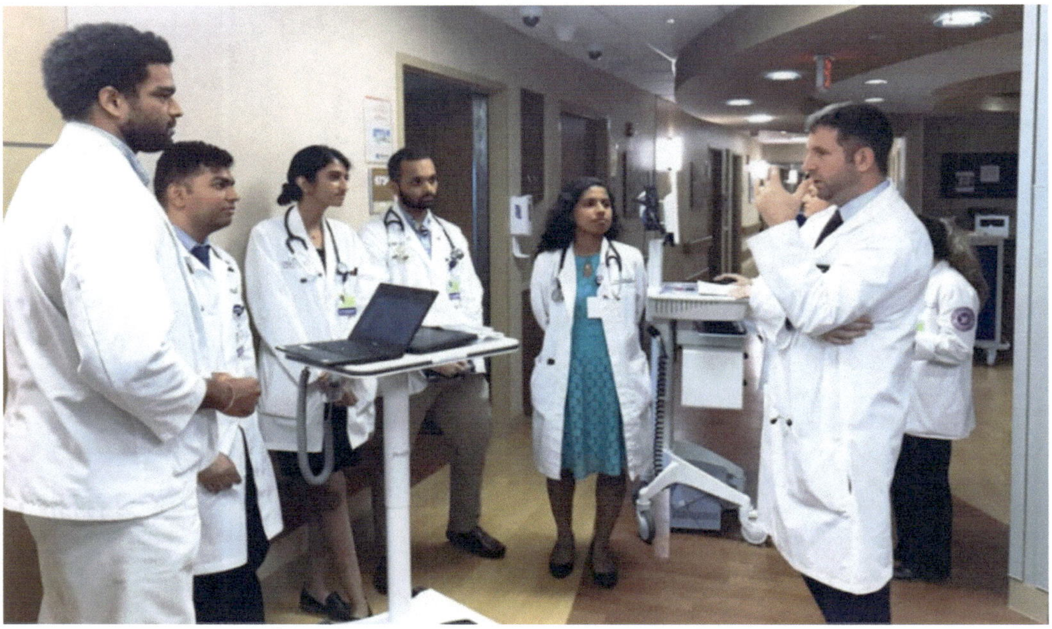

Figure 13.7. Training and education for community members.

Source: https://s3-prod.modernhealthcare.com/s3fs-public/styles/width_792/public/Memorial-Healthcare-System-edit.jpg.

By applying participatory methodologies, the program underscored the essential process of mutual learning in which the facilitators and members of the community were able to exchange experiences and share ideas. This allowed for greater levels of comprehension among participants about principles of resilience as well as operationalizing major levers like partnership and self-sufficiency. These strategies not only emphasized the incorporation of resilience measures into the community framework but also guaranteed an assurance of ongoing learning, emphasizing the critical incorporation of the voice of the community in crafting resilient measures to address emergencies (Bromley et al., 2017). Moreover, education frameworks constructed in accordance with international policies, such as the Hyogo Framework for Action (HFA), further emphasize the criticality of training in the reduction of disaster risks. The HFA emphasizes the role of the integration of education, innovation, and knowledge in the establishment of a culture of safety and resilience in all tiers of society. There are, however, differences in effective application of these training programs, particularly in higher learning institutions where future leaders are trained. The deficiency should be filled because effective disaster resilience education resonates with the principles of sustainability and empowerment for everyone, hence placing communities in a better position to contend with impending disasters. Along with the identified knowledge gaps, recommending integrated educational strategies will reinforce community capacity, enabling emergency preparedness to be an honored civic responsibility (Figure 13.7).

13.3. Role of Government in Emergency Preparedness

In emergency preparedness, the role of the government is pivotal in formulating frameworks that enhance community resilience. Effective emergency management is not only the coordination of resources in emergencies but also requires a pre-emptive process that addresses the threats that are imminent prior to these events taking place. This pre-emptive focus requires engagement with a cross-section of stakeholders, from members of the public through local organizations to private sectors. This partnership enhances planning in a way that it is now achievable to value risks from natural disasters and climate change more. Notably, there is movement towards inclusive pre-emergency planning that can demobilize the internal focus that typically limits UK emergency management, allowing for public preparedness and society resilience (O'Brien et al., 2008). Based on the need for multi-stakeholder engagement, government intervention is called upon to establish the concept of sectoral community resilience. Governments have a key role to play in actualizing resilience policy while clarifying the responsibility and roles of stakeholders. The complexity of risk assessment poses an intimidating challenge, particularly in addressing low probability-high impact events. This communication barrier can be slow in achieving effective readiness and become difficult in risk prioritization in situations where resources are limited. Through recent studies, an integrated process of stakeholder engagement can facilitate greater understanding and participation and contribute to enhanced emergency planning and action at the community level (Adekola et al., 2020). Furthermore, government agencies must cultivate a culture that views resilience-building as an ongoing process rather than an after-the-fact response. Such cultural change must involve regular training and education initiatives for both citizens and officials, emphasizing the importance of readiness in day-to-day life. Government leadership for such efforts can serve to significantly influence public mind-set and enable active community involvement in building resilience. By instilling an environment in which citizens feel empowered to make a contribution to readiness initiatives, the government can actually enhance overall community resilience. Finally, by integrating a forward-looking approach of collaborative planning, learning, and managing resources, communities will be better able to absorb, recover from, and deal with disasters while strengthening social cohesion in the process (O'Brien et al., 2008).

13.3.1. Federal, State, and Local Government Responsibilities

Effective emergency preparedness relies on intergovernmental cooperation with the federal, state, and local governments each playing distinctive but interconnected roles in developing community resilience. Federal government agencies such as the FEMA formulate overall policy at the federal level and provide funding support for disaster response, mitigation, and recovery operations. The Federal government also formulates national strategies for enhancing disaster resilience, as contained in the National Strategy for Disaster Resilience proposals. Such regulations offer a framework for cooperative work at various levels of government, depicting the importance of having a shared approach towards emergency management through coordinated resources and goals. As global warming and extreme weather events become more common, the importance of federal guidelines to influence forward-thinking approaches cannot be emphasized enough, emphasizing the importance these agencies hold in enabling communities to prepare against likely disruptions efficiently (Bergin et al., 2014). State governments are instrumental in transforming federal policies into practical programs designed to meet the specific requirements of their jurisdictions. They implement certain disaster management regulations that govern the organization and conduct of readiness preparations throughout the state. These include establishing the appropriate training, conducting risk assessment, and conducting statewide drills to enhance readiness levels throughout local communities. Importantly, state governments also support local governments by making necessary resources and technical assistance available, keeping municipal and county agencies in readiness to respond to disasters efficiently. These state-local government relationships foster a partnership culture and sense of shared responsibility where local governments take ownership of the disaster planning process in their jurisdictions. State agencies are therefore part of the emergency preparedness system, establishing a robust support system that enhances total community resilience (Bajracharya et al., 2010). Local governments themselves tend to be the first line of responders in case of emergencies, hence their role being crucial in fostering community resilience. Having direct access to citizens, local institutions stand to respond by putting disaster preparedness measures in place that are specifically tailored for their people—be it through community education, allocation of resources, or building resilient infrastructure. Their involvement tends to mean greater community awareness and involvement in disaster preparation initiatives. Subnational authorities adopt policies and principles that not only reflect national mandates but also define local threats and demands, and create tailor-made solutions to address emerging risks. However, there are problems of taking such policies into effective practice, as noted in studies into local government responses to documented disaster management policies. Local identification of and addressing implementation hurdles ensures that local institutions are in a position to effectively contribute to a community's overall resilience, supporting further the necessity of proper communication and coordination among all levels of government (Bajracharya et al., 2010).

13.3.2. Funding and Resources for Emergency Management

Adequate funding and resource allocation are critical to assist in enhancing emergency management and, by association, community resilience. Increasing frequency and severity of natural disasters necessitate an initial outlay in readiness initiatives that can enhance local capacity. Both regional and national governments must prioritize funding emergency management programs. That includes not only budgetary expenditure but also the fact that these are utilized in comprehensive training and infrastructure investments. When communities are well-funded, they are better placed to conduct risk assessment and preparedness. This creates a virtuous circle, as greater preparation leads to a greater perceived resilience within the community, which is important during emergencies. By adopting a multi-dimensioned financing approach, the stakeholders can better enable the sustained development of community resilience policies and guarantee equitable allocation of resources among diverse demographic and geographical populations (Adekola et al., 2020). Further, acknowledging interdependence among the various stakeholder groups supports maximizing resource utilization in emergency management systems. Coordination between local governments, non-profit groups, and private organizations can compound the effects of funding and provide a more integrated way of building disaster resilience. For example, money can be used for collaborative training exercises that unite stakeholders from different segments, building relationships that are crucial during actual emergencies. Breaking down communications barriers and perceptions of risk differences among stakeholders can create a more integrated emergency response plan. Such partnerships become essential as communities face low probability-high consequence events, when communication and coordination issues could daunt rapid response. Overcoming such issues is essential in order to enable the formation of an integrated support system, strengthening community resilience by empowering well-resourced and well-managed resources (Bergin et al., 2014). Strategic deployment of emergency management resources must also be aligned with long-term resilience aims. While projections indicate that the economic impacts of natural disasters will soar, governments have to establish strategic plans that target sustainable sources of funding. Initiatives such as hazard mitigation schemes, public awareness, and infrastructure improvement all require stable financial commitments spanning multiple fiscal cycles. Additionally, leveraging federal and state sources of funding can enhance local capacities so that communities are able to adapt and recover more efficiently. By setting priorities and allocating finance to resilience objectives, the community will be better placed to tackle challenges of increasing disaster risks. In this sense, a proactive funding strategy can develop a culture of preparedness, which ultimately leads to a collective improvement in communities' overall resilience to impending crises (Bergin et al., 2014) (Figure 13.8).

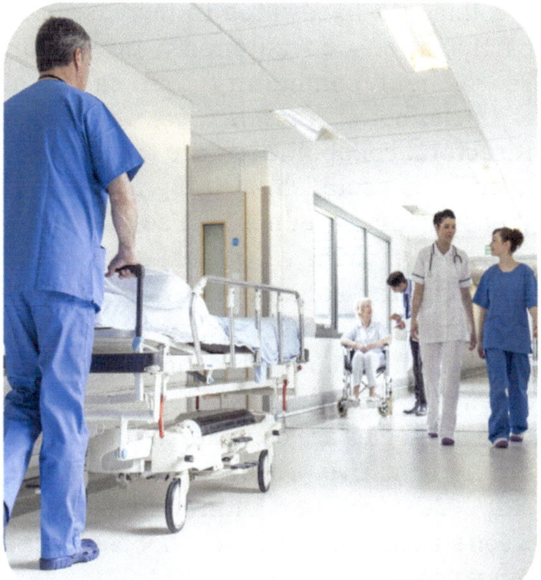

Figure 13.8. Funding and resources for emergency management.

Source: https://www.medxcel.com/getattachment/Resources/Expert-Advice/Funding-a-First-Class-Emergency-Management-Program/Funding-a-First-Class-Emergency-Response-Program-Blog-Graphic_Graphic.png.

13.3.3. Collaboration with Non-Governmental Organizations (NGOs)

Effective collaboration with NGOs is also important in establishing emergency preparedness as well as community resilience. NGOs possess unique strengths including local knowledge, existing trust among communities, and specialized skills in areas of health, disaster response, and social services. By these strengths, government and emergency management organizations can better tailor their policies to the requirements of populations with differences, particularly vulnerable populations who are more likely to be at risk during disasters. One example of this nature is seen through the LACCDR program, where collaborative partnerships were fostered between government agencies, community groups, and residents. This collaboration resulted in increased levels of participation and autonomy, developing a more resilient community that can handle emergencies better (Bromley et al., 2017). These multisectoral collaborations are the strength of teamwork in establishing integrated systems of disaster preparedness. Also, developing good relations with NGOs makes it possible to have greater community participation in building resilience. Involvement of community members in the planning and implementation of emergency preparedness strategies guarantees that the strategies are contextually relevant and culturally sensitive. Through having multiple voices, NGOs facilitate bidirectional learning between stakeholders with room for feedback and modification of strategies that cannot function in particular contexts. By making commitments to resilience principles, NGOs help mobilize community assets and resources. For instance, how the members of the coalition in the LACCDR initiative engaged vulnerable group members in resilience training brought to the forefront the importance of the role that tailored education and outreach measures play in enhancing the awareness and preparedness of communities (Bromley et al., 2017). Such a community arrangement makes it possible for communities to address disaster risk management proactively. Besides, the cooperative relationship between the government and NGOs addresses the multifaceted nature of disasters and the roles that the various actors should play in emergency management systems. With increased climatic uncertainty and increased threats from natural disasters, good governance is vital. FEMS, for example, have been studied in Europe, with varying success in integrating community preparation into the systems. Where NGOs are engaged, coordination and cooperation between actors operating towards flood resilience are improved. By incorporating lessons from NGOs' operating experiences, including people-centered processes of recovery and institutional learning, emergency management systems improve. The synergy of collaboration not only prepares communities for shock absorption but also long-term resilience through improved communal cohesion and resource networks.

13.4. Community Engagement and Involvement

Community involvement and engagement are essential factors in establishing emergency preparedness and community resilience. Active participation by members of the community in disaster planning and response initiatives may lead to more effective and tailored strategies that accommodate the specific needs and circumstances of local communities. Engaging residents not only produces a feeling of ownership of disaster preparedness activities but also allows mobilization of local resources. Public involvement in the development of emergency management plans produces strategies that not only happen to be pragmatic but are culturally sensitive as well. This participatory approach has been seen to significantly increase institutional trust between communities and enhance collaboration in times of emergencies, building a support system that becomes invaluable in times of disaster. The importance of community participation in effective disaster response is further highlighted by the need for participative communication channels. Studies highlight that societies with open and diverse channels of communication—e.g., town hall meetings, social networking websites, and multicultural media—are better able to pass on essential information in times of crisis.

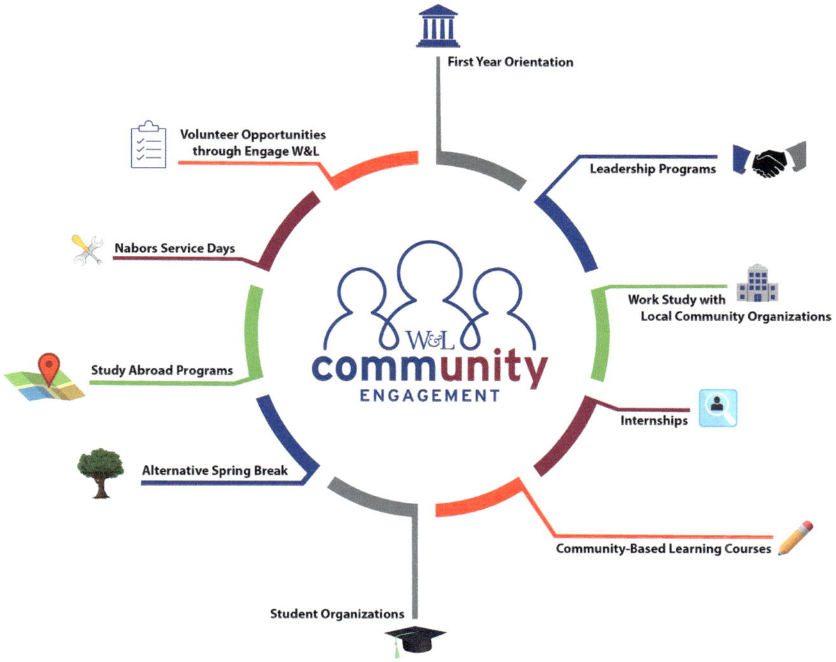

Figure 13.9. Community engagement and involvement.

Source: https://s3.amazonaws.com/assets1.wlu.edu/files/resources/cbl-graphic-no-2.png.

In addition, frequent interaction strengthens the ties between members of the society and therefore builds a shared identity that increases social solidarity. In cases of flooding and other disasters, pre-emptive release of information not only sensitizes people but also educates residents on how to take timely life-saving measures. This is in accordance with the notion that informed and participatory communities are far more resistant to adverse impacts of emergencies, as noted in analysis evaluating community responses to climatic variation and associated risks (Amaratunga et al., 2013a; Amaratunga et al., 2013b). In addition, community-based interventions can be a catalyst for building long-term resilience by the establishment of adaptive capacities among local populations. Through participatory workshops and simulations, individuals gain hands-on experience in emergency management and preparedness, reducing dependency on external aid. Programs of this type can benefit the poor by imparting to them knowledge and means that enhance their autonomy during crises. Furthermore, inter-organization collaboration with the government and citizens is the foundation of sustained community participation. Through stakeholder integration, collaborations can mobilize various types of expertise and resources, thereby constructing a community's resilience to face future crises. Overall, synergy enhanced through community participation not only enhances immediate responses but also lays the foundation for long-term resilience in case of unavoidable future problems (Figure 13.9).

13.4.1. Importance of Community Participation in Preparedness

Community participation is at the heart of enhanced emergency preparedness because it fosters a partnership environment where various perspectives and resources converge. Engaging individuals from the community not only empowers individuals to take responsibility for their security but also guarantees that critical information regarding potential threats and countermeasures reaches the people. Initiatives that utilize local knowledge and resources, such as the LACCDR program, demonstrate the efficacy of bottom-up efforts. With the facilitation of the government agencies, organizations, and residents in an organized manner, the LACCDR successfully executed resilience principles that boosted overall community preparedness, demonstrating that bidirectional learning and recolonization among stakeholders maximize preparedness processes (Bromley et al., 2017).

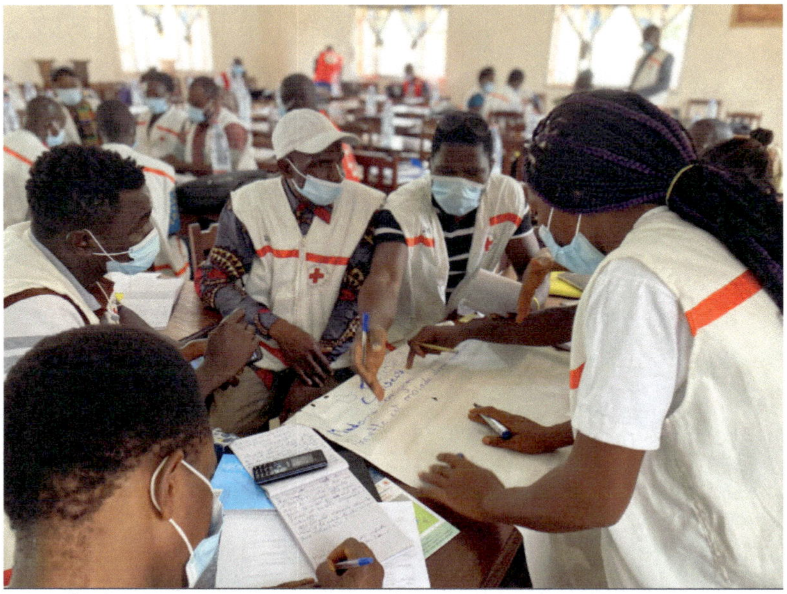

Figure 13.10. Importance of community participation in preparedness.

Source: https://preparecenter.org/wp-content/uploads/2023/01/Red-Cross-volunteers-receive-community-engagement-and-accountability-training-scaled.jpeg.

Integrating community participation in preparedness initiatives is more than just information sharing; it evokes a spirit of community and reciprocal responsibility among citizens. If individuals are motivated to engage proactively in conversation and choice-making regarding risk management, they are likely to understand the impacts of their decisions and contribute participatory efforts to community resilience. Furthermore, such an inclusive approach promotes equity by ensuring marginalized groups are included and matters of access to resources and support are considered. As evidenced in the LACCDR results, intervention efforts that include vulnerable groups can enhance equitable distribution of resources and support, hence enhancing community resilience (Bromley et al., 2017). In addition, the global perspective in terms of people's participation in preparedness highlights its ability to reverse the devastating effects of disasters. Global practice, i.e., what happened due to Typhoon Haiyan in the Philippines, testifies to the need for preventive measures in vulnerable areas. Investing in community readiness is not only an ethical imperative but also an economic investment, for every dollar spent on prevention having the potential to save multiple dollars in response cost. By making it easier for international partnership and sharing of information and knowledge in disaster management, communities everywhere can build up the competencies and infrastructures necessary to enhance their capacity to withstand future disasters. Hence, involvement by the community is an important aspect in weaving a cloth of preparedness that is robust and effective in dealing with the complex dynamics of emergency conditions (Figure 13.10).

13.4.2. Strategies for Effective Community Outreach

Successful community outreach strategies are critical in making emergency preparedness and overall community resilience. One of the key strategies is the establishment of multi-sector alliances that facilitate collaboration between the various stakeholders, including government agencies, non-profit groups, and communities. One such example is the Los Angeles County Community Disaster Resilience program, where coalitions of community players and organizations came together to apply the principles of resilience. Via participatory community practice, these coalitions engaged residents in two-way learning, not only informing them about preparedness but also allowing them to share useful insights and experiences. Such a sharing increases the stakeholders' trust and cooperation, with the principles of resilience being integrated into community practice successfully, hence augmenting the ability of the community to prepare more effectively against emergencies (Bromley et al., 2017). The second equally important strategy of effective outreach is the focus on self-sufficiency and education on a community level. Programs that give highest importance to educating residents about indigenous threats as well as the importance of readiness have an informed citizenry ready and capable of making proactive actions during emergencies. The practice of education may take the form of workshops, seminars, and distributing materials as per the special requirements of the community. Furthermore, such emphasis on knowledge sharing can lead to increased self-sufficiency since individuals are better able to prevent danger and respond effectively in the event of an emergency. When communities are empowered through knowledge, they not only build resilience but also create a culture of preparedness that encourages individuals to act collectively in times of crisis (N/A, 2011). The use of social media websites and technology in public participation has proved to be an efficient approach in emergency preparedness.

Through digital tools, information dissemination and communication in real time are provided, bridging the gaps between organizations and residents. Social media can also serve as a platform for live coverage, learning, and community engagement activities so the wider population will be informed and a sense of community will be felt by the residents, particularly during emergencies. In addition, such online platforms can also facilitate feedback mechanisms whereby the local leaders can identify community concerns and vary outreach accordingly. With technology being used, communities can amplify their outreach so that preparedness information is disseminated and tailored to meet the heterogenous needs of the populace. Thus, integration of technology can not only augment outreach efforts but also enhance the general resilience of communities in times of emergencies (Bromley et al., 2017).

13.4.3. Building Trust and Communication Among Residents

Good community communication lies at the center of emergency resilience. Residents who are engaged and informed tend to contribute to active measures, and this fosters a culture of preparedness. Trust-building among members of the community facilitates this communication, as citizens become more inclined to speak up and suggest solutions if they feel that they are being heard. The Living in Queensland Survey reflects the importance of residents' risk perception and capacity within a community, with enhanced communication augmenting a community action towards disaster preparedness. The survey evidently indicates that government and community trust has changed following crisis, demonstrating that more resilient communities are the ones that prioritize open communication and community learning processes among citizens (Antrobus et al., 2013). Moreover, establishing dependable relations extends beyond community relations; it also includes strong relations with local authorities and institutions.

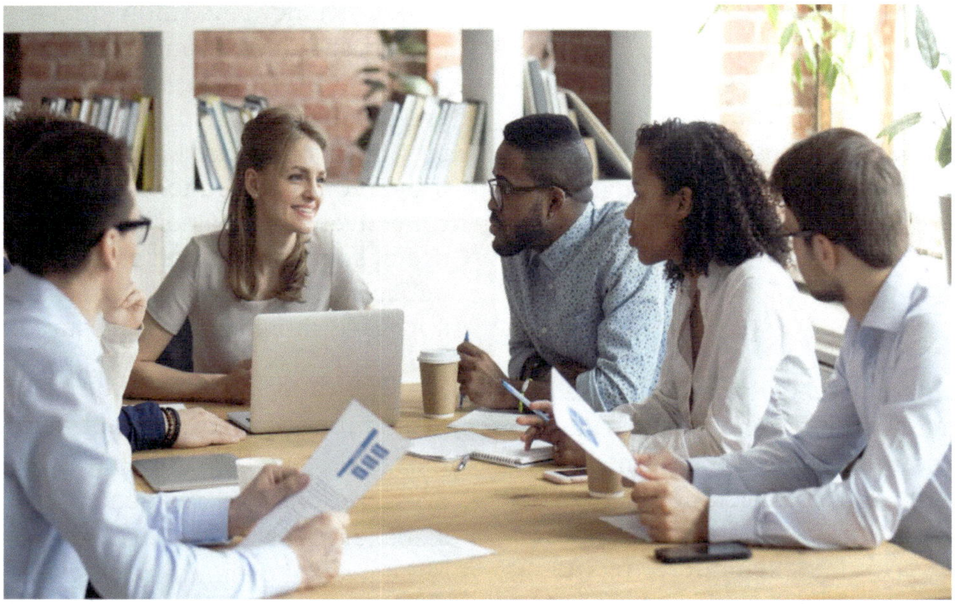

Figure 13.11. Building trust and communication among residents.

Source: https://trainingindustry.com/content/uploads/2019/07/Building-Trust-and-Improving-Communication-7.9.19.jpg.

Relations of local residents with local authorities are of the greatest importance in attaining a concerted emergency planning strategy. As is evident in comparative cases of flood-risk neighborhoods, effective management of the threats, including proactive measures for communications, is of vital importance in minimizing vulnerability. In the settings whose interagency collaboration is strong, like with the Edeytsys model, residents are also more assured regarding flood control and support mechanisms. The trust ensures that members of the public engage more in preparedness activities, an aspect that not only enhances resilience but also facilitates swift collective response to disaster situations, which, in effect, proves that strong communication lines have a direct correlation with improved emergency situation outcomes (Kontar et al., 2017). Moreover, creating avenues for open communication can facilitate overcoming generational and socioeconomic barriers within communities. Different groups are likely to have varying access to resources and information that can impede collective preparedness work. By leveraging community forums, workshops, and social media, local leaders can make certain that all citizens have important information on emergency preparedness. Such activities need to be crafted so as to create an enabling environment in which everyone feels empowered to contribute. As the Queensland survey indicates, increased awareness and understanding lead to better preparedness behaviors. Through participation in forums and programs, residents build confidence not only with their community members but also with the mechanisms in place to protect them. Such cooperative engagement strengthens interpersonal ties in the community and enhances disaster resilience in the future, demonstrating that communication and trust are crucial factors in building a more prepared society (Antrobus et al., 2013) (Figure 13.11).

13.5. Technology and Innovation in Emergency Preparedness

The use of technology and innovation in emergency preparedness has a revolutionizing potential that maximizes community resilience to disasters. As global warming enhances the frequency and intensity of weather-related events, societies are compelled to devise sophisticated strategies that utilize sophisticated technology. For instance, geographic information systems (GIS) can assist in mapping regions requiring mitigation such that disaster relief preparation is simplified and resources are easily distributed. Additionally, mobile applications have the potential to improve engagement between emergency service providers and civilians to give timely information and updates during an emergency. As noted by N/A (2017), the impact of climate change on water management and public health presents the value of incorporating these technologies in emergency response programs. By using data analytics for predictive modeling, communities can instill a culture of preparedness, thereby saving lives and property. Moreover, the incorporation of state-of-the-art technologies in education provides an essential route towards building a resolute community, particularly for disaster risk reduction. School can serve as a vehicle for the dissemination of information on emergency preparedness through integrated curricula that embrace cutting-edge technology. The Hyogo Framework for Action (HFA) highlights that it is essential to foster safety and culture of resilience at all levels of society, which could be achieved through disaster management education (Adeniyi et al., 2014). It not only enhances personal preparedness but also incites community engagement through awareness regarding the threats of disasters. Lastly, integrating technology in educational systems equips future generations with the competencies and knowledge required to address the complexities associated with upcoming threats. Finally, integration of government agencies, non-profit organizations, and the private sector is essential in propelling technology-driven solutions for emergency preparedness. Such a multi-factorial effort promotes sharing of resources and utilizing the specialization within sectors towards creating comprehensive strategies for disaster management. Through partnerships, the stakeholders can explore new technologies such as drones for aerial mapping, artificial intelligence for real-time analysis, and social media for outreach. Through such partnerships, the effectiveness of emergency plans can be significantly improved, as is evident through effective models all over the world. As populations are beset with increasingly sophisticated challenges brought on by climate change and changing threats, the merging of technology and innovation becomes a pillar of strength, informing overall efforts to promote safety and well-being for all citizens (Figure 13.12).

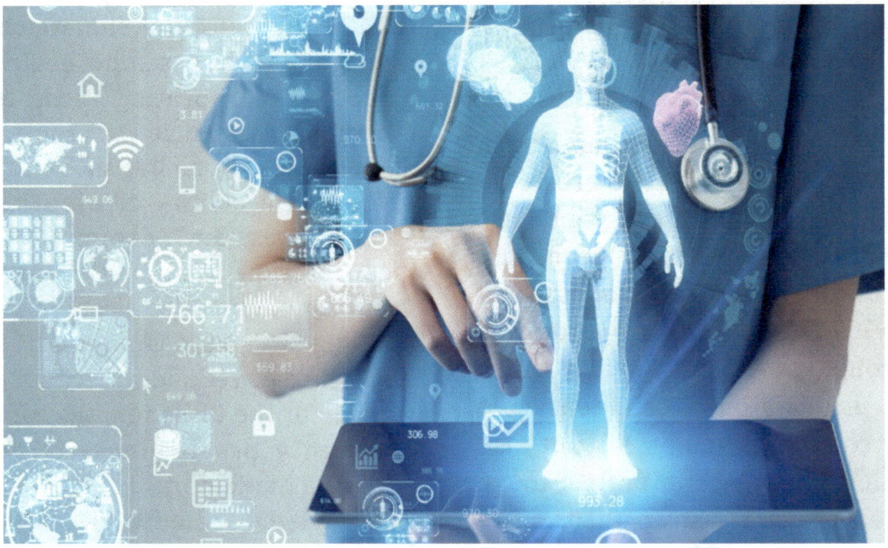

Figure 13.12. Technology and innovation in emergency preparedness.

Source: https://www.trendyonlinesolution.in/wp-content/uploads/2022/05/Benefits-of-Digital-Technology-in-Healthcare.jpg.

13.5.1. Use of Social Media for Information Dissemination

Social media has, in recent years, emerged as a key platform for information dissemination during emergencies, and it has significantly enhanced community resilience. The accessibility and velocity of platforms such as Twitter, Facebook, and Instagram have facilitated information to be disseminated easily by individuals and institutions on a timely basis. This makes a well-informed citizenry that is able to respond rapidly to emerging events. In addition, these sites make it possible to distribute widely safety advice, up-to-the-minute information, and alerts that can go far beyond geographical boundaries. Social media enables a twin-channel strategy where authorities convey messages to the public while at the same time allowing members of the community to post their own experiences, worries, and observations. All such interactions contribute to building an adaptive society in a position to mobilize solidarity and resources during emergencies, thereby transforming traditional methods of emergency communication and preparedness (Amaratunga et al., 2015). Secondly, the capacity of social media to disrupt traditional power relations in communication cannot be exaggerated. Social media, through information democratization of access, empowers individuals and societies to participate in decision-making related to their safety. In times of crisis, real-time information sharing minimizes reliance on centralized bodies and encourages a culture of risk management by citizens. Social media user-generated content is an important source of local knowledge and experience that might not always be reflected in official bulletins and warnings. With the youth around the globe having become more and more accustomed to using social media as the predominant medium of communication, the trend most likely enhances the spread and scope of emergency messages, further enhancing community resilience (Amaratunga et al., 2015). Its ability to tailor emergency messages for multitudes using social media is key in encouraging inclusive disaster preparedness approaches. Targeted communication campaigns can factor in various demographic segments such as gender and age so that the vulnerable segments are reached with appropriate information. Communication within segments of society through social media also offers a chance to encourage gender equality because men and women consume and interpret information in varying ways. By engaging with social media, organizations can develop specific measures to empower women and other vulnerable groups to become active participants in their community's resilience process. Lastly, strategic use of social media for information dissemination during emergencies not only enhances real-time response but also long-term community resilience (Amaratunga et al., 2015).

13.5.2. Advancements in Emergency Alert Systems

The recent advancements in emergency alert systems have significantly boosted community preparedness and resilience. The incorporation of multi-channel communication methods enables alerts to better reach multicultural communities by using text messaging, social media, and conventional media. This multi-channel framework not only enables a better possibility of information exchange during emergencies, but also facilitates access for the people with varied needs. For example, existing systems pay greater attention to visual warnings for the deaf and language localization, expanding the audience and mitigating potential dangers at the time of disasters. These accomplishments underscore the importance of inclusive planning that can facilitate a safety culture and culture of awareness for communities and, in turn, enhance their ability to respond to emergencies appropriately.

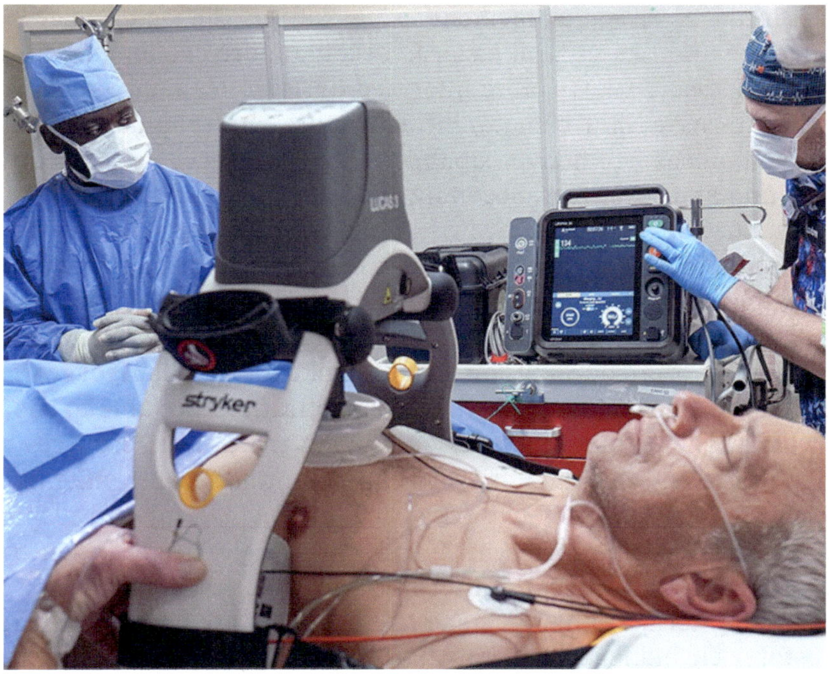

Figure 13.13. Advancements in emergency alert systems.

Source: https://media-assets.stryker.com/is/image/stryker/Hospital_Solutions_Product_Lifestyle_440x350?max_width_1440.

Accompanying technological advance is the transition in methods of emergency management which marks a historic shift in disaster preparedness at the community level. Development of the emergency management life cycle supports proactive methodologies through resilience and mitigation over mere response. Paradigm shift is necessary because it seeks to address strategies in a holistic manner and consider the involvement and participation of communities during the planning of disaster preparedness. Through simulation exercises and training, societies can establish the foundation for collective knowledge and resources to become more prepared. Furthermore, as Bennett et al. (2016) notes, there is increasing realization of the social, cultural, and political determinants of community responses, implying that successful preparedness initiatives must tackle these dimensions holistically in order to be effective. Nevertheless, the technological advance of emergency alert systems is fraught with challenges. Federal, state, and local budget limitations can make such programs less viable, as described in recent public health analyses (N/A, 2011). Budget cuts to emergency preparedness budgets disenable continued improvement in alert systems with the possibility of their effectiveness being reduced. Moreover, ensuring all community members, especially vulnerable populations, receive timely and accurate information remains an overreaching challenge. Ongoing investment in infrastructure, training, and technology is essential to keep up with resilience in the face of ever more natural and man-made catastrophes. Although societies try to integrate advanced alert systems, firm commitment to sustained funding and resources cannot be overstressed to provide a successful emergency preparedness climate (Figure 13.13).

13.5.3. Role of Data Analytics in Risk Management

Data analysis is essential to risk management, especially in the emergency preparedness and community resilience function. As natural hazards become more challenging for communities, the ability to analyze large datasets allows more informed decision-making. Sophisticated analysis can identify trends and patterns within climate, infrastructure, and population data. This combined framework not only enhances predictive capability but also serves to identify weak links that require immediate action and resources. Secondly, the integration of data analytics into emergency management infrastructure enables proactive risk reduction. Through the understanding of threats through rigorous analysis of data, communities can devise solutions that address specifically immediate and long-term threats, thereby enhancing their resilience and capacity to manage emergencies (Dunaway et al., 2017). Further, bringing together data analytics with the concept of risk management enhances the coordination among stakeholders like governments, non-profits, and communities. Through sharing data insights, such institutions are able to coordinate responses more effectively in emergency situations, thus optimizing the use of resources during crises. For instance, applying IoT data and live data analysis can potentially lead to intelligent infrastructure planning. Through this means, societies will be able to better plan for and respond to unexpected events, such as floods or heavy storms, which are increasingly being driven by climate change. Emphasizing data collection and interpretation not only aids in prompt response in emergency situations but also in long-term resilience plans to build capacity and sustainability (N/A, 2017). Data analytics use for risk management equally extends beyond the limitations of immediate response endeavors to encompass long-term public safety agendas. By applying advanced data analysis techniques, communities are able to simulate various emergency scenarios such that the leaders can develop effective contingency plans and procedures. The preparedness component makes the community members not only knowledgeable but also prepared to handle emergencies.

Continuous refinement of such models in accordance with the actual outcomes creates a cycle of improvement and adjustment that is critical under the influence of ever-changing environmental conditions. Finally, the best use of data analytics empowers communities to navigate through complexity created by crises, bolstering their ability to recover quickly and maintain social cohesion following disasters and, in the process, boost overall resilience at the community level (Dunaway et al., 2017) (Figure 13.14).

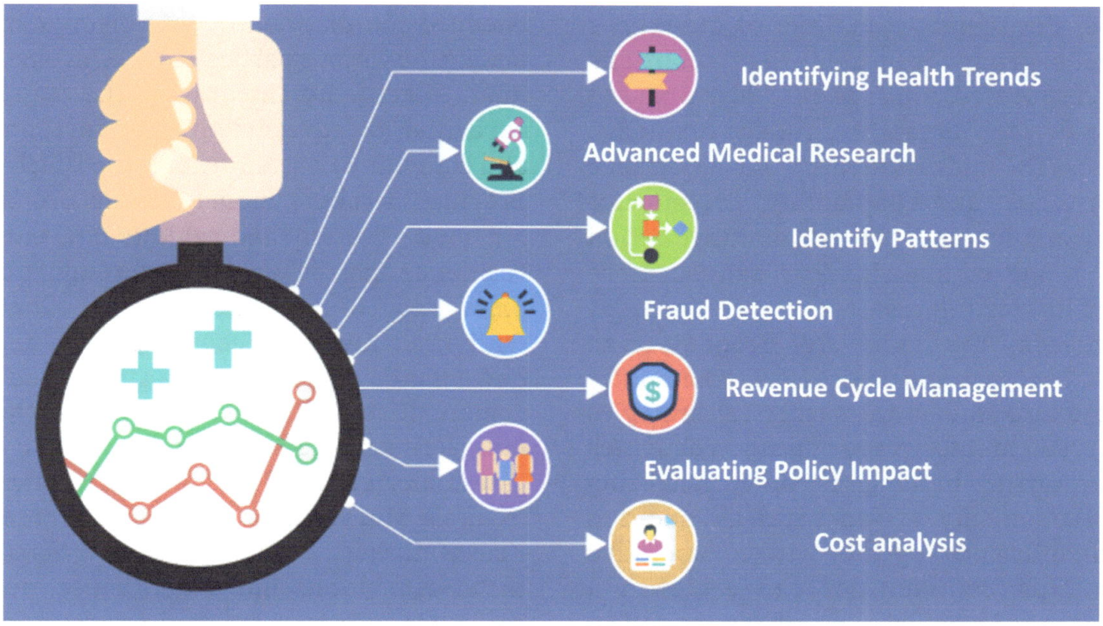

Figure 13.14. Role of data analytics in risk management.

Source: https://assets-global.website-files.com/634fa785d369cb60d80b6dd1/6439012643aa956a743a4760_Data%20Analytics%20Healthcare-4.webp.

13.6. Case Studies of Successful Community Resilience

Case studies of successful community resilience tell us a lot about the way that local areas can mitigate the impacts of disasters. For instance, those that have implemented Community Managed Disaster Risk Reduction (CMDRR) strategies have managed in some way to reduce climate change-related vulnerabilities. These systems draw on existing local capacities and knowledge, allowing communities to assess risks and develop tailor-made preparedness plans. These actions showcase not just a response to immediate threats but also an ongoing attempt to build resilience against coming harm. The urgency of climate-related issues makes CMDRR a necessity, since many communities remain open to increased risk due to inaction at the international level, as per N/A (2009). This case shows that community resilience has its foundation in active participation and grassroots empowerment. A good example of a well-functioning community resilience is the LACCDR program. This initiative, founded on the principles of community resilience, aims to build stronger partnerships among government agencies, local organizations, and residents through participatory methods. By randomizing 16 coalitions to either the Enhanced Standard Preparedness or Community Resilience approach for 24 months, the program facilitated a robust comparison of methodology. To their surprise, the thematic analysis of interviews and focus groups revealed that coalitions that incorporated bidirectional learning not only knew but actually applied resilience principles. The findings identify the importance of involvement and adaptability in resilience planning and forecast that collaborative action from a range of stakeholders can be more resilient in tackling disaster preparedness, as highlighted by the findings of Bromley et al. (2017). Through the successful community resilience case studies, the successful strategies are observed to interweave education activities with partnership building. By operationalizing levers of community resilience such as education and self-sufficiency together with collaborative partnerships, communities can establish a proactive and reactive web of support. The LACCDR initiative is used to demonstrate this, since coalitions were tested and finally achieved commitments to the principles of resilience through mutually reinforcing strategies. All these collective efforts demonstrate that resilience is not just a question of resource but also social solidarity and mutual support solidarity among the population. Through establishing these ties and carrying out integrative education, communities can potentially enhance their ability to recover and withstand the effects of disasters and thereby reiterate the importance of a systematic response to emergency preparedness and resilience.

13.6.1. Examples of Communities that Effectively Responded to Disasters

Preparedness by communities in responding to disasters is well captured by the practice of flood risk management by the Netherlands. It has adopted complete FEMS that emphasize resilience in the form of preemptive measures. By harmonizing high-level scientific research with local government, the Netherlands gets its communities ready to resist and recover from floods. This strategy also emphasizes the need for effective coordination by proper organizations among the various parties involved in emergency management. By integrating the aggregated capacities of government, non-governmental, and community organizations, the Dutch model provides a robust model for the preparation for flood adversity and exhibits how enhanced resilience can be achieved through effective emergency preparedness efforts. Compared with other European countries, such an active governance approach has increased local communities' resilience to natural disasters and mitigates adverse social and economic effects (Alexander et al., 2016). Another motivational example of a resilient response is Greensburg, Kansas, during the 2007 disastrous tornado. Upon the disaster, locals and leaders concentrated on resilience by reconstructing buildings as well as reinforcing communal bonds. Through an inclusive effort, the community engaged all stakeholders in renovating its infrastructure into a model of sustainable processes, placing particular emphasis on environmental concerns. This transformation was triggered by the understanding that vulnerability extends beyond immediate physical losses to include socio-economic concerns to be addressed. By weaving concepts of sustainability into their recovery plan, Greensburg residents demonstrated that disaster responses should include long-term measures for risk reduction and participation of the public, and illustrate how resilience in a community can be built from managing concerted efforts for addressing multiple aspects of vulnerability (Cannon et al., 2025). Similarly, Joplin, Missouri, municipality is a successful instance of community action for recovery from disaster with overall preparedness and response measures after a destruction-causing tornado in

2011. The immediate response was instant mobilization by the community, when citizens rallied to provide shelter, food, and relief to the victims. It was followed by institutional action on the part of the local government and volunteer organizations, which established systems for facilitating long-term recovery. Joplins recovery plan involved not just the rehabilitation of the physical infrastructure but also the setting up of structures for mental health services and social services to address the inclusive needs of its people. The example of Joplin illustrates how communities are able to utilize direct response and long-range planning toward enhancing resilience, ultimately making their disaster strategy a tool for constructing social networks and governing communities (Cannon et al., 2025).

13.6.2. Analysis of Resilience-Building Initiatives

Resilience building is vital in reducing community preparedness for emergencies, particularly in the context of increasing natural disasters due to climate change. Resilience-building efforts include various measures to enhance the capacity of communities to prepare against shocks. Cultural heritage integration in disaster risk reduction is one of the core strategies. Cultural heritage, now understood to include not just monumental landscapes but living landscapes and intangible practices, can be a rich asset in enhancing resilience. Employing insights derived from history and community relations integrated into cultural practices, these projects can improve social cohesion, the most significant of which is required during emergencies. Heritage use not only guards against disaster impacts but also strengthens the identity of the community and renders it stronger in resisting future disasters, as in Albrito et al. (2013). CMDRR is also an enabling mechanism in the construction of resilience programs.

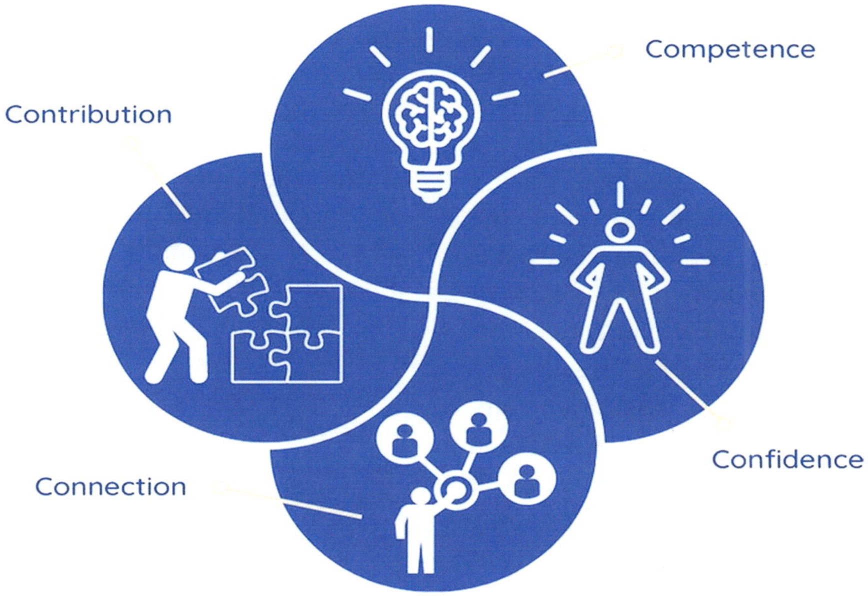

Figure 13.15. Analysis of resilience-building initiatives.

Source: https://static.wixstatic.com/media/e817ab_d6859322ca2a4652aad2e7cf36c91330~mv2.jpg/v1/fill/w_1000,h_645,al_c,q_85,usm_0.66_1.00_0.01/e817ab_d6859322ca2a4652aad2e7cf36c91330~mv2.jpg.

The bottom-up approach is led by the local community, with members of the community fully involved in disaster risk reduction and mitigation processes. By providing communities with more autonomy over decision-making and resource management, CMDRR addresses local vulnerabilities and incentivizes sustainable responses sensitive to distinctive issues affecting groups at the vanguard of climate change. Unfortunately, as reported in N/A (2009), the global reaction to these urgent issues usually proves too late, with too little aid being given to beleaguered communities. Effective CMDRR on top of building the capacity of local communities to respond to disaster risks promotes a stronger culture of preparedness and adaptation, thus on the foundation of community resilience. Integration of resilience programs into mainstream emergency preparedness policy is crucial for addressing cross-cutting risks that communities face. This necessitates deep understanding intersectoral collaboration including government institutions, non-governmental organizations, and local institutions. Engaging the diverse stakeholders serves to provide an enabling platform for risk and resilience understanding, as well as the sharing of knowledge and information. Through this, collaborative efforts are able to lead to the development of contextualized emergency plans that are culturally responsive and effectively applicable, thus enhancing their effectiveness. Moreover, programs should take precedence in making use of continuous assessment and modification to ensure they remain effective in addressing changing risk. The cumulative impact of robust resilience-building activities not only prepares communities for forecasted disasters, but also creates an anticipatory culture that supports sustainability and interdependence in the context of expected uncertainties, as emphasized in Albrito et al. (2013) (Figure 13.15).

13.6.3. Impact of Community-led Recovery Efforts

Locally initiated recovery processes play a crucial role in determining local disaster resilience, particularly flood disaster resilience, which increases with each climatic change. These interventions allow the locals to own their recovery, hence establishing ownership and empowerment, which has the potential to build the capacity of the community to withstand future disasters. For instance, effective community engagement implies that recovery strategies are tailored to the individual socio-economic and cultural conditions of the affected groups, as reflected in the growing preoccupation with resilience discourse in public policy. Such a localized approach not only enables efficient resource deployment but also sustains social solidarity among local communities, allowing them to better confront and adapt to future arising difficulties, which aligns well with the new paradigms of FEMS in Europe (Alexander et al., 2016). Moreover, community-based initiatives manage to bridge gaps between institutional action and local demands, effectively integrating local knowledge into disaster management policy. Case studies illustrate how, as active participants in the recovery process, communities are better positioned to innovate and devise means of overcoming their challenges rather than through top-down interventions. The recovery from flooding at Cockermouth, UK, for example, illustrates how local stakeholders collaborated with government agencies to create flood management plans that addressed not only immediate requirements but also long-term resilience (Amaratunga et al., 2013). Such collaborative efforts are central in fostering a culture of citizen voice and engagement, confirming the perception that sustainable recovery is indeed a collective effort that will lead to improved governance and future readiness. Finally, the impacts of community-led recovery go beyond rapid disaster response;

it builds a culture of resilience that finds its way into all spheres of community life. This model of building resilience is dependent on long-term institutional knowledge growth and knowledge exchange within societies. Effective recovery of societies is always coupled with learning and enhancing public awareness of disaster preparedness, hence promoting proactive attitudes among inhabitants. By emphasizing public participation and collective responsibility, societies are able to absorb floods' shocks and stresses more effectively and hence improve their overall emergency preparedness system. Building these capacities and consciousness not only consolidates current capacity but also lays the foundation for eventual resilience, further underscoring the vital importance of locally led intervention to long-term recovery (Alexander et al., 2016; Amaratunga et al., 2013).

SUMMARY

Emergency preparedness and community resilience are directly related, calling to mind the imperative to use planning and engagement by all interested parties in society. Proactive preparedness cannot be overstressed, as it forms the foundation for effective response during times of crises. A robust emergency management system engages the people, fostering a culture of awareness and readiness that transcends actions by the government. Indeed, community participation in the preparation process leads to enhanced application of resources and greater social cohesion, vital during disasters. As conversations on various academic platforms, such as the seminar in Kathmandu on climate change and disaster risk reduction, highlight, creating a resilient society requires collective action and shared responsibility among all the members in order to possess effective risk management and response (Aryal et al., 2008). Moreover, examination of emergency management practices, particularly in climate change, reveals that changing the paradigm is essential for developing resilience. The inwardly directed tactics that have been applied in the past can limit the extent to which communities can prepare for and respond to emergencies. Taking an outward, proactive stance towards participation can open doors to involving the public, optimizing communal readiness and fostering a sense of ownership of risk management programs. Lessons learned from UK emergency management practice illustrate this imperative; as highlighted, a participatory approach placing social engagement as primary is not only optimized for mobilization of resources but also increases community understanding of emergency processes (O'Brien et al., 2008). In summary, embedment of emergency preparedness in the life of communities is pivotal in reinforcing resilience to crises. Understanding the interdependence of the various stakeholders—like the government, non-profits, and the general public—increases the overall capacity of the community to mitigate risks associated with disasters. Facilitating inclusive planning processes allows for a more informed understanding of the unique vulnerabilities and capacities of various communities. Therefore, the conjoining of these elements is central because active communities putting money into emergency preparedness are ultimately better equipped to withstand and bounce back from adversity, and invite a more resilient future.

The literature on emergency preparedness and community resilience acknowledges the importance of facilitating multi-sector partnerships to establish more capable community-level capacities for coping with disasters. A good case in point is the LACCDR initiative, which applies community participatory methods to bring about the ideas of resilience. Randomly, coalitions in communities engage government agencies, organizations, and residents, allowing for two-way learning that amplifies greater knowledge towards resilience. Thematic analysis of the focus group and interview data highlights successful approaches that enhance resilience drivers such as engagement and education, thereby eliciting community commitment to actions of preparedness. They not only foster a culture of collective work but also address specific vulnerabilities of vulnerable communities in the community (Bromley et al., 2017). In a different geographical context, the Napier City emergency preparedness policy in New Zealand focuses on the need for response systems in case of seismic hazards. The city vulnerable to earthquakes and tsunamis has developed an evacuation plan that focuses on quick action after the occurrence of a strong or prolonged earthquake. A survey among residents of Napier Hill showed willingness to assist evacuees in a calamity; there was a problem, though, with the access to resources and agency support needed for effective aid. The findings of this research provide critical input to the planning strategies of local governments, guiding policy actions that are translated to individual readiness and community-level resilience to natural disasters (Becker et al., 2019). Overall, community participation, strategic partnerships, and efficient response mechanisms are the pillars leading to enhanced emergency readiness and resilience. Both LACCDR project and Napier City research exhibit how use of local knowledge and collaborative labor could potentially increase community disaster-readiness. Both projects reflect on the significance of preparing disaster strategies to conditions in a particular location and yet being bound by principles of equity and inclusiveness. By establishing connections among different sectors and understanding the unique needs of each community, municipalities can establish resilience that not only endures the immediate impacts of disaster but also brings about long-term development and recovery after emergencies.

KEY TERMS FROM THIS CHAPTER

Disaster Preparedness	Emergency Response	Community Resilience
Risk Assessment	Crisis Communication	Emergency Planning
Vulnerability Assessment	Continuity of Operations	Resilience Building
Public Health Emergencies	First Responders	Surge Capacity
Disaster Risk Reduction	Evacuation Planning	Emergency Drills
Community-Based Response	Early Warning Systems	Natural Disasters
Preparedness Training	Mental Health Support	Resource Mobilization
Post-Disaster Recovery	Health System Preparedness	

CLOSER LOOK

GENERAL GOAL OF COMMUNITY RESILIENCE

A closer look at the general goal of community resilience reveals a fundamental aim to strengthen a community's ability to prepare for, respond to, recover from, and adapt to adverse situations such as natural disasters, economic shocks, public health crises, or social disruptions. Community resilience is not just about bouncing back from hardship—it's about bouncing forward, using challenges as opportunities for growth, transformation, and long-term sustainability. The overarching goal is to empower communities to become more self-reliant, cohesive, and adaptable in the face of uncertainty. This involves building strong social networks, fostering inclusive decision-making, ensuring access to essential resources, and promoting equity so that all members—especially vulnerable populations—are supported during crises. Resilient communities invest in infrastructure that can withstand environmental and social stresses, develop robust emergency response systems, and create education and communication strategies that keep the public informed and engaged. They also promote mental health, economic stability, and environmental stewardship as foundational components of resilience. Importantly, the goal of community resilience is not solely reactive; it involves proactive planning, capacity building, and learning from past experiences to mitigate future risks. Collaborative efforts between governments, non-profits, local businesses, and residents are central to creating resilient systems that reflect the unique values and needs of the community. By focusing on both physical and social capital—such as trust, leadership, and mutual support—resilient communities are better equipped to handle adversity without long-term harm. Ultimately, the general goal of community resilience is to ensure that communities are not only able to survive disruptions but also to emerge stronger, more connected, and better prepared for future challenges. It is a continuous process that supports the well-being and sustainability of communities across all sectors and at every level.

REFERENCES

1. Adekola, J., Fischbacher-Smith, D., & Fischbacher-Smith, M. (2020). Inherent complexities of a multi-stakeholder approach to building community resilience. https://core.ac.uk/download/293868637.pdf (accessed on 26th June 2025).
2. Adeniyi, O., Jayawickrama, J., Perera, S., Zhou, Q., et al. (2014). The implication of Hyogo Framework for Action for disaster resilience education. https://core.ac.uk/download/41071264.pdf (accessed on 26th June 2025).
3. Albrito, P., Boccardi, G., Dolcemascolo, G., Douglas, I., et al. (2013). Heritage and resilience: Issues and opportunities for reducing disaster risks. https://core.ac.uk/download/20544501.pdf (accessed on 26th June 2025).
4. Alexander, M., Bruzzone, S., Gilissen, H. K., Matczak, P., et al. (2016). A framework for evaluating the effectiveness of flood emergency management systems in Europe. https://core.ac.uk/download/287602598.pdf (accessed on 26th June 2025).
5. Amaratunga, D., & Ingirige, B. (2013). Minimizing flood risk accumulation through effective private and public sector engagement. https://core.ac.uk/download/30733249.pdf (accessed on 26th June 2025).
6. Amaratunga, D., De Silva, K., & Haigh, R. (2015). Third revolution digital technology in disaster early warning. https://core.ac.uk/download/30734699.pdf (accessed on 26th June 2025).
7. Antrobus, E., Ramirez, S., & Williamson, H. (2013). Living in Queensland: Preparing for and communicating in disasters and emergencies. https://core.ac.uk/download/18443725.pdf (accessed on 26th June 2025).
8. Aryal, K., & Gadema, Z. (2008). Climate change and disaster impact reduction. https://core.ac.uk/download/9304445.pdf (accessed on 26th June 2025).
9. Asrat, S. (2015). Urban flood response planning: Building urban resilience in Calgary and Toronto. https://core.ac.uk/download/143687631.pdf (accessed on 26th June 2025).
10. Bajracharya, B., Childs, I., Godber, A., Hastings, P., et al. (2010). Policy into practice: Adoption of hazard mitigation measures by local government in Queensland: A collaborative research project between Queensland University of Technology and Emergency Management Queensland in association with Local Government of Queensland Disaster Management Alliance. https://core.ac.uk/download/196605722.pdf (accessed on 26th June 2025).
11. Becker, J., Kaiser, L., & Payne, B. (2019). Understanding residents' capacities to support evacuated populations: A study of earthquake and tsunami evacuation for Napier Hill, Napier, Aotearoa New Zealand. https://core.ac.uk/download/304655507.pdf (accessed on 26th June 2025).
12. Bennett, D. M., Davis, E., & Phillips, B. D. (2016). The future of accessibility in disaster conditions: How wireless technologies will transform the life cycle of emergency management. https://core.ac.uk/download/232772595.pdf (accessed on 26th June 2025).
13. Bergin, A., Nichola, D., & Barnes, P. (2014). Working as one: A road map to disaster resilience for Australia. https://core.ac.uk/download/pdf/30673432.pdf (accessed on 26th June 2025).
14. Bromley, E., Chandra, A., Eisenman, D. P., Kim, Y., et al. (2017). How do communities use a participatory public health approach to build resilience? The Los Angeles County Community

Disaster Resilience Project. https://core.ac.uk/download/323077313.pdf (accessed on 26th June 2025).

15. Cannon, T. (2025). Reducing people's vulnerability to natural hazards: Communities and resilience. https://core.ac.uk/download/pdf/6379948.pdf (accessed on 26th June 2025).
16. Deeming, H., Medd, W., & Whittle, R. (2011). Recommendations for changes in UK National Recovery Guidance (NRG) and associated guidance from the perspective of Lancaster University's Hull Flood Studies. https://core.ac.uk/download/1556070.pdf (accessed on 26th June 2025).
17. Drager, K. H., & Robertson, T. V. (2014). Global response for capacity building of disaster preparedness: A TIEMS initiative. https://core.ac.uk/download/77936177.pdf (accessed on 26th June 2025).
18. Dunaway, M., Lopresti, D., Murphy, R., Palen, L., et al. (2017). Research agenda in intelligent infrastructure to enhance disaster management, community resilience and public safety. https://arxiv.org/abs/1705.01985 (accessed on 26th June 2025).
19. Federici, F., & O'Brien, S. (2019). Crisis translation: Considering language needs in multilingual disaster settings. https://core.ac.uk/download/294759802.pdf (accessed on 26th June 2025).
20. Kontar, Y. Y., Контарь, E. E. (2017). Comparative analysis of spring flood risk reduction measures in Alaska, United States and the Sakha Republic, Russia. https://core.ac.uk/download/286607717.pdf (accessed on 26th June 2025).
21. Mabaso, E., & Manyena, B. (2013). Contingency planning in southern Africa: Events rather than processes? https://core.ac.uk/download/41071138.pdf (accessed on 26th June 2025).
22. O'Brien, G. (2008). UK emergency preparedness: A holistic local response? https://core.ac.uk/download/4146907.pdf (accessed on 26th June 2025).

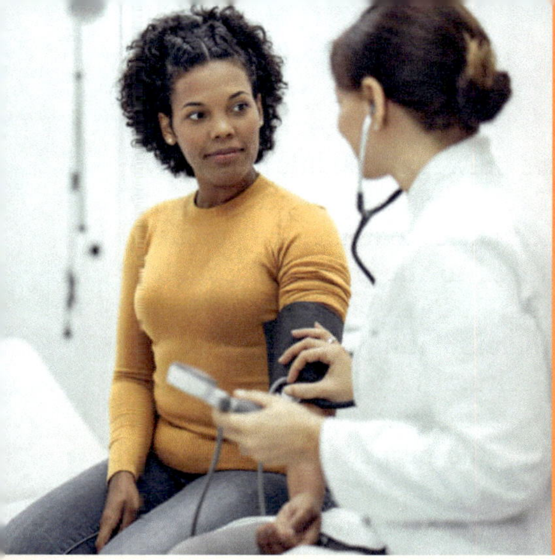

Chapter 14

SPECIAL POPULATIONS IN COMMUNITY HEALTH

Contents

Introduction

Over the past few years, the importance to meet the special populations' health disparities in community health has grown significantly. Special populations have long included marginalized groups with unique challenges such as racial and ethnic minorities, low-income groups, and those with disabilities. These groups experience a disparate burden of disease, have limited access to health care services, and experience poorer health outcomes compared to the broader population. Emphasis on these disparities is relevant to the formulation of efficacious interventions in public health that affect health equity. Emphasis on targeted needs enables clinicians and policymakers to formulate strategies that bridge the gaps in care, offer resource distribution, and advance overall community health outcomes for these populations. The Mountain West Clinical Translational Research Infrastructure Network (CTR-IN) Program has been a model program that has been effective in developing the research capacity to address health disparities among special populations. The broad geographical scope that encompasses numerous institutions unites an array of research disciplines to work together, eventually resulting in improved health outcomes in the Mountain West region. Piloting a number of grant programs, the initiative brings attention to critical health issues, such as disparities between Hispanic and Native American populations as they relate to ischemic stroke patients. These targeted studies not only create additional research but also shape evidence-based practices and policies that have the potential to reverse health inequity trends. This collective effort bears witness to the power of people's participation, inter-disciplinary efforts, and a robust support system in being able to effectively tackle health disparities among special groups. At the center of understanding the complexities of health disparities is the recognition of the socio-economic and cultural factors that guarantee their perpetuation. There is evidence to conclude that entrenched poverty, political instability, and inferior healthcare infrastructure have much to do with guaranteeing the perpetuation of special populations' ills. Social determinants of health, such as education, income, and access to care, act in a dynamic manner to enhance or diminish vulnerabilities. The effect of neglected tropical diseases, say, must be met with an integrated approach that incorporates these determinants, as Danso-Appiah et al. (2009) cites. Through the application of methods from a variety of social sciences, from population and behavioral studies, these scholars can enhance measurement of the interplay of such determinants and develop integrated strategies to disease prevention and health promotion. Finally, an accurate picture of these dynamics is important in enabling effective intervention with regard to the exact needs of special populations in community health (Figure 14.1).

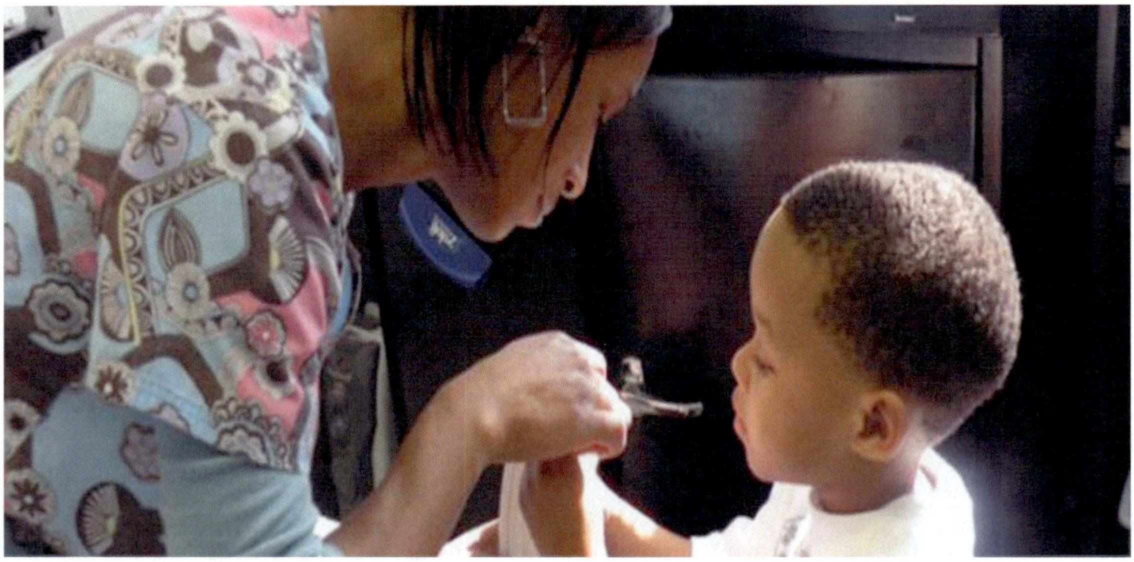

Figure 14.1. Special populations in community health.

Source: https://www.chcchronicles.org/sites/default/files/styles/thumbnail_1200x467/public/specialpopulations_healthcarefor.jpg?itok=q5WtyHvC.

Definition of Special Populations

The concept of special populations of community health is a heterogeneous group of populations with unique social, economic, and health-related problems. Special populations can include, but are not limited to, racial and ethnic minorities, people with disabilities, older adults, low-income households, and the uninsured. These populations are prone to structural barriers of access to health care, stigmatization, and health disparities. It is imperative to comprehend the intricacy of definitions and attributes of these populations as a precursor to formulating effective public health interventions appropriate to their specific needs. Moreover, success in community health programs often lies in being able to identify and engage these special populations effectively to reduce disparities as well as maximize overall health outcomes. There is a need to understand the definition of special populations in executing effective community health interventions to improve outcomes among marginalized communities. Special populations are not only characterized by their demographic features, but also by their unique health needs and health care barriers. For instance, racial and ethnic minorities are exposed to healthcare disparities due to socioeconomic disparities as well as culturally incompetent health care systems. In addition, the disabled have unique needs for accessible health care services and can be discriminated against in health-related settings. Activities that have been created in order to develop medical homes, such as the ones discussed in the projects presented by Takach et al. (2009), illustrate how holistic and integrated models of care can address the complex needs of special populations and thereby enhance their health outcomes. More significantly, the definition of special populations also includes those subjected to geographic factors, social determinants of health, and altering community dynamics. In the case of diasporas, for example, communities have close relationships with their countries of origin and they influence their resource access and health-seeking behaviors. It is vital to learn about these forces in an effort to develop sustainable health programs. Insights from studies that examine the contributions made by the diasporas to their homelands are that it is possible to access improved health practices and outcomes as pointed out in Johnson (2007). By comprehending the multidimensional and dynamic character of special populations, healthcare providers can design outreach efforts not only to address their immediate needs but also to equip them to more successfully use the healthcare system.

Importance of Addressing Health Disparities

The importance of eliminating health disparities in special populations cannot be overstated as they are typically fueled by complex socio-economic determinants, including education level, socioeconomic status, and access to health care. Health disparities disproportionately affect marginalized groups, leading to worse outcomes and quality of life. For instance, those living in neighborhoods that are "Health Equity Zones" (HEZs) face extreme barriers to accessing healthcare, in addition to systemic disparities (RIDOH). The impact of these disparities not only is felt on an individual level but also has a downstream effect on communities, leading to increased healthcare costs and lost productivity. Resolution of these problems through the use of focused interventions sensitive to the particular needs of each population is crucial in order to provide health equality. Moreover, the role culturally competent communication plays in the closing of health disparities is at the center. Health systems that do not create mechanisms to observe and react to cultural differences may actually perpetuate disparities the very systems aim to eliminate. Fostering effective communication among providers, health plans, and communities can potentially optimize the quality of care delivered to diverse populations. Recent initiatives toward improving cultural competency have shown the promise to decrease racial and ethnic disparities in healthcare access and quality. Evidence indicates that when healthcare practitioners engage with patients using a culturally sensitive approach, outcomes are significantly improved, hence the importance of systems reform to address inclusivity in care delivery (Lurie et al., 2004). Programs that foster such practices will help in bridging barriers that have long hindered equitable access to healthcare. Activation of community-based interventions is crucial towards achieving disparities in health effectively (Lurie et al., 2004).

Programs written in collaboration with local communities, such as those funded by the Rhode Island Department of Health, demonstrate a successful model for intervening in the root causes of health inequities. In developing localized Health Equity Zones, these programs provide communities with the ability to identify their own unique challenges and collectively develop responsive solutions. These approaches not only increase the access of healthcare but also increase feelings of ownership among citizens, thereby increasing efforts in health improvement in the long run (Alexander-Scott et al., 2017). Ultimately, reduction of health disparities by community involvement not only increases health outcomes but also social cohesion and resilience among susceptible groups, exemplifying the interdependence of health, social justice, and empowerment of communities (Figure 14.2).

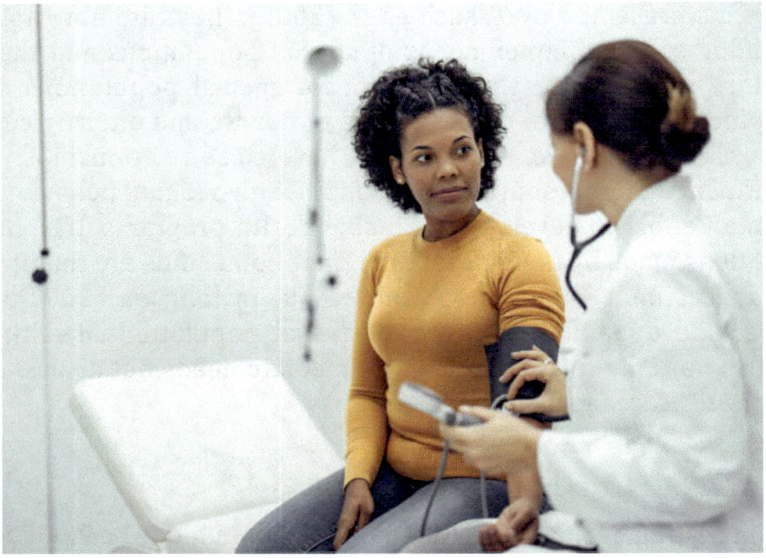

Figure 14.2. Importance of addressing health disparities.

Source: https://www.verywellhealth.com/thmb/28zhufSBRwb6RpQo2TPPie9tu8U=/750x0/filters:no_upscale():max_bytes(150000):strip_icc()/health-disparities-4173220_v1-e8914773af574e3d9f02b08d86835de5.jpg.

Overview of Community Health Initiatives

Community health programs are critical to address the unique needs of special populations, emphasizing holistic healthcare that transcends traditional medical models. Community health programs typically entail a variety of approaches including preventive care, health education, and outreach activities specifically directed at reaching vulnerable populations. Focusing such efforts on specific groups, such as adolescents, racial and ethnic minorities, or individuals with socioeconomic issues, enhances their effectiveness. Through encouraging alliances among government agencies, healthcare providers, and community organizations, stakeholders are able to streamline resources in an effective manner to aim at health disparities. As this collaborative approach expands, measuring the success of these programs in improving healthier outcomes becomes more critical, with the need to make evidence-based modifications to better impact vulnerable populations. Certain health concerns of special populations dominate community health programs. Mental health, alcohol and drug abuse, and chronic diseases are among the illnesses that disproportionately affect specific groups and demand particular interventions to achieve health equity. For instance, increasingly, programs focus on youth development and provide an intervention to assist at-risk adolescents in making effective transitions to adulthood. The "disconnectedness" is the susceptibility of such individuals and demands certain responses in order to foster resilience. Further, programs with protective factors, as evident in the federal overview of youth policy, prevent adverse outcomes for high-risk youth. Through understanding such challenges and instituting comprehensive interventions, community health programs can benefit special populations more effectively, promoting overall welfare and resilience among such populations. The success of community health programs largely relies on the degree of participation and empowerment among communities. Participation of local stakeholders in the planning and implementation processes instills a sense of ownership, thereby increasing the likelihood of sustained commitment and support. Community capacity-building programs are essential for making projects context-relevant and culturally sensitive, catering to special populations' unique needs and predispositions. Furthermore, ongoing evaluation and feedback processes are essential to the identification of successes and pitfalls. Data-driven decision-making and feedback mechanisms can help ensure that projects develop and change in response to shifting community forces. By assigning utmost importance to participation of the community and creating a cycle of continuous betterment, health initiatives can create a more equitable healthcare space for marginalized groups, going step by step towards the achievement of total health equity (Figure 14.3).

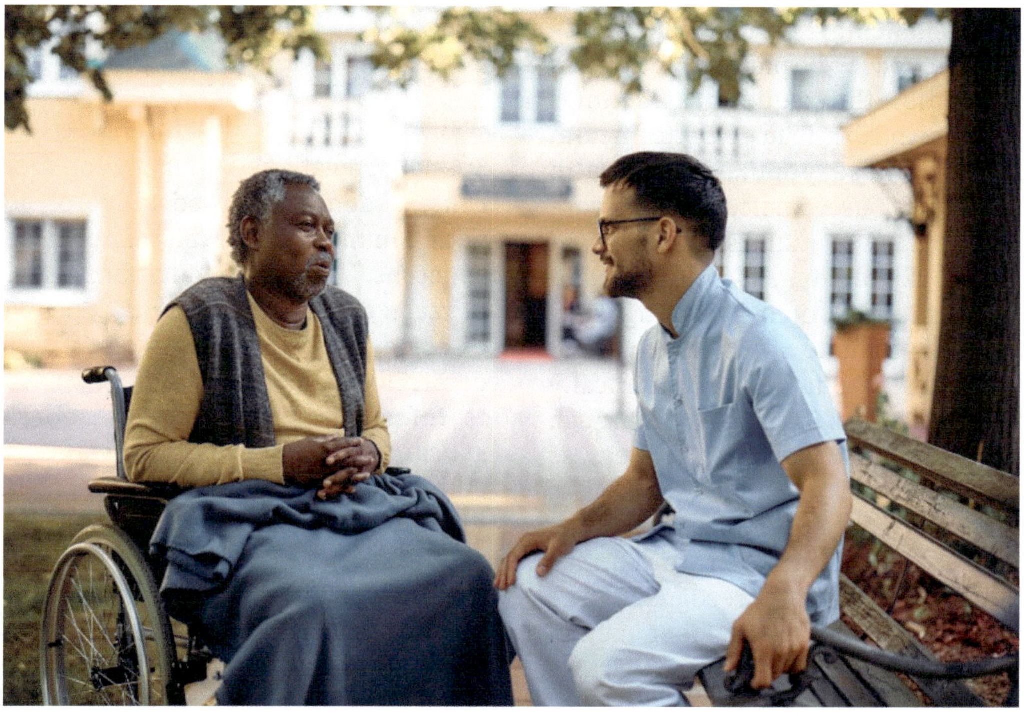

Figure 14.3. Overview of community health initiatives.

Source: https://online-learning-college.com/wp-content/uploads/2024/01/Community-Health-Initiatives-Promoting-Wellness-Locally-1.jpg.

14.1. Identifying Special Populations

Special populations identification is a crucial aspect of community health that requires a balanced understanding of the diverse challenges and needs of various groups. Special populations are generally groups of individuals who are marginalized by social determinants of health, chronic illnesses, or socioeconomic factors. The complexities involved in these factors can lead to delayed intervention and diagnosis, creating health disparities. For instance, limited access to health services and screenings in time are typical for poor families, for whom direct policy recommendations have to be developed for its increased involvement in healthcare systems. Such policies as the increase in Medicaid and Childrens Health Insurance Program coverage, according to Kenney et al. (2010), can become significant in enhancing efforts toward early detection. Moreover, well-planned outreach programs can offer the required screenings and referrals that in turn lead to better health outcomes among these populations. Health and economic status are particularly relevant in assessing populations that have significant barriers to work or health engagement. Programs with the aim of overcoming such barriers can offer holistic solutions that not only focus on health but also economically empower the populations. For instance, thorough employment programs for former offenders, as evaluated in programs outlined by Redcross et al. (2007), show how specific interventions can have positive impacts on both work status and overall health statuses. By recognizing the interdependence between employment, mental health, and physical health, such programs advocate a concerted approach. This approach ensures that health policies are not doing things in isolation but rather in conjunction with socioeconomic assistance mechanisms set out to deal with the unique challenges of such populations. To properly identify and provide for special populations, there has to be the implementation of evidence-based policies that monitor and quantify the precise needs of such communities. Recurrent data analysis and collection can be employed to inform the development of responsive programs that are attentive to the socioeconomic and demographic profiles of special groups in a community. For example, leveraging data to improve access to well-child visits and screenings can be employed to address the barriers discussed in the recommendations of Kenney et al. (2010). In addition, evaluation frameworks may be utilized to recognize emerging needs in varied populations, thereby facilitating timely modification of health interventions. By improving continuously in service provision, the public health system may offer special populations the tailored care that they need in order to improve their health outcomes and overall quality of life.

14.1.1. Characteristics of Special Populations

Special populations, within the community health context, denote a broad range of populations with common vulnerabilities or special health concerns. The said populations usually consist of racial and ethnic minorities, people who are disabled, and poor households. Awareness of the determinants of such populations is essential to inform intervention that addresses their specific health needs. For instance, racial and ethnic minorities may suffer from higher chronic disease rates, prompted by socioeconomic conditions and limited access to health care services. Therefore, public health interventions must address not only medical treatment but also socioeconomic factors that affect health. Recognition of such features allows healthcare providers and policy-makers to modify their activities so that intervention efforts can be successful and fair among differing demographic groups. The health problems of special populations are often compounded by structural barriers, including inadequate access to healthcare and social services. The majority of members of these groups rely on community health centers, which are a primary source of closing gaps in care for the uninsured, publicly insured, and underinsured. Scientific evidence has shown that community health centers are adept at delivering culturally competent care and addressing the unique needs of their patient population. They are, however, plagued every step of the way by problems of funding, staffing, and their ability to add services. Delving into the funding realities of health centers reveals that the viability of such valuable services depends on legislation and adequate funding, as has occurred with the 2008 community health center reauthorization legislation (Finnegan et al., 2009). Therefore, the nature of the special populations is necessarily tied to the infrastructure that exists to care for them. Furthermore, the epidemiology of many of the health concerns that affect special populations necessarily determines the methods of intervention and treatment taken. For instance, infectious disease control programs for onchocerciasis in West Africa illustrate how specific approaches are customized based on the detail of a population's characteristics and geographical setting (Alley et al., 2017). These programs must consider various factors, including the intensity of disease transmission and local patterns of disease vector migratory routes. Such a nuanced comprehension places value on decision-making based on data in public health. By learning about the epidemiological patterns and the specific behaviors of special populations, health programs can develop specific strategies that optimize health results and address the specific challenges of these populations (Figure 14.4).

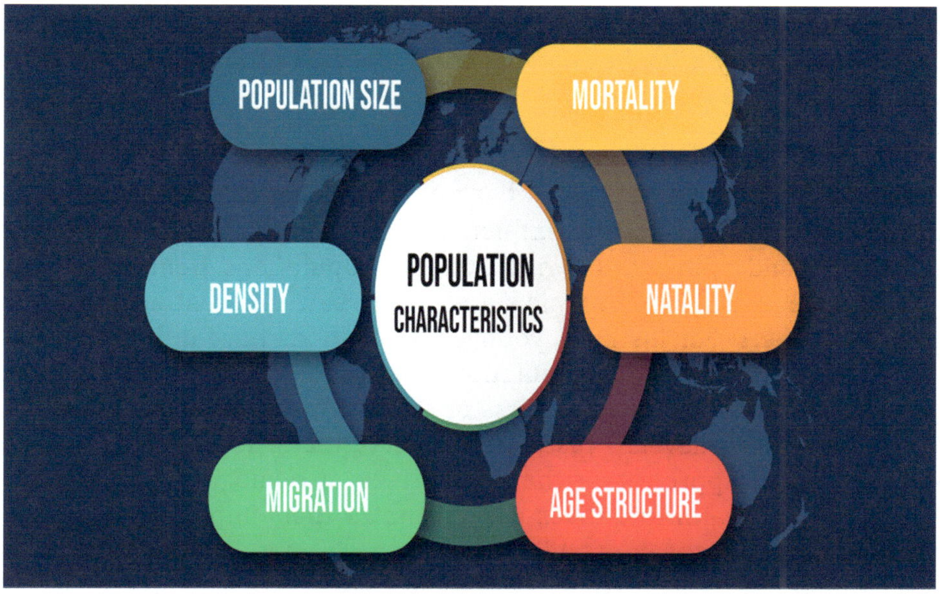

Figure 14.4. Characteristics of special populations.

Source: https://media.geeksforgeeks.org/wp-content/uploads/20230828180610/Characteristics-of-the-Population.png.

14.1.2. Examples of Special Populations (e.g., Elderly, Disabled, Minorities)

Understanding the complexities of special populations in community health requires a specialized investigation of specific groups, for instance, the elderly, the disabled, and minorities. All of these groups experience varying challenges that can have a powerful impact on their health outcomes. For instance, the elderly population loses physical function and cognitive ability, making them vulnerable to chronic illness. They might also lose social relationships as a result of challenges like mobility or loss of peers, affecting mental health. These topics emphasize the importance of creating specific health interventions based on the multiple aspects of aging, as argued in research works that focus on the quality of human relations in a community setting (N/A, 2009). The disabled constituency is also a critical group that requires extra attention in community health interventions. Individuals with disabilities typically encounter gigantic barriers, including physical barriers to health access and social stigma that may hinder their full participation in community life. As a result, they may endure higher levels of chronic illness and mental disorders compared to their able-bodied counterparts. It is imperative that health policies not only address the specific medical needs of disabled groups but also provide environments that promote inclusiveness and accompaniment. This requires comprehensive plans that accommodate healthcare provision to fit various disabilities while enhancing the overall quality of life for such individuals (N/A, 2009). Minorities represent another key special population for community health settings. These heterogenous populations are often faced with systemic inequities as well as historical marginalization that directly affect their health status. Social determinants of health such as income, education, and quality care are very uneven by racial and ethnic group. For instance, in California, successful interventions to address the growing needs of aging minority populations focus on the intersectionality of race, age, and socioeconomic status in health outcomes. Equal delivery of health services to meet the unique needs and issues of minorities is vital in order to increase their level of general well-being and health within community environments, thereby necessitating culturally sensitive care and outreach services.

14.1.3. The Role of Demographics in Community Health

Demographics play a significant role in influencing community health by determining health behavior, access to care, and health status within various populations. Demographic characteristics, such as age, gender, race, and socioeconomic status, can create different health profiles and needs among community members. For instance, younger populations have different issues, like mental illness and substance abuse, than older populations that usually suffer from chronic ailments that necessitate specialized treatment. An awareness of these demographic variations is important for health providers who want to develop customized interventions addressing the specific concerns of certain communities. In appreciating the crucial role of demographics in the forecasting of health trends, community health initiatives can maximize their impact and ensure overall well-being in the population. It has been established that special populations such as the sexual and gender minorities (SGM) and the economically disadvantaged are usually confronted with systemic impediments to equal healthcare access. The PRIDE Study accomplishes this by demonstrating the utility of inclusive research designs that collect demographic and health information from SGM individuals, who are underrepresented in most traditional healthcare studies (Bibbins-Domingo et al., 2019). Community health programs, on recognizing the specific health needs and concerns of these populations, can develop targeted interventions to bridge the gaps in care. This approach can generate a sense of empowerment and belonging, leading to larger participation in health programs and healthier consequences tailored to the demographic situation of the population. Furthermore, the impact of demographics extends to specific intervention in health, such as recurrent HIV testing for pregnant women in Kenya. Socio-demographic determinants of healthcare provider conduct and patient adherence may be realized to clarify barriers to effective service delivery (Bukusi et al., 2016). For example, disparate education, worldview, and information accessibility can dramatically affect willingness for receiving care and providers' capability to implement essential health guidelines. Demographic inequities may be worked towards through specifically targeted education and resource provision, thus facilitating enhanced health advice compliance and thus improved health in at-risk groups. Demographic variables are, thus, a fundamental factor in developing community health interventions that are effective, equitable, and accessible.

14.2. Health Disparities

In community health, health disparities are clearly evident in special populations, including racial and ethnic minorities, individuals with disabilities, and low socioeconomic status individuals. These groups experience greater rates of chronic diseases and their complications resulting from, in substantial part, systemic disparities in healthcare access and quality. The interventions need to be population-specific in order to address the unique needs and barriers that these populations entail. Implementation of evidence-based behavioral interventions (EBIs) has the potential to be the major strategy in reducing such disparities through the establishment of community-based support and the use of local resources. The challenge is the customization of such interventions for the specific contexts of the marginalized groups without compromising their effectiveness. Full understanding of the community dynamics is critical in ensuring effective adaptation and implementation of EBIs towards improving the health outcomes of marginalized communities (N/A, 2025).

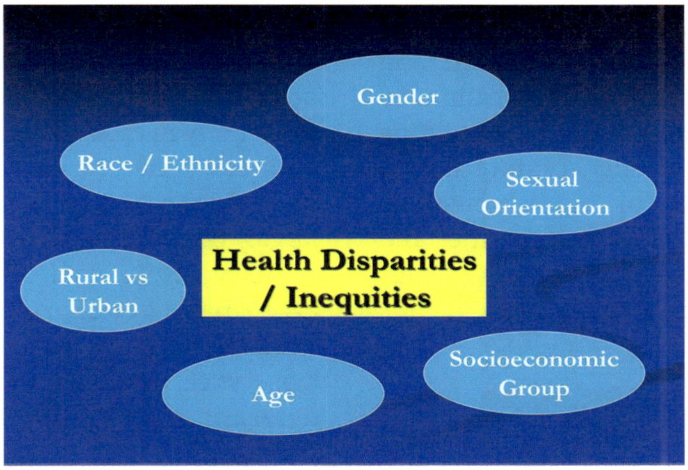

Figure 14.5. Health disparities.

Source: https://image3.slideserve.com/6313040/health-disparities-inequities5-l.jpg.

Chronic conditions still account for health inequalities, particularly among poorer groups with MCCs. There is a recognition of the level and nature of MCCs in such settings that is essential in formulating effective health policies. Literature emphasizes that the definition of MCCs should be expanded beyond the mere aggregation of clinical conditions to incorporate wider health-related factors influencing overall health. Taking this broader view, it is possible for researchers and policy makers to more accurately identify and intervene in these disparities particular to these groups. Additionally, this overall understanding can be employed to guide particular prevention-oriented and management interventions for MCCs, an ultimate goal put forth by the U.S. Department of Health and Human Services (Shadmi et al., 2013). Sealing these knowledge gaps is essential for the formulation of health policies that can adequately meet the needs of marginal groups. Effective community health programs addressing health disparities need to have high levels of prioritizing the establishment of strong infrastructure that enables interaction among researchers, practitioners, and residents. Such collaboration is essential in translation and implementation of evidence-based interventions that are applicable to the specific needs of special populations. The process entails a series of deliberate actions, such as compiling relevant information, adjusting program components, and securing local capacity to facilitate adoption and sustainability. By attending to these issues, health strategies can utilize community resources while retaining fidelity to EBIs. Finding the right balance between adapting interventions and retaining their core components is instrumental in optimizing their influence. Lastly, promoting community involvement and creating health interventions tailored for disenfranchised groups will ease existing health disparities and promote improved health equity across various populations (N/A, 2025) (Figure 14.5).

14.2.1. Factors Contributing to Health Disparities

Disparities in health are firmly grounded in a variety of socioeconomic factors that permeate the existence of marginalized communities. Money, education, and access to high-quality health care become determinants of paramount influence that affect health outcomes. The low-income population regularly faces limitations that prevent them from accessing medical care, thereby falling victim to disease prevalence and poor health status. Besides, educational disparities can affect health literacy, where it is hard for the individuals to make suitable decisions concerning their own health. The society of areas such as Appalachia illustrates how health-related socioeconomic status could lead to a situation of poor health outcomes. Specifically, ailing industries such as coal mining not only exacerbate economic insecurity but also cause serious health conditions, as illustrated in research focusing on chronic disease among coal-exposed populations (Meacham et al., 2013). It is important to tackle such underlying social determinants to alleviate inequalities in health. Cultural determinants are also crucial in health inequalities because they have an influence on behaviors, beliefs, and perceptions of health and wellness. For instance, cultural norms and health-seeking attitudes within specific ethnic groups can influence reception and response to health information. In indigenous groups, such as the Maori in New Zealand, research has demonstrated that cultural identity and conventional beliefs can affect health-seeking behavior and result in delayed presentation for treatment. Also, the quality of healthcare services obtained by these groups tends to be low, leading to inequity in their outcomes. For Maori patients with colon cancer, for example, the difference in survival rate with their non-Maori peers can largely be attributed to higher degrees of patient comorbidity as well as inadequate access to care (Blakely et al., 2010). This highlights the need for culturally appropriate interventions to close such disparities in care. Environmental determinants, particularly those caused by industrial processes, are significant drivers of health disparities among special groups. Areas that rely on industries such as mining have unique health issues caused by environmental deterioration and exposure to hazardous toxins. Coal mining in the Appalachian region, for instance, is associated with various chronic conditions, such as lung conditions and cancer, which exacerbate the existing health disparities within the area. The quality of environmental health and poor health outcomes have been found to have a positive relationship based on the literature review of chronic health conditions in such environmentally dependent coal communities (Meacham et al., 2013). Hence, solving environmental health hazards is as vital for maintaining ecological systems as it is to enhance public health among the vulnerable groups. Sustainable practice and policies to prevent environmental hazards can be an important driver in reducing health inequities.

14.2.2. Impact of Socioeconomic Status (SES) on Health

The role of SES in health is a multifaceted and layered factor that disproportionately affects vulnerable groups. Individuals of low SES have fewer options for seeking high-quality care, and this has the net impact of worse health. For instance, in the case of pediatric cancer in Ghana, the low-income children face significant barriers such as delayed diagnosis and lower availability of treatment, which are associated with lower survival rates compared to their affluent peers. This inequality not only indicates the expenses in terms of lower SES but also identifies the systemic concerns in healthcare systems that are not equitable. Hence, specific socioeconomic barriers require targeted interventions that can enhance health equity and ensure that children of all backgrounds get proper and prompt medical intervention (Agyapomaa, 2024). In addition, eating habits are significantly shaped by socioeconomic factors, which also impact overall health and nutrition. Latin American studies detail precipitous fluctuation in the quality of diet as a function of SES, indicating that the poor socioeconomic groups have less diverse and nutritionally inadequate diets. These individuals specifically eat fruits, vegetables, and whole grains in lesser quantities and eat more legumes. These dietary practices result in not only unhealthy health but also increased incidences of conditions such as obesity and related comorbidities. Consistent with the evidence, nutrition education and healthy food access must be promoted by health policy to overcome these disparities and build the health of low SES communities (Gómez et al., 2021). In addition to the problems brought in with nutrition and care access, the interplay between SES and health extends even further. Education level, employment status, and community infrastructure also have a strong impact on health. For instance, lower SES people are able to live in neighborhoods that lack large areas for recreational space, which assists in creating sedentary lifestyles and compromised health. Besides, poor health literacy will also exacerbate the determinants since the populations might not access available health facilities effectively. It is, thus, crucial to address these intertwined determinants in an effort to attain health equity among special populations, a sign of the need for comprehensive measures that involve medical care alongside social care, education, and community engagement (Agyapomaa, 2024).

14.2.3. Access to Healthcare Services Among Special Populations

One of the key aspects forming part of community health is availability of healthcare service amongst special populations. This primarily includes refugees, migrants, and other underprivileged groups. These groups of people tend to face serious challenges while seeking proper medical care. Language differences, culture, and socioeconomic inequalities have been described as some of the contributing factors towards these issues that hinder proper communication between patients and healthcare providers. In addition, immigration status-related concerns can also hinder access further as the majority of individuals fear deportation or legal repercussions when seeking medical care. Thus, special populations are likely to experience a higher prevalence of untreated disease, which exacerbates their vulnerabilities and further reinforces the need for targeted interventions within healthcare systems (Weiss et al., 2015).

Culturally competent care is paramount in meeting the unique needs of special populations. Increasing access to healthcare also involves removing physical barriers while enriching healthcare providers' ability for communication with diverse communities. Culturally competent communication can help establish trust and understanding, allowing for ease in patients' access to the healthcare system. Furthermore, there should be policies in healthcare facilities to support cultural awareness training for doctors, so they can more effectively treat the specific health concerns of different ethnic and racial groups. Such education campaigns can bridge the gap between medical professionals and patients and have been shown to be effective in eradicating health disparities over time (Lurie et al., 2004). Creative solutions that center on outreach to communities can further enhance special populations' access to health care. Partnerships with communities and community health workers are just two examples of how outreach can be simplified and made more accessible and familiar. Locating health resources in or adjacent to communities enables such programs to directly address obstacles to care, such as transportation difficulties and unfamiliarity with current services. Besides, interpreter services can further improve substantially the communication of non-native speakers, thereby allowing them access care without fear of misinterpretation or stigmatization. Ultimately, comprehensive strategies that solve the unique circumstances of special populations will be essential in facilitating equity in accessing health care services within community health facilities (Weiss et al., 2015).

14.3. Cultural Competence in Healthcare

Health cultural competence is a necessary element to provide special populations with equal and efficient medical care. As healthcare systems become increasingly diverse, healthcare providers are faced with the challenge of addressing unique culture, language, and social needs of their patients. This is crucial not only in efforts to improve health outcomes but also to sustain trust among patients and healthcare providers. Culturally competent care has the ability to significantly reduce healthcare access barriers, and it has the ability to lead to more timely and appropriate treatment for at-risk populations. Moreover, when healthcare providers exhibit cultural competence, this facilitates communication whereby patients are able to easily explain their concerns and preferences, thus leading to more accurate diagnoses and individualized treatment plans. The process of developing cultural competence actually recasts healthcare delivery into a responsive service to the diverse needs of the community. Efforts at building cultural competence in healthcare settings need to be structural and systemic, cutting across every level of the healthcare system. Effective efforts include specialized training of healthcare professionals, which equips them with the competencies to comprehend and communicate with diverse populations. In addition, healthcare organizations need to implement policies that prioritize cultural competence, where personnel receive ongoing education on the significance of cultural consciousness within the clinical setting. Such interventions are vital in responding to systemic differences typical of healthcare. In studies, it has been discovered that provider and institution level cultural competent communication is paramount in averting racial and ethnic disparities in the quality of care, as indicated by literature evidence (Lurie et al., 2004).

Successful interaction with cultural competency has the potential to trigger vast improvement in patient satisfaction as well as health outcomes. Moreover, organizations need to keep track of and update their processes on a continuous basis in order to become more culturally competent. This involves applying the use of assessment instruments to gauge the effectiveness of cultural and linguistic competency programs in all healthcare environments. With data collection on outcomes and patient experience, healthcare providers are in a position to identify areas of improvement, particularly among special populations, who are likely to suffer healthcare disparities. Reports, articles, training materials on cultural competence may be applied to facilitate the ongoing process of evaluation and improvement (Mason, 2007). Last but not least, the integration of cultural competence into healthcare delivery enhances health equity such that all patients, regardless of background, receive quality care to which he or she is entitled. This emphasis on continuous learning and adaptation is essential in promoting an inclusive healthcare culture that emphasizes the needs of all people in society.

14.3.1. Importance of Cultural Awareness in Health Services

Cultural competence in healthcare is especially important to improve the quality of care for special groups of people in community health settings. Cultural knowledge provides health practitioners with the ability to communicate with patients across different backgrounds, build trust, and enhance patient responses. Cultural insensitivity, on the other hand, will cause providers to unintentionally distance minority individuals from receiving proper services, contributing to disparities in healthcare utilization. Culturally sensitive care involves acceptance and respect for the differing beliefs and customs that influence health behavior and preference. An illustration includes a pamphlet by the VCU Institute for Women's Health that emphasizes the support role that inducting Latino cultures and belief systems into practice plays in helping providers deliver congruent health interventions that are relevant to specific populations (Virginia Commonwealth University, 2006). Besides, cultural sensitivity eliminates barriers to effective healthcare access. When health service is designed with the priorities of culture and language at the center of the population, it can reduce confusion and enhance patient involvement. Implementing policies for cultural competence, according to the guidelines for meeting patients' needs, provides a friendly environment in healthcare centers. These guidelines promote the collection of relevant information and the development of culture-aware services directed towards identifiable cultural groups. By placing these issues at the forefront, health care workers are able to attempt to eliminate healthcare disparities that typically target oppressed groups (Wilson-Stronks et al., 2008). Such attempts not only improve health outcomes but also empower the community because they validate their cultural identity. Finally, ongoing training and education in cultural competence among health care workers are essential components to the movement towards equal health care. With an ever-diversifying population, it is increasingly important that practitioners be educated in the cultural contexts that shape their patients' perceptions of health. Not only does this facilitate empathic care but it is also central to mitigating serious public health problems that disproportionately strike special populations. Self-reflection and working with community organizations are strategies that can enhance the knowledge of providers regarding the issues that prevail across various populations. Hence, this strategic process of cultural awareness can lead to improved interventions and ultimately better community health outcomes by promoting an inclusive vision of healthcare that respects and is sensitive to the diversity of patient backgrounds (Wilson-Stronks et al., 2008).

14.3.2. Strategies for Improving Cultural Competence

Growing cultural competence within community

health settings demands an multi-dimensional approach that includes education, policy modification, and direct contact with special populations. Perhaps the most vital strategy is integrating culturally responsive training modules into educational curricula for healthcare practitioners. These training programs can equip practitioners with the knowledge to decode disparate cultures and their influences on health outcomes and behaviors. By education and awareness, these initiatives can reduce biases and improve patient-clinician interactions. Health education must involve the populations being served so interventions are tailored to address the unique needs, values, and beliefs of specific cultural groups. These educational initiatives lay the groundwork for a healthier health environment that ultimately gives rise to equitable access to care. Policy reform is also a necessity for improving cultural competence in health care settings. Some state policies can promote the objective of equal access to quality health care by instituting the morality of cultural competency in all areas of the organization. This integrated approach entails reviewing current proposals for healthcare reform and ensuring that they are in conformity with equity standards intended to remove disparities among special populations. By implementing systemic reforms, health systems are able to deliver culturally sensitive services and establish universal access to them, creating a culture of inclusiveness that welcomes diversity. Moreover, as discussed in Fish-Parcham et al. (2008), universal and innovative solutions that strengthen universally accessible health insurance are critical towards developing a sustainable platform for health equity. This will be important to engage policymakers to ensure reforms do not only exist on paper but rather get actualized in real-life improvements in service delivery. Lastly, culturally competent communication cannot be overemphasized because it breaks barriers between heterogeneous populations and healthcare providers. Communication strategies need to be tweaked at different levels from a provider-patient interaction level to health plan goals and even institutional policies. By addressing these areas, organizations can improve the quality of care provided to racial and ethnic minorities, as illustrated in Lurie et al. (2004). These include systematic alterations such as providing language services and using cultural brokers who can interpret interactions. Besides that, health plans must also invest in internal training programs that emphasize the importance of culturally competent communication among all staff members. By addressing the nuance of communication, health organizations will be able to reduce noticeably the disparities and enhance overall care effectiveness delivered to special populations.

14.3.3. Case Studies of Successful Cultural Competence Initiatives

Cultural competence strategies used in community health programs are a prime method of providing improved health outcomes among diverse populations. A suitable case study example is in urban health clinics that adopted organized approaches toward enhancing the cultural appropriateness of service provision. By placing utmost emphasis on policies that enable cultural competence, those clinics were able to modify services to meet the specific needs of diverse ethnic groups. This entailed the development of in-house practices for the identification and handling of linguistic issues, in the process establishing a patient-friendly setting for patients with diverse backgrounds. Besides, the involved programs included regular self-assessment tools that enabled clinics to measure their performance in delivering culturally responsive care and thus increasing health equity among the underserved populations (Wilson-Stronks et al., 2008). Another compelling example of successful cultural competence programs is in collaborations among managed care organizations and community health champions. These initiatives have centered on the development of training programs designed to enhance providers communication skills and eliminate implicit biases. Targeting culturally competent communication at multiple levels—providers, institutions, and health plans—these initiatives are central to remedying disparities in care that racial and ethnic minorities face. These kinds of strategies not only enable improved patient-provider relationships but also aid in the overall quality enhancement of care offered by the healthcare system. Through these collaborative arrangements, managed care organizations are better able to understand and meet the unique challenges faced by special populations (Lurie et al., 2004). The effectiveness of community health programs depends on an ongoing investment in culturally competent practices that are attuned to the shifting needs of diverse populations. Effective case examples illustrate the worth of building an organizational culture committed to inclusivity, such as recruiting a diverse workforce representative of served communities. In addition, the inclusion of mechanisms for patient feedback allows health organizations to be continually responsive to the unique needs and wants of their customers. Continuous engagement with community stakeholders not only educates program developers but also sustains an accountability structure for health equity. As modeled by initiatives that emphasize cooperation and adaptability, the ongoing course toward cultural competence is a revolutionary plan for resolving the healthcare disparities faced by so many of the country's special populations (Lurie et al., 2004; Wilson-Stronks et al., 2008).

14.4. Mental Health Considerations

Mental health considerations are most important when addressing the needs of special populations in community health. The special populations like individuals with disabilities, oppressed groups, and the elderly tend to have unique mental issues with societal stigma, restricted access to healthcare, and system barriers. All efforts must be focused on raising mental health awareness and access to necessary services through universal settings. The link between generic health care services and disability-specific agencies, as established in the Collaboration Brief series, highlights the importance of valuing particular needs of such populations. Through improved understanding of goals and determinants of eligibility, agencies are better positioned to plan resources and offer the most optimal systems of support which are the backbone in countering mental health disparities in such populations (National Center on Workforce and Disability/Adult, 2007). Also, the incorporation of mental health services into mainstream healthcare systems has the ability to dramatically affect special populations' outcomes. Primary or community-based co-location can remove access barriers and enable more integrated treatment approaches. Simultaneous treatment of physical health and mental health can produce a more integrated picture of patients' needs, which can lead to better health outcomes in the long run. Studies highlight the benefits and probable drawbacks of this approach, laying down the condition that successful integration is planned meticulously and includes collaborative effort by different providers of services (Ginsburg, 2008). The recognition of the interdependence between physical and mental health encourages a unified framework that can be utilized with different populations, ensuring that mental health problems form part of community health programs. Finally, the value of focused intervention in promoting mental health in special populations cannot be overstated. Specialized interventions aimed at the particular stresses faced by these populations, such as economic insecurity, social isolation, and limited access to health care, are essential. Mental health care should be designed culturally and to various settings to be most effective. Also essential are educational interventions to heighten awareness and reduce stigma that support the promotion of mental health as a priority among communities. Focusing on collaborative methods and their establishment of partnerships among agencies, stakeholders are able to create environments that address the mental health issues of special populations integratively, ultimately towards healthier communities and improved public health outcomes.

14.4.1. Prevalence of Mental Health Issues in Special Populations

The interconnection between special populations and mental health disorders is complex and multidimensional. Inmates, for instance, represent a particularly vulnerable population wherein there exists a high prevalence of mental illness as compared to the larger population. Empirical evidence has revealed that a significant number of individuals who are incarcerated have mental disorders like depression, bipolar disorder, and schizophrenia. This prevalence requires specially targeted intervention within the prison setting to specifically address these specific issues. Furthermore, the prison experience can exacerbate existing mental health issues, rendering successful treatment challenging due to a range of compounding factors. Mental health courts have been proposed as effective intervention; however, their success can vary widely by location. Therefore, it is vital to ensure that mental health services in prisons are available and effective to help promote better results for offenders on release (Pacecca et al., 2013). Another special population that generates significant mental health problems is Asian American and Pacific Islander (API) youth, who sometimes experience unique cultural and societal stressors. A comprehensive study organized by the SAAY Consortium reports that API youth tend to experience mental health issues, including depression and anxiety, as further exacerbated by mental illness stigma within their communities. Over 300 Asian youths were interviewed and an alarming rate reported experiences of victimization, stress management difficulties, and use of drugs as coping strategies. These findings indicate the urgent need for culturally sensitive mental health services that acknowledge the distinctive experiences of API youth. Drawing upon supportive networks, such as the Asian Youth Advocacy Network, is a key element in enhancing mental health outcomes among this population, providing youth with the resources they require to surmount their adversity and flourish (N/A, 2004). Placing a focus on the prevalence of mental illness among various special populations highlights the importance of intersectionality in community health initiatives. The interplay between socioeconomic status and mental health continues to offer some of the most important data, particularly among vulnerable populations. For instance, individuals below the poverty line are at higher risk for prison as well as mental illness as evidenced by correlations achieved in research on these populations. Therefore, interventions in community health must adopt a holistic approach that takes into consideration the socio-economic determinants of mental well-being. Taking into account the interconnectedness of poverty and mental well-being, population-based interventions can design more appropriate interventions. These interventions must incorporate education outreach, resource access, and advocacy activities that address systemic inequalities, ensuring equality in the availability of mental health care for all special populations (N/A, 2004; Pacecca et al., 2013).

14.4.2. Barriers to Mental Health Care Access

Obtaining mental health services is increasingly recognized as a part of total health, yet numerous barriers to needed services reach special population members. Among these barriers are systemic barriers including inadequate funding for mental health programs, insufficient mental health professionals, and the pervasive stigma about mental illness. For example, marginalized groups, including racial and ethnic minorities, not only encounter monetary obstacles but also cultural obstacles that render accessible services unavailable or culturally insensitive. Consequently, their mental health problems fall beneath the radar and therefore go untreated with the passage of time, leading to deteriorating conditions, which are detrimental to the overall health and well-being of the population. Prison populations, particularly women, demonstrate the challenge of access to mental health care. Female inmates are subjected to a multifaceted array of health issues, mostly grounded on previous disorders that are also escalated while in prison. As discovered, female criminal justice system members suffer significantly from mental health disorders but receive insufficient services with a focus on their unique needs. The California case reveals the systemic gaps in the health care delivery system for these women, a vast majority of which are racial and ethnic minorities and are frequently provided culturally incompetent care. This improper provision of services continues to worsen health disparities and illustrates the need for an interagency strategy to expand access to mental health care for this vulnerable population (N/A, 2006). Also, when individuals, particularly ex-offenders, attempt to become re-established in society, they are subjected to a significant barrier of not accessing mental health care services, as cited in release planning discussions. Ex-prisoners released from prisons will often struggle with housing, work, and stigma, which may impede their ability to access suitable mental health care. Good release planning plays a significant role in bridging the gap between confinement and community reintegration, making mental health services responsive to the needs of such individuals (Davies et al., 2008). Through addressing the fundamental needs of parolees and fostering collaborations between corrections agencies and community organizations, it may be possible to promote a model of comprehensive care that finally improves mental health outcomes and reduces recidivism for these groups.

14.4.3. Community-based Mental Health Programs

Community-based mental health programs are significant in addressing special populations' unique needs through accessible, targeted care. These interventions are designed to deliver mental health services directly in the communities that the people reside in, thereby reducing travel, cost, and stigma barriers. Such interventions are most helpful for individuals who are marginalized, including low-income families, minorities, and others with poor access to mainstream healthcare resources. Through the promotion of an integrated strategy, community-based interventions may incorporate preventative interventions, early intervention, and long-term management of mental health disorders in order to promote an environment supportive of mental health. This local perspective not only deals with individual need but also with building community, forming a support network that is paramount to recovery and resilience in the population with mental health. While successful, community-based mental health programs are faced with several issues that can reverse their successes. Shortages in funding and available resources make it difficult to maintain the ability to provide services that address differences in levels of mental health needs. Furthermore, program operation may be hampered by bureaucratic barriers in the provision of services among public health, mental health, and substance abuse treatment programs. These subtleties render coordination of care difficult, particularly in developing seamless pathways that will lead to individuals receiving adequate interventions and care. As talked about in recent studies, these concerns necessitate new efforts of service provision, something whose significance is realized in the immediacy of required federal health reform and government services realignment towards successful delivery of mental health care in communities (Kelch, 2011). Breaking down such systemic barriers is vital to optimizing the effectiveness and reach of community-based mental health initiatives. Successful community-based mental health initiatives exhibit some characteristics that contribute to their overall success. Those programs with robust care coordination work to ensure that not only are the individuals receiving initial treatment but also follow-up and ongoing care. This inter-connected system permits the identification of potential intervention needs in children and adults, thus optimizing services to ensure maximum efficiency and promote health-enhancing outcomes. Inter-relations among community agencies, healthcare professionals, and policy-makers form an integral part of this system because they ensure a culture of inter-cooperation that maximizes service delivery. Additionally, feedback loops are needed to ensure continuous improvement and program responsiveness to meet evolving special population needs. Best practice lessons can be used to frame policy implications to enable integrated care systems that ultimately yield better community health results (Hagelow et al., 2010). These are imperative initiatives to address gaps left by traditional models of healthcare and ensure that all benefit from needed mental health care.

14.5. Policy and Advocacy

Policy and advocacy are crucial to respond to the healthcare needs disparities of special populations in community health initiatives. Effective policymaking relies on the determination of the diverse needs of such populations, especially the homeless and aged, who have multi-morbidities. Specific policies by stakeholders can be put in place to intervene against obstacles to access, shifting the emphasis from reactive to preventive care. A comprehensive approach demands collaboration among government agencies, health care providers, and community organizations in order to guarantee that the concerns of vulnerable populations are not only identified but actively addressed. A comprehensive approach enables the establishment of a more equitable health care system because it emphasizes the importance of individualized interventions that respond to the unique needs of older people and other socially excluded populations in society and therefore foster inclusivity and better health outcomes. Advocacy efforts are essential in enacting policy reforms that impact the health conditions of special populations. The voices of directly involved communities must be listened to so that their influence on policy makers and access to the resources they need can be realized. Take, for instance, getting to know the dynamics of the most vulnerable older states and how they contribute to bringing out innovative and effective approaches appropriate to their health concerns. By spotlighting research-based facts in advocacy campaigns, stakeholders can call for legislative action supporting funding services that enhance elderly health. The advocacy is not just focal on the compelling necessity for resource availability but also on the imperative of building programs responsive to the increasing demands of aging populations. This further underlines the need for constant engagement with affected communities to ensure that their contribution influences policy and healthcare agendas. Brought together also is the need for policy and advocacy in addressing homelessness, an overarching issue of community health that weighs heavily on marginalized populations. Research carried out by organizations like the Charles and Helen Schwab Foundation illustrates the complex relationship between homelessness and health, highlighting the necessity for policies that address the social determinants of health. Effective advocacy will have to try and sensitize the public to the systemic forces contributing to homelessness and lobby for policies with stable housing interventions and healthcare access. By funding strategic programs that meet immediate needs as well as long-term stability for homeless persons, policymakers can significantly enhance health outcomes. These efforts ultimately lead to a more comprehensive understanding of the health of the community, which acknowledges the value of stable living conditions as the underpinning element of health and well-being.

14.5.1. Role of Policy in Addressing Health Needs of Special Populations

Policies have a significant role in meeting the health needs of special populations, especially through the funding and establishment of community health centers. Such centers, which were reasserted through landmark legislation in 2008, are essential providers for the uninsured, publicly insured, and underinsured groups. The populations being treated in these facilities reflect the great diversity of health care needs among communities, highlighting the imperative for targeted health services to increase access and outcomes in vulnerable populations. Of significance, the ability to provide quality care in spite of adversity through unstable revenue streams is key to eliminating health disparities for special populations. Thus, supportive policy is instrumental in the sustainability and effectiveness of these vital health service providers so that they can keep providing services to the populations at highest risk (Finnegan et al., 2009). Another key policy framework that plays a significant role in determining the health outcomes of special populations is Medicaid and the Childrens Health Insurance Program (CHIP). These programs have been instrumental in getting health coverage for not just low-income families but also the vulnerable, like children with special needs. Medicaid and CHIP, by shielding access to primary health care and medication, have promoted overall health and financial stability for millions of individuals. Further, sustained protection against reductions in the budget is crucial for these populations, as decreasing funding can greatly hamper access to needed care. The role of these programs goes beyond economic assistance; they serve as a safety net that complements the ability of special populations to receive timely and adequate medical care, ultimately leading to improved better community health outcomes (N/A, 2011). Besides, the connection between special populations and health policy is strengthened by the strategic application of public health programs that are aimed at affecting specific social determinants of health. The programs target issues such as housing, education, and nutrition that have disproportionate effects on marginalized populations. Therefore, comprehensive policies need to recognize and address such interconnected problems in a bid to adequately work on the health inequities of special populations. Coordination between government institutions, community organizations, and health-care providers is critical to the development of integrated strategies unique to the particular needs of these populations. Through sensitive policies to the specific requirements for special populations, communities can facilitate environments for enhanced health gains, ultimately bringing the vision of equal health care for all within realization (Finnegan et al., 2009; N/A, 2011).

14.5.2. Advocacy Efforts for Equitable Health Care

Advocacy to bring equitable health care is imperative in dealing with the disparities of special populations in community health. Many grassroots organizations have been formed to give a voice to marginalized communities, advocating for policy reforms that provide access to relevant health care services. For example, San Francisco's Chinese Progressive Association (CPA) is a great example of successful community-based activism. By mobilizing low-income Chinese immigrants for over four decades, the CPA spearheaded the campaign for the Health Care Security Ordinance (HCSO), which has had a near-universal access to health care program since 2006 implementation. Not only did the program expand access to health care but also proved how community organizing can harvest dramatic policy dividends as a vehicle to tackle larger concerns like economic inequality and gentrification, providing a blueprint toward equitable health care for underserved populations (Fang et al., 2018). The coalition-building role cannot be overstressed in health advocacy. Collaborative efforts, as seen in the case of the CPA's participation in the HCSO coalition, project the potential of united fronts in enhancing advocacy effectiveness. Communication among various stakeholders—among residents in a local level and other health organizations—gives rise to a mutual understanding of health care disparities and inspires collective action. These coalitions are central to shaping policy conversations around health equity, so that the particular needs of diverse populations are at the table. The outcomes of these efforts suggest that advocacy is more than one issue in terms of organizing support, but also in the creation of lasting alliances that can assist in shaping systemic change. As the State of Health Equity Movement report notes, the cooperative strategies employed by advocacy agencies reflect the key aspect in maintaining health equity for marginalized populations (Birnbaum et al., 2011). The effective advocacy also entails ongoing monitoring and adaptation to keep pace with the changing set of community health needs. Organizations need to learn from the achievements and failures of their campaigns. For instance, the CPA's experience with the HCSO is instructive in the matter of dynamic relations between local organizing and more extensive political contexts. From this knowledge of the origins of inequalities, such as economic shifts and policy limitations, is a more knowledgeable development of targeted strategies for future advocacy campaigns. Frequent contact with the community provides a model of participation, in that advocacy is adapted to shifting priorities of the individuals it aims to advocate for. Lastly, the health advocacy platform for equitable healthcare must be fluid since it constantly adapts to address the diverse challenges that face special populations, thereby evidencing the commitment towards health equity for all (Fang et al., 2018).

14.5.3. Impact of Legislation on Community Health Initiatives

The intersection of legislation and community health programs significantly shapes health outcomes for various populations. Legislative action aimed at promoting fair access to quality health care is the foundation for constructing successful community health programs. By offering policy frameworks that promote health equity, such legislations can have a direct impact on the availability of resources, funding, and innovative practice aimed at targeting underserved populations. For example, legislation that identifies and encourages certain health equity initiatives can create channels for innovative action responsive to the needs of the local community, hence enhancing insurance coverage in terms of accessibility and inclusivity. These initiatives are especially vital for special populations because they help to remove disparities and provide coordinated care. Also, federal health reforms overflow outside of policy-making to impact operational procedures states must use to get individuals to required health care. Reforms enable health care system coordination and integration when special populations, particularly those who handle difficult health conditions, obtain integrated health care. By ensuring that states are incentivized to promote coordination among various health providers, federal law guarantees that there is a better smoother patient experience. This integration has the capability to bolster health outcomes as there emerge specialized programs to address the unique demands of marginalized populations. In support of well-crafted legislation, community health initiatives can develop into successful interventions that address chronic conditions as well as social determinants of health. The emphasis on results-oriented strategies in health legislation also supports efficiencies that significantly enhance community health initiatives. Where legislation is based on measurable outcomes, it compels organizations toward data-informed practices, eventually leading to improved service delivery and allocation of resources. For instance, states are able to employ legislation in issuing policies that strengthen the provision of services effectively in response to the needs of special populations. Regular revision of these policies helps ensure that health programs remain effective and responsive. Therefore, by adequate and well-designed legislation, community health programs not only solve immediate health problems but also establish foundations for long-term gains in health, particularly among the most vulnerable sectors in society, thus propelling the overall objective of health equity.

14.6. Community Engagement and Education

Community education and participation play master roles in addressing special populations' health differences, particularly among Indigenous people and underrepresented populations. Effective community engagement programs establish trust, respect, and collaboration, such that health interventions are culturally appropriate and meaningful. For instance, the inclusion of such groups in health education allows for the recognition of particular challenges and barriers that they face, thus the creation of education programs addressing their unique needs. Efforts like the Clinical Research Education in Genome Science (CREiGS) are one step in this direction by conducting genomic and statistical training for a broad segment of participants, including underrepresented group members. These efforts not only enhance the participants' skill sets but also allow participants to motivate their communities to engage in health-centric discussions, which ultimately leads to the attainment of health equity and informed decision-making within healthcare settings (Gomes et al., 2025). Among special populations, such as Indigenous people, awareness of distinctive health issues should be matched with specialized educational strategies. Soil-transmitted helminthiasis (STH), for example, is widespread among Indigenous people and illustrates the necessity of applying community expertise to health education interventions. Reduction in the burden of STH calls for more than frequent mass drug administration (MDA) but also the enhancement of WASH behavior. Strategies to educate populations about STH control measures should be concurrent with cultural systems of beliefs and access issues for highest impact. For example, interviews and focus group discussions with community leaders may uncover local perceptions about treatment safety and programmatic implementation difficulties, allowing the collaborative creation of culturally appropriate health education materials that resonate with community members (Ladia et al., 2024). Moreover, the need for ongoing monitoring and adaptation of community engagement and education strategies cannot be overstated. Stakeholder feedback is key to ascertaining the success of educational interventions and keeping these responsive to the evolving needs of special groups. For CREiGS, participants' competence and confidence were gauged, with areas where the training program could improve identified. Such assessments educate and inform subsequent cohorts and assist in developing an inclusive learning environment. Also, the framework employed to define the participation of Indigenous populations demonstrates ongoing efforts at dialogue between health authorities and the community members. Construction of strong feedback mechanisms allows populations to voice themselves and adapt strategies effectively, resulting in enhanced health as well as a sense of ownership over community health programs (Gomes et al., 2025; Ladia et al., 2024).

14.6.1. Importance of Community Involvement in Health Programs

Participatory role by the community plays a vital role in the effectiveness of healthcare programs, particularly for special populations with certain challenges. Enrolling community members enhances a feeling of ownership, which leads to active participation within programs for health. Involvement is especially vital in planning programs to meet the specific needs of distinct populations, such as homeless youth or youth within the juvenile justice system. There is evidence that these individuals are frequently faced with serious barriers, such as interrupted education and fluctuating housing, that will influence their health status negatively. By involving communities' voices in the design and implementation of health programs, the stakeholders will be in a better position to overcome these impediments, paving the way for interventions and preventive measures that are attractive to the target population, ultimately fostering better health outcomes and community resilience in the long run. Secondly, the success of transferring health programs to a community environment heavily relies on establishing partnership relations among residents, healthcare providers, and local agencies. These collaborations can enhance resource sharing, enable exchange of information, and help establish a supportive environment for special populations. Integrated program models with the leverage of varying community systems are an example. These can enhance public health programs' ability significantly. The coordinated efforts can facilitate easier access to mental health services, hence addressing the needs of youth being discharged from residential treatment programs. Community participation, therefore, becomes a force to drive the provision of comprehensive care that is tailored to meet special population individualized needs, finally leading to improved healthier outcomes and enhancing the general quality of life for the community. The combination of community participation and health programs also underscores the requirement of tailored interventions in addressing equity and overcoming systemic inequities. When communities are empowered to participate actively in health programs, they are capable of contributing ideas that translate to culturally relevant and accessible services. Such integration is especially crucial for marginalized communities who are likely to experience problems accessing healthcare compared to their non-marginalized peers. For example, programs for youth who are homeless can leverage community engagement to help them weather legal and social issues, and by doing so decrease their risk of entanglement with the juvenile justice system. In most cases, integrating community involvement in health programs makes the programs more effective and also an inclusive environment in which all its members are concerned about their health status, as shown in Pilnik (2017) and enhancing the general health infrastructure, as shown in Cameron et al. (2012).

14.6.2. Strategies for Effective Health Education

Effective health education is crucial to improving well-being in special populations because it addresses specific needs and issues of such populations. One of the basic strategies is the development of culturally appropriate materials that address the beliefs and values of the target groups. By considering the population's cultural setting, the health educator can achieve highest participation and better understand health concepts. Culturally responsive communication builds trust, and it also supports the transfer of important health information. To further increase this effect, health education programs need to be incorporated into community member feedback so the materials are tuned to their experiences and worldview. This strategy not only enables participants but also has a critical role in overall health initiative success in reducing disparities, as identified by the literature on health disparities that prioritizes the importance of culturally competent communication at different levels of the healthcare system (Lurie et al., 2004). Another possible method of health education among special populations is incorporating technology and digital media. The growing use of mobile and internet technology facilitates fresh approaches to reaching underserved groups. Web-based resources, cell phone apps, and social media marketing are among the methods employed by health educators to spread information and make contact with these populations. This approach not only expands the audience for health education but also enables instant communication and information sharing. It should be ensured that digital solutions are accessible and optimized to meet the precise requirements of the target group, keeping in mind aspects such as language proficiency and technical savvy. Furthermore, powerful data collection systems can track levels of engagement and health outcomes, enabling continuous improvement of health programs. Emphasis on the use of technology is aligned with frameworks that have effectively attempted to reduce disparities in health in managed care settings through espousing community outreach and education (Baquet et al., 2004). Lastly, developing partnerships among stakeholders is essential to optimizing the effectiveness of health education. Community agency collaboration with health providers and public health organizations is capable of leading to integrated health education programs that are attuned to the multiple reach of health disparities. These collaborations provide opportunities for resource sharing, cross-fertilization of skills, and the development of common approaches to health promotion. Joint efforts, for instance, can lead to the planning of health fairs, workshops, and training that are specifically designed to meet the unique needs of special groups. By leveraging the advantages of multi-organization alliances, health educators can optimize delivery of services and guarantee that health messages are not only aligned but also backed by multiple avenues. As observed in healthy community models, these collaborative models can significantly enhance reach and influence for health education, ultimately fostering enhanced health outcomes among vulnerable populations (Baquet et al., 2004).

14.6.3. Examples of Successful Community Engagement Initiatives

Effective community outreach interventions play a critical role in bridging health gaps among special populations. One excellent example can be seen in the endeavors of Rhode Island Department of Health (RIDOH), which used localized Health Equity Zones (HEZ). These HEZ focus on social determinants of health by providing financial support to 10 locally initiated collaboratives that offer strategies tailored to local needs. RIDOH's approach prioritizes evidence-based strategy augmented by bottom-up grassroots community involvement, which is necessary for the understanding and dismantling of the obstacles to health equity. Furthermore, the creation of the Health Equity Institute and an explicit HEZ Team provides sustainable assistance, introducing sustainable projects that are able to directly involve community stakeholders into interventions in health to improve the results among historically marginalized communities (Alexander-Scott et al., 2017). Another excellent example is the evolution of diaspora activism in health-focused giving among foreign-born communities. As diasporas come to play larger roles in influencing health conditions through philanthropy, institutions that aim to foster these patterns of giving have come into prominence. The evolution of strategic models has brought forth models that connect diaspora communities in America with home nations. These initiatives not only boost expenditure on health programs but also mobilize group action among people within communities, leading to innovative solutions to essential health demands. The impact of successful diaspora involvement is manifested in enhanced development of health infrastructure and enhanced access to health care for special populations, thus portraying effective community involvement (Johnson, 2007). Apart from these noted initiatives, the use of local voices in program planning and implementation of health programs cannot be emphasized enough. Effective community engagement programs tend to place a high value on transparency and inclusivity so that community members' concerns and input inform projects. The participatory nature of this process improves trust, which further encourages community members to participate actively in health promotion activities. For instance, community advisory boards have been shown to enhance the significance of projects by providing diverse ideas well-positioned to heal the conditions of special populations. Not only do these collaborative models empower individuals but also give them a sense of ownership of health outcomes, which argues in favor of effective engagement in a bid to attain health equity for all members of a community. Therefore, such efforts present a solid foundation for continuous dialogue and collaboration among healthcare organizations and the populations they serve.

SUMMARY

Hence, in addressing the health inequities faced by special populations, multi-dimensional and collaborative efforts are necessary. In making sense of the unique issues facing these populations, stakeholders can craft interventions that address the social determinants of health head-on. Programs such as HEZ are only a few examples of the means by which localized responses can unite communities in building sustainable health gains. Organizing funding for local collaboratives operating within the zones, organizations are able to instill a sense of ownership among the community, which eventually builds resilience and empowerment. The RIDOH serves as evidence of this approach in action since it lays the groundwork for effective community-based solutions with a concentration on data-driven strategies and the importance of involving grassroots perspectives in strengthening health outcomes (Alexander-Scott et al., 2017). Secondly, the incorporation of diverse leadership in nonprofit organizations is key to improving the capacity to effectively serve special populations. Financial investments, such as multiday grants to minority-serving entities, build infrastructure and ensure the participation of those traditionally left out of health discourse. With leadership diversity, health initiatives have a better chance to speak more profoundly to the populations they aim to serve. This shared commitment builds trust, an essential element of community health engagement. Breaking down systemic barriers to access of healthcare, such as economic limitations and cultural bias, is the most important approach towards long-term health equity (N/A, 2008). Finally, the journey towards health equity among special populations is a persistent process and requires persistent effort from all the concerned stakeholders. Policymakers, doctors, and community organizations must collaborate closely and assess and alter their strategies on an ongoing basis. Furthermore, encouraging a culture of measurement and responsiveness to community need will complement these efforts. Education and outreach can also increase awareness about health disparities, ensuring community members are informed and motivated to battle for their health. As communities evolve, so does our approach, once again affirming the importance of collaborative action guided by equity in ensuring the well-being of all groups.

In community health dynamics analysis, special populations that are likely to have special needs should be considered. These include individuals living in homelessness, low-income family groups, older adults, and those living with disabilities, who require special interventions to address their individual health care needs. The research points out that access to health services, affordability, and social determinants of health are the pivotal factors that affect health outcomes among these groups of people. Initiatives for improving community health must confront the multifaceted obstacles to health disparities, thereby assuring that such vulnerable groups are maximally assisted in their pursuit of health equity. Addressing these issues requires a concerted effort, merging the practice of public health and social welfare policies into an overarching scheme for improving community health. Food security is also a concern for special populations, particularly in emergencies when support networks are disrupted. Analytically, the vulnerable and low-income portions of the population are disproportionately affected by food insecurity where robust disaster preparedness programs are critically needed. The strategies must not only consider immediate response but also the long-term sustainability of the food system to enhance resiliency among impacted communities. Recommendations further underscore the importance of involving such communities in planning, particularly because they are likely to provide valuable information on their own particular needs and aspirations. Community participation can not only mitigate the impact of disasters but enhance overall health outcomes among people who otherwise tend to be marginalized in times of crisis (Bonini et al., 2014). Moreover, homelessness entails complexities that require holistic solutions that cross different segments of community health. There has been a commissioned study by the Charles and Helen Schwab Foundation that has made evident strategies by which the lives of the homeless can be improved, revealing that philanthropic intervention can play a vital role in building up health care services in this sector (Pontecorvo et al., 2002). The link between housing stability and health is profound; without a stable home, health will suffer. Thus, integrating health services with housing support can create a safety net that serves both immediate and long-term needs. Ultimately, community health programs must be fueled by cross-agency coordination among government agencies, non-profits, and the communities themselves to create solutions that endure for special populations.

KEY TERMS FROM THIS CHAPTER

- Vulnerable Populations
- Culturally Competent Care
- LGBTQ+ Health
- Homelessness
- People with Disabilities
- Maternal and Child Health
- Low-Income Populations
- Mental Health Services
- Community Outreach
- Incarcerated Individuals
- Health Literacy
- Access to Care
- Trauma-Informed Care
- Health Disparities
- Underserved Communities
- Rural Health
- Migrant and Refugee Health
- Elderly Population
- Minority Health
- Chronic Disease Management
- Language Access Services
- Immigrant Health
- Youth and Adolescents
- Social Inclusion
- Prevention Services

CLOSER LOOK

SEXUAL AND GENDER MINORITIES (SGM)

A closer look at sexual and gender minorities (SGM) highlights the diverse identities and experiences of individuals whose sexual orientation, gender identity, or gender expression differs from societal norms. This group includes, but is not limited to, lesbian, gay, bisexual, transgender, queer, intersex, asexual, and non-binary individuals. While sexual and gender diversity is a natural part of human identity, SGM populations often face significant social, legal, and health disparities due to systemic discrimination, stigma, and exclusion. These challenges can result in reduced access to healthcare, higher rates of mental health issues, increased risk of violence, and economic insecurity. Stigma and minority stress—caused by chronic exposure to discrimination—can negatively impact both physical and mental health, leading to outcomes such as depression, anxiety, substance use, and suicide. Moreover, in many regions, legal barriers and cultural taboos prevent SGM individuals from seeking support or receiving equitable care. To address these disparities, it is essential to create inclusive environments that affirm diverse identities and promote equal rights and protections. This includes implementing anti-discrimination laws, training healthcare providers in culturally competent care, and developing targeted public health programs that meet the specific needs of SGM communities. Education and awareness-raising are also critical for reducing prejudice and fostering acceptance in schools, workplaces, and public spaces. Importantly, meaningful inclusion of SGM voices in policy development, research, and service delivery ensures that interventions are both effective and respectful. Despite persistent challenges, SGM communities continue to show resilience, strength, and leadership in advocating for equity and social change. By acknowledging the unique struggles they face and actively working to remove structural barriers, society can move toward a future where all individuals—regardless of their sexual orientation or gender identity—can live with dignity, safety, and full participation in public life.

REFERENCES

1. Agyapomaa, M. (2024). Abstract B042: Socioeconomic and racial disparities in pediatric cancer outcomes in the Ghanaian health sector: Challenges and strategies for equitable care. *Cancer Research.* https://www.semanticscholar.org/paper/a83ce76dfeab43e60cb817bc262eaa6a3000370b (accessed on 26th June 2025).
2. Alexander-Scott, N., Ankoma, N., et al. (2017). Rhode Island's Health Equity Zones: Addressing local problems with local solutions. https://digitalscholarship.unlv.edu/cgi/viewcontent.cgi?article=1643&context=jhdrp (accessed on 26th June 2025).
3. Alley, E. S., Boatin, B., Christensen, O. W., Dadzie, K. Y., et al. (2017). Patterns of epidemiology and control of onchocerciasis in West Africa. https://core.ac.uk/download/85209667.pdf (accessed on 26th June 2025).
4. Baquet, C. R., Bengen-Seltzer, B., & Carter-Pokras, O. (2004). Healthcare disparities and models for change. https://core.ac.uk/download/pdf/17192976.pdf (accessed on 26th June 2025).
5. Bibbins-Domingo, K., Capriotti, M. R., Flentje, A., Frazier, L., et al. (2019). Using mobile technology to engage sexual and gender minorities in clinical research. https://core.ac.uk/download/323073814.pdf (accessed on 26th June 2025).
6. Birnbaum, N., Masterson, E., & Schoomaker, H. (2011). *State of Health Equity Movement, 2011 Update Part B: Catalog of Activities DRA Project Report No. 11–02.* https://core.ac.uk/download/pdf/18491811.pdf (accessed on 26th June 2025).
7. Blakely, T., Chen, J., Cormack, D., Cunningham, R., et al. (2010). Survival disparities in Indigenous and non-Indigenous New Zealanders with colon cancer: The role of patient comorbidity, treatment and health service factors. https://core.ac.uk/download/148643017.pdf (accessed on 26th June 2025).
8. Bonini, C., & Rapp, S. (2014). *San Francisco Disaster Food System Report.* https://core.ac.uk/download/75782845.pdf (accessed on 26th June 2025).
9. Bukusi, E. A., Cohen, C. R., Kwena, Z., Oyaro, P., et al. (2016). Implementation of repeat HIV testing during pregnancy in Kenya: A qualitative study. https://core.ac.uk/download/323308645.pdf (accessed on 26th June 2025).
10. Cameron, G., Frensch, K., & Smit-Quosai, T. (2012). *Improving Community Adaptation Outcomes for Youth Graduating from Residential Mental Health Programs: A Synthesis Review (FULL REPORT).* https://core.ac.uk/download/157835009.pdf (accessed on 26th June 2025).
11. Danso-Appiah, A., Utarini, A., Crampin, A. C., Pond, B., Paul, B. D., Babu, B. V., Braga, C., et al. (2009). Social research on neglected diseases of poverty: Continuing and emerging themes. https://core.ac.uk/download/338058.pdf (accessed on 26th June 2025).
12. Davies, E., La Vigne, N., Halberstadt, R., & Palmer, T. (2008). *Release Planning for Successful Reentry: A Guide for Corrections, Service Providers, And Community Groups.* https://core.ac.uk/download/71348466.pdf (accessed on 26th June 2025)
13. Estes, C. L., Yeo, G. W., Molina, L. C., Plumb, M., Hernandez, M., Goldberg, S., Wallace, S. P., et al. (2007). *Women, Health and Aging: Building A Statewide Movement.* https://core.ac.uk/download/71355916.pdf (accessed on 26th June 2025).
14. Fang, S., Ivey, S. L., Lee, E. J. M., Ly, M. H., et al. (2018). Closing the loophole: A case study of

organizing for more equitable and affordable access to health care in San Francisco. https://core.ac.uk/download/323310450.pdf (accessed on 26th June 2025)

15. Fernandes-Alcantara, A. L. (2012). *Vulnerable Youth: Background and Policies*. https://core.ac.uk/download/9347168.pdf (accessed on 26th June 2025)
16. Finnegan, B., Shin, P., & Rosenbaum, S. (2009). *Community Health Centers in An Era of Health System Reform and Economic Downturn: Prospects and Challenges*. https://core.ac.uk/download/71350331.pdf (accessed on 26th June 2025).
17. Fish-Parcham, C., Panares, R., & Adland, S. (2008). *Identifying and Evaluating Equity Provisions in State Health Care Reform*. https://core.ac.uk/download/71352106.pdf (accessed on 26th June 2025).
18. Ginsburg, S. (2008). *Collocating Health Services: A Way to Improve Coordination of Children's Health Care?* https://core.ac.uk/download/71350229.pdf (accessed on 26th June 2025).
19. Gomes, S., Crosby, L. E., Jacquez, F., Knapke, J., Michell, J., Meinzen-Derr, J., Buxo, C. J., et al. (2025). 209 The Clinical Research Education in Genome Science (CREiGS) short course: An innovative program for enhancing research capacity in genome science. *Journal of Clinical and Translational Science, 9*, 64–65. https://www.semanticscholar.org/paper/a6c4d0d282d8c14bb0d7ff32a9643e94f655fcf8 (accessed on 26th June 2025).
20. Gómez, G., Kovalskys, I., Leme, A. C., Quesada, D., Rigotti, A., Cortés Sanabria, L. Y., Yépez Garcia, M. Y., et al. (2021). Socioeconomic status impact on diet quality and body mass index in eight Latin American countries: ELANS study results. *Nutrients, 13*. https://www.semanticscholar.org/paper/65df4fb6f84cb4f58dad03a343a127dcdc5f3c31 (accessed on 26th June 2025)
21. Hagelow, G., & Silow-Carroll, S. (2010). *Systems of Care Coordination for Children: Lessons Learned Across State Models*. https://core.ac.uk/download/71355339.pdf (accessed on 26th June 2025).
22. Johnson, P. D. (2007). *Diaspora philanthropy: Influences, initiatives, and issues*. https://core.ac.uk/download/71350777.pdf (accessed on 26th June 2025).
23. Kelch, D. R. (2011). *The Crucial Role of Counties in The Health of Californians: An Overview*. https://core.ac.uk/download/71357956.pdf (accessed on 26th June 2025)
24. Kenney, G. M., & Pelletier, J. E. (2010). *Improving the Lives of Young Children: The Role of Developmental Screenings in Medicaid and CHIP*. https://core.ac.uk/download/71347983.pdf (accessed on 26th June 2025).
25. Kumar, P. (2019). Mountain West Clinical Translational Research-Infrastructure Network: Introduction. https://digitalscholarship.unlv.edu/cgi/viewcontent.cgi?article=1987&context=jhdrp (accessed on 26th June 2025).
26. Ladia, M. A., Belizario, V., Cubarrubias, D. L. P. F., & Agustin, A. M. D. L. (2024). Accessibility of soil-transmitted helminthiasis control strategies in selected Indigenous People communities in the Philippines. *Acta Medica Philippina, 58*, 25–33. https://www.semanticscholar.org/paper/d44060c7c9fad0d90a295f1c331eac64e93b1154 (accessed on 26th June 2025).
27. Lurie, N., & Taylor, S. L. (2004). The role of culturally competent communication in reducing ethnic and racial healthcare disparities. https://core.ac.uk/download/pdf/18491828.pdf (accessed on 26th June 2025).
28. Mason, M. A. (2007). *Equality in Health: An Annotated Bibliography with Resources on Health*

Disparities and Cultural and Linguistic Competency. https://core.ac.uk/download/71346571.pdf (accessed on 26th June 2025).

29. Meacham, S., Metzger, D., Sukpraput, T., et al. (2013). Publications on chronic disease in coal dependent communities in Central Appalachia. https://digitalscholarship.unlv.edu/cgi/viewcontent.cgi?article=1081&context=jhdrp (accessed on 26th June 2025).
30. N/A. (2004). *Moving Beyond Exclusion: Focusing on the Needs of Asian/Pacific Islander Youth in San Francisco*. https://core.ac.uk/download/71341912.pdf (accessed on 26th June 2025).
31. N/A. (2006). *The Spiral of Risk: Health Care Provision to Incarcerated Women*. https://core.ac.uk/download/71341837.pdf (accessed on 26th June 2025).
32. N/A. (2008). *Strengthening Nonprofit Minority Leadership and The Capacity of Minority-Led and Other Grassroots Community-Based Organizations*. https://core.ac.uk/download/71355260.pdf (accessed on 26th June 2025).
33. N/A. (2009). *Human Relations Report*. https://core.ac.uk/download/71346008.pdf (accessed on 26th June 2025).
34. N/A. (2011). *Medicaid Works: A Review of How Public Insurance Protects the Health and Finances of Children and Other Vulnerable Populations*. https://core.ac.uk/download/71358653.pdf (accessed on 26th June 2025).
35. N/A. (2025). *Prev Chronic Dis*. https://core.ac.uk/download/144195177.pdf (accessed on 26th June 2025).
36. National Center on Workforce and Disability/Adult. (2007). *Essential Considerations for Establishing Partnerships Among Agencies Addressing the Employment-Related Needs of Individuals with Disabilities*. https://core.ac.uk/download/5119015.pdf (accessed on 26th June 2025).
37. Pacecca, M. (2013). *Mental Illness in The Prison System: Exploring the Issues and Possible Solutions*. https://core.ac.uk/download/236292309.pdf (accessed on 26th June 2025).
38. Pilnik, L. (2017). *Addressing the Intersections of Juvenile Justice Involvement and Youth Homelessness: Principles for Change*. https://core.ac.uk/download/80510642.pdf (accessed on 26th June 2025).
39. Pontecorvo, D., & Putnam-Walkerly, K. (2002). *Homelessness: Key Findings and Grantmaking Strategies*. https://core.ac.uk/download/75778392.pdf (accessed on 26th June 2025).
40. Redcross, C., Bloom, D., Hsueh, J., Rich, S., & Martin, V. (2007). *Four Strategies to Overcome Barriers to Employment: An Introduction to The Enhanced Services for The Hard-To-Employ Demonstration and Evaluation Project*. https://core.ac.uk/download/71340912.pdf (accessed on 26th June 2025).
41. Shadmi, E. (2013). Disparities in multiple chronic conditions within populations. https://core.ac.uk/download/pdf/29572286.pdf (accessed on 26th June 2025).
42. Takach, M., & Kaye, N. (2009). *Building Medical Homes in State Medicaid and CHIP Programs*. https://core.ac.uk/download/71349689.pdf (accessed on 26th June 2025).
43. Virginia Commonwealth University. (2006). *Metro Richmond Latino Health Services & Resource Guide–2006*. https://core.ac.uk/download/51286596.pdf (accessed on 26th June 2025).
44. Weil, A., Gauthier, A. K., Cantrell, C., Justice, D., Scott, J., Witgert, K., Zemel, S., et al. (2009). *A*

State Policymakers' Guide to Federal Health Reform: Part I: Anticipating How Federal Health Reform Will Affect State Roles. https://core.ac.uk/download/71355186.pdf (accessed on 26th June 2025).

45. Weiss, R. (2015). *Confronting Cultural Challenges for Migrant Healthcare in Switzerland.* https://core.ac.uk/download/232737448.pdf (accessed on 26th June 2025).

46. Wilson-Stronks, A., Kopp, A. L., Cordero, C. L., Galvez, E., & Lee, K. K. (2008). *One Size Does Not Fit All: Meeting the Health Care Needs of Diverse Populations.* https://core.ac.uk/download/71353544.pdf (accessed on 26th June 2025).

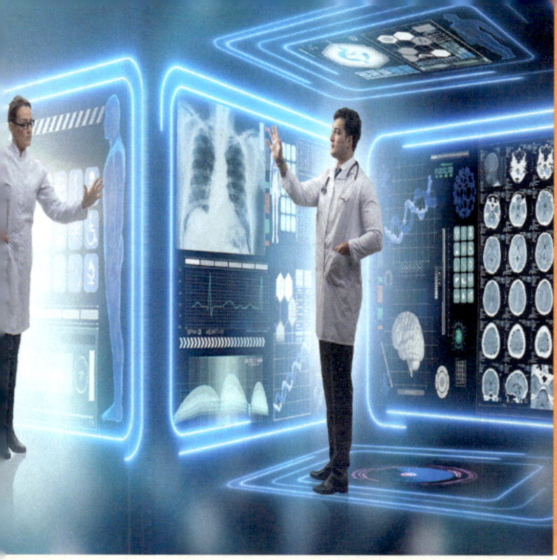

Chapter 15

EMERGING TRENDS AND FUTURE DIRECTIONS IN COMMUNITY HEALTH

Contents

Introduction

The social determinants of present-day community health have been radically altered by emerging trends that enhance the interdependence of public health interventions and social determinants. According to recent debates on health promotion, interventions at the population and community levels have played a crucial role in combating non-communicable diseases (NCDs) as well as promoting mental health outcomes. This integrated approach addresses not only the individual capacities, but also the broader socio-political and environmental determinants of health equity. The Shanghai Declaration reinforces the assumption that effective health promotion intervention should be evidence-based, sustainable, and context-appropriate to respond to the multi-dimensional needs of populations and prepare the grounds for intervention in community health in the future (Kilibarda, 2024). Collaborative efforts are needed in working on these determinants to build a stronger governance, expand health literacy, and enhance social mobilization towards more equitable health. In the rapidly digitalizing world, the role of technology in enhancing community health cannot be overstated. Social media has emerged as a viable platform for disseminating information and interacting with community members. Social media platforms such as Twitter and Facebook enable health workers to address the public directly, sharing significant information regarding disease prevention and health education. Democratization of medicine in platforms, as discussed under medical education, offers greater access to necessary health knowledge (Jain et al., 2024). As public health campaigns leverage such digital technologies, they can effectively disseminate vital messages about preventive measures and encourage participation among people, thus giving more overall awareness and participation in health. These tendencies indicate how technology can empower gaps in health communication and enable inclusive public health program participation. In the future, the future of community health will demand an adaptive approach that reflects the evolving character of challenges that come with globalization, environmental change, and socio-political tensions. The adjustment process for adapting health promotion for the response to challenges demands considerable sensitivity to emerging public health trends and how to anticipate shifts in the needs and trends of the community. A visionary methodology of health promotion coupled with an examination of existing health systems and policy frameworks will be critical in elucidating the dynamics of the contemporary health imperative. This visionary framework requires a convergence towards intersectoral action and collaboration among sectors to develop a comprehensive health model that encompasses not just medical care but also socio-economic health. Through the establishment of solid infrastructure for promoting health, communities are able to more effectively implement effective interventions that are responsive to changing health environments (Kilibarda, 2024) (Figure 15.1).

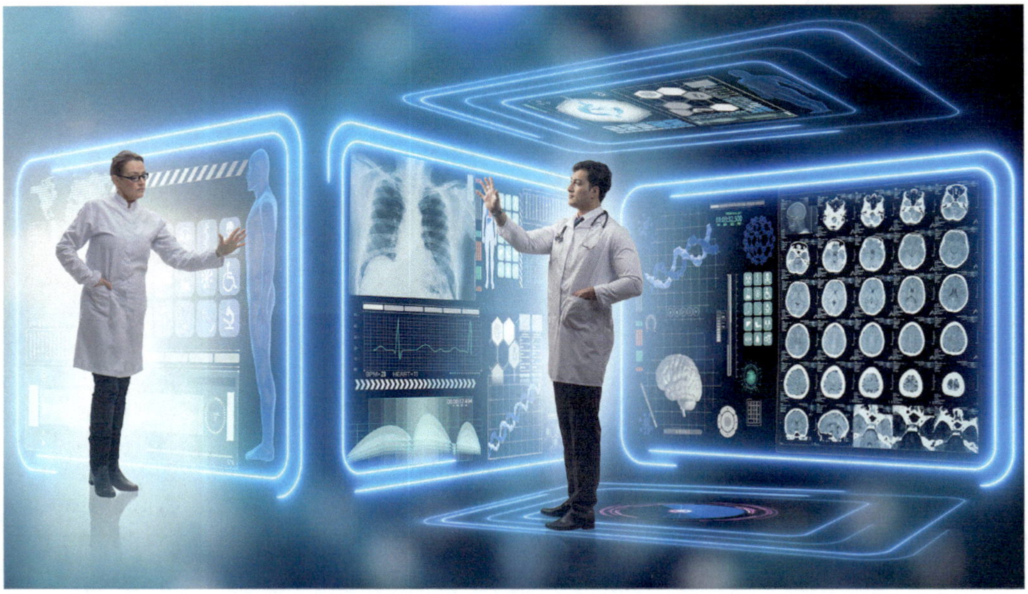

Figure 15.1. Emerging trends and future directions in community health.

Source: https://primesourcex.com/wp-content/uploads/2019/04/image007.jpg.

Definition of Community Health

Community health is increasingly described as a multidisciplinary body of knowledge focused on addressing the emotional, social, and physical health of populations in a specific geographic area.

Its ambit extends beyond merely curing sicknesses to include the broader social determinants of health, such as education, income, and access to healthcare services, which cumulatively shape the state of a community's health. The growing acknowledgment of these factors' interdependency gives rise to a shift in the way interventions for health are formulated and implemented. Such a determination of community health requires a delicate process, where the people in the community are asked by health practitioners what they desire and need specifically (Adger et al., 2016). Such a participatory model is compatible with prevailing trends that emphasize involvement of the community as a key element in health program development and policy-making, leading to better and sustainable health outcomes. As community health practice matures, innovative and creative methods through technology and data analysis are increasingly being seen. The use of electronic health tools provides a means of capturing real-time data on health outcome and behavior, hence making it possible to identify patterns and lacunae in health service delivery. Integration of health information systems into community health frameworks is encouraging collaborative approaches to disease prevention and health promotion (Ezz et al., 2013). Such transformation not only enhances the efficiency of health services but also encourages interdisciplinary collaboration that brings together public health officials, health care providers, and community members. The kinetic nature of such change calls for a rethink of traditional models of health service provision, causing community health programs to adopt adaptive, flexible strategies attuned to the particular challenges of populations. Moreover, the philosophy of community health increasingly complements a focus on environmental determinants and human-nature interaction as predictors of health. Current discussion suggests that environmental factors, including the prevalence of green areas and pollution, play a significant role in impacting community health, with interdisciplinary examination being central to addressing complex health issues (Adger et al., 2016). This broad framework calls upon stakeholders to embrace ecological sustainability as a fundamental component of community health initiatives. The integration of environmental health within models of community health allows for an overall outlook on health promotion in which community strategies can equally focus on limiting environmental risks and creating improved living conditions. In so doing, the term community health is not static; rather, it is expanding to encompass an increased understanding of how multiple factors, including environmental, social, and technological forces, influence the well-being of populations.

Importance of Community Health in Public Health

Community health is integral to the greater context of public health, keeping an emphasis on the importance of collective well-being and preventive medicine. By focusing on population health rather than health, community health programs address social determinants with significant effects on health outcomes. Such determinants, including socioeconomic status, education, and environment, are the causes of disparities in access to health and health outcomes across various populations. For instance, improving community health means not only treatment but also prevention interventions targeting high-risk groups, consequently reducing the disease burden. Embedding community health in public health policy encourages intersectoral collaboration to facilitate delivery of comprehensive health services that are culturally relevant and accessible, which is crucial considering that marginalized populations carry an unequal burden of health inequities. Furthermore, the advances in technology and data analysis are transforming community health. Telemedicine and mobile health apps are just a few of the instruments through which health services can be made more effective for disadvantaged populations. These trends in technology can help ensure timely dissemination of information on preventive health practices and disease management, ultimately developing healthier communities. Furthermore, the data acquired using these technologies offers valuable insight into community health patterns, enabling public health officers to develop evidence-based interventions. The WHO guidelines for physical activity and sedentary behavior 2020 also focus on building environments in support of an active lifestyle, which is crucial to community well-being. Strategies that harness technology can sufficiently address objectives that favor physical health across all age groups and abilities and therefore support physical activity as part of the social fabric of community daily life, as highlighted in the guidelines. The position of mental health among the health of communities cannot be exaggerated, particularly with recent global issues. Mental health issues are deeply embedded in the narrative of community health, impacting productivity, social coexistence, and overall wellbeing. Promoting sensitivity to mental health and establishing support groups among communities is crucial in bridging resilience and stigma against mental health conditions. Combining these elements with public health interventions enhances the integrated agenda advocated by various institutions of health to demonstrate the interconnectedness of physical and mental health. In line with the WHO 2020 guidelines, mental health community-based interventions benefit not only the person but also the achievement of overall health outcomes, such as improved learning and work performance. The focus on mental health highlights the necessity for robust public health programs that reflect the complexity of societal issues in modern times (Figure 15.2).

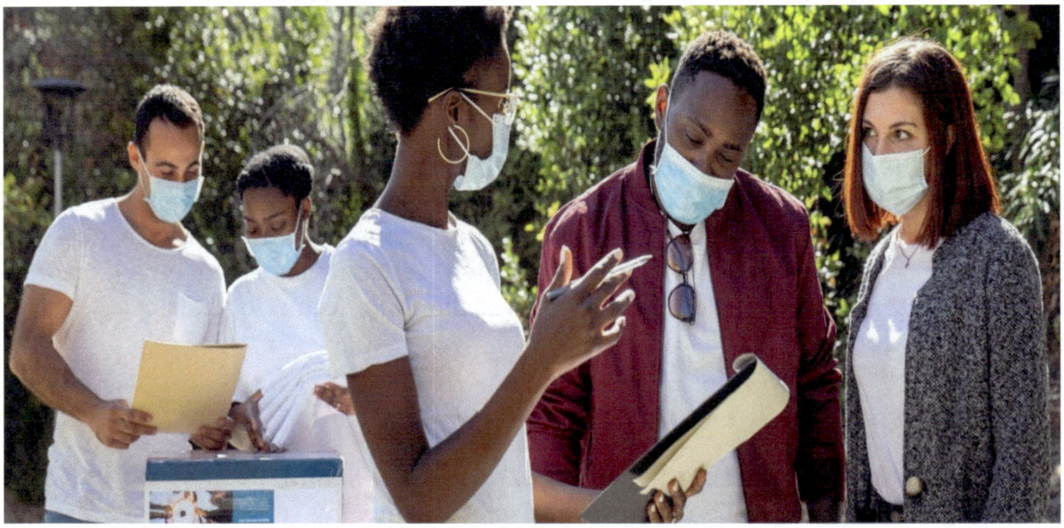

Figure 15.2. Importance of community health in public health.

Source: https://onlinepublichealth.gwu.edu/wp-content/uploads/sites/47/2021/10/Why-is-Public-Health-Important-3.jpg?resize=440.

Overview of Emerging Trends

Technological innovations in the field of community health have greatly transformed the arena of public health practices. The growing convergence of telemedicine, wearable health technology, and mobile health applications has transformed access to healthcare resources by communities. In addition to expanding patient engagement through the availability of tailored health management resources, the technologies advance the efficiency of health services. From the growing uptake evident, technology plays a central role in advancing health information communication and distant consultations, hence alleviating barriers to healthcare access. Moreover, the focus on evidence-based decision-making reflects a shift towards more inclusive and flexible health strategies. As communities leverage these technological assets, the need to bridge potential gaps in digital health equity is that much greater, so that benefits are realized across all groups of populations without driving additional inequities. Another influential trend emerging in community health is that of awareness and response to antimicrobial resistance (AMR), a significant global health issue that has garnered enormous attention over the past several years. Overuse and misuse of antibiotics-in human, animal, and environmental contexts-have driven the resistance crisis, complicating treatment possibilities and threatening public health interventions. The war against AMR not only requires new treatment methods but also strict policy measures to promote the judicious use of antibiotics. Multilateral action, such as the WHO Global Action Plan on AMR, highlights the importance of an intersectional response to the issue. Innovative solutions, including bacteriophage therapy and antimicrobial peptides, show promising avenues, but are met with insurmountable barriers in the way of economic disincentives and regulatory challenges. Effective control of AMR will thus demand convergent strategies that harmonize scientific research with expansive policy responses, focusing on a One Health approach. Furthermore, the transition towards decentralized healthcare models has emerged as a pointed reaction to the failure of traditional public health paradigms. The study of decentralization indicates a notable shift toward empowering local government in order to more adequately address local needs and health delivery. Such a transition is particularly fitting in the context of the present global crisis, such as the COVID-19 pandemic, which reinforced the demand for robust local health systems that are able to act swiftly in event of emergencies. The theme of decentralization requires emphasis on the dynamic equilibrium among health outcomes, community participation, and governance. Researchers note that with the advancing process of decentralization, it comes with chances and challenges that are in need of further study. Key questions arise regarding the roles and mandates of the decentralized institutions in managing public health crises, necessitating further debate on improvement of governance trends towards improved community health outcomes across different settings (Sajida et al., 2025).

15.1. Technological Advancements

Over the last few years, technological innovations have drastically impacted community health, especially with the adoption of Health Information Technology (HIT). This new field is defined by its capacity to improve medical resource availability, enhance quality of care, and narrow down health disparities. As technology improves through HIT, it offers innovative features that are instrumental in collecting improved data, thus enabling appropriate intervention strategies for public health. Such innovations can help to shape the provision of healthcare without leaving behind vulnerable communities. It is, nevertheless, important to implement HIT in a thoughtfully planned and informed manner to offer solutions for present disparities and improve the health system effectively. Without consideration for the needs of different communities, even it can augment, rather than diminish, health inequities among vulnerable populations, highlighting the importance of an inclusive health technology strategy (N/A, 2013). And yet another groundbreaking step ahead is brought by the advent of 5G wireless technology, which has the potential to transform global healthcare systems and transform community health paradigms. By offering high-throughput and low-latency wireless connectivity, 5G enables seamless interoperability of various emerging technologies like the Internet of Things (IoT), artificial intelligence, and big data analytics. These developments have the potential to considerably enhance the effectiveness of healthcare services by enabling real-time information exchange, remote patient monitoring, and enhanced communication between medical professionals. With healthcare systems adapting to accommodate these developments, there is growing optimism regarding their capacity to overcome chronic deficiencies in the current models. Yet, making this transition requires the strategic overcoming of potential technical challenges as well as systemic barriers to which the widespread implementation of 5G-enabled health solutions may be subjected (Farooq et al., 2017). The integration of advanced technologies not only has the capacity to maximize healthcare delivery but also stands to potentially democratize access to health information for all. By utilizing the technologies of cloud computing, artificial intelligence, and crowdsourcing data, communities can leverage great quantities of information to define patterns of health, influence public health policy, and deliver enhanced preventive care. The technologies enable individuals to take charge of their health by providing them with access to customized health information and support. Placing equitability first in the roll-out of technology aligns with global initiatives to make everyone's access to quality healthcare as encapsulated in the United Nations Sustainable Development Goals. With further technological innovations arising every day, thus, community health systems must be adaptable so that they can facilitate innovations to be beneficial for maintaining sustainable long-term health equity and improved outcomes for populations (Farooq et al., 2017) (Figure 15.3).

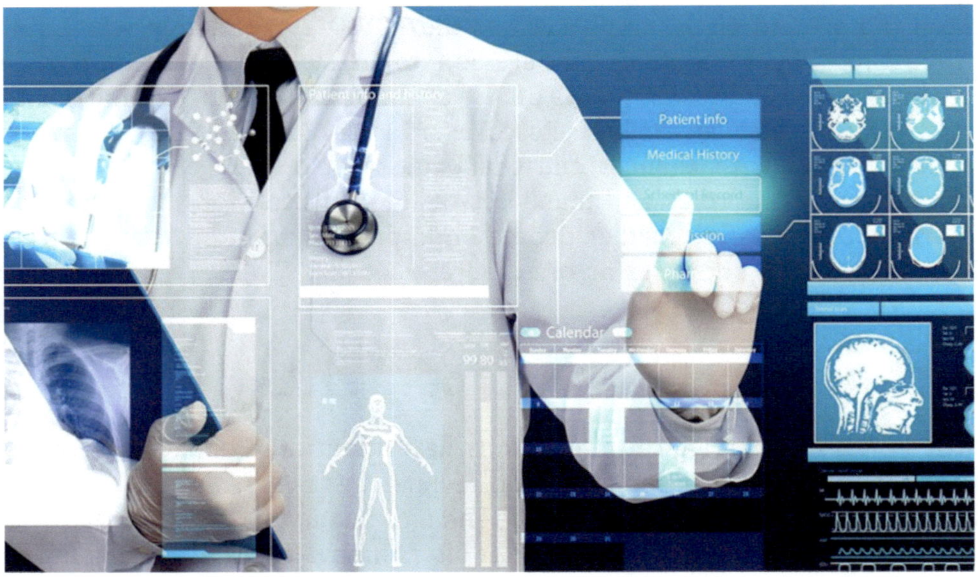

Figure 15.3. Technological advancements.

Source: https://www.pixelstech.net/article/images/health-technology.jpg.

15.1.1. Telehealth and Remote Patient Monitoring

Telehealth and remote patient monitoring are two of the most important emerging trends shaping the future of healthcare delivery. Telemedicine, or the electronic transmission of medical data over distances among hospitals, clinicians, and patients, ensures that medical care does not become inaccessible due to geographic location. Telehealth has been catalyzed by advances in digital communications and telecommunications and offers an unprecedented opportunity to provide quality care. This capacity helps healthcare systems reach out to underserved groups, allowing for timely intervention that can help transform patient outcomes as well as limit healthcare expenses. The emphasis on patient-centered care as well as comprehensive treatment plans arises, and with healthcare systems embracing these technologies, telehealth becomes a vital component in contemporary community health endeavors (Oliai et al., 2005).

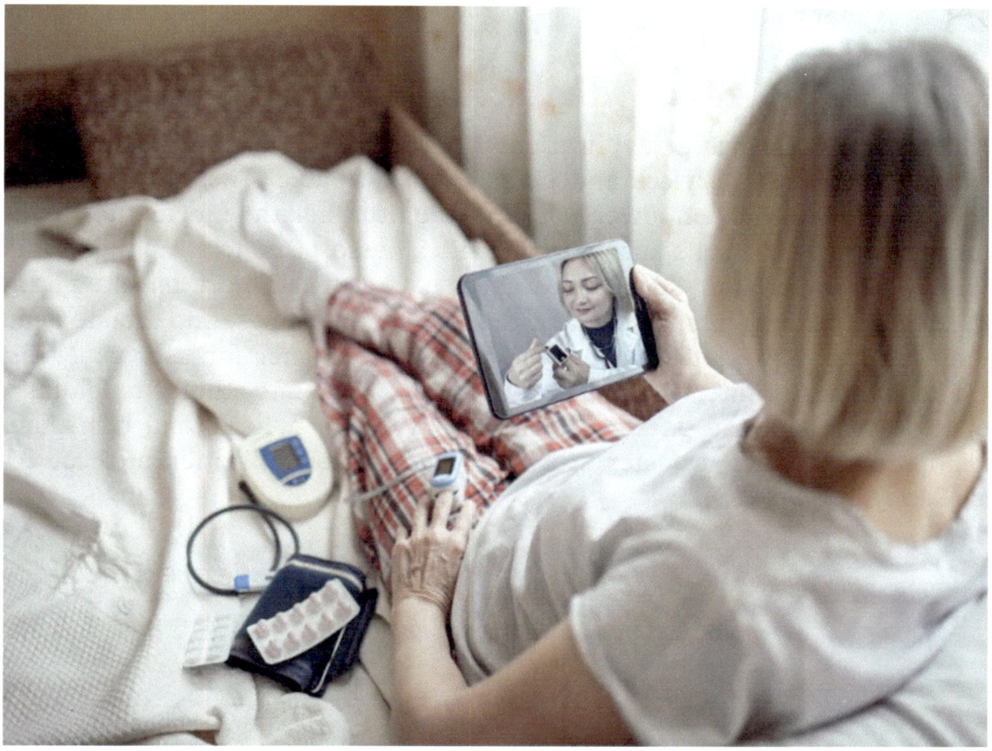

Figure 15.4. Technological advancements.

Source: https://summitwestcare.com/wp-content/uploads/2021/09/Unknown-18-1.png.

Remote patient monitoring (RPM), included in the telehealth package, enhances individual health management through the collection and interpretation of health data outside the traditional clinical setting. Real-time monitoring enables the individual to become the master of his or her own health by providing him or her with instant feedback on his or her vital statistics, enabling greater self-care and disease prevention. Additionally, RPM can improve chronic disease management through the delivery of timely and well-informed decisions from healthcare providers in real-time based on real-time data collected from patients. Improved treatment adherence and outcomes have been observed in RPM programs, thus reducing some of the pressure placed on health facilities through less in-person contact. As telehealth evolves, integrating RPM becomes an urgent endeavor to maximize individual and public health outcomes (Apesoa-Varano et al., 2020). Telehealth and remote patient monitoring have numerous strengths, but several challenges must be addressed for them to be put into action and utilized among different populations. Equity and access issues remain, as not everyone has the means and capability to utilize these systems in a productive way. Furthermore, privacy and data protection ethical issues cannot be sidestepped with increasing data sharing that jeopardizes patient confidentiality. Furthermore, political and regulatory factors such as technology standardization and interoperability pose extremely difficult hurdles in achieving the promise of telehealth. Overcoming these obstacles requires a collaborative effort that places inclusive design and equitable access to technology at center stage, so that telehealth solutions can empower every community and contribute positively to health outcomes (Apesoa-Varano et al., 2020; Oliai et al., 2005) (Figure 15.4).

15.1.2. Mobile Health (mHealth) Applications

The development of mobile health applications has transformed the landscape of community health by making healthcare services and information available. These programs leverage the prevalence of smartphones to empower users to monitor health information, access medical advice, and engage in the self-management of chronic illnesses. Due to a rapid growth in mHealth research paper publications after 2011, researchers have focused more on integrating emerging technologies, such as artificial intelligence and the Internet of Things, into mobile health systems. Such technology convergence not only sets the benchmark higher for user experience but also guides more effective health interventions in populations. With the studies unfolding, it becomes more crucial to learn about the effects of privacy protection policies and transparency during mHealth development in order to foster user trust and greater utilization of these digital health technologies (Zhang et al., 2025).

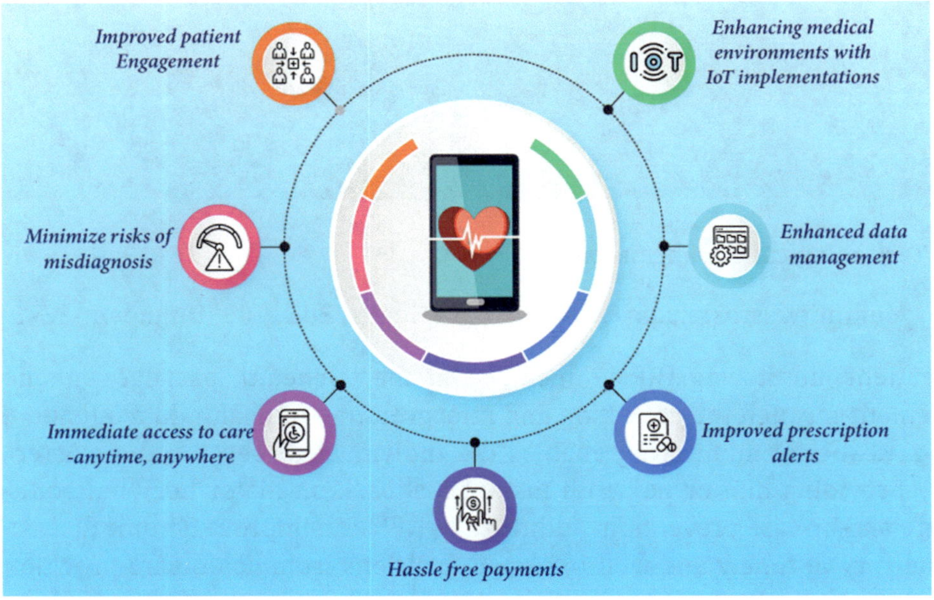

Figure 15.5. Mobile health applications.

Source: https://dkk4qeqny48s0.cloudfront.net/wp-content/uploads/2022/08/HealthcareApp.jpg.

Mobile health apps also play an important role in enhancing preventive care within community settings. By providing targeted health information, medication reminders, and chronic illness management tools, mobile health apps facilitate healthy behavior through active means. Future research indicates that mobile health apps can effectively enhance prevention healthcare activity with fidelity among historically underserved populations that have been avoided by health systems. For example, HIV self-testing apps have shown promising results in connecting users to critical health services upon a positive test (Mhando et al., 2024). The integration of chatbots and other digital health interventions facilitates care pathway navigation, thereby closing major gaps in the continuum of care (Mhando et al., 2024). This trend is one of the growing recognition of mHealth as a dynamic way of empowering people to take charge of their health and well-being. As mobile health expands, the paths that this field will follow in the future are likely to include integrating newer technologies and data analysis tools. Researchers are increasingly interested in leveraging big data to personalize user experiences and promote better health outcomes. Alongside, the use of blockchain technology in mobile health applications also provides enhanced data security and privacy measures, which are most critical in providing user trust in a digital platform of health. There will be a need for having cooperation between academia, health organizations, and technology developers in addressing the new challenges that will be present for mobile health applications. By adopting a holistic approach that integrates ongoing user and stakeholder input, the ability of mobile health applications to transform community health can be maximized, placing them at the forefront of contemporary healthcare delivery (Zhang et al., 2025) (Figure 15.5).

15.1.3. Data Analytics and Health Informatics

The past decade has seen the use of data analytics in health informatics as a transformative agent in community health. This technology-driven model provides healthcare professionals with access to vast amounts of patient data, whereby previously unachievable insights are made available. Advanced algorithms and analytics tools enable clinicians to see patterns and trends across populations of patients, enabling anticipatory interventions in population health initiatives. Such advancements not only increase the quality of care but also augment the efficiency of healthcare systems. In the long term, the capability of performing analysis of big data underpins more intelligent decision-making systems that empower personalized healthcare solutions catering to the specialized requirements of specific communities. While data-driven healthcare is about to become a reality, it is important to continuously analyze the implications and effectiveness of such technologies for the improvement of health outcomes among populations. Also, with increased use of digital healthcare solutions, teletherapy and mobile health applications are increasingly being accepted in community settings. These technologies reflect the application of data analysis in real-time, which allows individuals to manage their health in advance using tools. Through these platforms, healthcare providers are capable of monitoring patient behavior, adherence to treatment plans, and even social determinants of health influencing patient outcomes. Worth noting is the convergence of telepharmacy services and virtual consultations to enable communities to transcend geographical boundaries, thus enhancing accessibility to much-needed healthcare resources. With such technology, however, comes a concomitant challenge of data security and privacy. In mitigating such challenges, stakeholders have an obligation to ensure that ethical application of health informatics technology takes centre stage in championing equitable access to healthcare services while safeguarding patient data. Lastly, the contribution of data analytics towards building cooperation between stakeholders in healthcare cannot be overemphasized. Enhanced interoperability of electronic health records makes it simpler for patients' data to be shared among healthcare providers, facilitating effective communication and coordination of care. As highlighted, synergistic integration of data analytics and health informatics fosters collaborative learning and decision-making among patients, pharmacists, and doctors, significantly achieving enhanced health outcomes. Moreover, the use of sophisticated technologies like artificial intelligence can assist practitioners in developing predictive models that can be used to guide individual and community health strategies. Although these technologies offer enormous potential for community health, they also call for ongoing assessment of current policies and regulations to make them consistent with evolving trends. Hence, a systemic approach involving the cooperation of government agencies, medical professionals, and patients must be adopted to navigate the multi-dimensional landscape of data analytics and health informatics in community health (Figure 15.6).

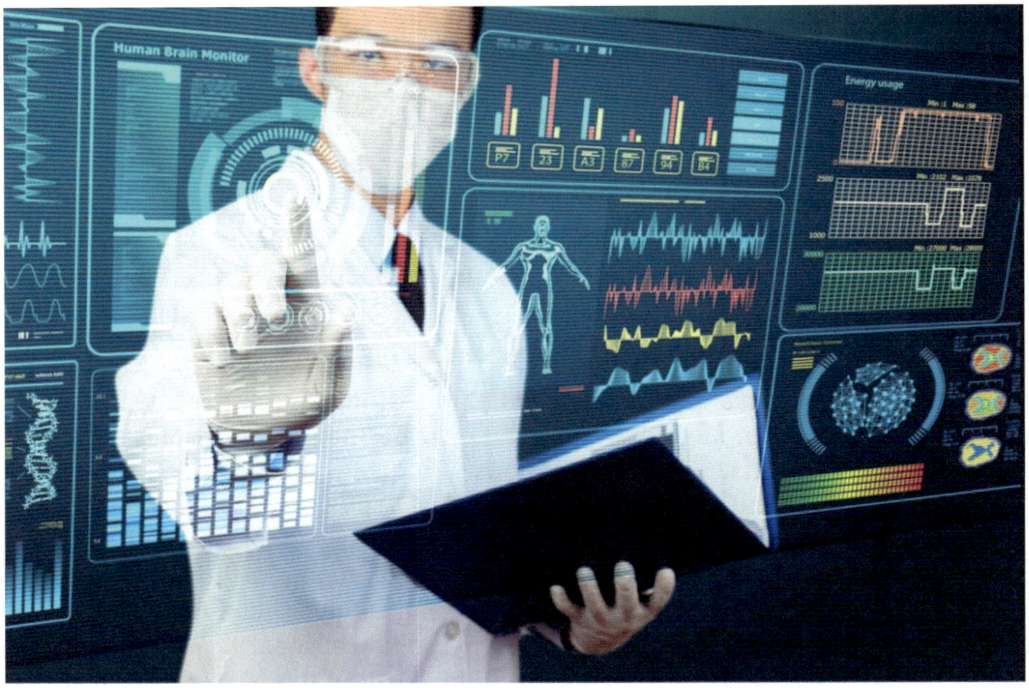

Figure 15.6. Data analytics and health informatics.

Source: https://www.lebigdata.fr/wp-content/uploads/2018/03/big-data-sante-bis-2025.jpg.

15.2. Social Determinants of Health (SDOH)

SDOH is a concept that has become highly relevant in community health discussions, highlighting the impact of non-medical factors on health outcomes. Determinants include a range of conditions like socioeconomic status, education, physical and neighborhood environment, employment, and social support networks. Research workers and healthcare professionals alike are increasingly acknowledging that the treatment of SDOH holds the key to enhancing population health as well as the realization of health equity. Being a key component of community health planning, an understanding of the intricate dynamics of SDOH enables stakeholders to better tailor interventions, wherein they can target the unique needs of various populations. This shift towards an expansive definition of health and wellness highlights the need for integrated models of care that extend beyond clinical settings, encouraging partnerships between sectors such as education, housing, and transportation that influence health outcomes at the community level. Furthermore, open discussion of SDOH highlights the necessity of interdisciplinary cooperation among policymakers, researchers, and healthcare professionals. This alliance promotes a holistic strategy toward the determinants causing health inequities. For instance, the health care providers and planners can implement interventions involving the community to avoid determinants like healthy food availability, job opportunities, and good education systems.

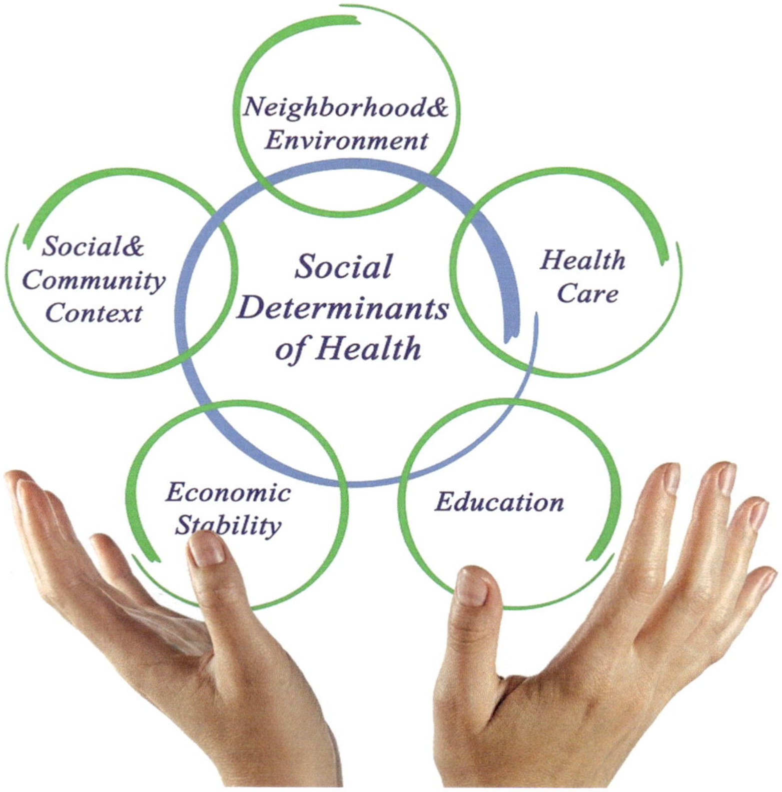

Figure 15.7. Social determinants of health (SDOH).

Source: https://cache.aapc.com/blog/wp-content/uploads/2019/12/04134330/SDOH.jpg.

The emerging trends project an incline towards an integrative model of health care in order to increase social equity and accountability. Simple strategies, such as developing dashboards for tracking community health measures, can offer insights and enhance the efficacy of interventions for SDOH. The incorporation of health equity into the core of health care reform activities is, therefore, essential, enabling more enhanced health outcomes and aligning with the aims of community health efforts focusing on sustainable, long-term health disparities effect (Acuff et al., 2017). In the future, the imperative for a paradigm-shifting research agenda responding to SDOH has also become more clearly apparent. Emerging evidence suggests that intersectoral research collaboration across sectors is crucial for creating all-encompassing solutions to health inequality. The Lowitja Institute's Aboriginal and Torres Strait Islander health and well-being project demonstrates the necessity of framing research that looks ahead to anticipate future trends in society and challenges. Deliberative workshops saw a critical need for innovative, integrative approaches to research that integrate community voices in constantly evolving fields of health policy. These approaches should inform public health policy that draws on knowledge across disciplines, making a system where research immediately informs practice and policy. The action call that arises from such discussions highlights the fact that SDOH mitigation not only enhances the effectiveness of health interventions but also furthers the greater good of fostering the achievement of health equity for all populations (Brands, 2014) (Figure 15.7).

15.2.1. Impact of Socioeconomic Status (SES)

The effect of SES on health in communities is substantial and multifaceted, with an influence that determines access to resources, healthcare, and overall well-being. People with higher SES tend to have better access to healthcare services, nutritious food, and conditions of safety. People from lower SES segments of society are more likely to face barriers that increase the gap of health disparities. These include limited finances, no transportation, and educational shortfalls, that impede the ability to access preventative health care. Furthermore, socioeconomic status is in close correlation with health literacy, that influences how individuals engage with health services and make informed decisions about their health. As local populations strive for improved health, it is essential that systemic inequalities are confronted in order that socioeconomically disadvantaged groups be offered properly individualized care and support.

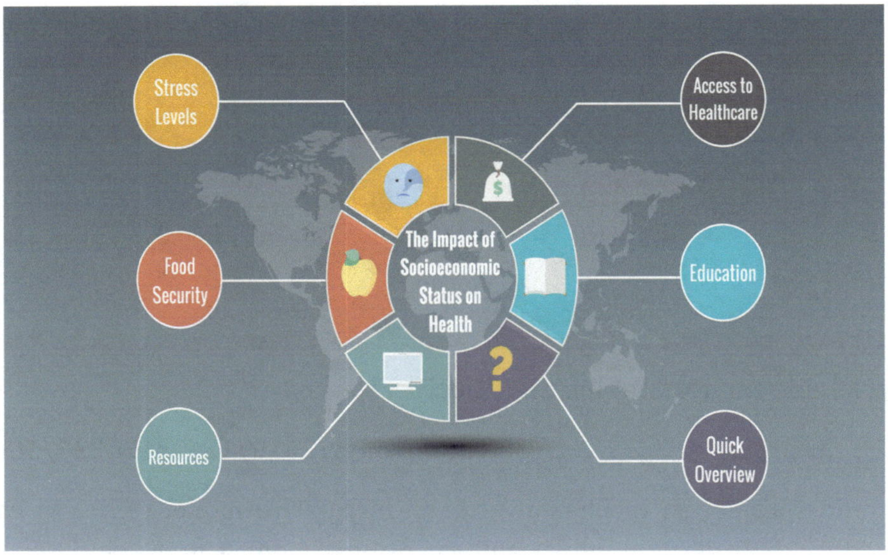

Figure 15.8. Impact of socioeconomic status (SES).

Source: https://0701.static.prezi.com/preview/v2/h5bm5tzd2dioj7uo5mumzuoybp6jc3sachvcdoaizecfr3dnitcq_3_0.png.

New evidence indicates the significant interaction between SES and specific health outcomes, above all regarding prevention and control of chronic diseases. Studies have established that lower SES correlates with higher levels of obesity, diabetes, and cardiovascular illnesses and is compounded by inadequate access to preventive care. Care of the same requires an integrated system of treatment that addresses not just the medical condition of the patient but also the social determinants of health that led to the condition. This calls for an understanding of how neighborhoods, employment prospects, and educational systems affect health behavior. Community health programs must thus utilize interventions that target vulnerable populations using resources and education to reverse the negative impacts of low socioeconomic status on well-being and health. With new public policies and guidelines coming out, such as those by the World Health Organization, there becomes an increasing need to incorporate socioeconomic considerations into community health planning and policy-making. The WHOs 2020 guidelines emphasize the importance of physical activity across all age categories and note in particular the disparities in recreational opportunities by income or socioeconomic status. For instance, lower SES individuals may lack access to secure parks or physical activity-promoting facilities and thus may adopt sedentary behaviors and allied disease conditions. Moreover, specific population groups like pregnant women and individuals suffering from chronic diseases have unique requirements that must be addressed on enacting community health policies. As we move towards holistic approaches to health, tailoring interventions to the realities of socioeconomic circumstance will be key to reducing health inequalities and building healthier communities for all, particularly for the marginalized who are worse off through the cumulative effects of socioeconomic disadvantage (Bull et al., 2020; Livingston et al., 2020) (Figure 15.8).

15.2.2. Role of Education and Employment

The linkage between work and education is crucial in addressing the challenges emanating from imminent trends in community health. Education equips one with the requisite information and skills to address the complexities of healthcare systems, which facilitates better entry into participatory decision-making for one's health. Additionally, levels of education significantly affect career opportunities, particularly in the health sector. As the demand for educated healthcare practitioners keeps growing, individuals with higher levels of education are likely to gain access to employment that not only guarantees their economic status but also good community health results. By fostering the educated workforce, communities can guarantee effective provision of health services, in the end, leading to improved standards of health among populations (N/A, 2019). Moreover, employment has a more significant effect on health and overall well-being. People who are in stable, paying jobs generally have better health through better access to health care, financial security, and improved mental health. However, changes in the job market such as the growth of gig economy jobs and non-traditional employment arrangements may pose challenges in maintaining these benefits. Workers in these kinds of jobs typically have restricted access to general health benefits, which would further exacerbate health disparity within the population. Addressing this issue requires strategic measures promoting job security but also giving more emphasis to collective bargaining and protection of labor. Implementing these structures can help ensure that all workers, but notably those who are in precarious work, have the facilities to facilitate their health and well-being (Kruk et al., 2018). Investments in education and workforce development programs can build a stronger public health system that is equipped to handle new challenges. Ensuring lifelong learning through training and adult education is important to maintaining the expertise of the workforce as health demands change. These programs not only equip workers to fill key positions within healthcare facilities but also improve their ability to work with and assist community-based health activities. Through the cultivation of a culture of continuous learning, communities are better placed to respond to emergent health priorities, and thus they are positioned to improve health outcomes in a sustainable way. Ensuring that education and employment are given high priority as central aspects of community health strategy is thus key to delivering the needs of an increasingly changing world (N/A, 2019).

15.2.3. Influence of Environment and Community Resources

Physical surroundings play a significant role in shaping the health of individuals and communities, a phenomenon enhanced by urbanization and shifting societal trends. Urban centers, generally comprising high population and resource deficit, present unique challenges and potential for public health. Wherever there is physical contact between wildlife and other carriers in an urban setting, infectious diseases may be generated. For instance, urban settings can offer interfaces between wildlife, livestock, and humans and thus facilitate the transmission of zoonotic disease. To design interventions that are effective at improving public health when urbanization is on an upward trajectory, understanding the way such interfaces are developed is critical (Bashshur et al., 2020). By analyzing the correspondence between environmental exposure and health outcomes, communities can be better prepared to face future health issues that environmental change will pose. Community resources like access to healthcare services, schooling, and social support networks are determinants of health outcomes. Distribution inequalities in resources tend to reproduce health inequities, particularly among vulnerable populations. Availability of local health services has a direct effect on health knowledge and behavior and impacts general community health. The rollout of telehealth solutions has been the leading response to the COVID-19 pandemic, bridging gaps where traditional mechanisms of delivering healthcare were lacking. Therefore, its function in enhancing community capabilities, such as telehealth infrastructure, not only aligns with health trends but is a key driver in addressing inequities in healthcare access. These advancements call for resolving resource limitations in an innovative manner that meets health equity and sustainability (Bashshur et al., 2020). In addition, the intersection of the environmental and community resources promotes a whole approach to health promotion. Wholeness practices, such as city green spaces and community gardens, can decrease stress levels and enhance mental health, in addition to providing the space for physical activity. These environments promote social solidarity in communities, cultivating resilience against health adversities. Second, as ongoing climate change impacts health, communities must use local environmental assets for successful adaptation. Green infrastructure can address both the environmental and health issues, offering sustainable models for communities. This approach is an exemplar of emerging trends in community health where an emphasis on environmental stewardship and resource optimization is a driver for public health initiatives, ultimately narrowing health inequities and enhancing community well-being (Hassell et al., 2016).

15.3. Health Equity and Access

Health equity principle is in the lead in addressing disparities in access to healthcare and its outcomes, particularly as communities seek to build more equitable health systems. For equitable healthcare to be realized, not only must individual health status be paid attention to, but also intervention in social determinants of health that frame people's lives. This involves addressing policy reforms, community, as well as empowering marginalized communities. The Shanghai Declaration emphasizes the need to tackle determinants of health and increase equity by promoting good governance and health literacy so that health is everyone's business. All stakeholders need to be included in community actions so that previously disenfranchised voices are right at the forefront of decision-making. This participatory approach can lead to lasting changes that foster equity between populations, ultimately leading to healthier communities better equipped to withstand public health emergencies (Kilibarda, 2024). Availability of healthcare remains a top issue for vulnerable populations that is often overridden by economic, geographic, and systemic factors. In all countries, including Brazil, historical inequities in the availability of healthcare are expressed in poorer health outcomes for certain groups, particularly women and children.

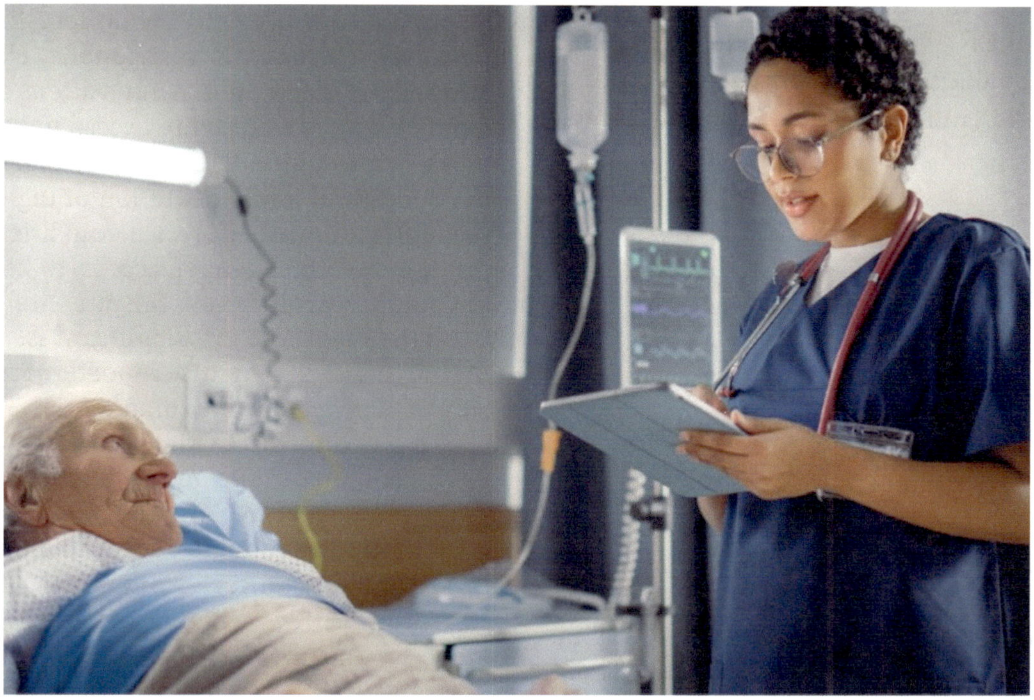

Figure 15.9. Health equity and access.

Source: https://www.nutritionpix.com/wp-content/uploads/2024/08/Paste-41.jpg.

The public healthcare system envisaged in the 1988 Constitution of Brazil was set up to ensure universal access and equity in health. Underfunding and inefficiency, however, have compromised those fundamental principles. Despite improvements in prenatal and maternal healthcare, gaps remain, particularly for marginalized populations like Indigenous and urban periphery populations. These gaps would require sustained investment in healthcare facilities, broad training of healthcare providers, and policies established to favor the most vulnerable segments of society. Guaranteeing equitable access to healthcare is important to foster not just community health, but also social justice (Vanderlei et al., 2016). In the future, strengthening health equity and access will need to adapt to address emerging global health challenges, including pandemics, climate change, and economic crises. This evolution needs new strategies that intersect health promotion with all areas of public policy, fostering intersectoral action that transcends the traditional limits of healthcare. Health in All Policies is a strategy that supports the integration of health considerations into policymaking in all sectors. By incorporating health equity into other areas such as education, housing, and transport, policymakers can create environments that facilitate better health for everyone. In addition, community engagement remains the critical factor in this process that allows local communities to actively participate in the building of health initiatives and policies. Thus, health equity along with access will demand collaborative effort from governments, organizations, and communities in establishing robust health systems that can respond to various populations' demands in the wake of a new world (Kilibarda, 2024) (Figure 15.9).

15.3.1. Disparities in Healthcare Access

The issue of disparity in healthcare access is a core issue in the paradigm of community health that not only impacts health outcomes of individuals but also overall public health. Varying factors determine the disparities in access to healthcare, including socioeconomic status, location, and culture. For instance, oppressed groups such as Native Hawaiians and Pacific Islanders (NHPI) have significantly higher mortality rates from specific cancers compared to their White peers, illustrating an alarming trend in healthcare disparity. These disparities are also heightened by system forces such as underrepresentation in clinical trials, which continues to drive disparities in effective therapies among diverse groups. As the health sector moves towards an inclusive paradigm, it is important to learn about these particular barriers in bridging the accessibility gap and realizing equivalent health outcomes across different groups. Technological innovations in digital health have the ability to address some of the health disparities in access, particularly among vulnerable populations. Telehealth and mHealth applications are becoming increasingly pivotal in delivering care to people with geographical and economic limitations. They enable remote access by healthcare professionals to patients, offering services that can range from medication management to mental health. Notably, as recent studies have indicated, incorporating digital health solutions can enable individuals to engage more actively in their own care, thereby encouraging health literacy and engagement. Apart from the above, the accessibility and convenience of digital platforms can help deal with issues related to transport and time constraints, particularly in the case of populations like NHPI, who face limitations because of economic restrictions. Hence, the adoption of digital health innovations allows for a major way of improving access to healthcare, along with equitable outcomes, too. However, the successful implementation of digital health technologies must address inequalities that can arise based on unequal access to technology and digital proficiency. Despite the potential of telehealth, there are significant issues about digital divides that disproportionately affect rural and lower-income communities, worsening existing health disparities. Insertion of digital health should be followed by targeted efforts to build infrastructure and educate patients and providers for equitable access to it. Initiatives like Roche-Genentech's Advancing Inclusive Research (AIR) initiative are three positive steps in the direction of engaging minority communities and mitigating participation barriers in clinical trials. With the creation of partnerships and investments in targeted community-directed strategies, stakeholders can begin filling the systemic barriers that prevent healthcare access. Ultimately, rectifying these inequalities is not simply a question of ethics but also a necessity for an equitable, healthier society, as emphasized by ongoing research initiatives seeking to understand and address the unique healthcare challenges in marginalized communities.

15.3.2. Strategies for Promoting Health Equity

Improving health equity demands a multi-faceted response, ultimately focused on social determinants of health disproportionately affecting marginalized communities. One of the successful strategies is to improve access to healthcare services through community-based efforts. Through mobile clinics and telehealth, healthcare providers can reach more underserved populations, thus reducing the problem of transportation and cost. Not only do these enhance access to healthcare, but they also build trust in the communities, ultimately enhancing health outcomes. Further, by using culturally competent care, these services can be improved significantly. Emphasizing the role of culturally responsive interventions, which respond to the local cultures in which different populations live, can lead to higher participation and adherence to health regimens and, hence, result in equitable health outcomes for all.

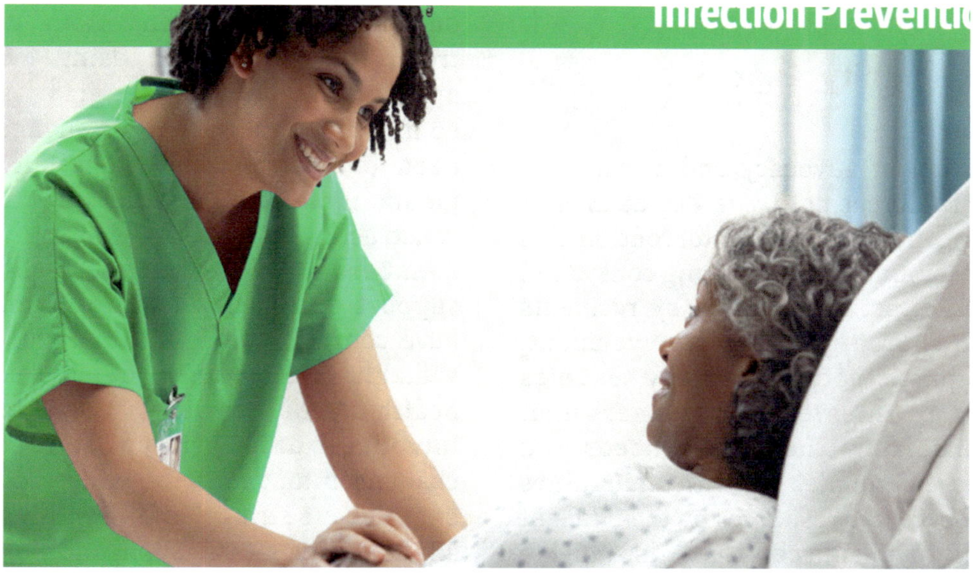

Figure 15.10. Strategies for promoting health equity.

Source: https://www.medline.com/wp-content/uploads/2023/11/BAN_LI_IP_Health-Equity_RGB.png .

Another key approach to being healthy being equal is the use of policy interventions that address inequities within organizations. Lobbying for policies on inexpensive housing, schooling, and employment can respond to the root causes of inequities in health. For instance, local government zoning codes can promote the development of low-cost housing and spending on public facilities in poor areas. This integrated approach ensures that populations are provided with the basic things needed for a healthy life. In addition to this, health organizations and social services that are in collaboration with one another can determine populations at risk, thus allowing one to plan intervention programs addressing the health issues of those populations. As observed in some of the programs, the combination of health promotion with social policy can produce sustainable health equity gains in a community. Medical technology is also becoming significant instruments in the struggle for health equity. The use of digital platforms and mobile applications can assist in bridging gaps in health access and information exchange. Using data analytics, healthcare organizations are able to establish health indicator patterns across different demographic groups so that interventions can be more focused. The metaverse as a virtual mode of engagement also holds potential for interactive health education and promotion that can target multiple audiences. With immersive experiences, users are better able to understand health issues and associated lifestyle modifications, especially in communities who may have been excluded in the past. Despite ongoing challenges regarding equal access to the technologies, the potential in promoting health equity through innovation is vast to further explore its significance for future community health intervention (Calvin et al., 2023; Dwivedi et al., 2022) (Figure 15.10).

15.3.3. Community Engagement and Advocacy

The conjunction of advocacy and community involvement is increasingly regarded as the key to maximizing public health interventions. In cases where communities are facing compound health issues, direct involvement by residents promotes ownership and empowerment. Grassroots participatory strategy enables stakeholders to intervene in manners that address immediately the unique needs and values of the community. Active communities are able to coordinate resources by the efficient mobilization of resources and also tackle transparency and establish trust between health organizations and populations they engage. Focusing on robust community engagement prioritizes efforts towards co-creating well-considered health policies informed by grassroots insights, considered practice that optimizes the relevance and efficacy of health interventions. This paradigm shift towards collaboration represents a departure from traditional top-down approaches and toward more participatory models that align with community dynamics. In addition, advocacy practice in community work cannot be overstated. Advocates serve as facilitators who amplify the voice of the people to ensure that they are heard in broader health debates regarding their concerns and priorities. Advocacy efforts can drive policy changes that target social determinants of health such as housing, education, and availability of healthcare services. These efforts emphasize long-term commitment by health agencies to sustain community partnerships leading to substantive change. Effective advocacy not only increases awareness of critical health issues but also generates impetus for systemic change that will improve health equity. Cooperative advocacy provides arenas in which individuals feel empowered and emboldened to demand response and accountability from policymakers, ultimately enhancing the collective health outcomes of populations. With future health trends suggesting increasing focus on the application of technological innovation, community measures of engagement will need to evolve. Innovations such as social media platforms provide new avenues for constructing dialogue and cooperation between members of populations. Technology can support outreach, enabling organizations to have constant communication while gathering valuable information about the community's health needs. However, these technologies introduce data privacy and accessibility challenges that must be addressed for digital engagement strategies to be fully available to all. Emphasizing the application of technology in community health will entail keeping a close eye on numerous different demographic factors, as digital divides can exacerbate current health inequities. As indicated in the most recent studies, technology and community advocacy intersection is a vital area for future research where learning about its significance would have far-reaching implications for informing public health approaches in the future (Lee et al., 2025; Mubdir et al., 2025).

15.4. Preventive Health Strategies

Preventive health strategies are coming more and more into the spotlight as key components of successful community health programs. Such interventions are targeted towards the reduction of disease and health condition incidence before actual incidence, hence enhancing the overall health of the general population. Prevention allows communities to utilize resources more effectively so that individuals receive what they require in time. Addition of preventive interventions into healthcare systems not only leads to better health but also helps keep the increased healthcare costs due to preventable disease treatment at bay. Moreover, the shift towards a preventive orientation of health is also an attempt to own one's health because such activities encompass exercise, proper diet, and periodic health check-ups. Preventive health programs in this context are not just a measure to save costs but also an integral component of a robust and resilient healthcare system. Conceptualization and implementation of preventive health interventions must be multi-dimensional in scope, encompassing various determinants of health. Successful interventions must consider social, economic, and environmental determinants of health inequity across communities. For instance, health policy that promotes healthy lifestyle choice has an immediate influence on community health outcomes. Community garden establishment, safe play area creation, and advocacy for healthy food access are a few of the measures that can significantly promote healthier behaviors. Secondly, mass public education campaigns favoring preventive care, for example, screening and immunization, can help eliminate prevalent myths and foster proactive health behaviors among broad groups of people. Lastly, a multi-faceted approach that addresses several determinants of health will be critical in the effectiveness of preventive health programs in addressing the community's needs. Merging the public health system with the health care system is essential to optimizing the effectiveness of preventive health activities. As elaborated, the Patient Protection and Affordable Care Act is an important step towards expanding healthcare accessibility but underscores the necessity of giving more priority to public health initiatives. Health systems and policies do not have to remain compartmentalized but must be converted into a network system favoring preventive care as the central tenet. Through the implementation of recommendations made that suggest public health infrastructure capacity is extended, policy-makers can further strengthen local health approaches and develop preventive intervention propagated effectively. Strategies such as collaborative cross-agency measures can facilitate the contexts in favor of healthier lifestyle patterns and reduce health inequities. Unless coordinated action is undertaken to bring together health care and public health, the full potential of preventive methods will be lost, limiting future gains in overall community health (Figure 15.11).

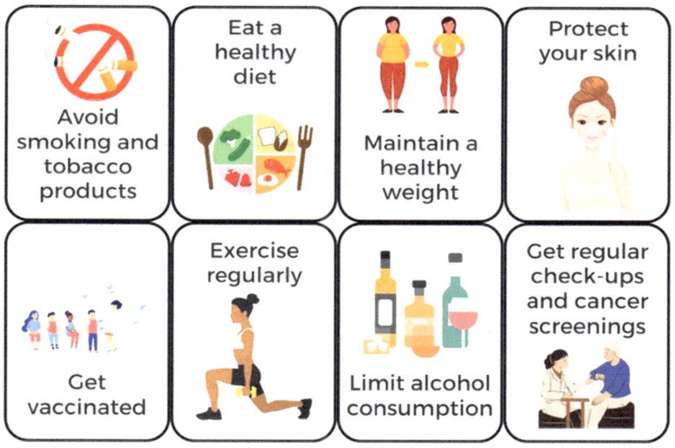

Figure 15.11. Preventive health strategies.

Source: https://vshospitals.b-cdn.net/wp-content/uploads/2023/08/infographic-1200-%C3%97-786-px-29-1024x671.webp.

15.4.1. Importance of Preventive Care

Preventive care is a key element in facilitating community health by detecting and intervening in illness early on, with final outcomes in enhanced health results and healthcare cost savings. The paradigm emphasizes proactive care, such as vaccinations, screenings, and health education, that minimizes the occurrence of chronic diseases and other ailments to a significant degree. Through investments in preventive care programs, communities are able to enjoy the advantages of decreased hospitalization and overall improved health. Furthermore, integration of preventive services within the healthcare system helps to add to a unifying process of health, resonating with the idea that effective health care and public health are interdependent though distinct aspects of a unified system, as borne out by the demand for fresh policy changes on this issue (Gostin et al., 2011). As populations evolve, emerging preventive care trends identify the importance of reacting to social determinants of health, which play a significant role in community and individual well-being. Environmental change interventions, such as increased healthy diet access and safe places for recreation, promote healthy behaviors in populations, enhancing the efficacy of traditional preventive measures. Organizations like TCWF are at the forefront in applying employment-based approaches to health disparities reduction and community health benefits enhancement (Yen et al., 2000).

Through creating partnerships with diverse sectors, incentive policies that promote healthy lifestyle can be effectively launched, with resulting system adjustments to facilitate preventive care approaches. These strategies not only contribute towards the improvement of individual health but also towards building a long-term sustainable health system, which endorses the central role played by preventive interventions in shaping public health.

Incorporation of preventive care within community health systems is particularly vital in the context of increasing healthcare costs and changing population dynamics. Changing towards a prevention focus can yield an enormous payback over the long term in economic as well as social terms. By addressing health prior to issues becoming too complex, health systems are able to decrease the stresses of maintaining multifaceted ailments that require great resources. Preventive care programs aren't merely beneficial; they are essential to creating strong communities that can maintain public health issues. Prioritizing prevention supports wider health reforms to enhance population health, making the case unequivocally that without proper investment in prevention activity, the population's health needs will remain inadequately served (Gostin et al., 2011). The future of community health unequivocally depends on a renewed focus on prevention as a core part of an equitable healthcare system (Figure 15.12).

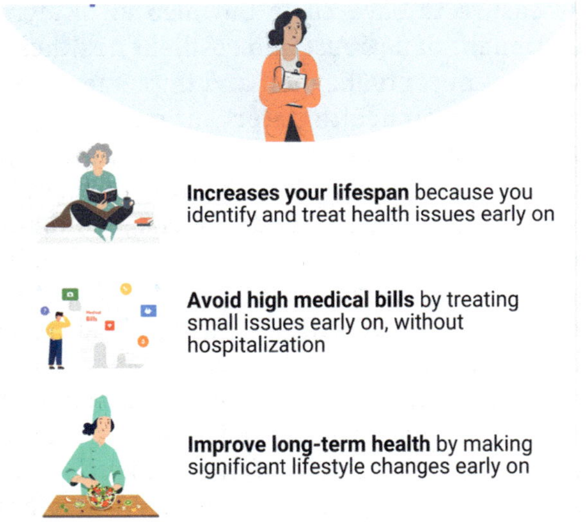

Figure 15.12. Importance of preventive care.

Source: https://assets-wp-cdn.onsurity.com/wp/wp-content/uploads/2021/03/27182620/Importance-of-Preventive-Care-1-1024x1024.png.

15.4.2. Community-Based Health Education Programs (CBHEPs)

CBHEPs are increasingly a key intervention in addressing public health problems, particularly in low- and middle-income countries (LMICs). CBHEPs emphasize the involvement of people from the community in health education to allow activities to be context-specific to the local culture and needs. By fostering dialogue and engagement between health authorities and community leaders, CBHEPs enhance health literacy and empower individuals to take control of their own health. Effective CBHEPs have been shown to improve health outcomes and strengthen community confidence in health systems, addressing systematic deficits in the quality of care that is so often found in LMICs, as evidenced in recent literature. Emphasizing local ownership and culturally responsive content, these programs support the vision of universal health coverage in that they address gaps in access and quality where traditional healthcare systems are bound to fall short (Kruk et al., 2018). Moreover, CBHEPs largely depend on a strong foundation that involves trained facilitators along with an integrated understanding of community dynamics. These models incorporate flexible and experiential teaching strategies that cater to the various means of learning for individuals. By applying complexity theory and empirical evidence to health education, practitioners are able to better understand the complexities of health behavior and results in populations. This approach promotes a platform for sustainable change, allowing community members to be engaged in and sustain health programs.

To this, the measure of the impact of CBHEPs is essential; establishing standards that equate to community engagement, improved health practices, and client satisfaction can assist in refining these programs and making them accountable (N/A, 2013). The implications of these measurements eventually guide the continuous development of CBHEPs, showing their relevance within the evolving context of community health. As health systems increasingly focus on equity and quality, CBHEPs are an essential strategy to address the unique needs of target groups. Not only do these programs educate individuals about health, but they create support networks that foster community resilience. Combining health education with advocacy for health rights, CBHEPs enable marginalized groups to voice their needs and negotiate the healthcare system more effectively. This empowerment is vital in ensuring that the human right to health is recognized and addressed, particularly for vulnerable groups who may experience obstacles towards accessing quality care. Thus, integrating CBHEPs in overall health plans indicates a commitment to improving health outcomes through collaboration. These programs are critical to address the bold health goals dreamed by global agencies, which require solutions that are both sustainable and inclusive in scope (Kruk et al., 2018).

15.4.3. Vaccination and Immunization Initiatives

The growth of immunization and vaccination programs is critical in addressing public health challenges as communities confront new diseases. Notably, cases of measles have increased in a number of states, exemplified by New York's patient zero who inadvertently infected 39 individuals in Michigan, demonstrating serious gaps in herd immunity due to vaccine hesitancy (Jain et al., 2024). These outbreaks emphasize the necessity for extensive vaccination programs extending to numerous communities, especially those in marginalized groups. Breaking down obstacles to immunization like socioeconomic factors and false information about vaccine safety is essential. Public health interventions have to facilitate cooperation with medical care providers and community leaders in establishing confidence. Lacking a concerted effort at increasing awareness and increasing access, the vaccination improvement programs will have no chance but fail, and populations will be vulnerable to vaccine-preventable disease. Social media plays a disruptive function in vaccination drives, having both clear benefits and demerits. On the positive side, social media sites such as Facebook and Twitter are capable of communicating accurate facts regarding vaccine safety and countering uninformed fiction that promotes vaccination hesitation (Jain et al., 2024). During health emergencies, social media serves as a rapid communication platform, through which public health organizations can share vital updates and educational content to masses. Social media, on the other hand, can be utilized to disseminate incorrect information, giving rise to public mistrust of vaccines, as witnessed in recent health pandemics. It is thus crucial that health communication utilizes the reach of social media but simultaneously monitors and counters misinformation. By the integration of new digital marketing approaches in immunization campaigns, public health players will be able to engage communities more effectively and tailor messages to suit their specific issues. Future directions in vaccination programs entail a multifaceted approach that strikes a balance between access and community mobilization. Mobile clinics and home-visiting programs can significantly increase immunization rates among the transport-barricaded population (Grewal et al., 2019). Beyond that, programs that incorporate community centers, churches, and schools can facilitate making contact and encouraging health workers to work with families in relaxed and familiar environments. Not only does this teach, but it addresses the psychosocial and cultural problems that are the substrates to acceptance of vaccines. As public health programs mature and progress, collaboration among family leaders, health professionals, and families will be central to achieving an educated populace that prioritizes preventive health. Ultimately, creating a community context that is supportive will be the most important factor for ensuring the success of immunization campaigns and maintaining public health (Figure 15.13).

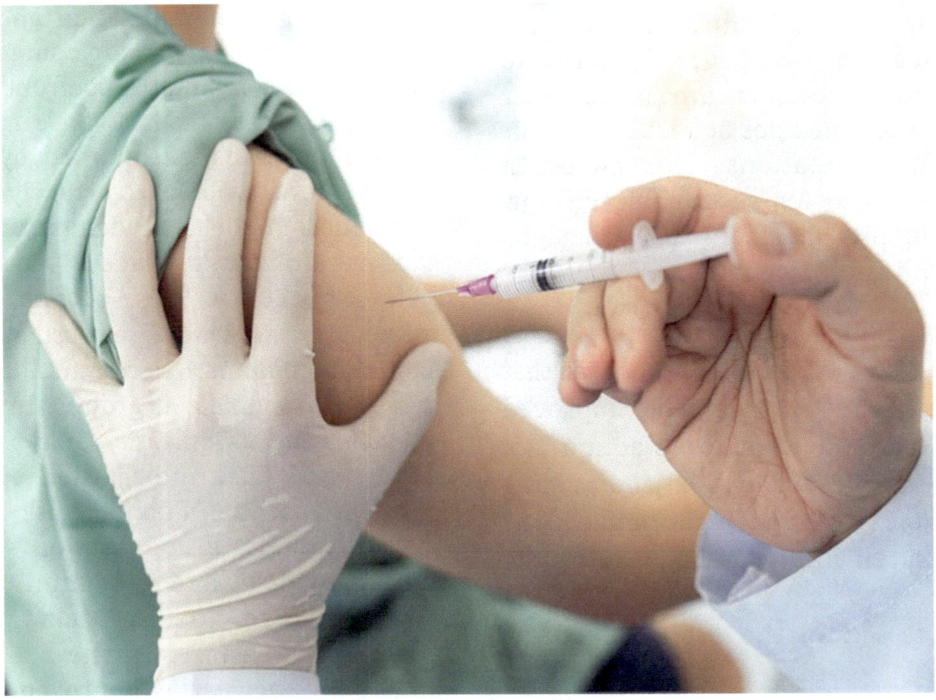

Figure 15.13. Vaccination and immunization initiatives.

Source: https://www.westtorrens.sa.gov.au/files/assets/public/v/1/services/health/immunisation.jpg?w=1080.

15.5. Mental Health Awareness

Heightened awareness of mental health awareness reiterates its crucial role in paradigms of community health. Mental health is increasingly viewed not only as the lack of disorder but also as a component of overall well-being that affects physical health, social functioning, and productivity. As society advances, more reference is made to mental health in conversations, with an emphasis on those aimed at reducing stigma and promoting access to care. This shift is strongest in schools, workplaces, and community agencies where open dialogue concerning mental health is encouraged. By raising mental health awareness, more individuals are able to access treatment and live healthier lives. These preventative measures can go a long way to significantly reducing the long-term cost of unchecked mental illness to society at large. Emerging trends in community health are necessitated by the urgency of integrating mental health awareness into public health and primary care strategies. Policymakers and health organizations increasingly recognize that mental and physical health results are intertwined in essence, an idea reinforced by initiatives aimed at mainstreaming mental health care into general health care strategies. For instance, physical activity interventions are linked to improved mental health corroborated by the WHOs 2020 guidelines, where adults should engage in regular physical activity and prescribe fewer sedentary behaviors. Mental health education initiatives equate to widespread community health interventions that entail prevention and intervention, shifting mental health perceptions, treatment, and management in community settings. This convergence brings forth improved accessibility and encourages prioritization of mental health as a core component of one's well-being. The future of community health must ensure sustained mental health awareness campaigns, recognizing its contribution to addressing pressing health inequalities. With the quickening pace of technology, telemedicine platforms are being used to enhance access to mental health care, enabling underserved populations to be addressed by mental health professionals remotely. This provides individuals the chance to seek assistance in a more accessible and less stigmatized way. In addition, community health interventions are becoming more targeted to integrated strategies that incorporate diverse groups, acknowledging differently subscribed cultural attitudes toward mental health. Meeting the specific needs of various communities is crucial for establishing culturally responsive interventions that resonate with the local populations. With increasing awareness regarding mental health, it is essential that programs for community health remain vibrant so they can cope with emerging issues in mental well-being while promoting overall well-being in society.

15.5.1. Increasing Recognition of Mental Health Issues

In recent years, increasing acceptance of mental health issues has emerged as a core aspect of the conversation regarding community health. This is representative of the acknowledgment that mental health is the same as physical health in the service of general well-being. The implementation of mental health awareness within public policy and community activism is an important step toward larger more inclusive care for health. This increased awareness has generated greater focus on stigma reduction so that people are able to seek assistance without social consequence. By making mental health a priority as a central component of public health, communities can build societies that not only assist those in need but also optimize overall resilience and productivity in society. Additionally, the intersectional overlap of mental health with other social determinants has been increasingly comprehended, further solidifying the need for comprehensive methods to address these complexities. Concerns such as poverty, education, and community safety closely intersect with mental health outcomes, emphasizing the requirement of an approach that is multi-dimensional. Studies and workshops have clarified the necessity for the reform of structures, whereby sectors such as education, justice, and local government come together to generate effective interventions. By the understanding of the interconnectedness of mental health and other social issues, community health models can be reinforced to provide more sustainable outcomes. Such integrative approaches are needed to enhance quality of life and close gaps for vulnerable groups to build a healthier nation. As greater recognition of mental health challenges sets the focus, trends are moving toward innovative practices and research capabilities to address these issues. The projects of the Lowitja Institutes mirror the necessity for forward-thinking strategies to look ahead to future demands in mental health research and services. Firstly, by generating a platform for debate around potential future contexts, stakeholders can identify priority research and delivery needs that respond to particular evolving needs of the community in terms of health. Secondly, through the focus on evidence-based interventions in mental health, especially preventative interventions, the urgency to develop programs that are targeted at particular community needs is increased. Since public health conversations are preeminently featuring mental health these days, it is crucial that ongoing practice and investigation in reality align with the interrelatedness of mental health with overall community well-being (Brands, 2014; Long et al., 2013) (Figure 15.14).

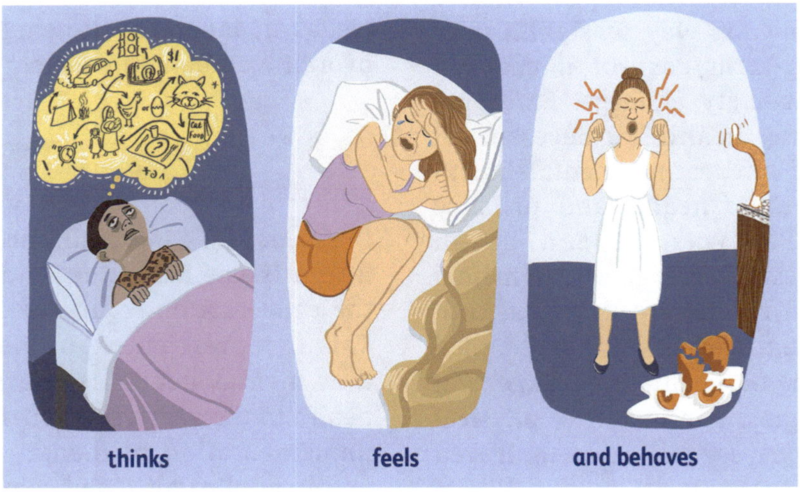

Figure 15.14. Increasing recognition of mental health issues.

Source: https://www.verywellmind.com/thmb/u_YyxyiUz6qeT5AtcsF41O42ngY=/1500x0/filters:no_upscale():max_bytes(150000):strip_icc()/definition-of-mental-illness-4587855-v1-cd7f9f37c61c49099ac8ede282db1e73.png.

15.5.2. Integration of Mental Health Services in Community Health

The integration of mental health treatment into a community health model is a significant shift in the provision of healthcare, one that results from an increasing awareness of the interconnection between mental and physical health. With urbanization comes the demographic consequences of increasingly diverse and complex populations, and so increasingly there is a need for an integrated approach addressing psychological as well as physical illness. Studies indicate that living in cities directly influences population health by reasons like social determinants and physical settings (Freudenberg et al., 2005). By having an integrated system with mental and physical health services, communities can improve access to treatment, reduce stigma, and gain a general improvement in health outcomes. This combined strategy facilitates preventive mental health management, which establishes early intervention strategies that are crucial in averting the development of chronic diseases as well as healthy populations at the individual level. Moreover, the emphasis on person-centered planning in mental health provision is critical in shaping fruitful community health outcomes.

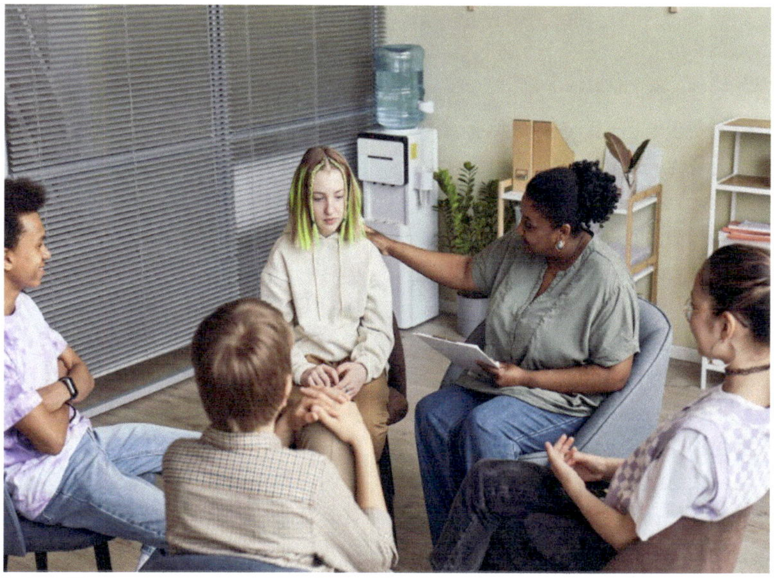

Figure 15.15. Integration of mental health services in community health.

Source: https://openminds.org.au/wp-content/uploads/2022/12/mental-health-support.jpeg.

The process prioritizes the individual's personal needs and preference to the highest extent, thus furnishing a more individualized healthcare service. Direct service workers with experience in heterogeneous service systems, such as schools and community agencies, cite the effectiveness of person-centered models to improve service outcomes for individuals with severe mental illnesses and developmental disabilities (Abery et al., 2006). The integration of mental health services under this framework not only enhances the quality of care but also ensures increased patient participation with resultant enhanced adherence to treatment regimens and ultimately better health outcomes. Such specific frameworks are crucial as they enhance participation by people in their own care, thus enhancing autonomy and empowerment in managing one's own mental health. Future trends in community health rely on the integration of mental health care, requiring collaboration among various stakeholders such as healthcare providers, local authorities, and community organizations. Through the consolidation of strengths in these heterogeneous entities, communities can establish supportive networks that endorse both mental and physical health programs. The collaborative model also facilitates resource-sharing and entrepreneurial approaches to suit individual needs, thus increasing overall population resilience. Due to the complexities of city life and its consequences on health, it is important to adopt a comprehensive strategy that integrates these complex problems (Freudenberg et al., 2005). By being active in addressing such issues, communities not only improve existing health statuses, but they also work towards creating lasting environments in which individuals not only thrive today but also in the years to come, in an unequivocal blueprint for future public health advancement (Figure 15.15).

15.5.3. Stigma Reduction Efforts

Stigma reduction is a crucial component in achieving health equity and optimizing community health outcomes. With the rising persistence of health disparities across various population groups, including racial and ethnic minorities, the socio-economically disadvantaged, and the LGBTQ+ population, targeted stigma reduction efforts are increasingly becoming important. These programs seek to inform communities about the health inequities that burden marginalized communities, making it a more inclusive place ultimately. By tackling myths and misconceptions in society, programs are able to make a huge change in how perceptions are perceived about some of these health issues, like HIV/AIDS or chronic diseases. This is not only an increase in access to health care but also encourages individuals to seek care without fear of judgment. As indicated, the urgent need for equitable health outcomes propels the worth of such efforts to combat stigma in addressing the systemic disparities that persist in access and quality of healthcare (Carlson et al., 2016). Aside from education, community stakeholder involvement in reducing stigma is important to effectiveness and sustainability. Collaborative models that bring in local leaders, healthcare providers, and affected populations have the possibility of enhancing the reach and efficacy of stigma reduction efforts. Programs that incorporate the voices of affected persons directly are particularly effective, as they provide authenticity and recognition to the message being transmitted. Such collaborations can lead to innovative solutions such as support groups that facilitate peer support and resilience among affected persons. Besides, community-based initiatives will be able to tackle cultural belief and practice resulting in stigma, hence the intervention will be contextually relevant. Such participatory interventions not only increase community ownership but also create long-term changes in attitude towards health and well-being, which go on to lead to improved health outcomes in general (N/A, 2007). Monitoring and evaluation in the long term are crucial to the success of stigma reduction activities within community health. Assessment of these interventions requires a broad understanding of the specific barriers to various populations and monitoring of the change created by interventions over time. Outcome indicators, such as access to health care, better literacy, and decreased reported cases of stigma, can provide valuable insights into the effectiveness of implemented strategies. Regular feedback from stakeholders on what is effective ensures that programs are able to adjust to new emerging needs. Through monitoring of the effectiveness of the stigma reduction work in a structured way, health organizations and policymakers can demonstrate progress and continue to invest in these key areas. Such dedication to measurement not only solidifies community confidence but also strengthens the integration of stigma reduction interventions into broader health care priorities, letting in an open public health future (Carlson et al., 2016).

15.6. Policy and Legislation

Community health is increasingly filled by the confluence of policy and legislation driven to enhance health outcomes for populations. New directions to universal health coverage (UHC) represent a watershed in health policy, with objectives not only to increase coverage for health care services but also to put a high value on the quality of these services. The recognition that excellent health systems will be based on a series of robust foundations, such as the ability to monitor and use health data, clearly points towards the necessity for legislation promoting these underlying principles. A comprehensive health policy reaction should emphasize equity, resilience, and efficiency and instill confidence in populations in their health systems. As the new frameworks articulate, the shift from merely expanding access to maintaining quality of care is paramount to solve the intricate health challenges of the populations, particularly those in low- and middle-income countries. Legislation to enhance community health services must also tackle social determinants of health, such as SES. Research more and more identifies the influence of SES on outcomes in health, with increased emphasis on chronic conditions, such as cardiovascular disease; income, education, and employment inequities highlight the need for focused interventions (Schultz et al., 2018). Such policies that incorporate these social determinants into a holistic health policy will assist in the mitigation of health inequalities. As such, good health policy should aim not just at healthcare provision but also at driving initiatives aimed at altering the wider determinants of health. For instance, community interventions that engage individuals of lower SES in structured physical activity programs are encouraging and highlight the potential for policy to foster intersectoral collaboration for the integrated health approach. Last but not least, the effectiveness of community health policies relies on strong governance and accountability mechanisms that guarantee transparency and civic participation. Empowering communities to demand accountability from health systems is needed to foster trust, especially in low-resource contexts where inefficiencies in the past could have eroded public trust. Legislation can enhance health system responsiveness by making the health system more responsive to the needs of diverse populations. High-quality care, as a political imperative and not just as a technical issue, needs broad-based support from policymakers, healthcare professionals, and their respective communities. With evolving health requirements and rising public expectations, the role of new models of policy cannot be overstated as they sit at the center of shaping the future direction of community health initiatives and securing long-term health gains throughout populations (Kruk et al., 2018).

15.6.1. Recent Legislative Changes Impacting Community Health

Moved by an increasing awareness of the role social determinants play in health, recent legislative reforms have led to heightened focus on addressing community health holistically. Policies that enhance access to care have gained traction with a special focus with an equity perspective aimed at eliminating disparities. Key among these advancements include those seeking to increase Medicaid eligibility and the level of funding for community health clinics, especially in areas of low health insurance coverage. These reforms not only seek to broaden insurance coverage but also support preventive care, a cornerstone to diffusing the cost of chronic diseases prevalent in low-income communities. With growing connectivity between populations and healthcare services, these efforts are at the forefront of building healthier environments where wellness is prioritized over treating illness, in alignment with trends that prioritize health at an integrated level. Furthermore, legislation regarding addiction treatment has undergone revolutionary transformations, which reflect the shifting trends toward a public health-oriented approach. Historically, addiction used to be treated with a penal orientation, but there is a shift in policies towards promoting harm reduction and integrating mental health services as part of community health. Implementation of specialty outpatient clinics and therapeutic community formation elucidate this legislative progress, presenting an embracing of addiction as a multifaceted health issue necessitating comprehensive treatment rather than stigmatized responses. Legislation has begun to incorporate behavioral health into primary care, showing greater understanding of the interdependence of physical and mental health. With populations grappling with heightened addiction rates, particularly during the COVID-19 pandemic, such law reforms are important strides in creating greater overall community resiliency and healthier outcomes (Besana et al., 2025). With a world increasingly shaped by the impact of climate change and worldwide geopolitical instability, new values in community health policy have arisen that focus on sustainable agriculture methods and environmental health. Debates among health practitioners today emphasize the integration of organic phosphorus research into broader health assessments, underscoring the need for inter-disciplinary cooperation in managing both health and environmental issues. Legislation is beginning to reflect these debates, signaling a commitment to promoting practices that secure food supplies while protecting environmental systems. Though the focus is more towards developing resilience to climate change effects, policies promoting soil health and sustainability will play a key role to ensure community health against impending global challenges. The alignment of policymakers, researchers, and communities is necessary to make these policy interventions worthwhile and widespread, resulting in healthier populations in the years to come (Lucas et al., 2025) (Figure 15.16).

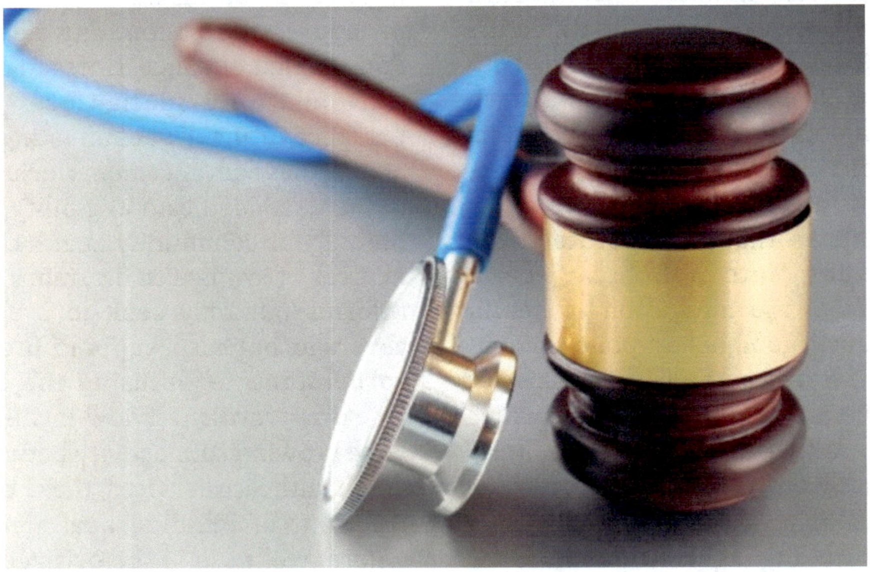

Figure 15.16. Recent legislative changes impacting community health.

Source: https://www.amnhealthcare.com/siteassets/candidate-blog/nursing/travel/healthcare-legislation.jpg.

15.6.2. Role of Government in Community Health Initiatives

Government's role in community health programs is significant, as it forms the platform for enhanced health and wellbeing of populations. Governments have the mandate of developing policies that efficiently respond to public health issues, from healthcare service access to the control of health risks such as epidemics. Besides, through the application of public finance and resource allocation, governments can promote disease prevention, health education, and health promotion programs. For example, investment in community health centers provides wider access for low-income communities and, thus, reduces health disparities. As new health trends emerge, indicating the requirement for preventive community action, governments are now more than ever obligated to take the lead and undertake efforts that bring stakeholders together to establish community-centered health approaches that address local issues. Governments must play a vital role in creating links between sectors such as business and education to further establish community health activities. Through collaboration with learning institutions, government agencies are able to combine resources to develop and implement training for prospective health care workers to ease the manpower shortages in the industry. Career pathway programs, for instance, that focus on career trajectories in health sciences not only prepare students to enter this vital sector but also address shifting workforce demands. This complementarity is especially pertinent in the case of states such as Alaska, where there exist special challenges of urban-rural disparities in healthcare access and delivery, which need special intervention by way of health education and training. This intersectoral collaboration increases the synergy of health interventions to ensure that they are sustainable and address the varied health needs of populations. Moreover, the government can enact policy and regulation that promotes health equity, which actively addresses socio-economic determinants of health outcomes. Policy to limit toxins in the environment or healthy food choices can lead to actual community health gains. The ability of governments to enact and enforce these kinds of policies is essential because they both protect the public health as well as promote behaviors leading to healthier lives. Emerging trends in health policy increasingly emphasize mainstreaming social determinants of health into public health programs with a suggestion of a drift toward broad paradigms. For example, reductions in food deserts and provision of healthy food options are pivotal in community health program support. Placing these at the top of the agenda, governments can achieve significant change in healthcare outcomes, emphasizing their relevance to overall success for community health initiatives (DeFeo et al., 2014 N/A, 2025).

15.6.3. Future Policy Directions for Community Health

The evolving nature of community health necessitates an anticipatory policy-making that is conscious of current and emerging problems. There must be a big focus on antimicrobial resistance (AMR), which is a gigantic threat to global health systems. The future direction of policies should entail embracing new therapeutic modalities, such as bacteriophage therapy and antimicrobial peptides, as well as regulatory guidelines that facilitate them to be introduced. According to recent research, effective interventions must entail collaborative international action and sustained finance agreements to foster research and development in this important area and render health policies at the community level sufficiently robust to combat the AMR menace while safeguarding public health (Senel et al., 2025). Policy makers also need to consider the socio-economic determinants of AMR and make attempts to implement fair access to new therapy, with health programs geared towards other public health goals. Community health policies, excluding AMR, also need to tackle safety issues that evolve in healthcare settings, with a particular focus on nursing practice. The evolving research landscape indicates increasing focus on patient safety culture and qualitative research methods, calling for integrative policies that respond to these trends. The potential future is to have environments that prioritize constant learning and improvement, ensuring that health professionals are equipped with the tools and training necessary to enhance patient outcomes. The results of the new research point to a shift in focus in research from reactive to preventive strategies, which must also be embodied in policy frameworks. Through the consideration of patient safety intricacies and integrating them into community health plans, policymakers are able to foster a more interdisciplinary approach that focuses not only on curing diseases but also on the health of communities in general (Lee et al., 2025). Lastly, a significant percentage of future policy for community health must address collaborative models including multiple actors within the healthcare system. Such an intervention can bridge hiatuses between scientific evidence, regulation, and practical intervention, leading to improved health outcomes. A more integrated One Health approach that combines human, animal, and environmental health could also do a lot to improve the policy endeavors to avert health emergencies, including AMR. Engaging local communities, health workers, and policymakers in a systematic conversation will support the identification of context-specific solutions and bear collective accountability. Through community health development, a concerted endeavor like this will be a determining factor in building strong and sustainable health systems capable of responding properly to new threats and sustaining maximum health among all members (Lee et al., 2025; Senel et al., 2025) (Figure 15.17).

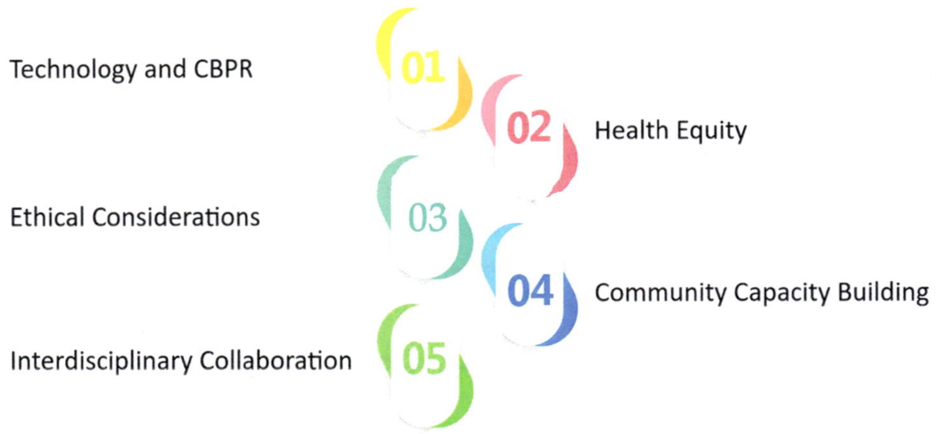

Figure 15.17. Future policy directions for community health.

Source: https://fastercapital.co/i/Advancing-Knowledge--CCPH-s-Impactful-Public-Health-Research--Future-Directions-for-Community-Based-Public-Health-Research.webp.

SUMMARY

Ultimately, the face of community health is undergoing revolutionary change with the power of new trends and modes of approaching. Research has highlighted a dramatic expansion in the field of patient safety in nursing practice, shifting the emphasis from traditional parameters like medical error analysis to more pervasive factors like patient safety culture and training. This advancement is an indicator of growing sensitization to the complexity of healthcare delivery and underscoring the requirement for extensive training for health personnel. As identified by studies using structural topic modeling, these innovations not only enhance patient care outcomes but also establish a safety culture that supports free communication and continuous learning in health institutions (Lee et al., 2025). While advancements are made in community health programs, it will be necessary to change with these developments as a way of guiding policy and practice in the future. The creation of AMR also emphasizes the need to resolve issues in community health. The application of literature on synthesizing novel therapies, such as bacteriophage therapy and novel antibiotic strategies, sits alongside the need to create effective policy frameworks that drive global health initiatives. Conclusion of the findings identifies significant barriers, scientific as well as economic, which impede fast evolution and application of solutions necessary. Along with this, usage of combined One Health interventions becomes inevitable in avoiding AMR, exemplifying the interconnectedness of human, animal, and environmental health. As explained in current literature, innovation in the development of diagnostic technologies and alternative funding schemes are essential in bridging the gaps in spearheading the collaboration of actors in the health sector (Senel et al., 2025). This multi-faceted approach entails addressing the threats that accompany AMR while enhancing the overall health of populations. In the future, the future of community health is based on unity among people and determination in addressing challenges that have been identified. As examined in contemporary scholarship, the intersection of various research agendas—varying from patient safety to resistance to antimicrobials—revels the complexity of community health context. The complexity necessitates a robust system of convergence among healthcare professionals, policymakers, and the community itself. Formulation of community health necessitates constant responsiveness and flexibility to emerging trends, such that interventions are both effective and just. By making sustainability in funding a priority, promoting innovative thinking, and embracing interdisciplinarity, the community health sector can address the issues of today effectively and safeguard public health for future generations. Institutionalizing these principles will be at the forefront of addressing the shift in paradigm in community health (Lee et al., 2025; Senel et al., 2025).

The fluid landscape of community health is being dramatically transformed by many critical trends that reflect broader changes in society. No trend may be more evident than the increased emphasis on more holistic health approaches that integrate physical, mental, and social health. As communities better understand the interconnectedness of these domains of health, programs aimed to promote all-around wellness are gaining traction. For instance, interventions that address social determinants of health, for instance, access to wholesome food and mental healthcare, are vital in reducing health disparities across marginalized groups. This development is also informed by trend reports from agencies that analyze trends in society, highlighting the need for community health programs to adjust their strategies so that they may address the complex issues of diverse populations (Gopal et al., 2012). Another deep trend is technological development in interventions for community health. The dissemination of mobile health apps and telemedicine coverage created new avenues of access to healthcare, particularly among the marginalized groups. This technological advancement enables real-time tracking of health and improves interoperability among providers of healthcare and community members to make the health infrastructure more reactive. Moreover, with technology advancements in data analysis and collection, there is increased ability to target health programs to address particular requirements and choices of communities. This targeted approach in health programs not only enhances response but also maximizes total health benefits, thereby positioning technology as an essential aspect of community health strategies in the future (Gilgoff et al., 2015). Moreover, community empowerment and community participation are increasingly emerging as significant trends in establishing good health models. Health programs emphasizing the active involvement of people in the community are likely to yield long-term outcomes. Involvement fosters ownership and accountability among individuals, leading to collective action towards common health goals. For example, programs that organize youth and communities of color to become involved in advocacy and decision-making activities are key to promoting equitable health outcomes. Utilizing the local knowledge and capacity of the area, these programs are more capable of being responsive to the local needs of different populations. Therefore, community engagement priority not only improves public health but also builds resilience among communities undergoing systemic inequalities, proving to be a crucial shift in public health practice (Gilgoff et al., 2015).

KEY TERMS FROM THIS CHAPTER

- Digital Health
- Artificial Intelligence (AI) in Health
- Data-Driven Decision Making
- Community-Based Technology
- Health Equity Innovation
- Global Health Security
- Mental Health Integration
- Health in All Policies (HiAP)
- Policy Innovation
- Big Data in Public Health
- Environmental Sustainability
- Behavioral Economics in Health
- Health Systems Strengthening
- Telehealth
- Precision Public Health
- Wearable Health Technology
- Social Prescribing
- Climate and Health Nexus
- Pandemic Preparedness
- Cross-Sector Collaboration
- Community-Led Interventions
- Population Health Management
- Mobile Health (mHealth)
- Culturally Tailored Interventions
- Decentralized Care Models

CLOSER LOOK

HEALTH INFORMATION TECHNOLOGY (HIT)

A closer look at Health Information Technology (HIT) reveals its critical role in transforming healthcare delivery, improving patient outcomes, and enhancing the efficiency of health systems. HIT encompasses a wide range of digital tools and systems used to store, manage, and exchange health information, including electronic health records (EHRs), e-prescribing, telemedicine platforms, health information exchanges (HIEs), and mobile health applications. At its core, HIT aims to streamline communication among healthcare providers, reduce medical errors, and empower patients to take a more active role in their care. By digitizing patient records, healthcare professionals gain faster, more accurate access to medical histories, lab results, and treatment plans, enabling better clinical decision-making and continuity of care. HIT also supports data analytics, which can identify trends, improve disease surveillance, and inform public health strategies. Moreover, HIT plays a vital role in patient safety, helping to flag drug interactions, track vaccinations, and reduce duplication of tests or procedures. With the rise of telehealth and mobile technologies, patients now have greater access to care, particularly in rural or underserved areas, enhancing equity and convenience. However, the implementation of HIT comes with challenges, including concerns about data privacy, interoperability, and the digital divide. Ensuring that health systems can securely share data across platforms while protecting patient confidentiality remains a top priority. Additionally, adequate training for healthcare professionals and user-friendly design are essential to maximize the benefits of HIT. Despite these hurdles, continued innovation and policy support have made HIT a cornerstone of modern healthcare infrastructure. It not only improves clinical efficiency and coordination but also empowers patients with greater transparency and control over their health information. In an increasingly digital world, HIT stands as a key driver in advancing high-quality, accessible, and patient-centered care.ss

REFERENCES

1. Abery, B., Allegretti-Freeman, J., Blessing, C., Osher, D., et al. (2006). *Learning from Other Communities*. https://core.ac.uk/download/5127278.pdf (accessed on 26th June 2025).
2. Acuff, C., Antonelli, R., Fox, D., Hirsch, G., et al. (2017). No equity, no triple aim: Strategic proposals to advance health equity in a volatile policy environment. https://core.ac.uk/download/142081335.pdf (accessed on 26th June 2025).
3. Adger, W. N., Ashford, L., Badyaev, A., Bahn, V., Baird, B., Barton, D., Baum, J., et al. (2016). The human–nature relationship and its impact on health: A critical review. https://core.ac.uk/download/163076696.pdf (accessed on 26th June 2025).
4. Ani, L. (2025). Access to emerging technologies and techniques in the Nigerian solid minerals sector: A cost-benefit analysis. *International Journal of Social Science and Education Research Studies*. https://www.semanticscholar.org/paper/f202eb32f859d1f17fefa50f625e991ba0ab42ab (accessed on 26th June 2025).
5. Apesoa-Varano, E. C., Gladstone, C., Kim, K. K., Lindeman, D., et al. (2020). Technology and caregiving: Emerging interventions and directions for research. https://core.ac.uk/download/323070528.pdf (accessed on 26th June 2025).
6. Bashshur, R. L., Doarn, C. R., Frenk, J., Kvedar, J. C., & Woolliscroft, J. O. (2020). Telemedicine and the COVID-19 pandemic: Lessons for the future. *Telemedicine Journal and e-Health, 26*, 571–573. https://doi.org/10.1089/tmj.2020.29040.rb (accessed on 26th June 2025).
7. Besana, F., Pasquariello, S., Costa, V., & Negri, A. (2025). The history of addiction clinics and treatment in Italy: An overview and future directions. *Histories*. https://www.semanticscholar.org/paper/c2607dcd6dc9633872199c111a3f09678a4a8e6f (accessed on 26th June 2025).
8. Brands, J. (2014). The shape of things to come: Visions for the future of Aboriginal and Torres Strait Islander health research. https://core.ac.uk/download/pdf/30674877.pdf (accessed on 26th June 2025).
9. Bull, F., Al-Ansari, S. S., Biddle, S., Borodulin, K., Buman, M. P., Cardon, G., Carty, C., et al. (2020). World Health Organization 2020 guidelines on physical activity and sedentary behavior. *British Journal of Sports Medicine, 54*, 1451–1462. https://doi.org/10.1136/bjsports-2020-102955 (accessed on 26th June 2025).
10. Calvin, K., Dasgupta, D., Krinner, G., Mukherji, A., Thorne, P., Trisos, C. H., Romero, J., et al. (2023). *IPCC, 2023: Climate Change 2023: Synthesis Report. Contribution of Working Groups I, II and III to the Sixth Assessment Report of the Intergovernmental Panel on Climate Change* [Core Writing Team, H. Lee and J. Romero (Eds.)]. IPCC, Geneva, Switzerland. https://doi.org/10.59327/ipcc/ar6-9789291691647 (accessed on 26th June 2025).
11. Carlson, C., Sholk, J., Nanni, J., Peterson, K., Smith, L. A., & Bhavaraju, N. (2016). *Breaking the Barriers to Specialty Care: Practical Ideas to Improve Health Equity and Reduce Cost–Striving for Equity in Specialty Care Full Report*. https://core.ac.uk/download/75785764.pdf (accessed on 26th June 2025).
12. DeFeo, D. J., Hirshberg, D., & LeCompte, C. (2014). *Alaska Career Pathways: A Baseline Analysis*. https://core.ac.uk/download/286999281.pdf (accessed on 26th June 2025).
13. Dwivedi, Y. K., Hughes, L., Baabdullah, A. M., Ribeiro-Navarrete, S., Giannakis, M., Al-Debei, M. M., Dennehy, D., et al. (2022). Metaverse beyond the hype: Multidisciplinary perspectives on

emerging challenges, opportunities, and agenda for research, practice and policy. *International Journal of Information Management, 66*, 102542–102542. https://doi.org/10.1016/j.ijinfomgt.2022.102542 (accessed on 26th June 2025).

14. Ezz, I., & Paul, R. (2013). The chaotic nature of healthcare information systems: The need for transdisciplinary collaboration. https://core.ac.uk/download/20089501.pdf (accessed on 26th June 2025).
15. Farooq, S., Imran, M. A., Latif, S., Qadir, J., et al. (2017). How 5G wireless (and concomitant technologies) will revolutionize healthcare? https://core.ac.uk/download/143476480.pdf (accessed on 26th June 2025).
16. Freudenberg, N., Galea, S., & Vlahov, D. (2005). Cities and population health. https://core.ac.uk/download/323072008.pdf (accessed on 26th June 2025).
17. Gilgoff, J., & Ginwright, S. (2015). *Toward More Equitable Outcomes: A Research Synthesis on Out-of-School Time Work with Boys and Young Men of Color*. https://core.ac.uk/download/75786240.pdf (accessed on 26th June 2025).
18. Gopal, S., & Najam, A. (2012). Connecting the dots: Information visualization and text analysis of the Searchlight Project newsletters. https://open.bu.edu/bitstream/2144/22895/1/Searchlight-Pardee-Report.pdf (accessed on 26th June 2025).
19. Gostin, L. O., Hardcastle, L. E., Jacobson, P. D., Record, K., et al. (2011). Restoring health to health reform: Integrating medicine and public health to advance the population's wellbeing. https://core.ac.uk/download/70374138.pdf (accessed on 26th June 2025).
20. Grewal, M., Singh, T., & Chopra, T. (2019). Measles crises in Detroit: Zero to 44, each one is one too many! *Infection Control & Hospital Epidemiology, 40*, 1176–1177. https://www.semanticscholar.org/paper/ebf6671353b38c95f368bf5cfc7e18fbe0e46148 (accessed on 26th June 2025).
21. Hassell, J. M., Begon, M., Ward, M. J., & Fèvre, E. M. (2016). Urbanization and disease emergence: Dynamics at the wildlife–livestock–human interface. *Trends in Ecology & Evolution, 32*, 55–67. https://doi.org/10.1016/j.tree.2016.09.012 (accessed on 26th June 2025).
22. Intergovernmental Panel on Climate Change. (2023). *Climate Change 2022–Impacts, Adaptation and Vulnerability*. https://doi.org/10.1017/9781009325844 (accessed on 26th June 2025).
23. Jain, M., Sharma, P. K., Kamboj, K., & Shyam, A. (2024). The impact of social media on medical education and health-care communication. *Journal of Orthopedic Case Reports, 14*, 1–3. https://www.semanticscholar.org/paper/b9b5922328e2fd5143d1e3ebd84cc77faed07afd (accessed on 26th June 2025).
24. Jonassen, D., & Driscoll, M. (2013). *Handbook of Research on Educational Communications and Technology*. Routledge eBooks. https://doi.org/10.4324/9781410609519 (accessed on 26th June 2025).
25. Kilibarda, B. (2024). Global challenges and opportunities in health promotion. *Proceedings of the International Congress Public Health–Achievements and Challenges–zbornik radova*. https://www.semanticscholar.org/paper/bce0d1aea33eb6a60140ae55c6a164aab5840c49 (accessed on 26th June 2025).
26. Kruk, M. E., Gage, A., Arsenault, C., Jordan, K., Leslie, H. H., Roder-DeWan, S., Adeyi, O., et al. (2018). High-quality health systems in the Sustainable Development Goals era: Time for

a revolution. *The Lancet Global Health, 6*, e1196–e1252. https://doi.org/10.1016/s2214-109x(18)30386-3 (accessed on 26th June 2025).

27. Lee, N. J., & Kim, N. (2025). A comprehensive analysis of patient safety research in nursing: Trends, topics, and future directions. *Journal of Patient Safety, 21*, e29–e39. https://www.semanticscholar.org/paper/7a1e361100837e514670ccf1a38fb52913e7853e (accessed on 26th June 2025).
28. Livingston, G., Huntley, J., Sommerlad, A., Ames, D., Ballard, C., Banerjee, S., Brayne, C., et al. (2020). Dementia prevention, intervention, and care: 2020 report of the Lancet Commission. *The Lancet, 396*, 413–446. https://doi.org/10.1016/s0140-6736(20)30367-6 (accessed on 26th June 2025).
29. Long, J., & Vages, N. (2013). *A Critical Scan of Four Key Topics for the Philanthropic Sector: A Study by the Rockefeller Foundation and Accenture Development Partnerships*. https://core.ac.uk/download/71362647.pdf (accessed on 26th June 2025).
30. Lucas, E. R., Nguyen, N. D., Celi, L., Condron, L., Fraser, T. D., George, T. S., Mora, M. L. D. L., et al. (2025). Organic phosphorus in the terrestrial environment: An update on current research and future directions. *Journal of Soil Science and Plant Nutrition*. https://www.semanticscholar.org/paper/a2895678b64e4ab50ff68217faa607bcae1000f3 (accessed on 26th June 2025).
31. Mhando, F., Nyankomo, M., Hall, C., Olughu, K. N., Hlongwa, M., Janson, S., Idahosa, L., et al. (2024). Digital intervention services to promote HIV self-testing and linkage to care services: A bibliometric and content analysis—Global trends and future directions. *Public Health Reviews, 45*. https://www.semanticscholar.org/paper/8fc49f95ec95e4c3d7b31cc6b7f96672f993351b (accessed on 26th June 2025).
32. Mubdir, G. A., Hashim, S., Ayob, A., & Rosli, N. (2025). Exploring customer engagement in social commerce: A literature review of frameworks, pathways, and emerging trends. *Engineering, Technology & Applied Science Research*. https://www.semanticscholar.org/paper/3597c8054700693a7eb14e7987476a692fac5cbc (accessed on 26th June 2025).
33. N/A. (2002). *Professional development for conservators in the United States: Report of the Directors' Retreat for the Advancement of Conservation Education*. https://core.ac.uk/download/71354022.pdf (accessed on 26th June 2025).
34. N/A. (2007). *Bringing HIV Prevention to Scale: An Urgent Global Priority*. https://core.ac.uk/download/71349645.pdf (accessed on 26th June 2025).
35. N/A. (2013). *Equity in the Digital Age: How Health Information Technology Can Reduce Disparities*. https://core.ac.uk/download/71361135.pdf (accessed on 26th June 2025).
36. N/A. (2025). *Building Australia's Comparative Advantages*. https://core.ac.uk/download/pdf/30672005.pdf (accessed on 26th June 2025).
37. Nwokedi, C. N. N., Olowe, K. J., Alli, O. I., & Iguma, D. R. (2025). The role of digital health in modern pharmacy: A review of emerging trends and patient impacts. *International Journal of Science and Research Archive*. https://www.semanticscholar.org/paper/018d6d3b745bbd5966df3dd695806e398ee61c56 (accessed on 26th June 2025).
38. Oliai, S. (2005). *Economic Environment and Applications of Telemedicine*. https://core.ac.uk/download/10685681.pdf (accessed on 26th June 2025).
39. Organisation for Economic Co-operation and Development (OECD). (2019). *OECD Employment*

Outlook 2019. OECD Employment Outlook. https://doi.org/10.1787/9ee00155-en (accessed on 26th June 2025).

40. Sajida, M., Muluk, S., & Durrety, S. (2025). Trends, issues, and future directions of decentralization in unitary state research: Bibliometric analyses from 1975–2024. *KnE Social Sciences*. https://www.semanticscholar.org/paper/b499e579ec11e5d5c0177b80a7451cc2af17e9e3 (accessed on 26th June 2025).
41. Schultz, W. M., Kelli, H. M., Lisko, J., Varghese, T., Shen, J., Sandesara, P. B., Quyyumi, A. A., et al. (2018). Socioeconomic status and cardiovascular outcomes. *Circulation, 137*, 2166–2178. https://doi.org/10.1161/circulationaha.117.029652 (accessed on 26th June 2025).
42. Senel, B., & Beka, H. (2025). Innovative strategies to combat antibiotic resistance: Emerging trends and future directions. *International Journal of Health Management and Tourism*. https://www.semanticscholar.org/paper/eb5f75c62dc7de4c9919a5419afbe76eb2b0a02d (accessed on 26th June 2025).
43. Shippy, K., Theodore, P., Di Felice, V., Mohan, S. V., & McKenzie, M. (2025). Maintaining momentum in cancer health equity: Examining Native Hawaiian and Pacific Islander US cancer mortality trends (1999–2024) and mechanisms for enhancing representation in oncology clinical trials. *Journal of Clinical Oncology*. https://www.semanticscholar.org/paper/0da531290345418db30a1967de0cdbb5d523507b (accessed on 26th June 2025).
44. Vanderlei, L. C., & Frias, P. (2016). Uncertainties in the Brazilian scenario and its implications in mother and child health. *16*, 375–376. https://www.semanticscholar.org/paper/60364e2965c935c3d1469e1005a7d46803cafc04 (accessed on 26th June 2025).
45. Yen, I., & Brousseau, R. T. (2000). Reflections on the connections between work and health. https://core.ac.uk/download/71354325.pdf (accessed on 26th June 2025).
46. Zhang, R., & Wang, H. (2025). Insights into the technological evolution and research trends of mobile health: Bibliometric analysis. *Healthcare, 13*. https://www.semanticscholar.org/paper/d9975f1ce0dc91309cf84aeafd9a2cd91e09e798 (accessed on 26th June 2025).

INDEX

F

G

H

I

L

M

T

U

V

W